Textbook of Three-Dimensional Echocardiography

Luigi P. Badano • Roberto M. Lang
Denisa Muraru
Editors

Textbook of Three-Dimensional Echocardiography

Second Edition

Springer

Editors
Luigi P. Badano
University of Milano-Bicocca
and Istituto Auxologico Italiano
IRCCS, San Luca Hospital
Milano
Italy

Roberto M. Lang
Department of Medicine
University of Chicago Medical Center
Chicago, IL
USA

Denisa Muraru
University of Milano-Bicocca
and Istituto Auxologico Italiano
IRCCS, San Luca Hospital
Milano
Italy

ISBN 978-3-030-14030-4 ISBN 978-3-030-14032-8 (eBook)
https://doi.org/10.1007/978-3-030-14032-8

This Springer imprint is published by the registered company Springer Nature Switzerland AG
The registered company address is: Gewerbestrasse 11, 6330 Cham, Switzerland

Preface

Three-dimensional echocardiography has completed its transition from a research tool to a clinically useful imaging modality able to provide additional and unique information to assist in the diagnosis, clinical management, and decision-making of patients with a wide range of cardiovascular diseases. In addition to the studies performed in the echocardiography laboratory, three-dimensional echocardiography is currently extensively used in the operating room and in the catheterization laboratory to help plan cardiac surgeries and guide interventional procedures.

This textbook on three-dimensional echocardiography is intended to be read by echocardiographers who are new to this technique, those who are interested in updating their knowledge in three-dimensional echocardiography, and also cardiac surgeons and clinical and interventional cardiologists who want to learn what additional information three-dimensional echocardiography can add to their clinical practice.

After introductory chapters describing the evolution of three-dimensional echocardiography, the physics supporting this technique, and how to implement its use from both the transthoracic and transesophageal approaches, we also included a chapter on "how to implement three-dimensional echocardiography in the routine workflow of a busy clinical laboratory." In this chapter, we tried to address all the issues that are still limiting its routine use despite the clear evidence of added value, compared to conventional two-dimensional and Doppler echocardiography. The remainder of the book's chapters are organized by cardiac structures and their respective diseases (i.e., the normal mitral valve followed by congenital abnormalities and stenosis, degenerative and functional mitral regurgitation, assessment during and after surgery, or interventional procedures on the mitral valve) emphasizing the technical aspects of three-dimensional echocardiography as well as the added value of this technique compared to conventional two-dimensional and Doppler echocardiography. At the end of these chapters, selected clinical cases were included to better illustrate the added diagnostic value provided by the three-dimensional echocardiography. The chapters are illustrated by over 1101 figures and 229 videos to help the reader become familiar with the different displays of three-dimensional data sets, the related anatomy as imaged with this technique, and how to postprocess data sets. At the end of each chapter, a selected list of annotated references is included. These references are suggestions for the reader who may be interested in reading more about a particular topic.

The first edition of the *Textbook of Three-Dimensional Echocardiography*, one of the first books on the topic, was published in 2011. Since the first edition, three-dimensional echocardiography technology has evolved dramatically, image quality has improved, and new software packages have been developed to provide improved postprocessing and near-automated quantitative analysis of the three-dimensional data sets. In addition, since our previous book, hundreds of publications which have contributed to broaden our knowledge of this echocardiographic technique have been published.

We have thoroughly revised this new edition to reflect these multiple changes. Denisa Muraru, MD, PhD, has joined our editorial team, and, in addition to writing several new chapters, she has overseen the illustration content of this book. The number of chapters has increased from 18 to 25, and 18 chapters are entirely new. The chapters which have been carried over from the first edition have undergone extensive update to broaden their content and highlight technical advances and clinical utility. In this new edition of our book, there are 31 new authors, all of them true experts on the topic they have written.

It should be emphasized that this textbook should be the starting point or frame of reference to start learning three-dimensional echocardiography. Appropriate training in three-dimensional echocardiography includes competency in the acquisition and postprocessing of high-quality data sets and knowledge of cardiac anatomy and pathophysiology of heart diseases. A textbook can only supplement the experience gained when attending “live” three-dimensional echocardiographic courses and when acquiring studies on patients with a wide range of heart diseases under expert guidance. Although this textbook cannot be a substitute for appropriate training and clinical experience, we hope that the superior quality of the three-dimensional echocardiography illustrations and videos, as well as the quality of the accompanying text, will enhance the learning experience of colleagues who are new to this technique and provide a useful update for those who are already experts.

Milano, Italy — Luigi P. Badano
Chicago, IL, USA — Roberto M. Lang
Milano, Italy — Denisa Muraru

Acknowledgements

Special thanks to the cardiac sonographers at the University of Padua, School of Medicine (Chiara Palermo and Federica Sambugaro), and the University of Chicago (Lynn Weinert, RDCS; Eric Kruse, RDCS; and Meghan Yamat, RDCS). The quality of most of the images and videos is due to their skill, commitment, and passion.

The many changes in the content and structure of the chapters in this second edition of the textbook are the results of the discussions we had with our sonographers and the researchers who joined us from all over the world to learn three-dimensional echocardiography and expand its clinical applications. Special appreciation are due to Sorina Mihaila Baldea (from Romania), Marcelo Haertel Miglioranza (from Brazil), Hoda Shehata (from Egypt), Elena Surkova (from Russia), Alex Felix (from Brazil), Hugo Zanella-Rodriguez (from Mexico), Csaba Jenei (from Hungary), Monica Luiza de Alcantara (from Brazil), Jurate Bidviene (from Lithuania), Ana Paula Siciliano (from Brazil), Attila Kovacs (from Hungary), Arnaldo Rabischoffsky (from Brazil), and Jonan Liao (from Taipei).

A special thanks to Prof. Cristina Basso, MD, PhD, from Cardiovascular Pathology Unit, University of Padua, School of Medicine, who generously provided the anatomy specimens.

Finally, our special thanks go to our colleagues in the echocardiography laboratory who provided many cases and whose comments and suggestions allowed us to better understand the place of three-dimensional echocardiography in the workflow of the laboratory.

Contents

About the Editors

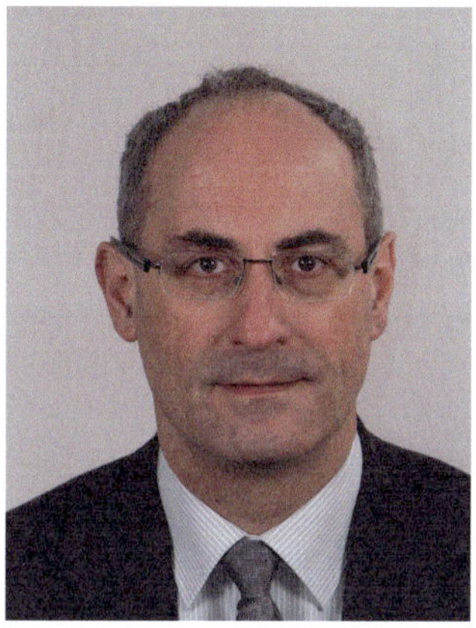

Luigi P. Badano, MD, PhD, FESC, FACC currently serves as director of the cardiovascular imaging laboratory at the Istituto Auxologico Italiano, IRCCS, San Luca Hospital, and professor of cardiology at the University of Milano-Bicocca, Milan, Italy.

His clinical interests include native and prosthetic valvular heart disease and right ventricular and atrial function, with research interests in three-dimensional and deformation imaging by echocardiography and cardiac mechanics.

He is member of the Italian Society of Cardiology, Italian Society of Cardiovascular Ultrasound, European Society of Cardiology, European Association of Cardiovascular Imaging, American College of Cardiology, and American Society of Echocardiography (ASE) and serves as fellow of the European Society of Cardiology and the American College of Cardiology.

He is a regular lecturer at ESC, ACC, ASE, and EuroEcho scientific meetings. He has published more than 290 peer-reviewed full papers and authored 9 books about echocardiography and cardiovascular imaging. He is honorary member of the British Society of Echocardiography and Romanian, Hungarian, and Korean societies of cardiology. From 2010 to 2012, he served as president of the European Association of Cardiovascular Imaging. In 2013, he was awarded with the silver medal of the European Society of Cardiology for his clinical and research activity and his services as president of the European Association of Cardiovascular Imaging.

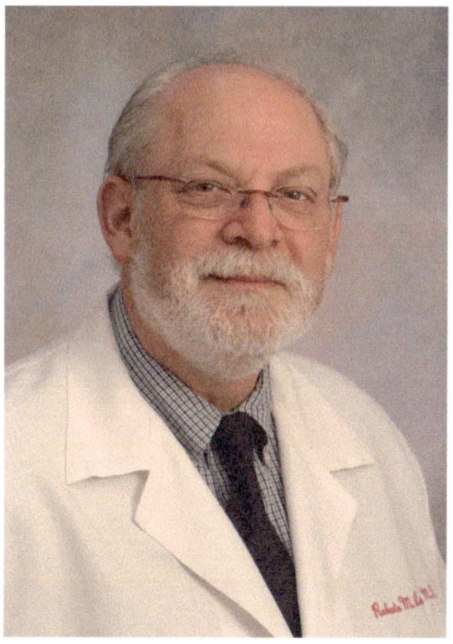

Roberto M. Lang, MD, FACC, FASE, FAHA, FRCP is currently the director of the Noninvasive Cardiac Imaging Laboratories at the University of Chicago and associate director of the Cardiology Fellowship Training Program. He is a professor of medicine and radiology at the University of Chicago Medical Center. He has published more than 570 manuscripts on cardiac imaging and physiology during his career as well as 10 books and 110 book chapters. He has been a pioneer in the development of three-dimensional transthoracic and transesophageal echocardiography, a noninvasive technique that is currently used worldwide to diagnose heart disease. He serves as a manuscript review consultant for most cardiology peer-reviewed journals and on the editorial boards of the *Journal of the American College of Cardiology*, *Echocardiography*, *Journal of the American Society of Echocardiography*, *Circulation Cardiovascular Imaging*, and *Journal of Echocardiography*, the official journal of the

Japanese Society of Echocardiography. His major research interests are the clinical utility of noninvasive techniques in assessing left ventricular contractile state/myocardial perfusion and three-dimensional echocardiography. He was the president of the American Society of Echocardiography and has recently given the Edler Lecture in the last Scientific Sessions of the American Society of Echocardiography and the Honorary Euro-Lecture of the European Society of Cardiovascular Imaging.

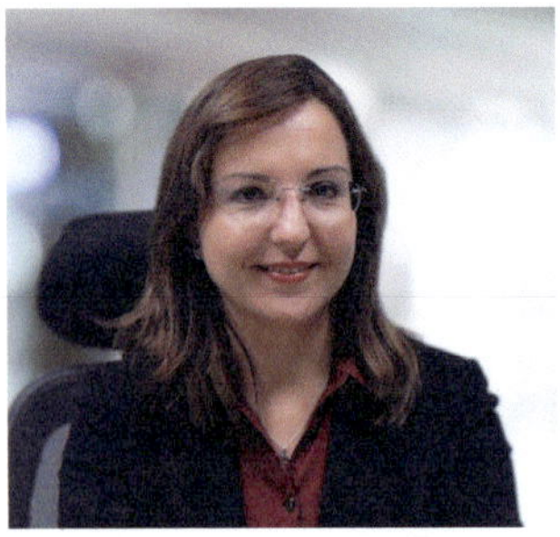

Denisa Muraru, MD, PhD, FESC, FACC, FASE is a cardiologist, currently working as a researcher at the University of Padua (Italy). She graduated from the "Carol Davila" University of Medicine and Pharmacy in Bucharest (Romania). In 2011, she moved to the University of Padua in order to perform clinical research in the field of 3D echocardiography and received her PhD degree in 2013. She has an *h*-index of 26 (Scopus 2019). Her main research interests are ventricular function and mechanics, valvular heart disease, and clinical implementation of 3D echocardiography (software validation, reference values, outcome). She has been co-director of several teaching courses and scientific meetings on 3D echocardiography organized by the University of Padua since 2012. She chaired the Education Committee of the European Association of Cardiovascular Imaging (EACVI) between 2016 and 2020.

The Evolution of Three-Dimensional Echocardiography: From the Initial Concept to Real-Time Imaging

1

Victor Mor-Avi, Bernhard Mumm, and Roberto M. Lang

Abstract

For decades, cardiac ultrasound had an important advantage over computed tomography and magnetic resonance imaging by virtue of its dynamic nature resulting in anatomically correct cross-sectional views of the beating heart. Nevertheless, it has remained limited to a single cut-plane at a time, necessitating sequential imaging of multiple views and considerable expertise to mentally align them in order to visualize the complex three-dimensional cardiac anatomy and detect abnormalities. Recent technological developments resulted in real-time three-dimensional ultrasound imaging of the heart, which is quickly conquering the clinical arena and adds unprecedented new dimensions to the diagnosis of heart disease. The goal of this chapter is to review the evolution of 3D echocardiography and describe the milestones this technology has gone through, and to highlight the promises and setbacks that drive the technological development towards the realization of its full potential.

Keywords

Three-dimensional imaging · Ultrasound imaging · Transthoracic echocardiography · Transesophageal echocardiography · Real-time imaging

V. Mor-Avi
Department of Medicine/Section of Cardiology, University of Chicago Medical Center, Chicago, IL, USA
e-mail: vmoravi@bsd.uchicago.edu

B. Mumm
TomTec Imaging Systems, Unterschleissheim, Germany
e-mail: bmumm@tomtec.de

R. M. Lang (✉)
Noninvasive Cardiac Imaging Laboratories, Department of Medicine/Section of Cardiology, University of Chicago Medical Center, Chicago, IL, USA
e-mail: rlang@bsd.uchicago.edu, rlang@medicine.bsd.uchicago.edu

Introduction

From the early days of medical imaging, the concept of three-dimensional (3D) imaging was indisputably perceived as desirable based on the wide recognition that depicting complex 3D systems of the human body in less than three dimensions severely limited the diagnostic value of the information gleaned from these images. Over the last half of the twentieth century, we have witnessed continuous technological developments driven by strong demand from the medical community that allowed the transition from fuzzy single-projection x-ray films to multi-slice tomographic images of exquisite quality depicting anatomical details previously seen only in anatomy atlases. The ability to visualize these details in a living patient had spurred revolutionary changes in how physicians understand disease processes and resulted in new standards in the diagnosis of disease. Today, the diagnosis of multiple disease states heavily relies on information obtained from noninvasive imaging. The ability to virtually slice and dice the human body in any desired plane has boosted the diagnostic accuracy and confidence by orders of magnitude.

Despite the broad appeal of computed tomography (CT) and magnetic resonance imaging (MRI), for several decades, heart disease has remained outside the scope of these sophisticated technologies because of the constant motion of the beating heart. While imaging of stationary organs was conceptually easy to solve by collecting information from different parts or from different angles consecutively, imaging of the beating heart required data collection to occur virtually in real time. While for decades, ultrasound imaging had this edge over CT and MRI, it remained limited to a single cut-plane. In fact, one may find in textbooks from the early 1970s explanations why real-time 2D imaging of a beating heart is an enormous technological advancement that is unsurpassable because of the limitations imposed by the speed at which sound waves travel inside the human body. Nevertheless, despite the fact that the speed of sound has

L. P. Badano et al. (eds.), *Textbook of Three-Dimensional Echocardiography*, https://doi.org/10.1007/978-3-030-14032-8_1

not changed since then, the combination of the meteoric rise of computing technology with ingenious engineering solutions that increased the efficiency of the process of image formation from ultrasound reflections dispelled this tenet. In the 1990s, we witnessed the increase in imaging frame rates from a crawling few to a blazing hundreds per second, paving the way to 3D echocardiography [1]. The concept behind this new imaging modality was that it should be possible to image multiple planes in real time, albeit at lower frame rates, similar to those of earlier versions of 2D imaging.

This vision turned into reality rather quickly, and today real-time 3D echocardiography is booming and has secured an important place in the noninvasive clinical assessment of cardiac anatomy and function [2–5]. The purpose of this chapter is to review the evolution of 3D echocardiography and describe the milestones this technology has gone through, and to highlight the promises and setbacks that propelled the technological development into the race for the next "base" in the understanding of its full potential.

Linear Multiplane Scanning

Before technology necessary for real-time scanning of multiple planes was in place, attempts for 3D reconstruction of the heart from echocardiographic images were based on the use of linear step-by-step motion, wherein the transducer was mechanically advanced between acquisitions using a motorized driving device [6]. However, this simple solution was not applicable for transthoracic echocardiography, because of the need to find inter-costal acoustic windows for each acquisition step. This approach was also implemented in a pull-back transesophageal echocardiography (TEE) transducer, known as "lobster tail" probe (Fig. 1.1).

Gated Sequential Acquisition

One developmental aspect crucial for the success of 3D reconstruction from multiplane acquisition was the registration of the different planes, so that they could be combined together to create a 3D image of the heart. This was achieved by sequential gated acquisition, wherein different cut-planes were acquired one-by-one with gating designed to minimize artifacts. To minimize spatial misalignment of slices because of respiration, respiratory gating was used, such that only cardiac cycles coinciding with a certain phase of the respiratory cycle were captured. Similarly, to minimize temporal misalignment because of heart rate variability, ECG gating was used, such that only cardiac cycles within preset limits of R-R interval were included. This methodology became standard in both transthoracic and transesophageal multiplane imaging aimed at 3D reconstruction and was widely used until real-time 3D imaging became possible.

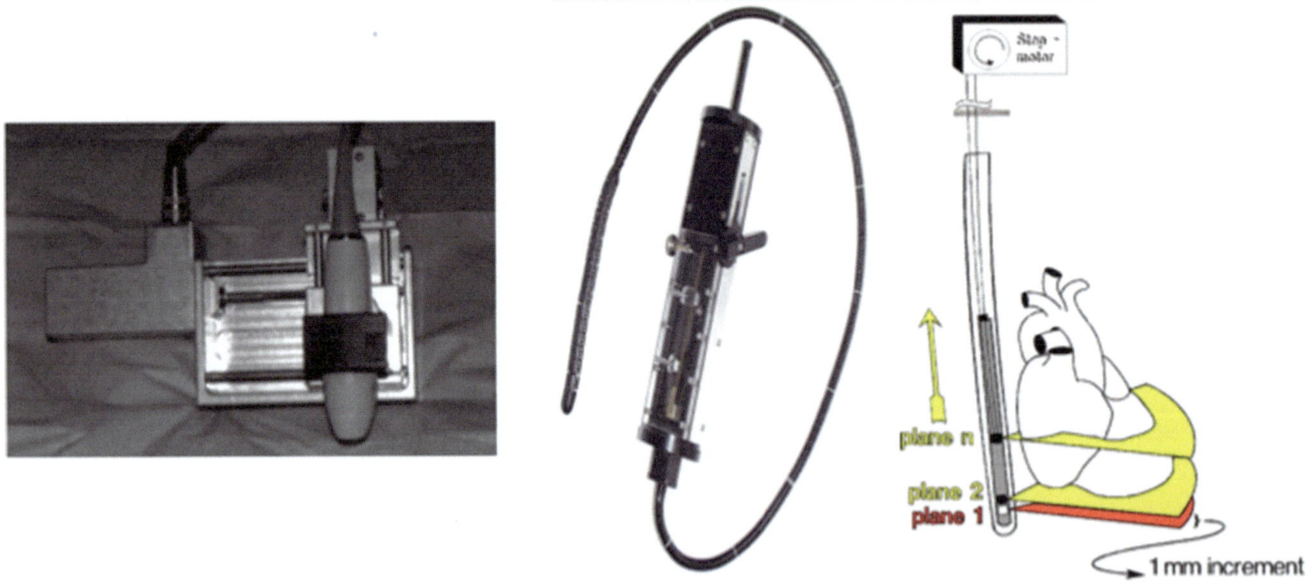

Fig. 1.1 Motorized linear-motion device used to acquire parallel cut planes for reconstructing 3D images using linear step-by-step transducer motion (left panel). Pull back transoesophageal probe that employed the same approach of linear motion (right panel) [7]. Reprinted by permission from Springer Nature, Muraru D, Badano LP. Physical and Technical Aspects and Overview of 3D-Echocardiography. In: Manual of Echocardiography, Casas Rojo E, Fernandez-Golfin C, Zamorano J. (eds). Springer, Cham, 2017, pages 1–44

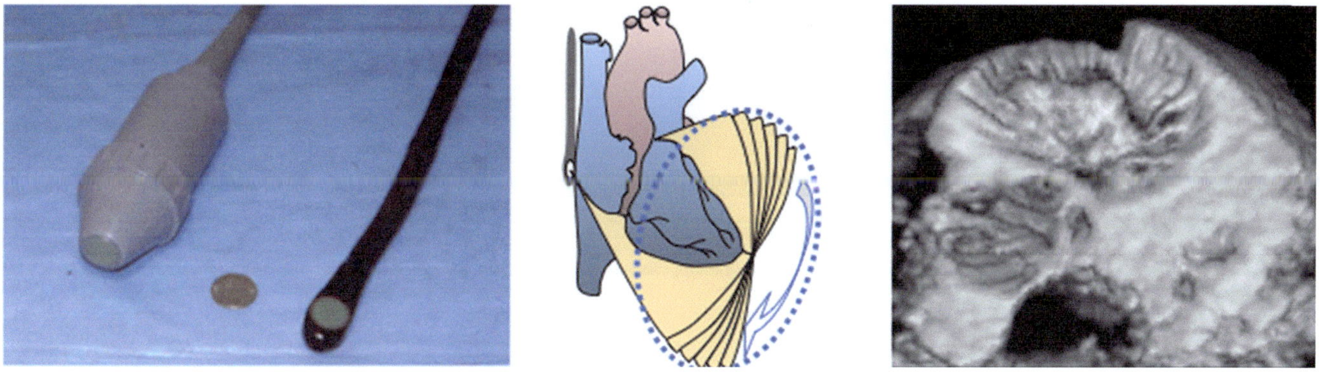

Fig. 1.2 Rotational approach implemented into a transoesophageal multiplane transducer (left panel). Schematic drawing of sequential ultrasound images obtained by progressive rotation of the transducer in a prespecified fashion (central panel). Example of a 3D image of the mitral valve with anterior leaflet prolapse from multiplane images acquired using this transducer (right panel) [7]. Reprinted by permission from Springer Nature, Muraru D, Badano LP. Physical and Technical Aspects and Overview of 3D-Echocardiography. In: Manual of Echocardiography, Casas Rojo E, Fernandez-Golfin C, Zamorano J. (eds). Springer, Cham, 2017, pages 1–44

Transesophageal Rotational Imaging

An alternative approach to linear scanning was to keep the transducer in a fixed position corresponding to an optimal acoustic window, and rotate the imaging plane by internally steering the imaging element in different directions (Fig. 1.2, **Central panel**). This concept of rotational scanning in combination with gated sequential scanning was implemented in TEE technology and resulted in a probe (Fig. 1.2, **Left panel**) that has subsequently become the main source of multiplane images used for 3D reconstruction, both for research and clinical practice [8, 9]. This approach provided 3D reconstructions of reasonably good quality due to the high quality of the original 2D images and the fact that the TEE probe is relatively well "anchored" in its position throughout image acquisition, especially in sedated patients. Nevertheless, cardiac structures, such as valve leaflets appeared jagged as a result of stitch artifacts (Fig. 1.2, **Right panel**), reflecting the contributions of individual imaging planes that could not be perfectly aligned during reconstruction, despite the ECG and respiratory gating. Multiple studies demonstrated the clinical usefulness of this approach mostly in the context of the evaluation of valvular heart disease.

Transthoracic Rotational Imaging

An early transthoracic implementation of rotational approach consisted of a motorized device that contained a conventional transducer, which was mechanically rotated several degrees at a time, resulting in first transthoracic gated sequential multiplane acquisitions suitable for 3D reconstruction of the heart [10–12]. A later, more sophisticated implementation used a multiplane TEE transducer that was repackaged into a casing suitable for transthoracic imaging (Fig. 1.2, **Left panel**). Despite the previously unseen 3D transthoracic echocardiographic images that excited so many, it quickly became clear that this methodology was destined to remain limited to the research arena because image acquisition was too time-consuming and tedious for clinical use. In addition, the quality of the reconstructed images was limited.

Transthoracic Free-Hand Imaging

An alternative approach for transthoracic 3D echocardiography is known as free-hand scanning [12–14]. This methodology is based on the use of spatial locators, conceptually similar to the global positioning system, widely known today as GPS, except these devices were communicating with a receiver unit located in the exam room, rather than on a satellite revolving around the Earth. Initially, these locators used acoustic technology known as "spark gaps" (Fig. 1.3), which was based on precise measurements of the differences in travel time of sounds emitted by three different sources mounted on the transducer. Subsequently, an electromagnetic version of this technology was used, based on phase differences of signals originating from different sources (Fig. 1.4). Regardless of the underlying technology, these devices could accurately determine the location and orientation of the transducer at any moment. This information was translated into precise location of the imaging plane, allowing the sonographer to image from any identifiable good acoustic window. These images could be added to the data set eventually used for 3D reconstruction, thus eliminating the problem of using suboptimal images obtained from poor acoustic windows.

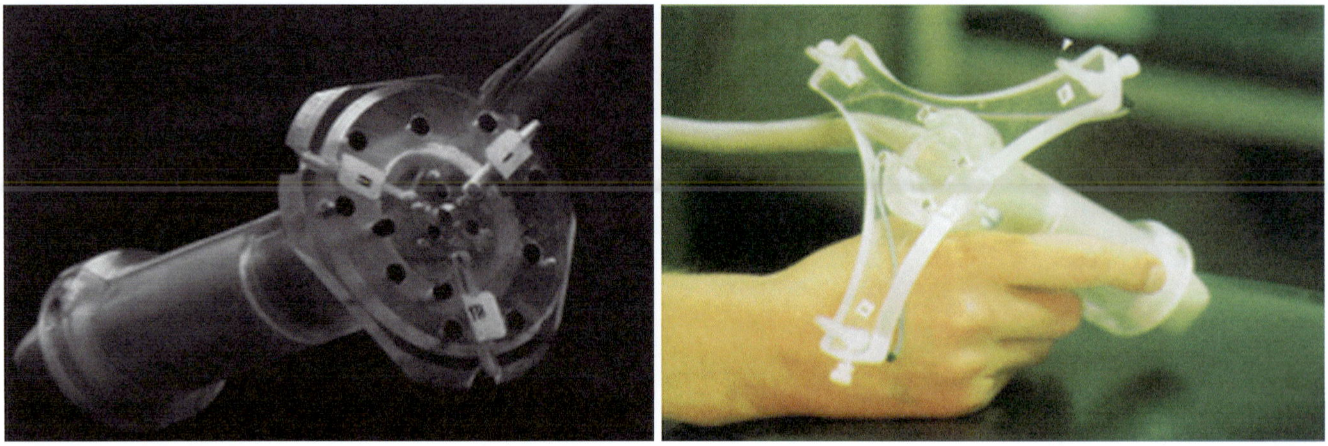

Fig. 1.3 Acoustic locator or "spar-gaps". The ultrasound probe position is tracked by a means similar to radar technology [7]. Reprinted by permission from Springer Nature, Muraru D, Badano LP. Physical and Technical Aspects and Overview of 3D-Echocardiography. In: Manual of Echocardiography, Casas Rojo E, Fernandez-Golfin C, Zamorano J. (eds). Springer, Cham, 2017, pages 1–44

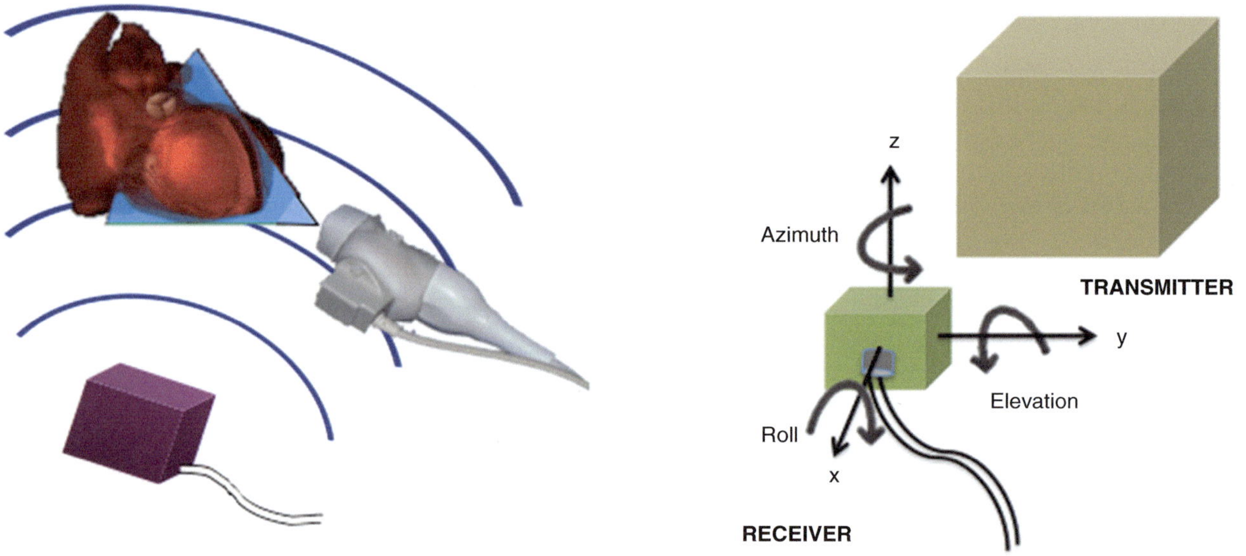

Fig. 1.4 Freehand scanning. A modified ultrasound probe is tracked in 3D space using an electromagnetic locator system (left panel). Schematic drawing of the receiver and transmitting device and the Cartesian coordinate system for tracking the location of the transducer (right panel). Images then may be reconstructed off-line to create 3D data sets [7]. Reprinted by permission from Springer Nature, Muraru D, Badano LP. Physical and Technical Aspects and Overview of 3D-Echocardiography. In: Manual of Echocardiography, Casas Rojo E, Fernandez-Golfin C, Zamorano J. (eds). Springer, Cham, 2017, pages 1–44

Since the number of planes typically acquired using this approach was relatively small (3–8), but nevertheless sufficient for 3D reconstruction of heart chambers and volume quantification, the acquisition was relatively quick. However, the downside of this high-speed acquisition was that there was not enough information to create detailed 3D views of the valves. Another drawback of this methodology was that while the acquired cut-planes could be perfectly aligned in the fixed room coordinates, they were not necessarily aligned anatomically, whenever any patient's body movement occurred between the consecutive acquisitions of individual cut-planes. The result again was motion artifacts that frequently necessitated repeated acquisition. Another factor that has limited the use of this methodology in the clinical practice was the relative lack of portability of the locator devices, although conceivably they could be incorporated into the imaging system.

Transthoracic Real-Time 3D Imaging

The collective experience and the limitations of the gated sequential acquisition and offline 3D reconstruction gradually led developers to the understanding that scanning volumes rather than isolated cut-planes would intrinsically resolve many of these limitations [15, 16]. This revolutionary idea led to the development of the first system equipped with a phased-array transducer (Fig. 1.5), in which piezoelectric elements were arranged in multiple rows, rather than one row, allowing fast sequential scanning of multiple planes. The phased array technology, that has been an integral part of the 2D transducers for decades, was modified to electronically change the direction of the beam not only within a single plane to create a fan-shaped scan, but also in the lateral direction to generate a series of such scans. Importantly this was achieved without any mechanical motion, allowing the speeds necessary for volumetric real-time imaging.

The first generation of real-time 3D transducers was bulky due to unprecedented number of electrical connections to the individual crystals, despite the relatively small number of elements in each row. This sparse array matrix transducer consisted of 256 non-simultaneously firing elements and had large footprint, which did not allow good coupling with the chest wall for optimal acoustic windows, and produced 3D images that were suboptimal in any selected plane, when compared to the quality of standard at the time 2D echocardiographic images. Nevertheless, the mere fact of successful real-time 3D imaging was a huge technological breakthrough.

The subsequent generations of fully sampled matrix array transducers differed from this prototype first and foremost in the considerably larger number of elements per row, with a total of approximately 3000 elements. This dramatic increase in the number of elements was accompanied by progressive miniaturization of electronic connections, resulting in 3D transducers with footprints comparable to those of conventional 2D transducers, capable of providing high 3D resolution images (Fig. 1.6). Today, cut-planes extracted from these 3D datasets are similar in their quality to 2D images obtained using state of the art 2D transducers.

From Gated to Single-Beat Acquisition

Because of the limited size of the 3D scan volume, ECG-gated "full-volume" acquisition mode was used to capture the entire left ventricle section-by-section over several

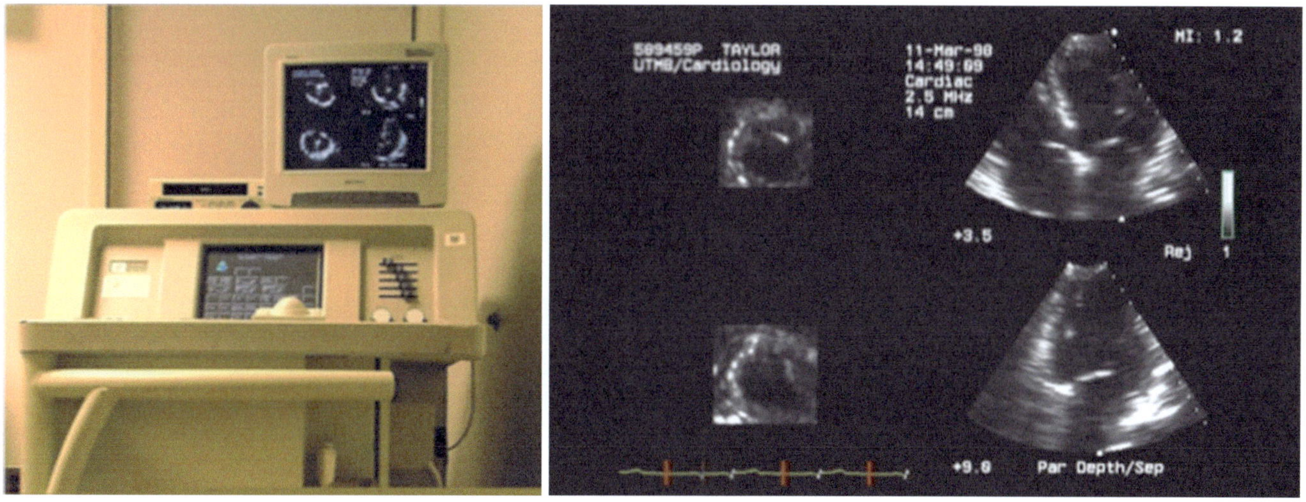

Fig. 1.5 The first real-time 3D echocardiography system (C-scan, Volumetrics, Inc.) equipped with a sparse matrix array transducer (left panel). In the right panel the images which can be obtained with that system (simultaneous display of multiple tomographic planes extracted from the real-time data) are shown: apical views of the heart on the right (four-chamber on top, and two-chamber of the left ventricle on the bottom), and short axis, or C scans, of the LV derived from perpendicular cuts through the apical views on the left [7]. Reprinted by permission from Springer Nature, Muraru D, Badano LP. Physical and Technical Aspects and Overview of 3D-Echocardiography. In: Manual of Echocardiography, Casas Rojo E, Fernandez-Golfin C, Zamorano J. (eds). Springer, Cham, 2017, pages 1–44

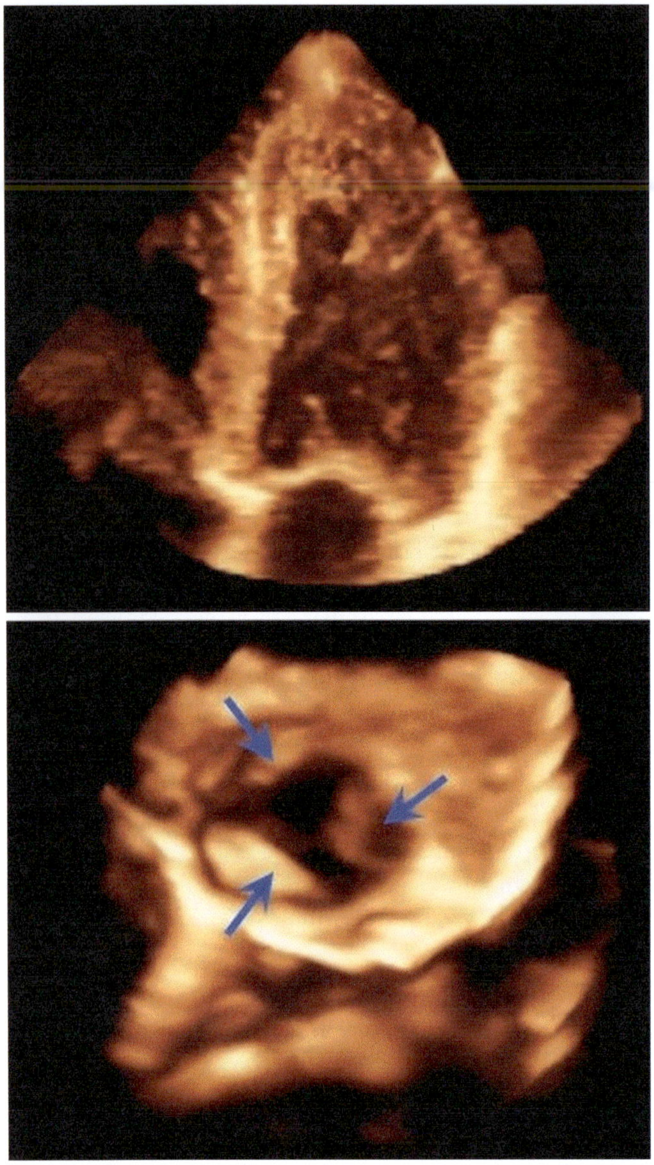

Fig. 1.6 Transthoracic real-time 3DE images of the heart extracted from the pyramidal datasets: apical four-chamber cross-sectional view obtained from a full-volume acquisition (top), and zoomed acquisition of the aortic valve in early systole shown from the left ventricular perspective depicting the three aortic valve leaflets (bottom, arrows)

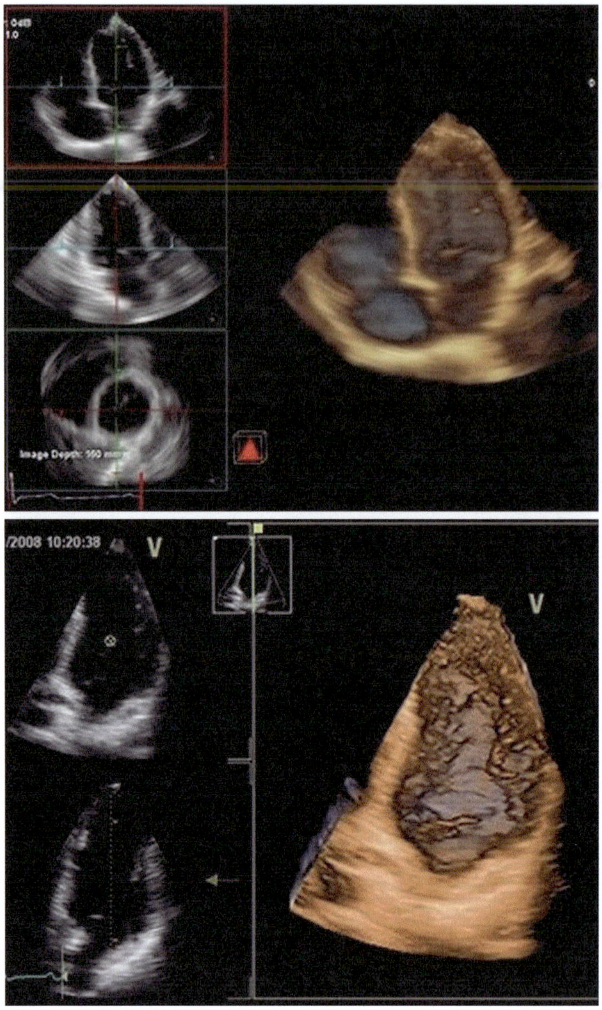

Fig. 1.7 Single-beat acquisition mode, currently available from several vendors (left and right panels), is time saving not only because the entire beating left ventricle can be captured in a single cardiac cycle, but because it reduces motion artifacts, thus eliminating the need for repeated acquisition

cardiac cycles. The major drawback of this approach was misregistration of the subvolumes, manifesting itself as "stitch artifacts" as a result of irregular heart rhythm, respiration, or any movement of the patient or transducer during image acquisition, which frequently needed to be repeated to obtain a high quality dataset. Subsequent technological developments resulted in the capability to capture the entire heart in a single cardiac cycle (Fig. 1.7). This approach further improved the ease of real-time 3D echocardiographic evaluation of the left ventricle by improving the speed of acquisition and reducing artifacts.

Transesophageal Real-Time Imaging

More recently, transesophageal imaging has also undergone the transition from gated sequential multiplane acquisition and off-line reconstruction to real-time volumetric scanning. Technological advances have allowed the miniaturization of matrix-array transducers by using integrated circuits that perform most of the beam forming within the transducer, rather than in the imaging system (Fig. 1.8). This modification allowed fitting thousands of piezoelectric elements into the tip of the TEE transducer, resulting in unprecedented views of the heart valves and unparalleled level of anatomic detail virtually in every patient [17, 18]. Over the last few years, this methodology has assumed a leading role in perioperative assessment of patients with valve disease.

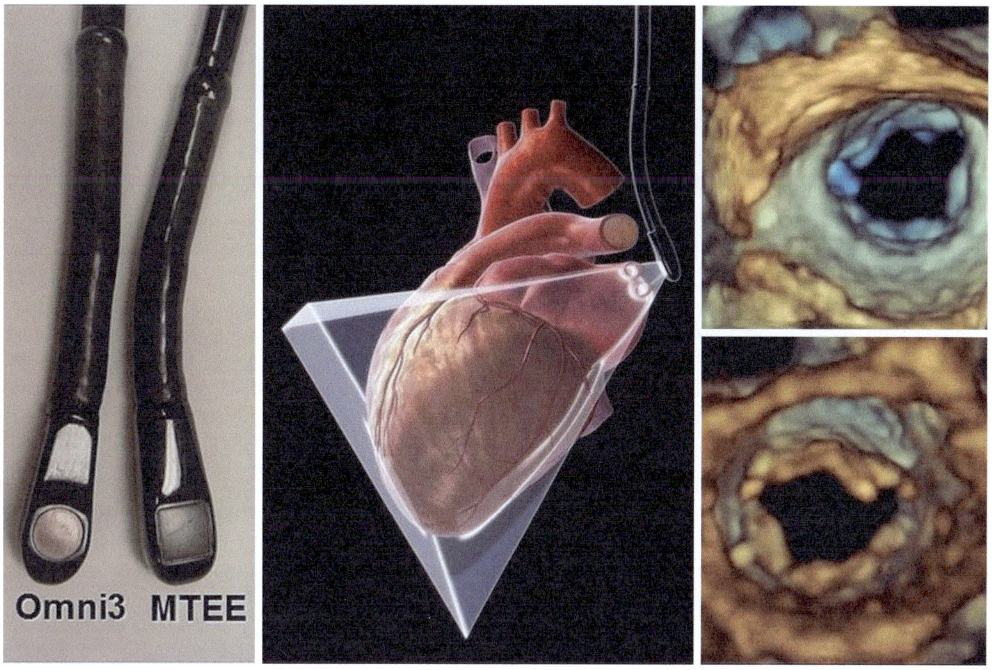

Fig. 1.8 Multiplane Omni-3 and matrix array transesophageal (MTEE) transducers shown side-by-side (left). While the dimensions of both transducers are similar, the MTEE probe that utilizes miniaturized beam-forming technology that allows fitting of near 3000 piezoelectric elements into the head of the probe and thus provides real-time 3D images of the heart (middle). Example of 3D TEE views of the mitral valve from the left atrial (right, top) and left ventricular (right, bottom) perspectives obtained during diastole

Display of 3D Image Information

Another important part of 3D echocardiography, which has gone through its own developmental phases, is the display of the 3D information. Regardless of the mode of acquisition, multi-plane reconstruction or real-time imaging, the information needs to be displayed in a way understandable to the user, which should be suited to a specific clinical goal in each case. Thus, evaluation of valvular pathology requires detailed dynamic 3D rendering of the annulus and leaflet surface and an ability to easily manipulate the rendered image in terms of view angle [9]. The assessment of the spatial relationships in complex congenital heart disease relies on accurate visualization of anatomic detail as well [19], but also requires extensive capabilities of changing the dynamic range of colors and opacity. In contrast, the evaluation of chamber size and function requires a dynamic display of the detected endocardial surface [20, 21], from which chamber volume can be calculated over time and regional abnormalities can be visualized, but understandably does not require the same level of anatomic detail as valve imaging. These specific applications branched off of the original display of simple planes selected from the 3D dataset, and each of them has gone over the last decade through multiple improvements, finally resulting in vivid images tailored to answer a variety of diagnostic questions [22].

Volumetric Quantification

It is widely accepted today that quantitative measurements replacing subjective visual interpretation are of significant clinical value, because they allow serial evaluation of the effects of therapy in individual patients as well as inter-subject comparisons essential for objective detection of abnormalities. Nevertheless, the development of quantitative tools for analysis of 3D echocardiographic images has initially been lagging behind the continuous progress in the imaging technology. There are several reasons for this, including: (1) analysis tools emerge only after imaging capabilities are tested and proven, (2) developing and testing new analysis tools requires time and resources, (3) proving the clinical usefulness of such tools through publications takes time as initial reports are confirmed by multiple investigators and collective experience is gathered. Also, historically, the manufacturers of ultrasound imaging equipments did not have the resources necessary to develop and market software tools. However, this picture has changed dramatically over the last decade, as most manufacturers, having realized the need for such tools, provide today more and more comprehensive software tools for analysis of 3D echocardiographic images with their imaging equipment. These tools allow anatomic measurements that aid clinicians in the diagnosis of disease processes, and researchers in collecting information that eventually constitutes the scientific basis for official guidelines and standards.

Summary

In summary, over the last two decades, echocardiographic community has witnessed technological developments and breakthroughs that have propelled 3D echocardiographic imaging from an initial concept requiring more advanced technology than available at the time, to a widespread clinically useful imaging modality. Today, 3D echocardiography has established itself as the preferred diagnostic method in many clinical scenarios, in which continuing technological refinements steadily improve the user's confidence and lead to better patient outcomes [4, 5]. This process is an example of technological development driven by clinical demand that evolves in turn with each increment in technology and pushes the envelope of addressing new, more complex clinical questions.

References

1. Levine RA, Weyman AE, Handschumacher MD. Three-dimensional echocardiography: techniques and applications. Am J Cardiol. 1992;69:121H–30H.
2. Roelandt JR. Three-dimensional echocardiography: new views from old windows. Br Heart J. 1995;74:4–6.
3. de Castro S, Yao J, Pandian NG. Three-dimensional echocardiography: clinical relevance and application. Am J Cardiol. 1998;81:96G–102G.
4. Lang RM, Mor-Avi V, Sugeng L, Nieman PS, Sahn DJ. Three-dimensional echocardiography: the benefits of the additional dimension. J Am Coll Cardiol. 2006;48:2053–69.
5. Mor-Avi V, Sugeng L, Lang RM. Real-time 3D echocardiography: an integral component of the routine echocardiographic examination in adult patients? Circulation. 2009;119:314–29.
6. Matsumoto M, Inoue M, Tamura S, Tanaka K, Abe H. Three-dimensional echocardiography for spatial visualization and volume calculation of cardiac structures. J Clin Ultrasound. 1981;9:157–65.
7. Muraru D, Badano LP. Physical and technical aspects and overview of 3D-echocardiography. I. In: Casas Rojo E, Fernandez-Golfin C, Zamorano J, editors. Manual of echocardiography. Cham: Springer; 2017. p. 1–44.
8. Pandian NG, Nanda NC, Schwartz SL, Fan P, Cao QL, Sanyal R, et al. Three-dimensional and four-dimensional transesophageal echocardiographic imaging of the heart and aorta in humans using a computed tomographic imaging probe. Echocardiography. 1992;9:677–87.
9. Flachskampf FA, Franke A, Job FP, Krebs W, Terstegge A, Klues HG, Hanrath P. Three-dimensional reconstruction of cardiac structures from transesophageal echocardiography. Am J Card Imaging. 1995;9:141–7.
10. Vogel M, Losch S. Dynamic three-dimensional echocardiography with a computed tomography imaging probe: initial clinical experience with transthoracic application in infants and children with congenital heart defects. Br Heart J. 1994;71:462–7.
11. Ludomirsky A, Vermilion R, Nesser J, Marx G, Vogel M, Derman R, Pandian N. Transthoracic real-time three-dimensional echocardiography using the rotational scanning approach for data acquisition. Echocardiography. 1994;11:599–606.
12. Kupferwasser I, Mohr-Kahaly S, Stahr P, Rupprecht HJ, Nixdorff U, Fenster M, et al. Transthoracic three-dimensional echocardiographic volumetry of distorted left ventricles using rotational scanning. J Am Soc Echocardiogr. 1997;10:840–52.
13. Levine RA, Handschumacher MD, Sanfilippo AJ, Hagege AA, Harrigan P, Marshall JE, Weyman AE. Three-dimensional echocardiographic reconstruction of the mitral valve, with implications for the diagnosis of mitral valve prolapse. Circulation. 1989;80:589–98.
14. Gopal AS, Schnellbaecher MJ, Shen Z, Boxt LM, Katz J, King DL. Freehand three-dimensional echocardiography for determination of left ventricular volume and mass in patients with abnormal ventricles: comparison with magnetic resonance imaging. J Am Soc Echocardiogr. 1997;10:853–61.
15. von Ramm OT, Smith SW. Real time volumetric ultrasound imaging system. J Digit Imaging. 1990;3:261–6.
16. Sheikh K, Smith SW, von Ramm OT, Kisslo J. Real-time, three-dimensional echocardiography: feasibility and initial use. Echocardiography. 1991;8:119–25.
17. Sugeng L, Shernan SK, Salgo IS, Weinert L, Shook D, Raman J, et al. Live three-dimensional transesophageal echocardiography: initial experience using the fully-sampled matrix array probe. J Am Coll Cardiol. 2008;52:446–9.
18. Sugeng L, Shernan SK, Salgo IS, Weinert L, Shook D, Raman J. Jet al. Real-time 3D transesophageal echocardiography in valve disease: comparison with surgical findings and evaluation of prosthetic valves. J Am Soc Echocardiogr. 2008;21:1347–54.
19. Magni G, Cao QL, Sugeng L, Delabays A, Marx G, Ludomirski A, et al. Volume-rendered, three-dimensional echocardiographic determination of the size, shape, and position of atrial septal defects: validation in an in vitro model. Am Heart J. 1996;132:376–81.
20. Gopal AS, Keller AM, Rigling R, King DL Jr, King DL. Left ventricular volume and endocardial surface area by three-dimensional echocardiography: comparison with two-dimensional echocardiography and nuclear magnetic resonance imaging in normal subjects. J Am Coll Cardiol. 1993;22:258–70.
21. Mele D, Maehle J, Pedini I, Alboni P, Levine RA. Three-dimensional echocardiographic reconstruction: description and applications of a simplified technique for quantitative assessment of left ventricular size and function. Am J Cardiol. 1998;81:107G–10G.
22. Lang RM, Badano LP, Tsang W, Adams DH, Agricola E, Buck T, et al. EAE/ASE recommendations for image acquisition and display using three-dimensional echocardiography. J Am Soc Echocardiogr. 2012;25:3–46.

Physics and Technical Principles of Three-Dimensional Echocardiography

2

Denisa Muraru and Luigi P. Badano

Abstract

The backbone of the three-dimensional echocardiography (3DE) technology is the transducer. Understanding the physics of 3DE and the way the matrix transducer works is pivotal for successful acquisition of good quality 3DE data sets. Different 3DE acquisition modalities are available (real-time/live, multi-beat, zoom, full-volume, color) to adapt to the different clinical needs. Once acquired, 3DE data sets should be postprocessed by cropping, rotating and slicing them in order to obtain the images that are needed to meet the clinical or research needs. Different ways of displaying the data sets are also available: volume rendering (to show anatomy), wireframe or solid surface rendering (for quantitative analysis) and multislice (for analysis of regional function and anatomy and 2D quantitative analysis). Moreover, new display modalities (such as stereoscopic vision, 3D printing and holography) are entering the clinical arena to provide an actual 3D appreciation and manipulation of images.

Keywords

Three-dimensional echocardiography · Physics · Probe · Transducer · Spatial resolution · Temporal resolution · Parallel beamforming · Multibeat acquisition · Data set acquisition · Real-time · Full-volume · Cropping · Rotating · Slicing · Volume rendering · Surface rendering · Multislice · Stereoscopic vision · 3D printing · Holography

Electronic Supplementary Material The online version of this chapter (https://doi.org/10.1007/978-3-030-14032-8_2) contains supplementary material, which is available to authorized users.

D. Muraru · L. P. Badano (✉)
University of Milano-Bicocca, and Istituto Auxologico Italiano, IRCCS, San Luca Hospital, Milano, Italy
e-mail: denisa.muraru@unimib.it; luigi.badano@unimib.it

The milestone in the history of three-dimensional echocardiography (3DE) has been the development of fully-sampled matrix array transthoracic transducers based on advanced digital processing and improved image formation algorithms which allowed the operators to obtain on cart transthoracic real-time volumetric imaging with short acquisition time, high spatial and temporal resolution (see also Chap. 1). Further technological developments (i.e. advances in miniaturization of the electronics and in element interconnection technology) have made possible to insert a full matrix array into the tip of a transesophageal probe and provide transesophageal real-time volumetric imaging (see also Chap. 3).

In addition to transducer engineering, exponential increase of computer processing power and the availability of dedicated software packages for both on- and off-line analysis have allowed 3DE to become a practical clinical tool.

In this chapter, we will describe the differences between two-dimensional (2DE) and 3DE transducers, review the main concepts about the physics of 3DE imaging which are useful to understand the various acquisition modes, describe the currently used acquisition modalities and their main clinical uses as well as the conventional techniques used to display the 3DE data sets. Finally, new, emerging modalities to display the 3DE data sets are also described.

Comparison Between 2DE and 3DE Ultrasound Transducers

The backbone of the 3DE technology is the transducer. A conventional 2D phased array transducer is composed by 128 piezoelectric elements, electrically isolated from each other, arranged in a single row (Fig. 2.1, left). Each ultrasound wave front is generated by firing individual elements in a specific sequence with a delay in phase with respect to the transmit initiation time. Each element adds and subtracts

L. P. Badano et al. (eds.), *Textbook of Three-Dimensional Echocardiography*, https://doi.org/10.1007/978-3-030-14032-8_2

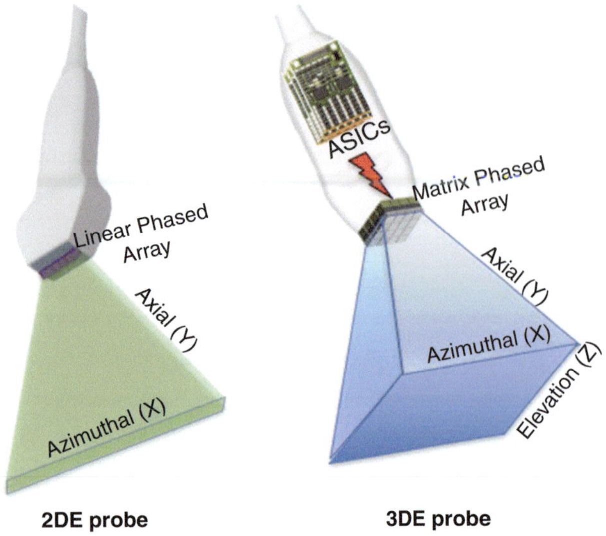

Fig. 2.1 Two- and three-dimensional echocardiography transducers. Schematic drawing showing the main differences between a two- (*left*) and a three-dimensional (*right*) probe. Since in the 2DE probe (*left*), the piezoelectric elements are arranged in a single row, the ultrasound beam can be steered in two dimensions only—axial and azimuthal—whereas the resolution in the elevation axis (i.e. the thickness of the tomographic slice) is related to the thickness of the piezoelectric elements. Current 3DE probes (*right*) are composed by around 3000 fully sampled piezoelectric crystals arranged in rows and columns to form a rectangular grid (matrix configuration) within the transducer. The phasic firing of the elements in that matrix is controlled by electronic boards within the probe to generate a scan line that propagates radially (y or axial direction) and can be steered both laterally (x or azimuthal direction) as well as in elevation (z direction) in order to acquire a volumetric pyramid of data. See text for details [1]

pulses to generate a single ultrasound wave with a specific direction that constitutes a radially propagating scan line (Fig. 2.2).

Currently, 3DE matrix-array transducers are composed of about 3000 individually connected and simultaneously active (fully sampled) piezoelectric elements with operating frequencies ranging from 2 to 4 MHz and 5 to 7 MHz for transthoracic and transesophageal transducers, respectively. To steer the ultrasound beam in 3D, a 3D array of piezoelectric elements needs to be used in the probe, therefore piezoelectric elements are arranged in rows and columns (e.g. 52 × 52) to form a rectangular grid (matrix configuration) within the transducer (Fig. 2.1, right). The electronically controlled phasic firing of the elements in that matrix generates a scan line that propagates radially (y or axial direction) and can be steered both laterally (x or azimuthal direction) as well as in elevation (z direction) in order to acquire a pyramid-shaped volume with a curved base.

By selectively activating specific lines of piezoelectric elements, matrix array probes can also provide real-time multiple simultaneous 2D views, at high frame rate, oriented in predefined or user-selected plane orientations (Fig. 2.3, Videos 2.1a and 2.1b). The main technological breakthrough which allowed manufacturers to develop fully sampled matrix transducers has been the miniaturization of electronics that allowed the development of individual electrical interconnections for every piezoelectric element which could be independently controlled, both in transmission and in reception.

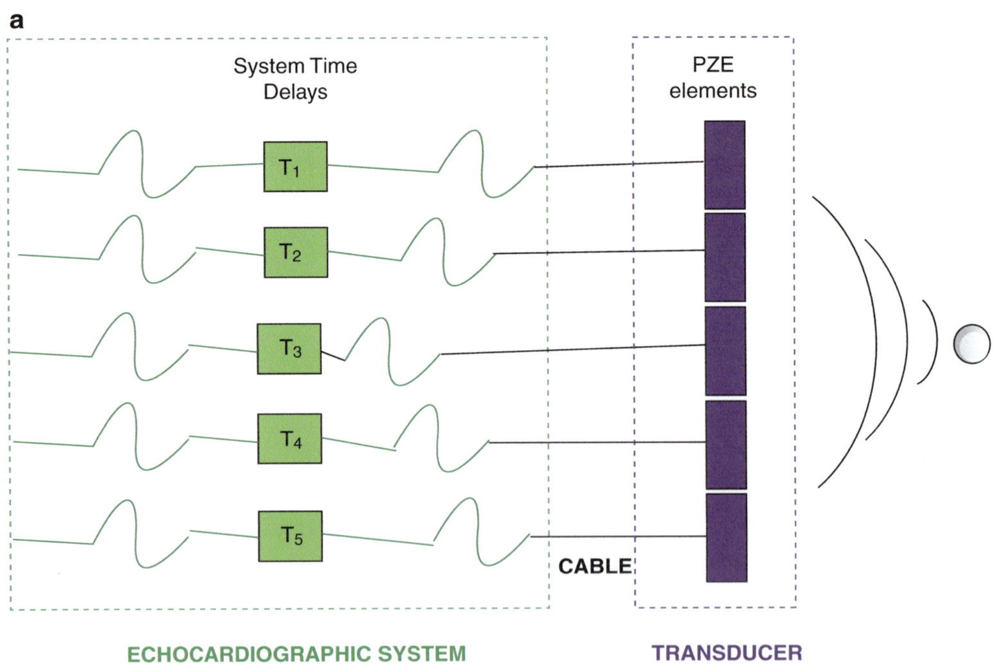

Fig. 2.2 Two-dimensional beamforming. Schematic drawing of beamforming using a conventional 2D phased array transducer. During transmission (**a**), focused beams of ultrasound are produced by pulsing each piezoelectric element (PZE) with pre-calculated time delays (i.e. phasing). During reception (**b**), focusing is achieved by applying selective delays at echo signals received by the different piezoelectric elements in order to create isophasic signals that will be summed in a coherent way [1]. Adapted from Badano L. The clinical benefits of adding a third dimension to assess the left ventricle with echocardiography. Scientifica (Cairo) 2014; 2014: 897431

Fig. 2.2 (continued)

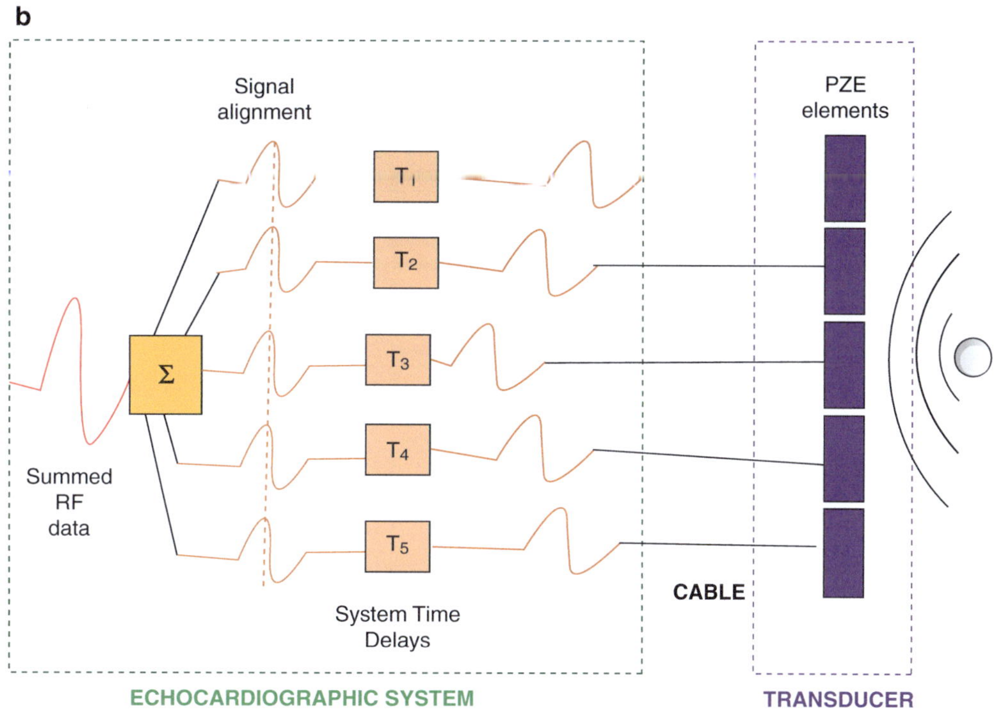

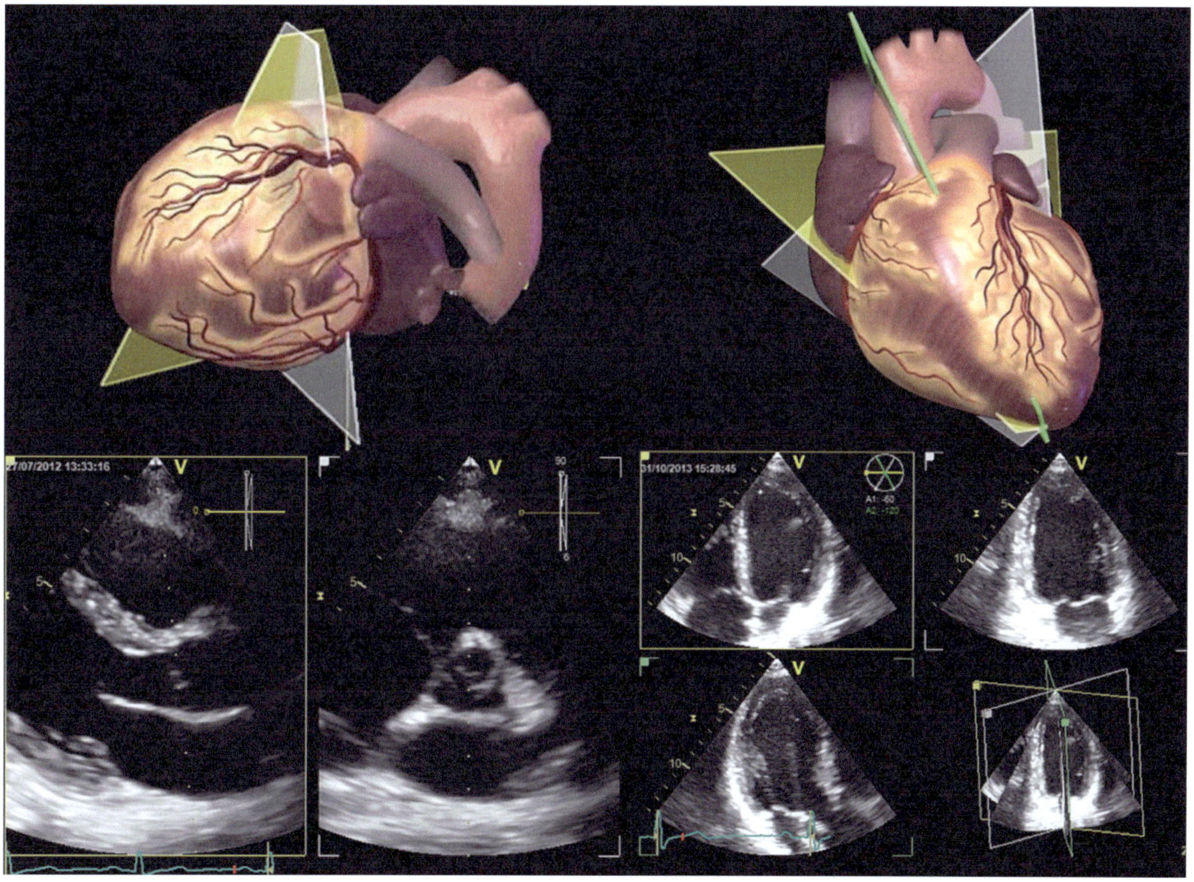

Fig. 2.3 Multiplane acquisition using the matrix array transducer. Bi-plane (left panel, Video 2.1a) and tri-plane (right panel, Video 2.1b) acquisitions with matrix array transducers. Simultaneous 2D views from a single heart beat can be obtained by selectively firing single lines of piezoelectric elements of the matrix transducer. The spatial orientation (angle of rotation) of the 2D views can be adjusted by the operator before the acquisition [3]. Reprinted by permission from Springer Nature, Muraru D, Badano LP. Physical and Technical Aspects and Overview of 3D-Echocardiography. In: Manual of Echocardiography, Casas Rojo E, Fernandez-Golfin C, Zamorano J. (eds). Springer, Cham, 2017, pages 1–44

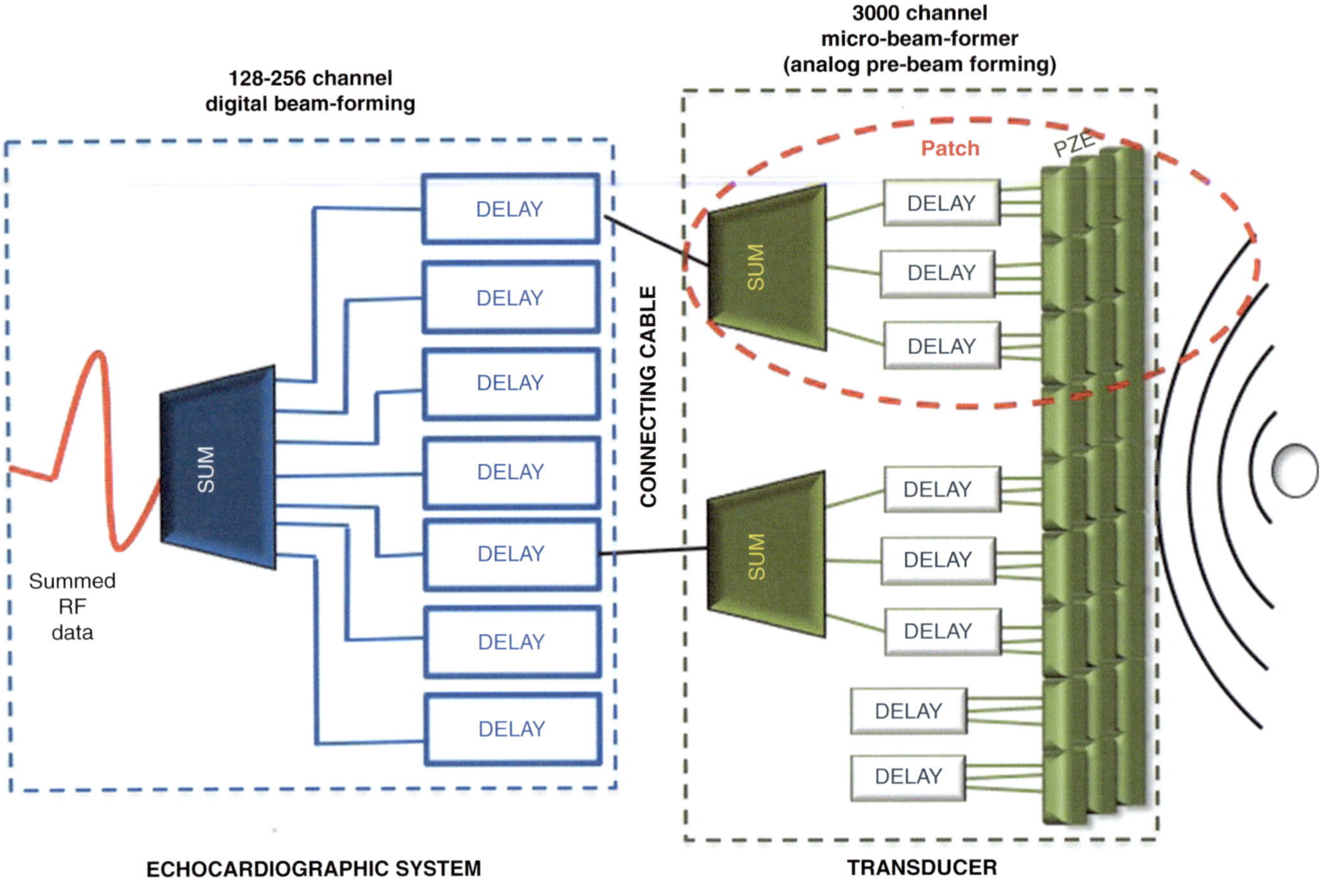

Fig. 2.4 Three-dimensional beamforming. Beamforming with 3D matrix array transducers has been split in two levels: the transducer and the ultrasound machine levels. At the transducer level, interconnection technology and integrated analog circuits (DELAY) control transmit and receive signals using different subsection of the matrix (patches) to perform analog pre-beamforming and fine steering. Signals from each patch are summed to reduce the number of digital lines in the coaxial cable that connects the transducer to the ultrasound system from 3000 to the conventional 128–256 channels. At the ultrasound machine level, analog-to-digital (A/D) convertors amplify, filter and digitize the elements signals which are then focused (coarse steering) using digital delay (DELAY) circuitry and summed together (Ξ) to form the received signal from the imaged object [1]. Adapted from Badano L. The clinical benefits of adding a third dimension to assess the left ventricle with echocardiography. Scientifica (Cairo) 2014; 2014: 897431

Beamforming is a technique used to process signals in order to produce directionally or spatially selected signals sent or received from arrays of sensors. In 2DE, all the electronic components for the beamforming (high-voltage transmitters, low-noise receivers, analog-to-digital converter, digital controllers, digital delay lines) are inside the echocardiography machine and consume a lot of power (around 100 W and 1500 cm^2 of personal computer electronics board area). If the same beamforming approach would have been used for matrix array transducers used in 3DE, it would require around 4 kW power consumption and a huge personal computer board area to accommodate all the needed electronics. To reduce both power consumption and the size of the connecting cable, several miniaturized circuit boards have been incorporated into the transducer, allowing partial beamforming to be performed within the probe (Fig. 2.4). This unique circuit design results in an active probe which allows microbeamforming of the signal with reduced power consumption (<1 W) and avoids to connect every piezoelectric element to the ultrasound machine. The 3000 channel circuit boards within the transducer control the fine steering by delaying and summing signals within subsections of the matrix, known as patches (Fig. 2.4). This microbeamforming allows to reduce the number of the digital channels to be put into the cable that connects the probe to the ultrasound system from 3000 (which would make the cabling too heavy for practical use) to the conventional 128–256 allowing the same size of the 2D cable to be used with 3D probes. Coarse steering is controlled by the ultrasound system where the analog-to-digital conversion occurs using digital delay lines (Fig. 2.4).

However, the electronics inside the probe produce heat and its amount is directly proportional to the mechanical index used during imaging, therefore the engineering of active 3DE transducers should include thermal management.

Finally, new and advanced crystal manufacturing processes produced single crystal materials with homogeneous solid state technology and unique piezoelectric properties. These new crystals result in reduced heating production by increasing the efficiency of the transduction process which improves the conversion of transmit power into ultrasound energy and of received ultrasound energy into electrical power. Increased efficiency of the transduction process, together with a wider bandwidth, result in increased ultrasound penetration and resolution which improve image quality with the additional benefits of reducing artifacts, lowering power consumption and increase Doppler sensitivity.

Further developments in transducer technology have resulted in a smaller transducer footprint, improved side-lobe suppression, increased sensitivity and penetration, and the implementation of harmonic capabilities that can be used for both gray-scale and contrast imaging. The last generation of matrix transducers are significantly smaller than the previous ones and the quality of 2D and 3D imaging has improved significantly, allowing a single transducer to acquire both 2D and 3DE studies, as well as of acquiring the whole left ventricular cavity in a single beat.

3D Echocardiography Physics

3DE is an ultrasound technique and the physical limitation of the constant speed of ultrasounds in human body tissues (approximately 1540 m/s in myocardial tissue and blood) cannot be overcome. The speed of sound in human tissues divided by the distance a single pulse has to travel forth and back (determined by the image depth) results in the maximum number of pulses that can be fired each second without producing interferences. Based on the acquired pyramidal angular width and the desired beam spacing in each dimension (spatial resolution), this number is related to the volumes per second that can be imaged (temporal resolution). Therefore, similar to 2DE imaging, in 3DE imaging there is an inverse relationship between the volume rate (temporal resolution), the size of the acquisition volume and the number of scan lines (spatial resolution). Any increase in one of these factors will cause a decrease in the other two.

The relation between volume rate, number of parallel receive beams, sector width, depth, and line density can be described by the following equation:

$$\text{Volume rate} = \frac{1540 \times \text{No.of parallel received beams}}{2 \times (\text{volume width / lateral resolution})^2 \times \text{Volume depth}}$$

Therefore, the volume rate can be adjusted to the specific needs by either changing the volume width or depth, or by decreasing or increasing the density of scan lines. The 3D system allows the user to control the lateral resolution by changing the density of the scan lines in the pyramidal sector too. However, a decrease in spatial resolution also affects the contrast of the image. Volume rate can also be increased by increasing the number of parallel receive beams, but in this way the signal-to-noise ratio and the image quality will be affected.

To put all this in perspective let us assume that we want to image up to 16 cm depth in the body and acquire a 60° × 60° degrees pyramidal volume. Since the speed of sound is approximately 1540 m/s and each pulse has to propagate 16 cm × 2 (to go forth and come back to the transducer), 1540/0.32 = 4812 pulses may be fired per second without getting interference between the pulses. Assuming that 1° beam spacing in both X and Z dimension is a sufficient spatial resolution we would need 3600 beams (60 × 60) to spatially resolve the 60° × 60° pyramidal volume. As a result, the temporal resolution (volume rate) of the acquired data set will be 4812/3600 = 1.3 volume per second, which is practically useless in clinical echocardiography.

The example above shows why the fixed speed of sound in body tissues has been one of the major challenges to the development of 3DE imaging. Manufacturers have developed several techniques such as parallel receive beamforming, multi-beat imaging and zoom acquisition to cope with this challenge but, in practice, this is usually achieved by selecting the most appropriate acquisition modality for different imaging purposes (Fig. 2.5).

Parallel receive beamforming or multiline acquisition is a technique where the system transmits one wide beam and receives multiple narrow beams in parallel. In this way the volume rate (temporal resolution) is increased by a factor equal to the number of the received beams (Fig. 2.6). Each beamformer focuses along a slightly different direction that was insonated by the broad transmit pulse. As an example, to obtain a 90° × 90°, 16-cm depth pyramidal volume at 25 vps, the system needs to receive 200,000 lines/s. Since the emission rate is around 5000 pulsed/s, the system should receive 42 beams in parallel for each emitted pulse. However, increasing the number of parallel beams to increase temporal resolution leads to an increase in size, costs and power consumption of the beamforming electronics, and deterioration in the signal-to-noise ratio and in contrast resolution. With this technique of processing the received data, multiple scan lines can be sampled in the amount of time a conventional scanner would take for a single line, at the expense of reduced signal strength and resolution as the receive beams are steered farther and farther away from the center of the transmit beam (Fig. 2.6, right panel).

Another technique used to increase the size of the pyramidal volume and maintain the volume rate (or the reverse, e.g. maintain volume rate while increasing the pyramidal volume) is the multi-beat acquisition. With this technique, a

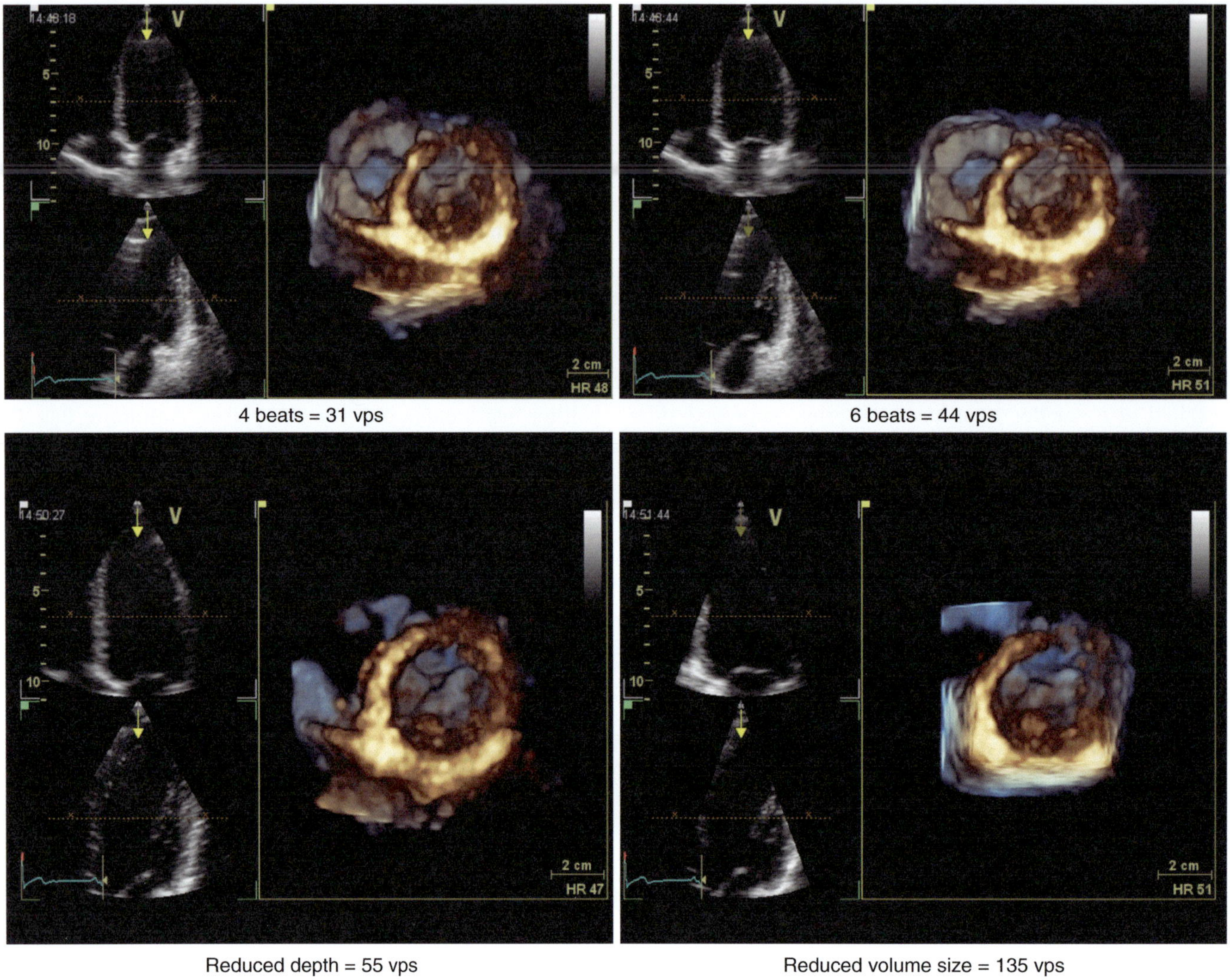

Fig. 2.5 Effects of acquisition settings on 3D data set resolution. Using a 60° × 60° volume size and a depth of 15 cm, a four-beat full volume acquisition will provide a temporal resolution of 31 volumes per second (vps) (*upper left*). Without changing volume size and depth, an increase of the acquired cardiac cycles from 4 to 6 will determine an increase of the temporal resolution from 31 to 44 vps (*upper right*). However, if we are interested to quantitate the left ventricular size, we do not need to acquire the left atrium too. By reducing the depth (the distance the ultrasound beam has to travel forward and backward) from 15 to 10 cm we can increase the temporal resolution from 44 to 55 vps by acquiring the same volume size and number of cardiac cycles (*lower left*). If we are interested to visualize the mitral valve (instead of quantitating the left ventricle) we can reduce the volume size from 60° to 45° and obtaining a much higher temporal resolution (135 vps) while acquiring the same number of cardiac cycles (6 beats) at the same depth (10 cm) (*lower right*)

number of ECG-gated sub-volumes acquired from consecutive cardiac cycles are stitched together to build up the final pyramidal volume (Fig. 2.7). Multi-beat acquisition will be effective only if the different sub-volumes will be constant in position and size, therefore any transducer movement, cardiac translation motion due to respiration, change in cardiac cycle length, or change of patient position will create sub-volume malalignment and stitching artifacts (Fig. 2.8, Videos 2.2a and 2.2b).

Zoom acquisition is obtained by adjusting the acquisition volume with the minimum lateral and elevation width. The ultrasound system automatically crops the adjacent structures to provide a small volume with high spatial and temporal resolution. This technique is ideal for the study of a restricted structure of interest (usually, valve structures or congenital defects) with high spatial and temporal resolution. Usually, the zoom acquisition is real-time. However, if the structure of interest is large, the temporal resolution can be further increased by using a multi-beat zoom acquisition [2].

Finally, the quality of the images of the cardiac structures which can be obtained by a 3DE data set will be affected by the point spread function of the system. The point spread function describes the imaging system response to a point input. A point input, represented as a single pixel in the "ideal" image, will be reproduced as something other than a single pixel in the "real" image (Fig. 2.9). The degree of spreading (blurring) of any point object varies according to the dimension employed. In

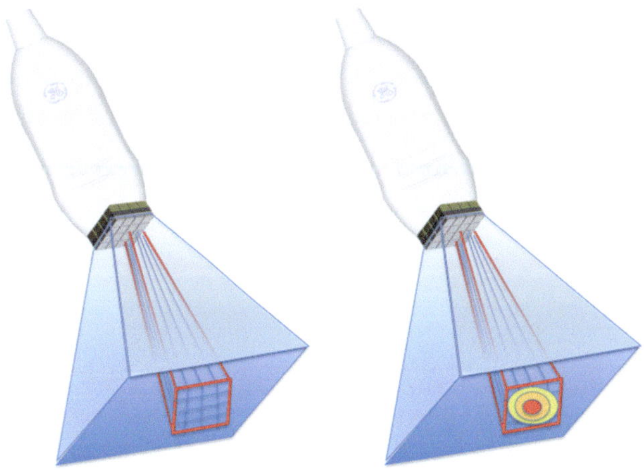

Fig. 2.6 Parallel receive beamforming. Schematic representation of the parallel receive or multiline beamforming technique receiving multiple (16 in the left image) beams (blue lines) for each broad transmit pulse (red pyramid). The right image shows the degradation of the power and resolution of the signal (from red maximal to bright yellow minimal) from the parallel receiving beams steered farther away from the center of the transmit beam [1]. Adapted from Badano L. The clinical benefits of adding a third dimension to assess the left ventricle with echocardiography. Scientifica (Cairo) 2014; 2014: 897431

current 3DE systems it will be around 0.5 mm in the axial (y) dimension, around 2.5 mm in the lateral (x) dimension, and around 3 mm in the elevation (z) dimension. As a result we will obtain the best images (less degree of blurring, i.e. distortion) when using the axial dimension and the worst (greatest degree of spreading) when we use the elevation dimension.

These concepts have an immediate practical application in the choice of the best approach to image a cardiac structure. According to the point spread function of 3DE, the best results are expected to be obtained by using the parasternal approach because structures are mostly imaged by the axial and lateral dimensions. Conversely, the worst result is expected to be obtained by the apical approach which mostly uses the lateral and elevation dimensions.

Image Acquisition and Display

Currently, 3D data set acquisition can be easily implemented into standard echocardiographic examination by either switching among 2D and 3D probes or, with the newest

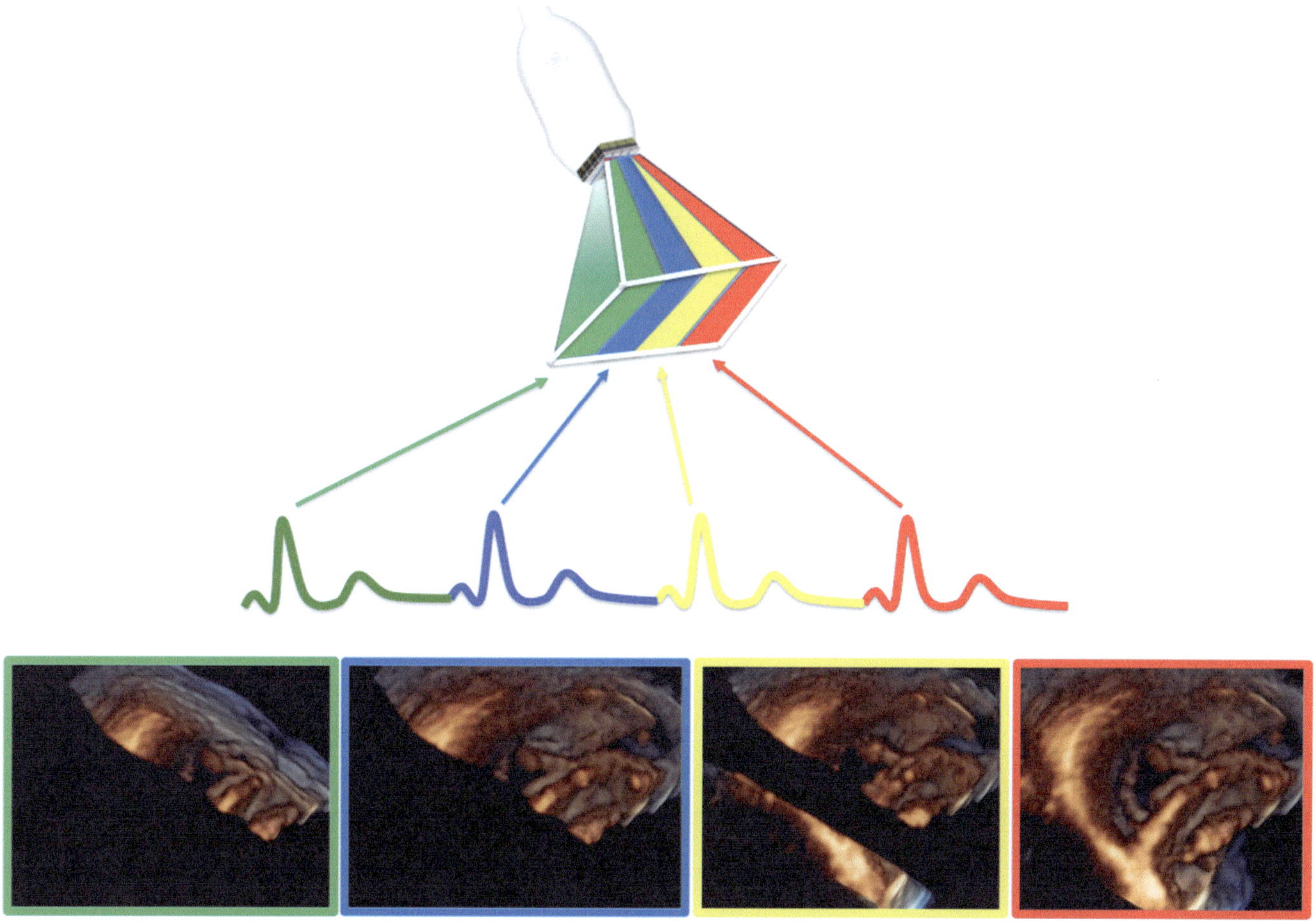

Fig. 2.7 Multibeat acquisition. Three-dimensional volume rendered imaging of the tricuspid valve from the ventricular perspective obtained from a four-beat full-volume acquisition (the colors show the relationships between the pyramidal subvolumes, the ECG beats and the way the 3D data set has been built up in the lower part of the figure) [1]. Adapted from Badano L. The clinical benefits of adding a third dimension to assess the left ventricle with echocardiography. Scientifica (Cairo) 2014; 2014: 897431

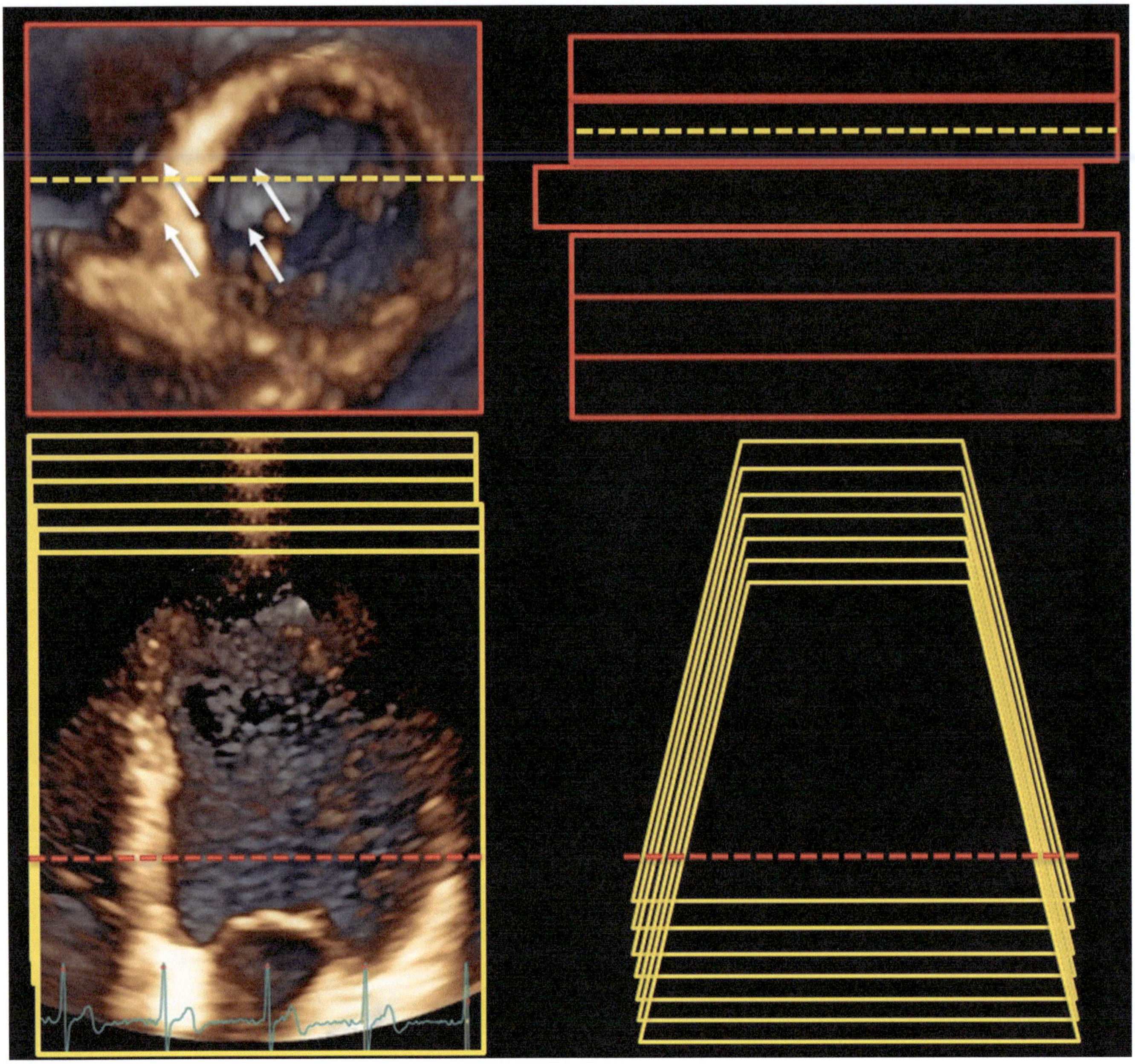

Fig. 2.8 Stitching artifacts. Six-beat full-volume data set and volume-rendered image displayed with stitching artifacts (white arrows, upper panel, Video 2.2a). The red lines highlight the misalignment of the pyramidal subvolumes. Since the data set has been acquired from the apical approach, the stitching artifacts cannot be seen in the longitudinal cut planes (lower panel, Video 2.2b) because the subvolumes are one in front of the other. To see the stitching artifacts, the cut-plane should be orthogonal to the direction of the acquisition (in this example, transversal cut planes). The red and the yellow dashed lines show the relative positions of the volume rendered images. Video 2.2a: Stitching artifacts. Transversal cut plane of the left ventricle acquired while the patient was breathing. The misalignment of the fourth subvolume can be clearly seen. Video 2.2b: Stitching artifacts. Longitudinal cut-plane from the same 3DE data set of Video 2.2a. Since the multibeat data set has been acquired from the apical approach the stitching artifact cannot be seen using this cut-plane

all-in-one-probes, by switching between the 2D and the 3D modalities available in the same probe. The latter probes are also capable to provide single-beat full-volume acquisition, as well as real-time 3D color Doppler imaging.

At present, three different methods for 3D data set acquisition are available [2]:

- multiplane imaging
- "real-time" (or "live") 3D imaging
- multi-beat ECG-gated imaging

In the multiplane mode, multiple, simultaneous 2D views can be acquired at high frame rate using predefined or user-

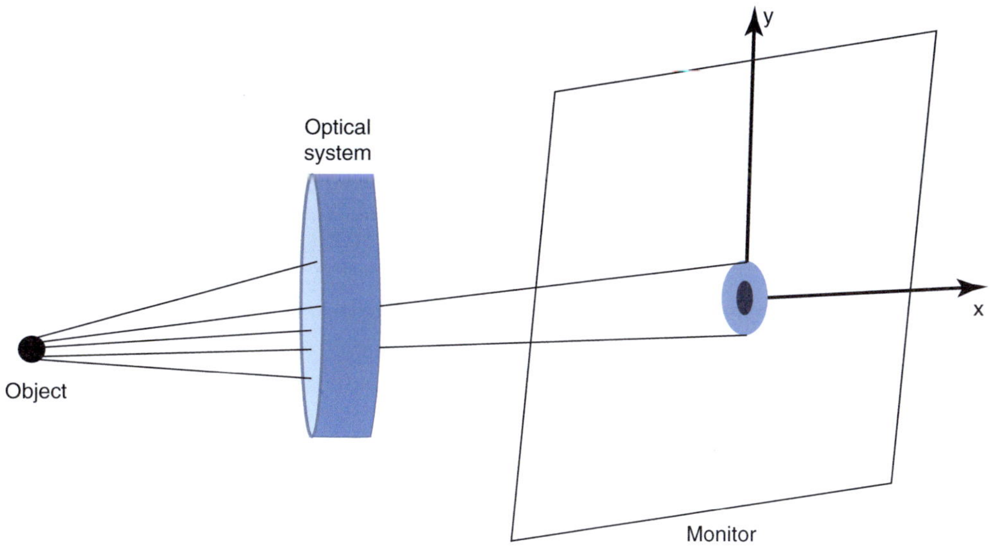

Fig. 2.9 Point spread function. Graphical representation of the extent of degradation (blur) of a point passing through an optical system [1]

selected plane orientations and displayed using the split screen option (Fig. 2.3, Videos 2.1a and 2.1b). The first view on the left is usually the reference plane that is oriented by adjusting the probe position while the other views represents views obtained from the reference view by simply tilting and/or rotating the secondary imaging planes. Multiplane imaging is a real time acquisition and, because it is obtained by selective firing of single lines of piezoelectric elements, secondary imaging planes can only be selected during acquisition. Doppler color flow can be superimposed on multiplane 2D images and in some systems both tissue Doppler and speckle tracking analysis can be performed. Although strictly not a 3D acquisition, this imaging mode is particularly useful in clinical conditions in which the availability of multiple views from the same cardiac cycle is critical (e.g. atrial fibrillation or other irregular arrhythmias, stress echo, evaluation of intraventricular dyssynchrony, etc.).

In the real-time mode, a pyramidal 3D volumetric data set is obtained from each cardiac cycle and visualized live, beat after beat as during conventional 2D scanning. As the data set is updated in real-time, image orientation and plane can be changed by rotating or tilting the probe. Analysis can be done with limited post-processing and the data set can be rotated (independent of the transducer position) to view the heart from different orientations. Heart dynamics is shown in a realistic way, with instantaneous on-line volume rendered reconstruction. It allows fast acquisition of dynamic pyramidal data structures from a single acoustic view that can encompass the entire heart without the need of reference system, electrocardiographic (ECG) and respiratory gating. Real-time imaging is time-saving both for data acquisition and analysis. Although this acquisition mode overcomes rhythm disturbances or respiratory motion limitations, it still suffers of relatively poor temporal and spatial resolution. Real-time imaging can be acquired in the following modes:

(a) Live 3D. Once the desired cardiac structure has been imaged in 2DE it can be converted to a 3D image by pressing a specific button in the control panel. The 3D system automatically switch to a narrow sector acquisition (approximately 30° × 60° pyramidal volume) to preserve spatial and temporal resolution. The size of the pyramidal volume can be increased to visualize larger structures, but both scan line density (spatial resolution) and volume rate (temporal resolution) will drop down. 3D live imaging mode is used to: (1) guide full-volume acquisition; (2) visualize small structures (aortic valve, masses etc.); (3) recording short-lived events (i.e. bubble passage, catheter positioning); (4) in patients with irregular rhythm/dyspnea that prevent full-volume acquisition; (5) monitor interventional procedures.
(b) Live 3D color. Color flow can be superimposed on a live 3D data set to visualize blood flow in real time. Temporal resolution is usually very low.
(c) 3D zoom. This imaging mode is an extension of live 3D and allows a focused real time view of the structure of interest. A crop box is placed on a 2D single- or multiplane image to allow the operator to adjust lateral and elevation width to include the structure of interest in the final data set, then the system automatically crops the adjacent structures to provide a real time display of the structure of interest with high spatial and temporal resolution. The draw-back of the 3D zoom mode is that the operator loses the relationships of the structure of interest with surrounding structures. Mainly used during transesophageal studies for detailed anatomical analysis of specific structure of interest.

(d) Full-volume. The full-volume mode has the largest acquisition volume possible (usually 60° × 60° degrees). Real-time (or "single-beat") full-volume acquisition is affected by low spatial and temporal resolution and it is used for quantification of cardiac chambers when multi-beat ECG gated acquisition is not possible (e.g. irregular cardiac rhythm, patient unable to cooperate for breath-holding)

In contrast to real-time/live 3D imaging, multi-beat acquisition is obtained from sequential acquisitions of narrow smaller volumes captured from several ECG-gated consecutive heart cycles (from 2 to 6) that are subsequently stitched together to create a single volumetric data set (Fig. 2.7). Once acquired, the data set cannot be changed by manipulating the probe like in live 3D imaging and analysis requires off-line slicing, rotation and cropping of the acquired data set. It provides large data sets with high temporal and spatial resolution that can be used for quantitating cardiac chamber size and function or to assess spatial relationships among cardiac structures. However, this 3D imaging mode has the disadvantage of the ECG-gating, as the images are acquired over several cardiac cycles and the final data set is available to be visualized by the operator only after the last cardiac cycle has been acquired ("*near real-time*" imaging) and it is prone to stitch artifacts due to patient or respiratory motion or irregular cardiac rhythms. Multi-beat imaging can be acquired with or without color flow mapping and usually more cardiac cycles are required for 3D color data sets.

After data acquisition, data are streamed through a random access memory for temporary data storage within the computer on the ultrasound machine to maintain data flow to the next step of data processing. Data storage allows immediate (on-line) data acquisition, storage, and processing within the ultrasound machine. The transformation of the scanned raw data for a specific volume into a 3D data set necessary to generate a 3D object is called data processing. Typically, data processing consists of two sequential processes: conversion and interpolation. These two steps are separate for the 2D technique, but they are fully integrated for the 3D technique. During conversion, all acquired raw data are placed into a Cartesian volume with each point assigned x-y-z coordinates and an echo intensity value. As a result, a group of points with distinctive echogenic characteristics and a known position in space is generated. Interpolation fills the gaps between all the known points in space with data points of similar characteristics. Interpolation generates a 3D data set made of voxels or volume elements for a specific volume in space. A voxel is a (vo)lume of pi(xels) that encrypts the physical characteristics and location of the smallest cube in a dataset, which is used for 3D display. The quality of the 3D image depends on the size of the voxel (similar to pixel size in 2D image resolution). Larger voxels are generated when raw data are available for fewer points in the space and there are wider gaps to be filed with interpolation.

The 3D technique generates a data stream using the computer random access memory and creates voxels while scanning, with near simultaneous conversion and interpolation.

Since 3D data sets contain all the voxels of the 3D object, they can be sectioned in several planes and rotated in order to visualize the cardiac structure of interest from any desired perspective, irrespective of its orientation and position within the heart (electronic dissection, similar to what the anatomist does in the anatomical theatre during autopsy). This allows the operator to easily obtain unique visualizations of cardiac structures that may be difficult or impossible to achieve using conventional 2DE (e.g. surgical views of the aortic and mitral valves, *en-face* views of the tricuspid valve or cardiac defects). Three main actions are undertaken by the operator to obtain any desired view from a 3D volumetric data set: cropping, slicing and rotating. Similarly to what the anatomists or the surgeons do, the echocardiographer should remove the surrounding chamber walls to expose an anatomic structure within a 3DE data set. This process of virtually removing the irrelevant neighboring tissue is called cropping (Fig. 2.10, Video 2.3), and can be performed either during or after the acquisition. In contrast with 2D images, displaying a cropped image requires also data set rotation (Fig. 2.10, Video 2.3) and the definition of the viewing perspective (i.e. since the same 3D structure can be visualized *en face* either from above or below, as well as from any desired view angle) [2]. Any volume-rendered 3D object can be freely rotated on the display screen to be viewed in any orientation either as a still or a moving data set. A moving (dynamic) 3D data set is often referred to as 4D, with time considered the fourth dimension.

Slicing refers to a virtual "cutting" of the 3D data set into one or more (currently, up to 12) 2D (tomographic) grey-scale images (Fig. 2.11, Videos 2.4a, 2.4b, 2.4c, and 2.4d).

Finally, irrespective of its acquisition window, a cropped or a sliced image should be displayed according to the anatomical orientation of the heart within the human body and this is usually obtained by rotating the selected images.

Acquisition of volumetric images generates the technical problem of rendering the depth perception on a flat, 2D monitor. 3D images can be visualized using three display modalities (Fig. 2.12):

- volume rendering,
- surface rendering
- tomographic slices

The volume rendering technique uses different types of algorithms to preserve all 3DE information and to project it onto 2D monitors for manipulation and viewing [2]. These

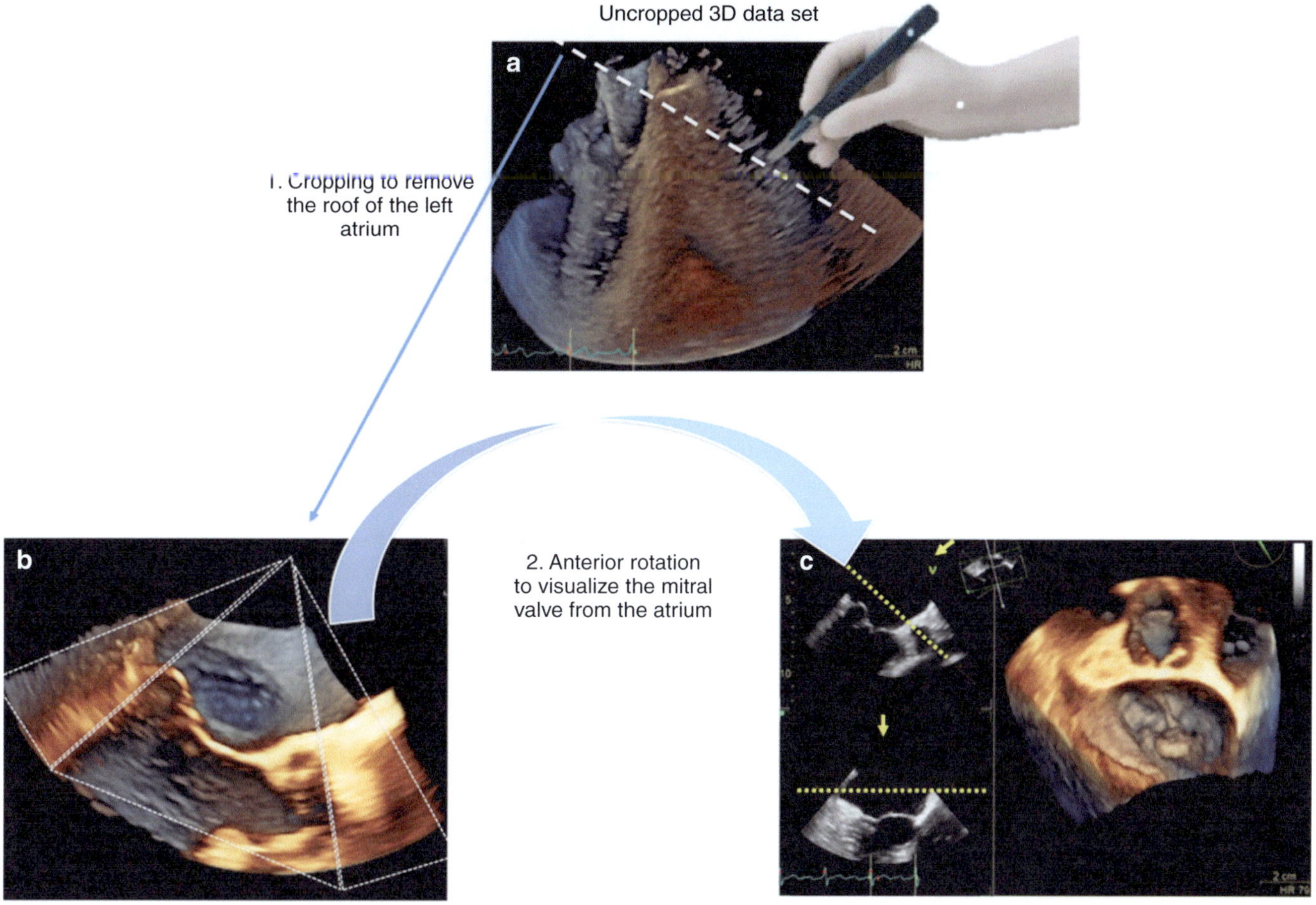

Fig. 2.10 Example of data set cropping and rotation. To display the mitral valve from the left atrial perspective (surgical view) a full-volume pyramidal data set (**a**) has been cropped to remove part of the left atrium from above. Then, the remaining data set (**b**) has been rotated to the desired perspective and to put the cardiac structures in an anatomical sound position (**c**). In this data set (**c**), the position of the observer is shown in the 2D views by the broken yellow line and the direction of view by the yellow arrow (Video 2.3)

algorithms cast a light beam through the collected voxels, then the voxels are weighted to obtain a voxel gradient intensity that, integrated with different levels of opacification and shadowing, allow the structures to appear solid (i.e. tissue) or transparent (i.e. blood pool). In addition, various color maps are applied to convey the depth perception to the observer. Generally, lighter shades (e.g. bronze, Fig. 2.5) are used for structures closer to the observer, while darker shades (e.g. blue, Fig. 2.5) are used for deeper structures. As opposed to 2D tomographic images, the tissue characterization is lost when displaying structures in the volume-rendered mode (e.g. presence of calcium or fibrous tissue is easier to assess using 2D imaging), in which various color shades depend exclusively on the depth of the structure relative to the cropping plane and of the total depth of the volume dataset in which the structure is contained (i.e. higher color gradient for smaller volume depths). Volume-rendering displays a 3D object with a rendered surface and details of its inner structure and it is commonly used to visualize cardiac anatomy, in particular the structures with complex morphology like heart valves or congenital defects, which require greater anatomical detail for clinically meaningful imaging.

Surface rendering modality (Fig. 2.12, right) displays the 3D surface of cardiac structures, identified either by manual tracing or by using automated endocardial border detection algorithms on multiple 2D cross-sectional images of the structure/cavity of interest. This stereoscopic approach is useful for the assessment of shape and for a better appreciation of geometry and dynamic function during the cardiac cycle.

Wireframe rendering (Fig. 2.13, left) is the simplest of the available surface rendering techniques. It identifies equidistant points on the surface of a 3D object obtained from manual tracing, or using semiautomatic border detection algorithms, to trace the endocardial contour in cross-sectional images and then connect these points using lines

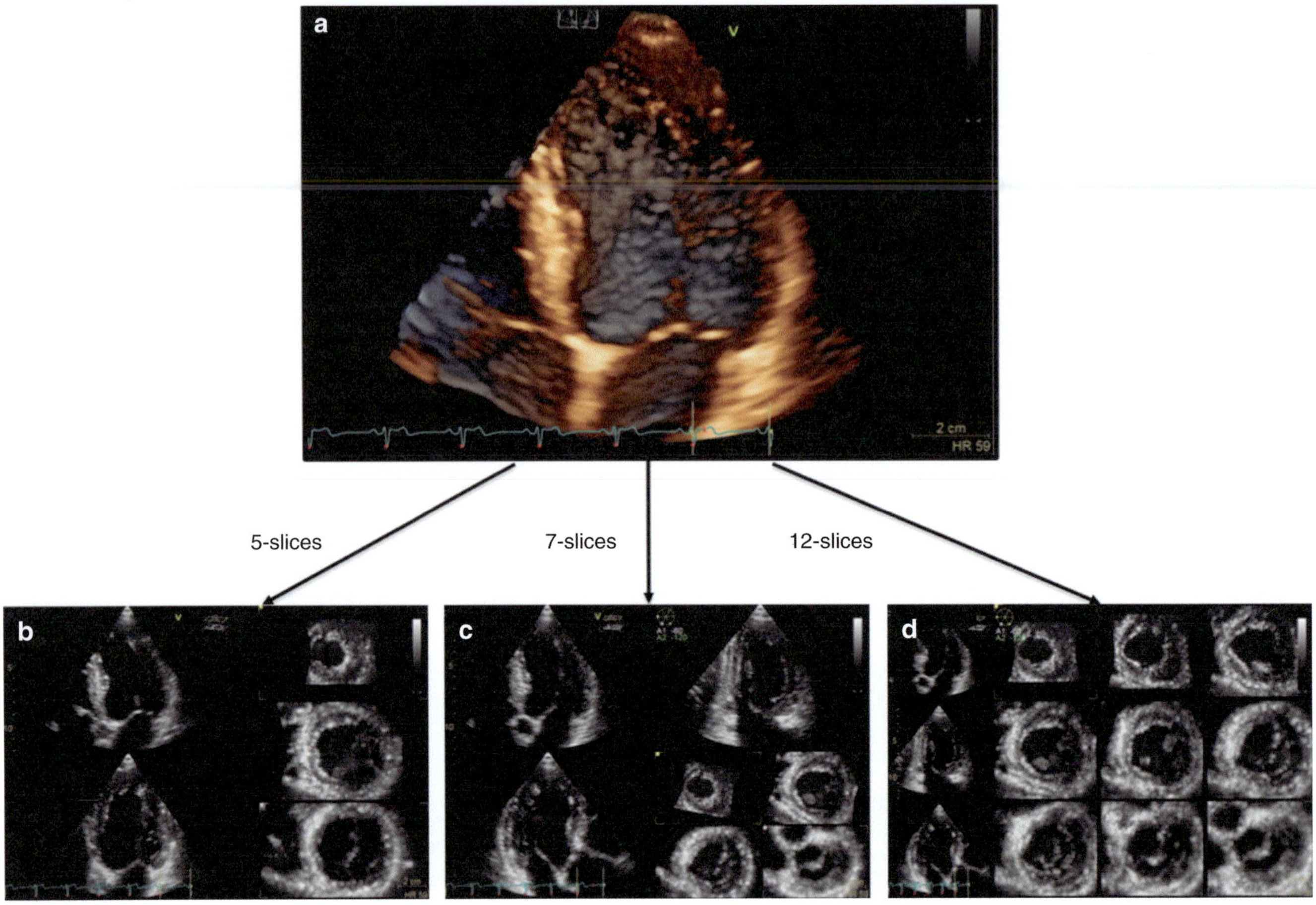

Fig. 2.11 Data set slicing. A full-volume data set (***Panel A,*** Video 2.4a LV full volume) can be sliced in several ways. Two longitudinal (four-chamber and the orthogonal view) plus three transversal (short-axes) planes (***Panel B***) (Video 2.4b 5 slices). Three longitudinal (four- and two chamber, plus the long-axis apical views) and four transversal slices of the left ventricle from the mitral valve (MV) to the apical (Apex) level (***Panel C***) (Video 2.4c 7 slices). Three longitudinal (four- and two-chamber plus the long-axis apical views) and nine transversal planes (**Panel D**) (Video 2.4d 12 slices). The position of the lowest and the highest transversal planes are adjustable by the operator both during acquisition and post processing, and the slices in between are automatically repositioned to be equidistant. Video 2.4d: 12 slices. Same concepts as in Video 2.4c 7 slices. In this display, the number of the transversal cut planes is 9, and all of them are equidistant from each other

(wires) to create a mesh of little polygonal tiles. Smoothing algorithms are used to smooth angles and give a realistic appearance to the structure of interest. This rendering technique processes a relatively low amount of data and it is used for relatively flat endocardial boundaries such as the cardiac chamber walls. This stereoscopic approach is useful for the assessment of shape and for better visualization of chambers volume and function during the cardiac cycle. Conversely, wireframe cannot be used to display structures with complex shapes, such as the cardiac valves that require greater anatomic detail for meaningful analysis.

The surface-rendering technique is very similar to the wireframe technique but identifies many more points on the surface of the structure of interest and the lines joining the points become indistinguishable (Fig. 2.13, left). It displays in detail the surfaces of the analyzed object facing the observer as a solid structure. The combination of solid and wireframe surface-rendering techniques can be useful to appreciate cardiac structure geometry and motion, such as right or left ventricular volume changes during the cardiac cycle.

Finally, the volumetric data set can be sliced or cropped to obtain multiple simultaneous 2D views of the same 3D structure (Figs. 2.11 and 2.12). Cut planes can be orthogonal, parallel or free (any given plane orientation), selected as desired by the echocardiographer for obtaining optimized cross-sections of the heart in order to answer specific clinical questions and to perform accurate and reproducible measurements. This method allows the observation of any cutting plane from any acoustic window, overcoming the limitations of conventional 2DE. The optimized cross-sectional planes of the heart provide accurate measurements of chamber dimensions and valve areas, as well as improved evaluation of the morphology and function. This functionality can also be used at the time of image acquisition, because it allows the evaluation of several 2DE views simultaneously during the study, thus allowing to check that the structure of interest is completely included in the data set.

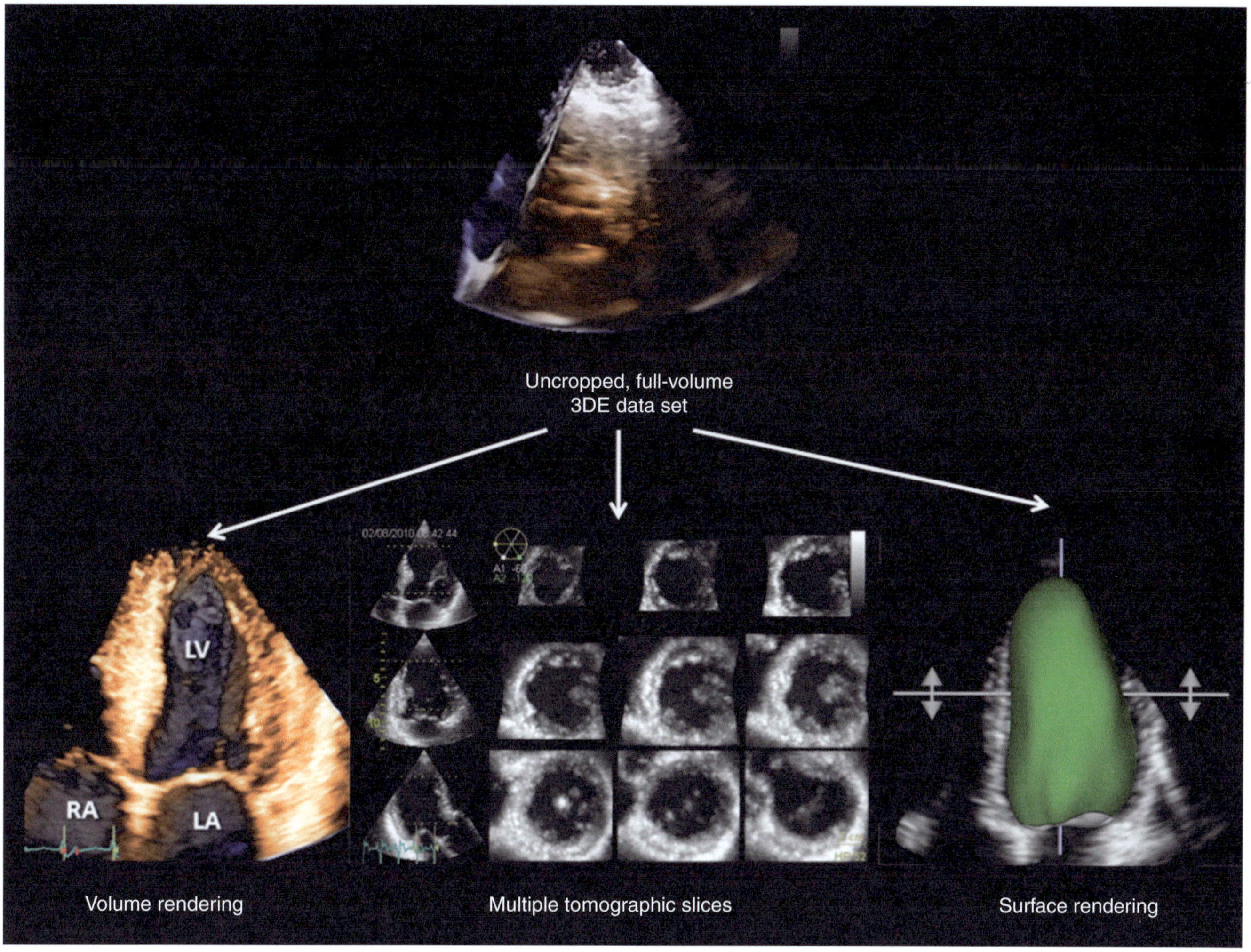

Fig. 2.12 Three-dimensional data set display. From the same three-dimensional data set, the left ventricle can be visualized using different display modalities: volume rendering, to visualize anatomy and spatial relationships among adjacent structures; surface-rendering, for quantitative purposes; and multi-slice (multiple two-dimensional tomographic planes extracted automatically from a single 3D data set) for morphological and functional (wall motion) analysis at different regional levels [3]. Reprinted by permission from Springer Nature, Muraru D, Badano LP. Physical and Technical Aspects and Overview of 3D-Echocardiography. In: Manual of Echocardiography, Casas Rojo E, Fernandez-Golfin C, Zamorano J. (eds). Springer, Cham, 2017, pages 1–44

The current software tools for 3DE volume segmentation along the three axes (x, y, z) can be used in real-time or during post-processing for qualitative assessment, as well as for linear and area measurements.

Advanced Display Modalities

Currently available modalities display the 3D volumetric data on 2D screens which restricts the image to a single plane of view, does not allow any direct interaction with the image and limits the perception of depth and spatial relationships among cardiac structures which can be critically important when guiding surgical or interventional procedures. Accordingly new ways of displaying the 3DE data sets like stereoscopic visualization, 3D printing or holographic display of cardiac structures have been explored.

The polar vision option is a new stereo vision technology combining polarized stereo with depth rendering displayed on a dedicated 3D monitor. This technology could be useful during interventional procedures in the catheterization laboratory to allow the interventional cardiologists to appreciate the spatial relationships and the actual distance among the cardiac structures, and the relative position of catheters and devices [4, 5]. However this approach is limited by the inability to interact directly with the data set and typically the need to use or wear ancillary equipment such as dedicated glasses, headgear or goggles (Fig. 2.14).

3D printing is a relatively new technology (also referred to as "rapid prototyping", "additive manufacturing" and "stereolithography") that allows to convert a 3D model created by a computer into an actual physical object. There are different ways of obtaining a 3D printing model: laying down additional layers of material (plastic, metal, etc.)

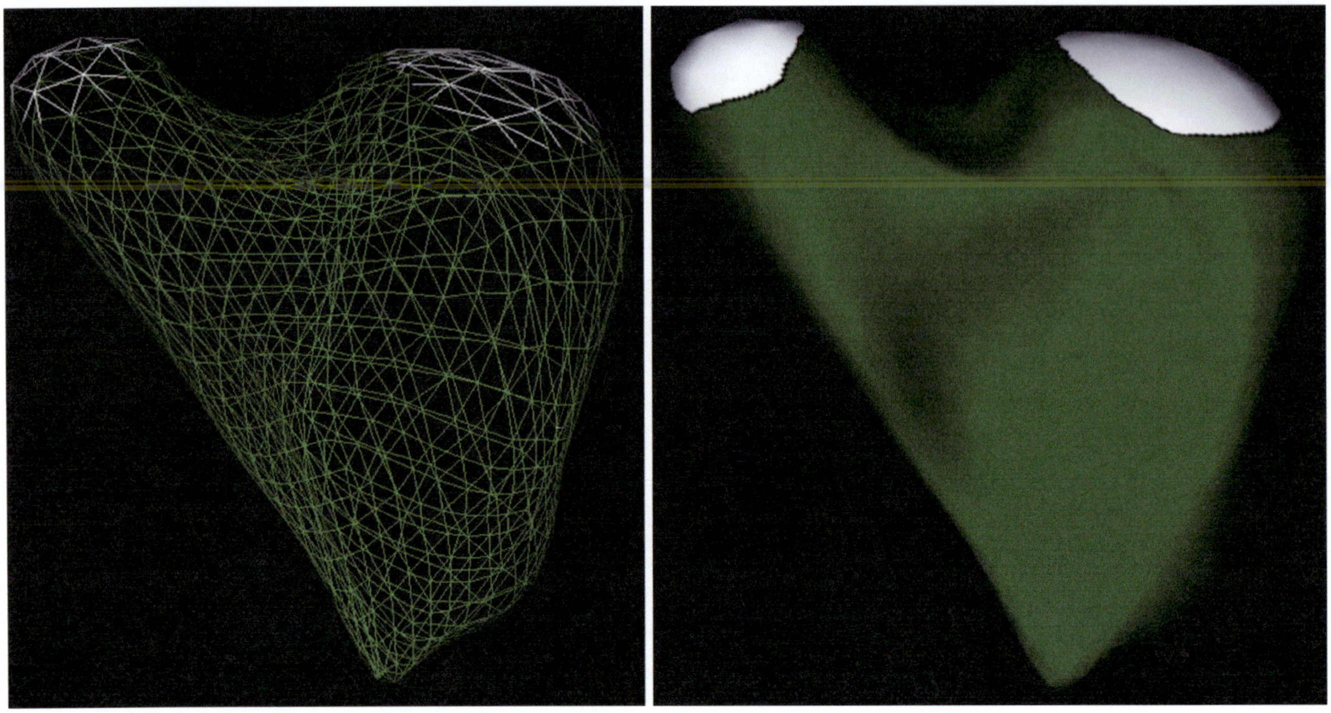

Fig. 2.13 Surface rendering of the right ventricle. Both wireframe (left panel) and solid (right panel) surface rendering display are shown for the same 3DE data set of the left ventricle [3]. Reprinted by permission from Springer Nature, Muraru D, Badano LP. Physical and Technical Aspects and Overview of 3D-Echocardiography. In: Manual of Echocardiography, Casas Rojo E, Fernandez-Golfin C, Zamorano J. (eds). Springer, Cham, 2017, pages 1–44

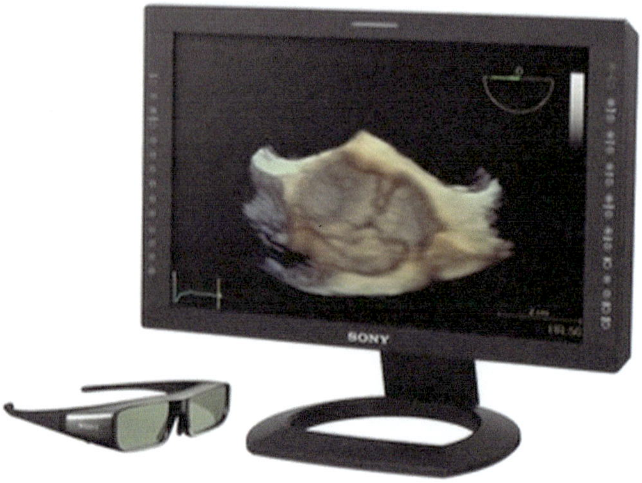

Fig. 2.14 4D polar vision. See text for details

onto a platform until a 3D model is complete; using a laser as the power source to bind powdered materials, ranging from nylon to steel, to create a solid structure; or using the inkjet technology to jet materials through print heads while being cured by an ultraviolet light into a 3D object. Three-dimensional printing technology has significantly advanced in the past 10 years [6, 7]. Three-dimensional printers now have the capability to print at any scale from nearly any type of material [8]. They have been used in various biomedical applications from prosthesis manufacture [6, 9–11] to cell and tissue culture [8, 12–14]. They have incredible spatial resolution to pick up on microscopic details. There is an emerging field involving the use of 3D simulation data in education [15–17] and pre-procedural planning [18], demonstrating excellent results in general [11, 19], including the cardiology and cardiovascular surgery fields [18, 20–22]. Beyond just visualizing the pathologic anatomy, 3D printing allows doctors to actually test an approach to repair [23, 24]. Shiraishi et al. [25] reported about feasibility and effectiveness of 3D printing full hearts of patients with congenital heart disease, including hypoplastic left heart syndrome and total anomalous pulmonary venous return, in a flexible material. The printed hearts were used to simulate the surgical repair, for example with a Norwood procedure in the patient with hypoplastic left heart syndrome. This has the potential to change completely education and practical training in both surgical and interventional fields, particularly for rare or relatively rare cardiac conditions. Since multiple copies of the same model could be printed and distributed to trainees to practice the repair, the lack of a specific type of pathology at a certain center will not be any more an issue leading to inadequate hands-on experience for trainees.

In the majority of the reports about the medical use of 3D printing, data were obtained by cardiac magnetic resonance imaging or computed tomographic are used to print high-quality cardiac reconstructions, which may involve intravenous contrast, sedation, and ionizing radiation. There are few reports of 3D printing of transesophageal echocardiography-based data sets of mitral valves, ventricular septal defects and peri-valvular leaks [21–23]. However, this technology is becoming more and more available and also the quality of transthoracic 3D data sets is gradually improving allowing the first report of the 3D printing of the tricuspid valve using a 3D data set acquired from transthoracic approach [26].

The steps in creating a 3D virtual model for the purpose of rapid prototyping start with the acquisition of a good quality (i.e. good blood pool to myocardial or valve structure contrast). Usually, 3DE images are post-processed to optimize the gain and eliminate any drop-out artefact. This is a critical step to reduce the time required to create a 3D virtual model and improve its quality. Segmentation, the process by which we designate the range of gray values that highlights our area of interest, becomes much faster with optimized data sets. Although 3DE data sets do not allow us to encompass the whole heart, acquiring only the volume of interest simplifies the process and makes it less time consuming and labor intensive. Once the data set has been optimized, dedicated image-processing software packages create a 3D structure (.STL file) that can be saved and then printed on a 3D printer to create a physical cardiac replica (Fig. 2.15). Depending on the size of the structure to be printed and on the 3D printer performance, the actual 3D printing process can require a few hours.

Three-dimensional printing is not the only method by which we could visualize structural anatomy in three dimensions and interact with the data sets. The advent of holography also allows similar display and interaction with cardiac

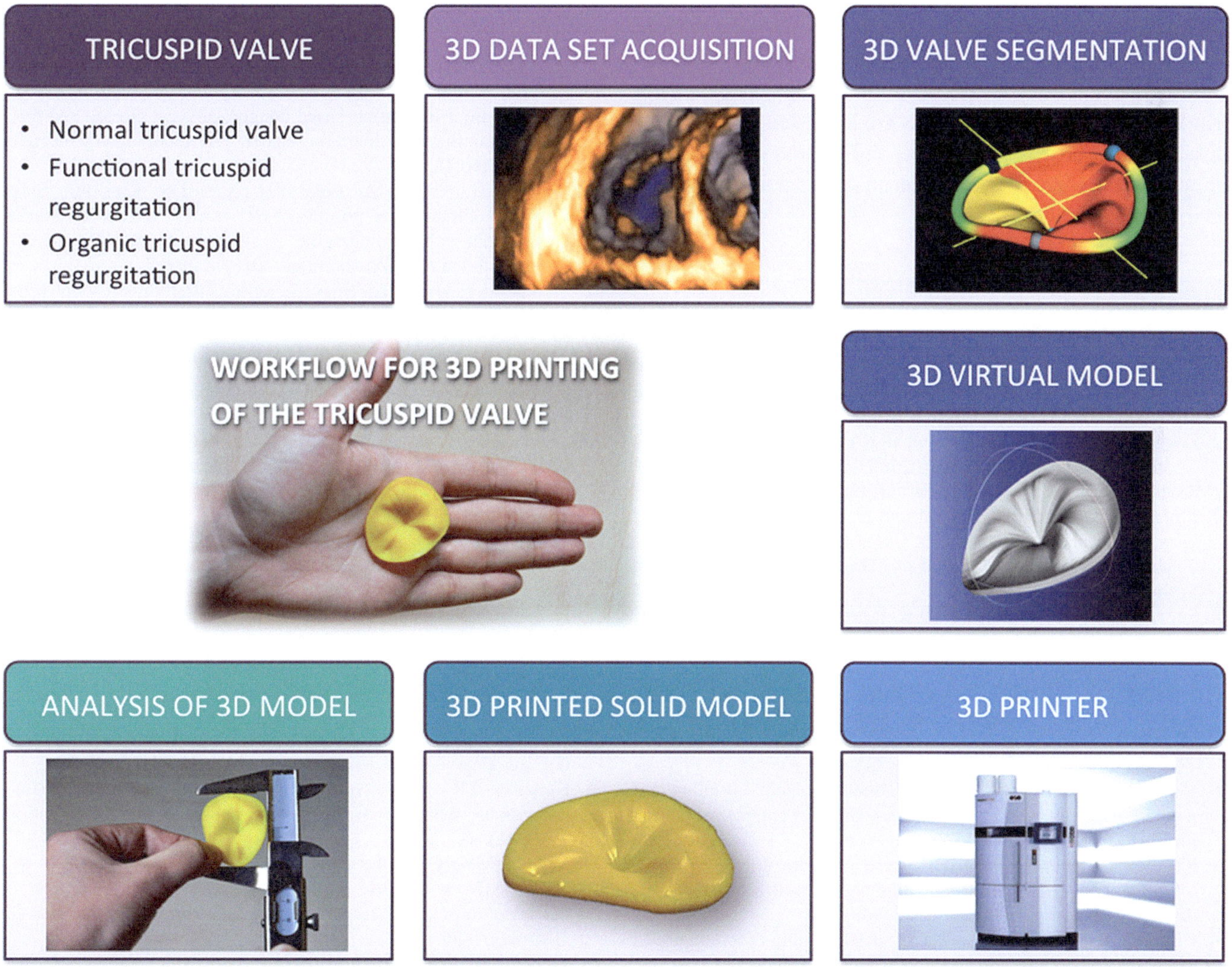

Fig. 2.15 Workflow associated with printing a 3D solid model of the tricuspid valve. A sample of workflow is shown diagrammatically from the transthoracic acquisition of the three-dimensional echocardiography data set, to its segmentation, creation of a virtual 3D model and stereolithographic file that can be printed using any commercially available 3D printer. The 3D solid model of the valve can be used to appreciate valve morphology and perform qualitative and quantitative analysis useful for pre-procedural (surgical or interventional) planning and teaching (see details in Muraru et al. [26]). Reprinted from Muraru D, Veronesi F, Maddalozzo A, Dequal D, Frajhof L, Rabischoffskky A, et al. 3D printing of normal and pathologic tricuspid valves from transthoracic 3D echocardiography data sets. European Heart Journal—Cardiovascular Imaging, © 2017, Vol. 18, Issue 7, pages 802–808, by permission of Oxford University Press/European Society of Cardiology

structures. Holography (whole drawing) is a technique that can provide an exact visual representation of a cardiac structure in three physical dimensions using light [27]. A holographic display of patients' 3D data is potentially useful in the clinical setting by providing the physician with a 3D image which is a true and spatially accurate representation of the patient's anatomy, having all the visual depth cues. Each point of light in the generated hologram is a separate physical entity in real 3D space and therefore direct interaction with the displayed structure is possible mimicking interventions performed on the patient's organ, since the image represents the precise anatomical coordinates of the patient. Holographic images have been used of the mitral valve, for example, allowing true assessment of mitral valve pathology in three dimensions before planning for an interventional procedure [28, 29].

However, both 3D printing and digital computer-generated holography provide only static 3D images from 3D volumetric data. The advantages of holography over 3D printing is that it obviates the need for specialized and costly printable material and that images are immediately available. Disadvantages are the higher costs and the loss of the consistency of the structure that could be an issue for surgeons who need training [30–32].

References

1. Badano L. The clinical benefits of adding a third dimension to assess the left ventricle with echocardiography. Scientifica (Cairo). 2014;2014:897431, for figs 2, 4, 6, 7.
2. Lang RM, Badano LP, Tsang W, et al. EAE/ASE recommendations for image acquisition and display using three-dimensional echocardiography. Eur Heart J Cardiovasc Imaging. 2012;13:1–46.
3. Muraru D, Badano LP. Physical and technical aspects and overview of 3D-echocardiography. In: Casas Rojo E, Fernandez-Golfin C, Zamorano J, editors. Manual of 3D echocardiography. Cham: Springer; 2017. p. 1–44.
4. Settergren M, Back M, Shahgaldi K, Jacobsen P, Winter R. 3D TEE with stereovision for guidance of the transcatheter mitral valve repair. JACC Cardiovasc Imaging. 2012;5:1066–9.
5. Vasilyev NV, Novotny PM, Martinez JF, et al. Stereoscopic vision display technology in real-time three-dimensional echocardiography-guided intracardiac beating-heart surgery. J Thorac Cardiovasc Surg. 2008;135:1334–41.
6. Marro A, Bandukwala T, Mak W. Three-dimensional printing and medical imaging: a review of the methods and applications. Curr Probl Diagn Radiol. 2016;45:2–9.
7. Kim MS, Hansgen AR, Wink O, Quaife RA, Carroll JD. Rapid prototyping: a new tool in understanding and treating structural heart disease. Circulation. 2008;117:2388–94.
8. Chia HN, Wu BM. Recent advances in 3D printing of biomaterials. J Biol Eng. 2015;9:4.
9. Yun PY. The application of three-dimensional printing techniques in the field of oral and maxillofacial surgery. J Korean Assoc Oral Maxillofac Surg. 2015;41:169–70.
10. Malik HH, Darwood AR, Shaunak S, et al. Three-dimensional printing in surgery: a review of current surgical applications. J Surg Res. 2015;199:512–22.
11. AlAli AB, Griffin MF, Butler PE. Three-dimensional printing surgical applications. Eplasty. 2015;15:e37.
12. Hsieh FY, Lin HH, Hsu SH. 3D bioprinting of neural stem cell-laden thermoresponsive biodegradable polyurethane hydrogel and potential in central nervous system repair. Biomaterials. 2015;71:48–57.
13. Collins SF. Bioprinting is changing regenerative medicine forever. Stem Cells Dev. 2014;23(Suppl 1):79–82.
14. Murphy SV, Atala A. 3D bioprinting of tissues and organs. Nat Biotechnol. 2014;32:773–85.
15. Liew Y, Beveridge E, Demetriades AK, Hughes MA. 3D printing of patient-specific anatomy: a tool to improve patient consent and enhance imaging interpretation by trainees. Br J Neurosurg. 2015;29:712–4.
16. Mahmoud A, Bennett M. Introducing 3-dimensional printing of a human anatomic pathology specimen: potential benefits for undergraduate and postgraduate education and anatomic pathology practice. Arch Pathol Lab Med. 2015;139:1048–51.
17. Bernhard JC, Isotani S, Matsugasumi T, et al. Personalized 3D printed model of kidney and tumor anatomy: a useful tool for patient education. World J Urol. 2016;34:337–45.
18. Farooqi KM, Saeed O, Zaidi A, et al. 3D printing to guide ventricular assist device placement in adults with congenital heart disease and heart failure. JACC Heart Fail. 2016;4:301–11.
19. Dickinson KJ, Matsumoto J, Cassivi SD, et al. Individualizing management of complex esophageal pathology using three-dimensional printed models. Ann Thorac Surg. 2015;100:692–7.
20. Costello JP, Olivieri LJ, Su L, et al. Incorporating three-dimensional printing into a simulation-based congenital heart disease and critical care training curriculum for resident physicians. Congenit Heart Dis. 2015;10:185–90.
21. Olivieri LJ, Krieger A, Loke YH, Nath DS, Kim PC, Sable CA. Three-dimensional printing of intracardiac defects from three-dimensional echocardiographic images: feasibility and relative accuracy. J Am Soc Echocardiogr. 2015;28:392–7.
22. Mahmood F, Owais K, Taylor C, et al. Three-dimensional printing of mitral valve using echocardiographic data. JACC Cardiovasc Imaging. 2015;8:227–9.
23. Vukicevic M, Puperi DS, Jane Grande-Allen K, Little SH. 3D printed modeling of the mitral valve for catheter-based structural interventions. Ann Biomed Eng. 2017;45:508–19.
24. Little SH, Vukicevic M, Avenatti E, Ramchandani M, Barker CM. 3D printed modeling for patient-specific mitral valve intervention: repair with a clip and a plug. JACC Cardiovasc Interv. 2016;9:973–5.
25. Shiraishi I, Yamagishi M, Hamaoka K, Fukuzawa M, Yagihara T. Simulative operation on congenital heart disease using rubber-like urethane stereolithographic biomodels based on 3D datasets of multislice computed tomography. Eur J Cardiothorac Surg. 2010;37:302–6.
26. Muraru D, Veronesi F, Maddalozzo A, et al. 3D printing of normal and pathologic tricuspid valves from transthoracic 3D echocardiography data sets. Eur Heart J Cardiovasc Imaging. 2017;18:802–8.
27. Bruckheimer E, Rotschild C, Dagan T, et al. Computer-generated real-time digital holography: first time use in clinical medical imaging. Eur Heart J Cardiovasc Imaging. 2016;17:845–9.
28. Hunziker PR, Smith S, Scherrer-Crosbie M, et al. Dynamic holographic imaging of the beating human heart. Circulation. 1999;99:1–6.
29. Vannan MA, Cao QL, Pandian NG, Sugeng L, Schwartz SL, Dalton MN. Volumetric multiplexed transmission holography of the heart with echocardiographic data. J Am Soc Echocardiogr. 1995;8:567–75.
30. Skolnick AA. New holographic process provides noninvasive 3-D anatomic views. JAMA. 1994;271:5–8.
31. Ko K, Webster J. Holographic imaging of human brain preparations—a step toward virtual medicine. Surg Neurol. 1995;44:428–32.
32. Erickson RR. Holographic medical imaging: the laser as a visual scalpel—issues and observations on 3-D display. IEEE J Quantum Electron. 1996;2:1–8.

Technical Principles of Transesophageal Three-Dimensional Echocardiography

3

Marcelo Luiz Campos Vieira
and Ricardo Ernesto Ronderos

Abstract

The advent of three-dimensional (3D) acquisition has been an important development in transesophageal echocardiography (TEE). This imaging technique entered the clinical arena during the first decade of the new century, when the expansion of the computing power of computers and the development of nanotechnology have made possible to insert a full matrix array into the tip of a transesophageal probe, providing TEE real-time volumetric imaging and prompting the use of 3D TEE in different cardiological, clinical, and research settings. Currently, major clinical applications of 3D TEE are left ventricular volume and ejection fraction measurement, assessment of heart valve anatomy and function, preoperative planning and monitoring different interventional procedures in the catheterization laboratory and hybrid surgical theatres.

Keywords

Echocardiography · Transesophageal echocardiography · Three-dimensional echocardiography · Diagnosis · Ultrasonography

Electronic Supplementary Material The online version of this chapter (https://doi.org/10.1007/978-3-030-14032-8_3) contains supplementary material, which is available to authorized users.

M. L. C. Vieira
Department of Echocardiography, Heart Institute (InCor), São Paulo University Medical School, São Paulo, Brazil

Hospital Israelita Albert Einstein, São Paulo, Brazil

R. E. Ronderos (✉)
Cardiac Imaging Department, Instituto Cardiovascular de Buenos Aires, Buenos Aires, Argentina

Instituto de Cardiologia La Plata, La Plata, Argentina

La Plata National University, School of Medicine, La Plata, Argentina
e-mail: rronderos@icba.com.ar

Introduction

The clinical application of three-dimensional (3D) transesophageal echocardiography has followed a slow path. Despite the first prototypes of 3D transesophageal probes appeared in 1981, the implementation of the technique in the clinical routine was not finalized till the beginning of the twenty-first century when nanotechnology with electronic miniaturization allowed the development of matrix transducers and real-time acquisition of 3D echocardiography data sets.

The first 3D echocardiographic systems used different modes of multiple tomographic images acquisition, always as a sequential manner (fan like, rotational, linear, etc.), followed by boring and long time off line imaging reconstruction of 3D data sets (see also Chap. 1) to obtain only several simultaneous left ventricular views and, later on, low spatial and temporal resolution 3D images (Figs. 3.1 and 3.2). The transesophageal approach was the main approach to obtain the first 3D images.

To obtain real-time 3D echocardiography, transducers had to change from the original 128 piezo-electric crystals arranged as phased array, to more than 3000 piezo-electric crystals arranged in a matrix array (see also Chap. 2). At the same time, the size of the transducer had to be miniaturized to become so small to be mounted in the tip of a conventional transesophageal probe [1, 2] (Fig. 3.3).

Principles of 3D Imaging

Appreciation of the 3D anatomy of cardiac structures displayed on a two-dimensional (flat) monitor requires the use volume rendering techniques (Fig. 3.4).

There are three parameters to include and understand in the process to visualize 3D images in a 2D format: (1) Shadowing, far objects are represented by shadows to give the aspect of solid objects. (2) Transparency, how good an object could be visualized through another in front of it and,

L. P. Badano et al. (eds.), *Textbook of Three-Dimensional Echocardiography*, https://doi.org/10.1007/978-3-030-14032-8_3

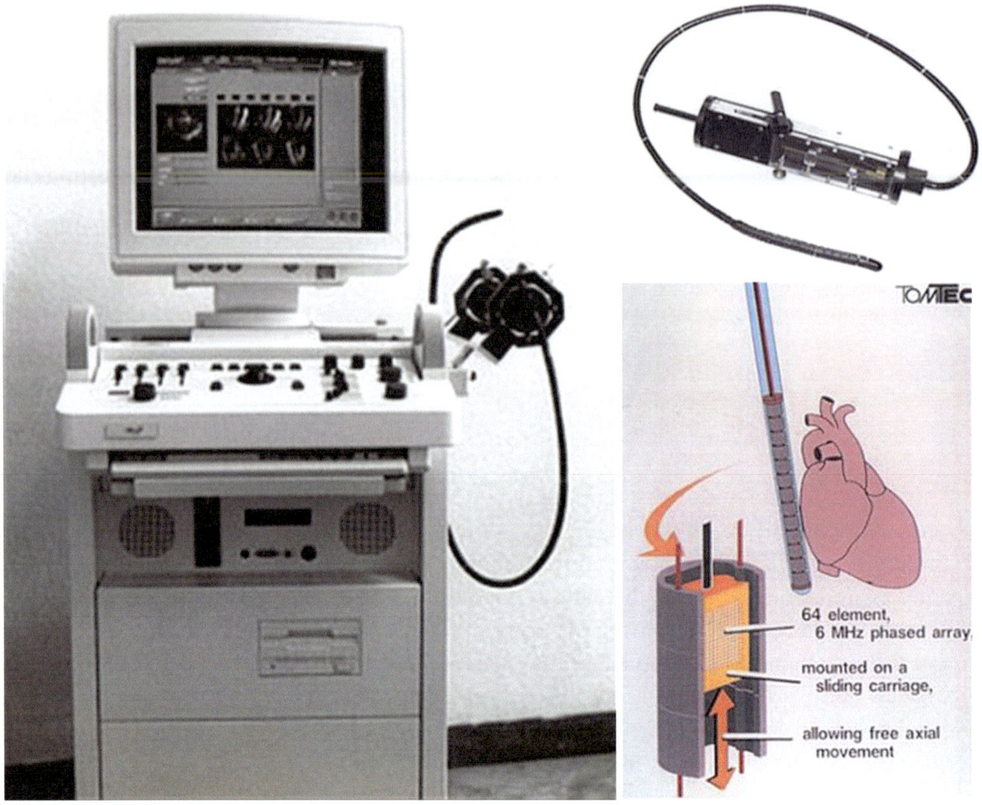

Fig. 3.1 Image of the first transesophageal echocardiography system (called "*the lobster tail*") for three-dimensional acquisitions using the transesophageal approach. Acquisition were obtained by parallel planes triggered by the EKG and respiration. Published by permission of Ediciones Journal, Ronderos R, Ecocardiografia tridimensional Ed Journal Buenos Aires, Argentina, 2016

finally, (3) Opacity, Objects opposite others get dark the far objects [2]. Combination of voxels and shadowing, transparency and opacity allow the visualization of the whole heart looking inside the volume of the voxels, depicting cardiac anatomy far than anatomy visualize in 2D cut planes (Fig. 3.4).

Technology

The main challenge in the process for the construction of miniaturized real time 3D transesophageal echocardiography probes was to develop all the electronics to control more than 3000 crystals arranged in a matrix manner and to miniaturize everything in order to be included in the small space available in a conventional transesophageal probe (Fig. 3.3).

Current 3D transesophageal transducers are reliable, with relatively good spatial and temporal resolution at acceptable costs, allowing 360° ultrasound beam and theoretically infinite cut planes to visualize the cardiac structures.

The last generation of 3D transesophageal echocardiography probes provides high quality images in volume rendering as well as simultaneous tomographic planes (multiplane display, Fig. 3.5, Videos 3.1a and 3.1b) [2].

Physics

Broadly, 3D transesophageal echocardiography follows the same principles discussed in Chap. 2. However, there are some peculiarities of this echocardiographic technique that has to be known by the operators to optimize the acquired data sets.

As we discussed in Chap. 2, 3D ultrasound imaging is still subject to the laws of acoustic physics. First, aperture is an important determinant of image quality. Larger apertures allow better beamforming from a focus point of view. Unlike abdominal echography, transthoracic echocardiography is limited by the ultrasound aperture that can fit in the space between the ribs. In transesophageal echocardiography, the aperture is limited by the size of the transducer that can be accommodated inside an adult esophagus. Transesophageal transducers generally employ higher frequencies than its transthoracic counterparts. This allows better image resolution for a given aperture size (the higher the transducer frequency, the better the ultrasound beam can focus but this comes at the expense of reduced penetration). Since the transesophageal approach is not limited by significant chest wall acoustic aberration, the higher frequencies and better acoustic substrate allow higher resolution data sets than those obtained from the transthoracic approach. Next, artifacts

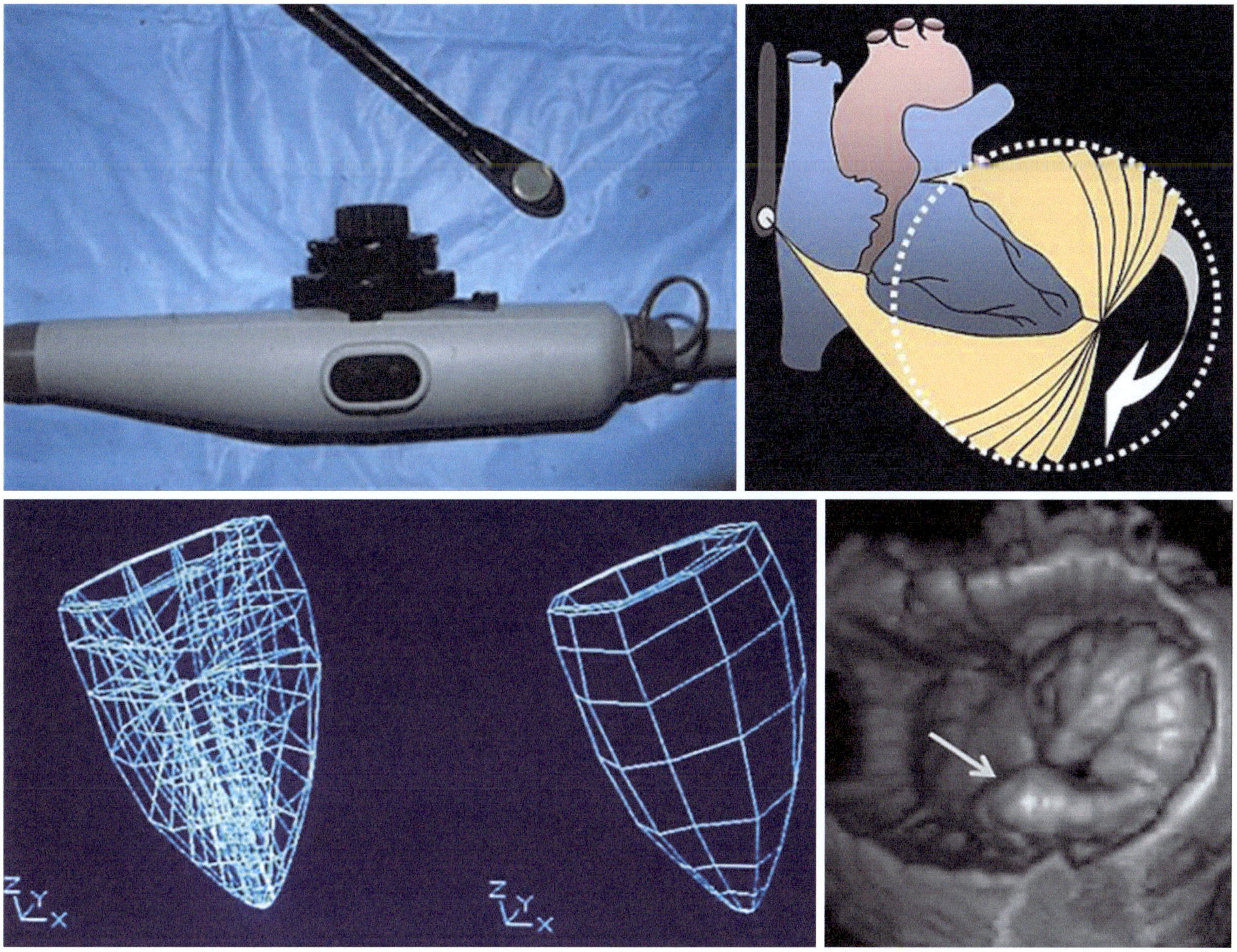

Fig. 3.2 Advanced transesophageal probe system using the omniplane transducer by Hewlett Packard. The cartoon shows the electronic planes of the rotational acquisition sequence. After the acquisitions, different display modalities were available: wire frame models of the left ventricle (bottom left) and 3D rendering of the mitral valve prolapse visualized from the left atrial perspective (white arrow). Published by permission of Ediciones Journal, Ronderos R, Ecocardiografia tridimensional Ed Journal Buenos Aires, Argentina, 2016

such as shadowing, reverberations, multi-path transmission and aberration play a role in degrading the ultrasound image. As with 2D echocardiography, 3D ultrasound cannot image through metallic or highly calcified objects. Moreover, the transesophageal approach has a "blind-spot" in visualizing the aortic arch due to limitations from the airway.

The relative image degradation that occurs by acquiring data sets from the transthoracic approach is due mainly to two phenomena: aberration and multipath reflection. Aberration originates from wavefronts traveling through different media with different velocities of sound. Multiple tissue layers create a distortion of the traveling wavefronts. This can be partially corrected by accounting for the varying speeds of sound. The layers of the chest wall contain varying degrees of adipose and connective tissue. This creates aberration but also multipath degradation. As an ultrasound wave get diverted to altering paths of propagation, the superposition of transmitted and returning echo signals consists of wavefronts of both desired and nondesired targets. Unwanted but real signals are defined clutter. However, since the esophagus represents a thin wall consisting of a stratified squamous epithelium and smooth muscle, this multipath degradation do not occur in 3D transesophageal echocardiography that produces higher image quality and lower cluttering.

Acquisition and Display

Pivotal, for a proper clinical application of 3D transesophageal echocardiography, it is the knowledge of advantages and disadvantages of the different modalities for 3D acquisition. Depending on the focus of the study, different modali-

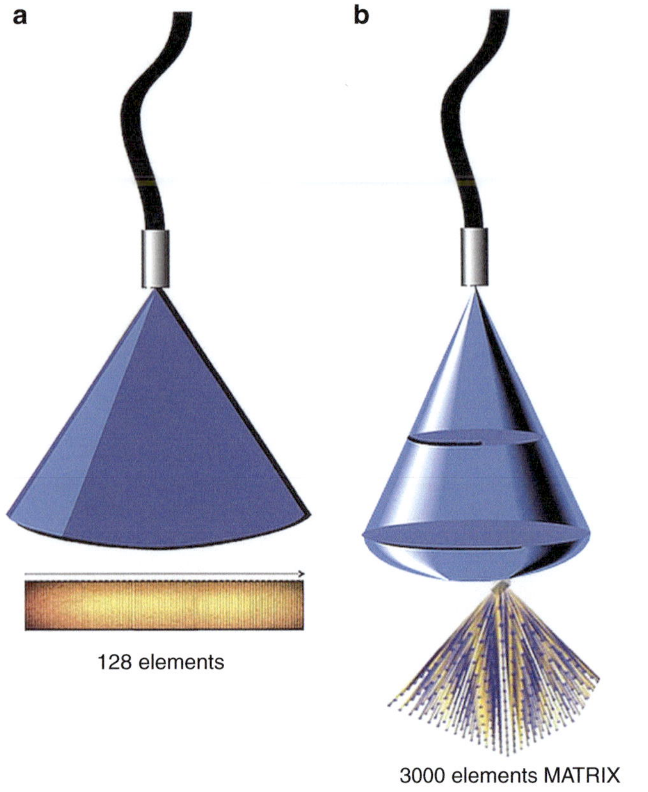

Fig. 3.3 Schematic representation of the difference between a 2D (**a**) and a 3D (**b**) transesophageal echocardiography transducer (see text) [2]

ties of 3D imaging will be better suited to the specific clinical question to answer.

Biplane Mode

To provide biplane imaging, two lines of the piezoelectric elements of the matrix transducer are simultaneously activated to display two simultaneous two-dimensional views from the same heart beat (Figs. 3.6 and 3.7). The track ball on the main control panel is used to change the position and the orientation of the plane of the second view.

Monitoring of interventional procedures such as left atrial appendage closure has greatly benefited by the use of biplane imaging [3, 4]. The landing zone of the occluder device has to be identified paying attention at the left circumflex coronary artery at a point which is 10 mm below the isthmus between the left atrial appendage and the upper left pulmonary vein. Using only a single 2D view, it would be difficult to align the device according to both landmarks. The biplane mode allows to see both landmarks simultaneously and facilitates the proper landing of the device. Biplane display can be used also in color Doppler mode, allowing the visualization of a regurgitant jet from different perspectives for a better understanding of the direction of the jet in space as well as the shape of the PISA.

Fig. 3.4 Top, schematic representation of the multiple ultrasound beams generated by a matrix array probe to obtain a volumetric 3D data set. Bottom, volumetric rendering of a mitral stenosis viewed from the left ventricular perspective. Published by permission of Ediciones Journal, Ronderos R, Ecocardiografia tridimensional Ed Journal Buenos Aires, Argentina, 2016

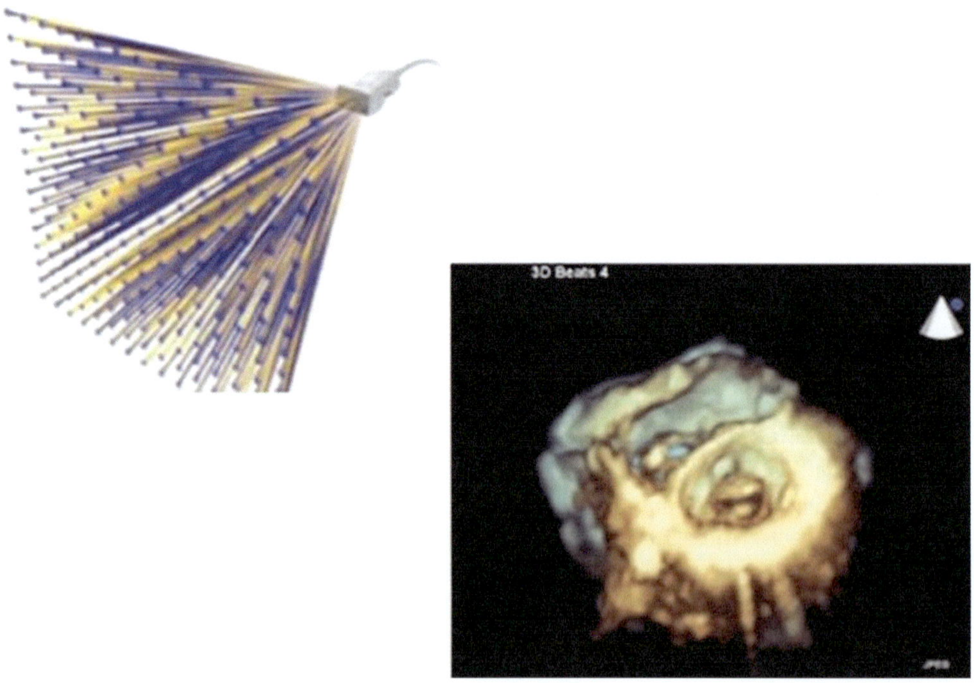

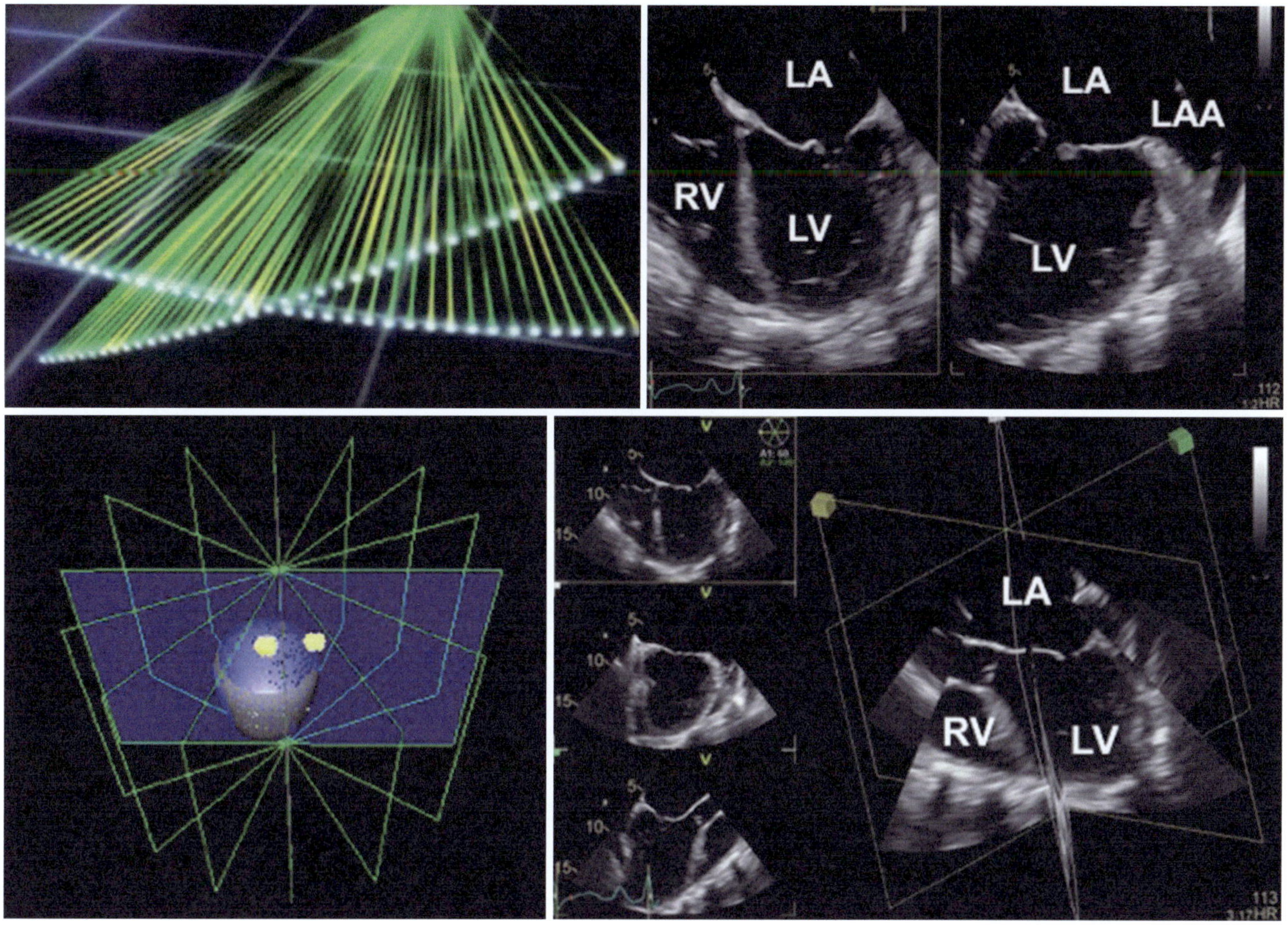

Fig. 3.5 *Upper panels*. Schematic representation of the generation of the biplane display modality with 3D probe, the secondary plane can be oriented from 0° to 180° using the trackball and the primary view as reference. In the example the primary plane is the apical four-chamber view and the secondary is the apical two-chamber view (Video 3.1a). *Lower panels*. Multiplane display (in the example triplane imaging) of the left ventricle (Video 3.1b). By default, the angles of the secondary planes are set at 60° and 120° from the acquisition plane. The orientation of the secondary planes can be adjusted by the echocardiographer. However, since changing the plane angle will fire a different line of piezoelectric elements, scan plane angle orientation can be adjusted only during acquisition

Volume Rendering

Real-Time Narrow Volume

Real-time narrow volume 3D acquisition is usually used to optimize the settings (sizing the acquisition volume, set the gain and compression) before starting the acquisition of the cardiac structure of interest. In addition, real-time narrow volume acquisition may also be used during monitoring of interventional procedures, when quick views and answers are needed, or to monitor rapidly occurring events like passage of bubbles through a patent foramen ovale during a bubble test. However, this acquisition modality does not allow to acquire large data sets and therefore is not useful to assess spatial relationships among cardiac structures or for quantitation.

Real-Time Color Doppler 3D

The limitations of real-time narrow volume 3D imaging have been described in the previous paragraph. Adding color Doppler will only further decrease both temporal and spatial resolution. Flow is important to be evaluated in dynamic manner and live color Doppler is still low temporal resolution, with the exception of few companies as Siemens who has a better temporal resolution but lower spatial resolution.

Real-Time Zoom 3D

Zoom 3D seems to be the most convenient acquisition modality for real-time 3D transesophageal echocardiography. There are many practical advantages to use this acquisition modality. First, 3D zoom is a real-time imaging. Of course, both temporal and spatial resolutions of the 3D data

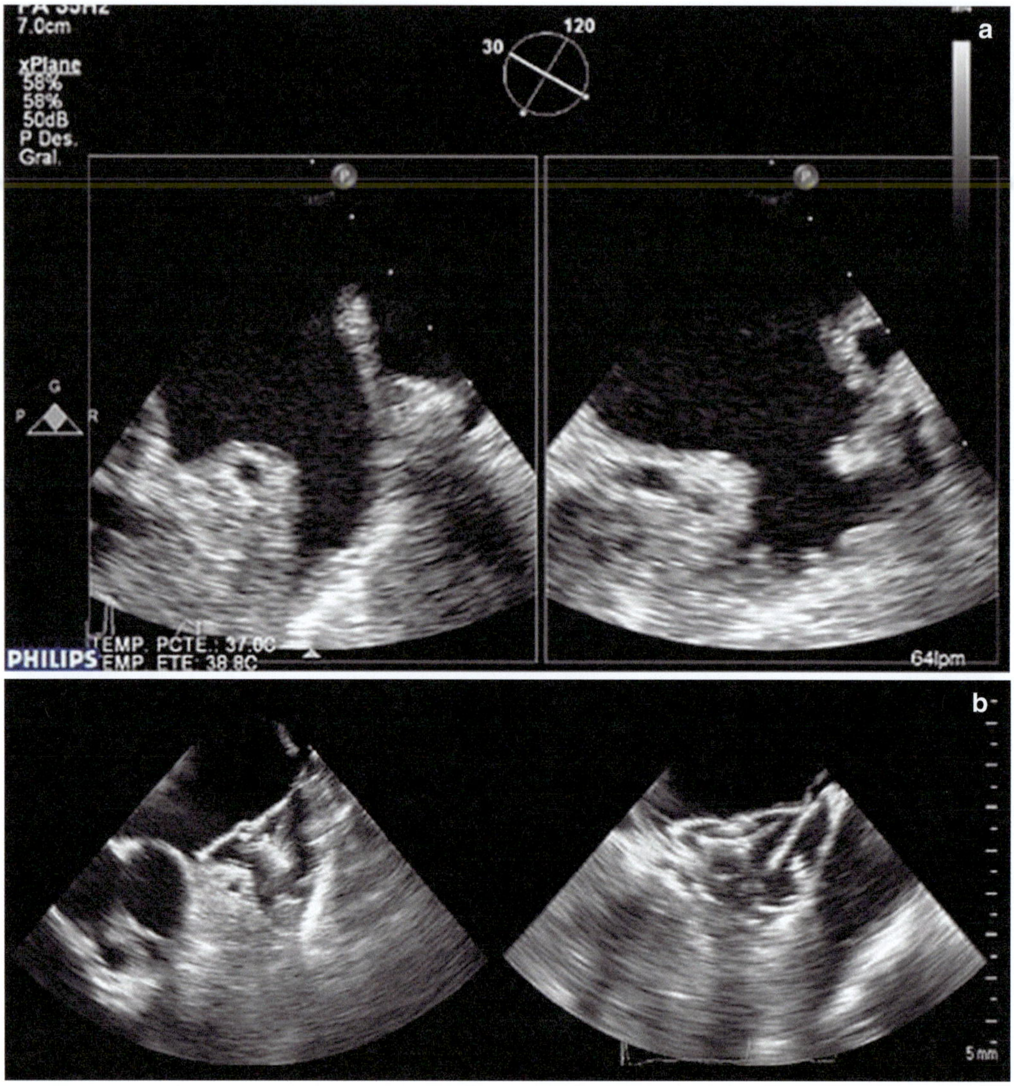

Fig. 3.6 Orthogonal biplane display of the left atrial appendage (LAA). To obtain the best view LAA the reference plane was rotated by 30°. The orthogonal plane allows the visualization of a bilobulated LAA (**a**). Occlusion of the LAA using an Amplatzer occluder. The biplane mode allows the simultaneous visualization of the LAA in two different, simultaneous two-dimensional views to check the proper landing of the device (**b**). Published by permission of Ediciones Journal, Ronderos R, Ecocardiografia tridimensional Ed Journal Buenos Aires, Argentina, 2016

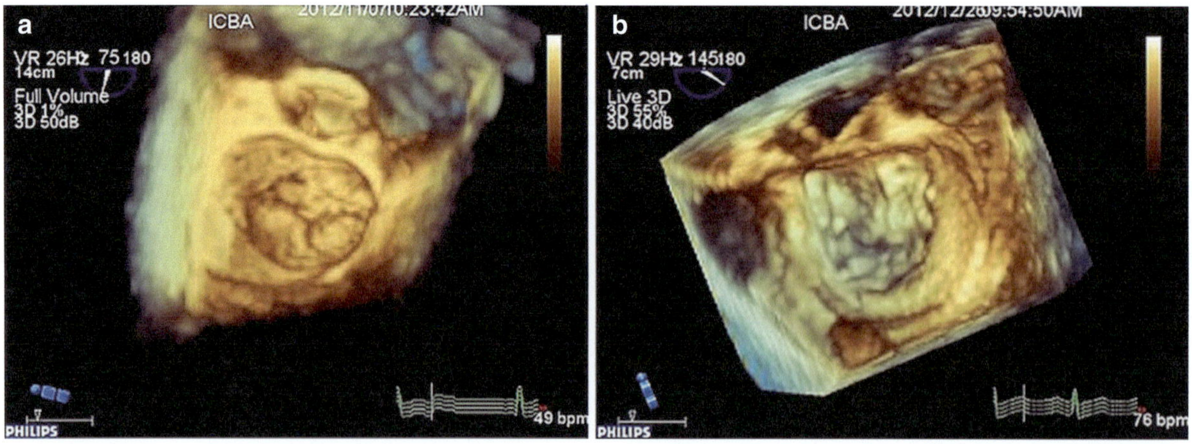

Fig. 3.7 Full volume (**a**) and zoom 3D acquisition modes (**b**) in two patients with Barlow's disease. Despite the similar temporal resolution using the four-beat acquisition in both modes, the full volume data set shows narrower near field than the data set acquired in zoom mode. Published by permission of Ediciones Journal, Ronderos R, Ecocardiografia tridimensional Ed Journal Buenos Aires, Argentina, 2016

set can be improved by acquiring two or four cardiac beats (multi-beat acquisition), but if multi-beat acquisition is not an option (uncooperative patient, or badly tolerated procedure), the small acquisition volume (usually 30° × 30°) of the zoom mode, the low depth and the high frequency of the transesophageal probe allow relatively good temporal and spatial resolutions to provide high quality 3D data sets. Both the shape and the size of the zoom volume can be controlled by the operator.

One potential limitation of the zoom mode acquisition is that it is usually employed to acquire data sets of single cardiac structures. Therefore, the anatomical relationships of the cardiac structure of interest with the surrounding structures are usually lost. As a consequence, the orientation of the structures in space is easier to obtain during the acquisition than during the post-processing of the data set after the end of the study.

Multi-beat Full Volume

Multi-beat full volume acquisition allows to obtain the largest amount of data with acceptable temporal and spatial resolution in the 3D data set. However, it is not real time, requires patient cooperation and stitching artifacts may occur due to respiration and/or arrhythmias. Therefore, this acquisition modality is not used to monitor interventional procedures or as the first approach when 3D transesophageal echocardiography is needed. On the other end, a full volume acquisition may be needed to visualize the whole mitral valve apparatus and to examine the papillary muscles together with the chordae and the leaflets. One limitation against the use of full volume acquisitions in patients with mitral valve or atrial septal defects, is the fact that the near field is very small and it may impair image quality when the left atrium is not enlarged. Whereas, using the 3D zoom acquisition it is possible to obtain a wider near field image (Fig. 3.7).

Multi-beat Full Volume Color Doppler

Despite the many advances in 3D echocardiography technology, 3D color Doppler data sets still show poor resolution, particularly temporal resolution. During transesophageal studies, this limitation is even more impressive than in transthoracic studies, when compared with the high quality of the volume rendering. To obtain data set of diagnostic quality a multi-beat acquisition is usually needed.

Multiplane Display

Either single- or multi-beat full volume data sets can be sliced in several longitudinal and transversal tomographic views. Multiplane display is mainly used for quantitative purposes (Fig. 3.8), to assess regional wall motion (multi-beat full volume acquisition) and to monitor left ventricular function during high-risk surgical or interventional procedures (single beat continuous monitoring).

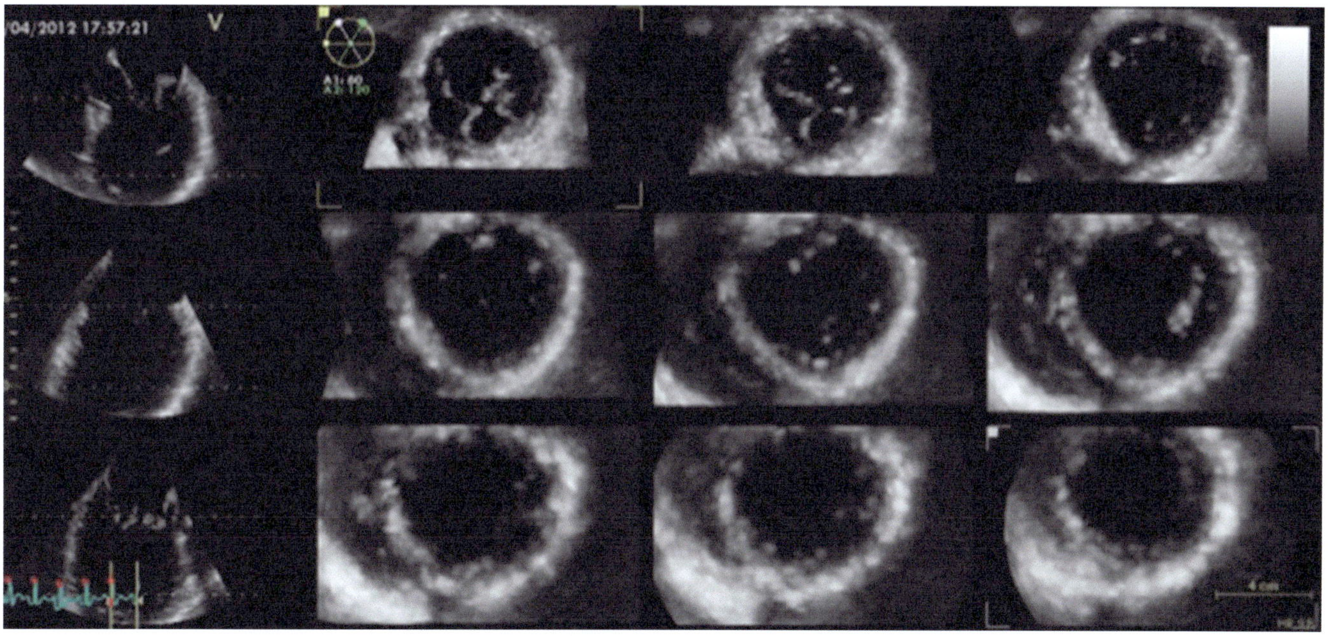

Fig. 3.8 Multi-slice display of a full volume data set of the left ventricle. The software package has sliced the data set in three longitudinal views (left panels) and nine transversal (short axis) views. The longitudinal views includes a four-chamber view (left upper panel) and, by default, two views obtained at 60° and 120°, respectively. However, the orientation of the secondary views can be adjusted by the operator to obtain true bicommissural and long axis views. For the transversal views, only the position of the apical and the basal slice can be controlled and oriented in order to obtain views perpendicular to the left ventricular long axis, by moving and tilting the dotted lines on the longitudinal views. Then, the remaining seven slices will be automatically repositioned between the apical and the bottom slices

Added Clinical Value of Three-Dimensional Transesophageal Echocardiography

Despite an extensive protocol for a complete 3D transesophageal examination has been described [5], this is very time consuming and unpractical to use in the clinical routine. Currently, 3D echocardiography is a technique that complements but does not replace 2D echocardiography. The most cost-effective use 3D transesophageal echocardiography is as a focused acquisition to address specific clinical questions rather than performing a comprehensive 3D examination.

One of the most significant advantages of 3D transesophageal echocardiography is that it provides high resolution, anatomically sound images of the cardiac structures in the beating heart to provide the anatomical basis of cardiac diseases and facilitate the communication among healthcare professionals (Figs. 3.9 and 3.10).

Moreover, high quality images that encompass the 3D complexity of cardiac structures are particularly useful to quantitate the geometry of these structures without assumptions about their shape. In addition to the visualization of the anatomy of cardiac structures in their true stereoscopic geometry, many echocardiographers believe that a significant added value of 3D echocardiography is the possibility to quantify. Myocardial and valvular motion occurs along three dimensions in space but traditional 2D views do not capture the entire motion as cardiac structures exit the scan plan during the cardiac cycle. Quantifying implies *segmenting* structures of interest from the 3D voxel set. Whereas voxels themselves can be tagged, for example coloring right ventricular voxels separately from left ventricular ones, computer vision techniques frequently employ methods that define an interface, for example the left ventricular endocardial border. This interface is typically constructed as a mesh of points and lines and displayed by a process known as *surface rendering* (see Chap. 2).

3D electronically steered transesophageal transducers yield high quality ultrasound images of cardiac structures (such as the mitral valve, Fig. 3.7) in the beating heart. This also allows the cardiac chambers and the valve structures to be segmented at end-systole with great accuracy and measured (Figs. 3.11, 3.12, and 3.13).

Finally, an expanding role of 3D transesophageal echocardiography is to plan and monitoring procedures to treat structural heart defects.

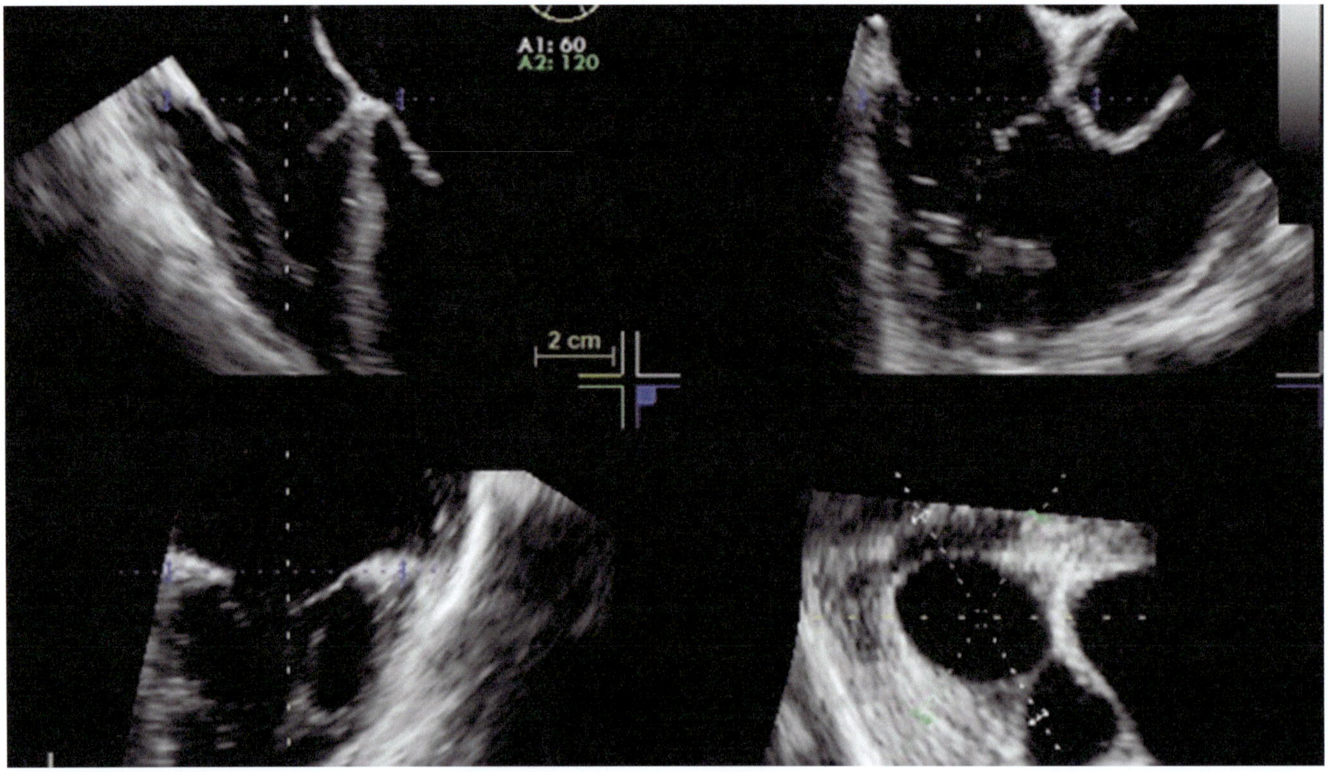

Fig. 3.9 Multi-slice of a full volume 3D data set of the right ventricle with careful orientation of the transversal plane (horizontal dotted line on the longitudinal planes) to obtain a transversal (short-axis) plane at the level of the tricuspid annulus (lower right panel) to planimeter tricuspid annulus area

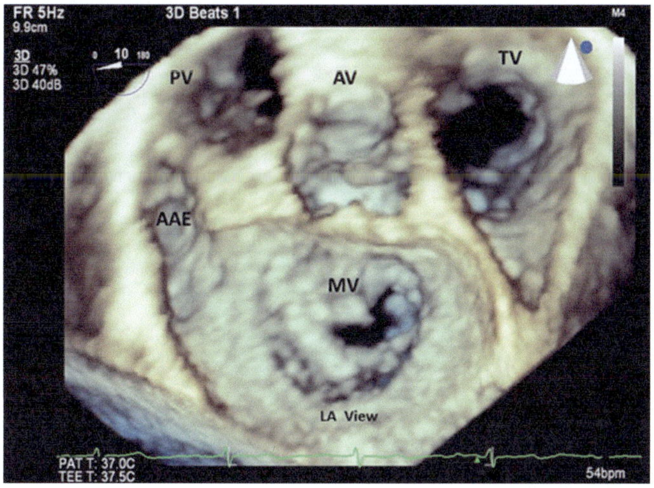

Fig. 3.10 Three-dimensional transesophageal echocardiography (full volume acquisition) cropped to visualize the anatomy of the base of the heart in a patient with mitral valve stenosis. *PV* pulmonary valve, *AV* aortic valve, *MV* mitral valve *TV* tricuspid valve, *LAA* left atrial appendage, *LA* left atrium. Published by permission of Ediciones Journal, Ronderos R, Ecocardiografia tridimensional Ed Journal Buenos Aires, Argentina, 2016

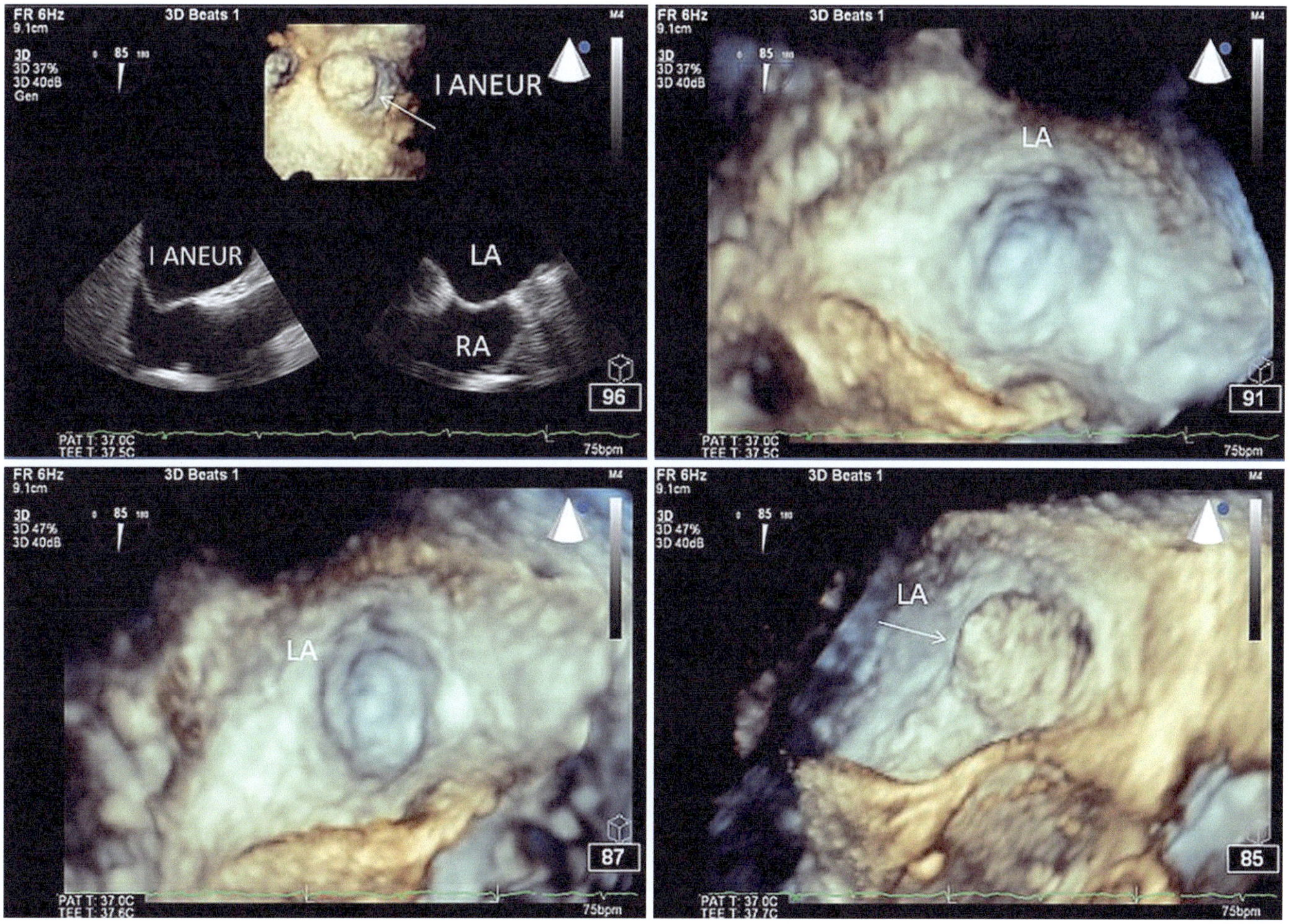

Fig. 3.11 Three-dimensional transesophageal echocardiography (3D zoom acquisition) in a patient with interatrial septum aneurysm (arrow). *ANEU* interatrial septum aneurysm, *LA* left atrium, *RA* right atrium. Published by permission of Ediciones Journal, Ronderos R, Ecocardiografia tridimensional Ed Journal Buenos Aires, Argentina, 2016

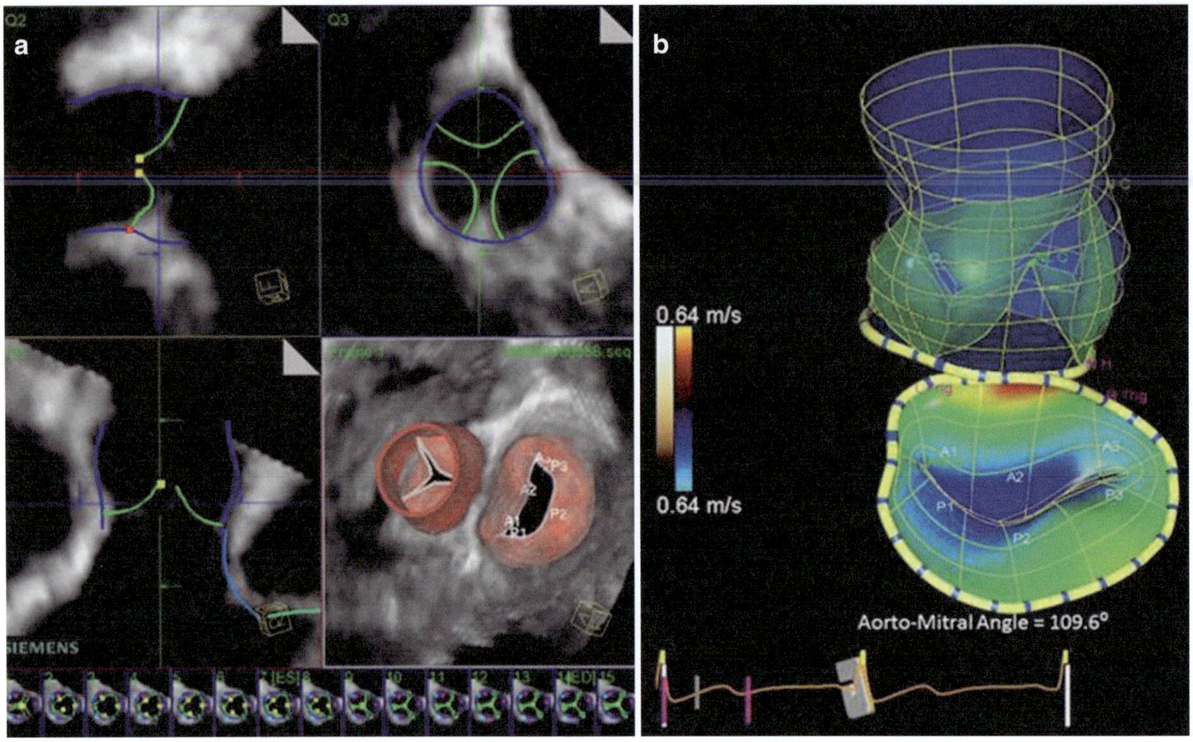

Fig. 3.12 Automated surface rendering and quantitative 3D modeling of the aortic root and mitral valve using data sets obtained with transesophageal 3D echocardiography

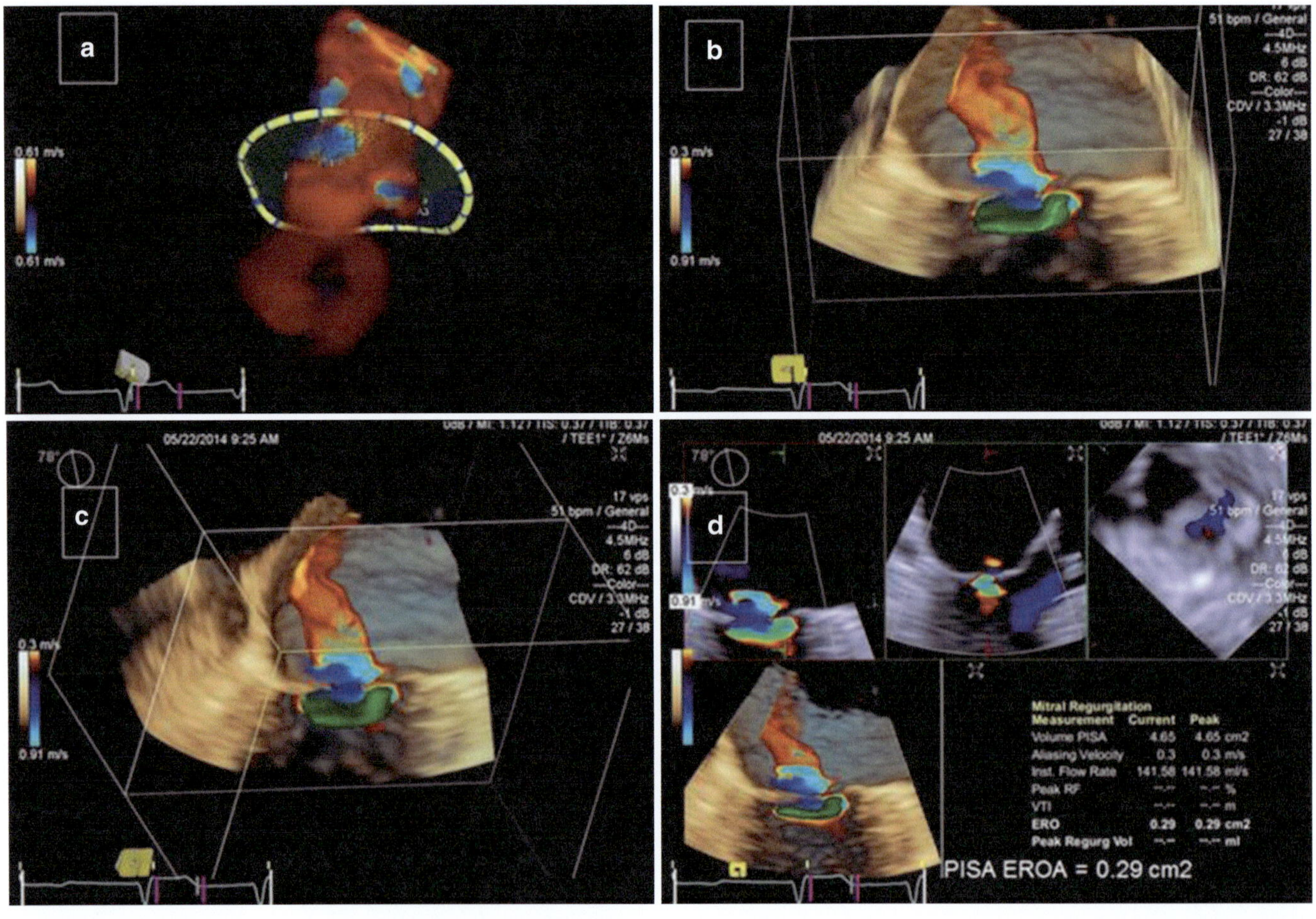

Fig. 3.13 3D quantitative measurement of mitral effective regurgitant orifice area and volume without geometric assumptions about the shape of the proximal isovelocity surface and regurgitant orifice

References

1. Ronderos R. Ecocardiografia tridimensional Ed Journal Buenos Aires, Argentina, Ediciones Journal. ISBN 978-987-1981-83-0, 2016.
2. Vegas A, Meineri M. Core review: three-dimensional transesophageal echocardiography is a major advance for intraoperative clinical management of patients undergoing cardiac surgery: a core review. Anesth Analg. 2010;110:1548–73.
3. Perk G, Lang RM, Garcia-Fernandez MA, et al. Use of real time three-dimensional transesophageal echocardiography in intracardiac catheter based interventions. J Am Soc Echocardiogr. 2009;22:865–82.
4. Zamorano JL, Badano LP, Bruce C, et al. EAE/ASE recommendations for the use of echocardiography in new transcatheter interventions for valvular heart disease. Eur Heart J. 2011;32:2189–214.
5. Lang RM, Badano LP, Tsang W, et al. EAE/ASE recommendations for image acquisition and display using three-dimensional echocardiography. Eur Heart J Cardiovasc Imaging. 2012;13:1–46.

How to Implement Three-Dimensional Echocardiography in the Routine of the Echocardiography Laboratory

4

Denisa Muraru and Luigi P. Badano

Abstract

The advent of three-dimensional echocardiography (3DE) represented a real breakthrough in cardiovascular ultrasound. Major advancements in computer and transducer technology allow to acquire 3D data sets with adequate spatial and temporal resolution for assessing the functional anatomy of cardiac structures in most of cardiac pathologies. Compared to conventional two-dimensional echocardiographic (2DE) imaging, 3DE allows the operator to visualize the cardiac structures from virtually any perspective, providing a more anatomically sound and intuitive display, as well as an accurate quantitative evaluation of anatomy and function of heart valves. In addition, 3DE overcomes geometric assumptions and enables an accurate quantitative and reproducible evaluation of cardiac chambers, thus offering solid elements for patient management. Furthermore, 3DE is the only imaging technique based on volumetric scanning able to show moving structures in the beating heart, in contrast to cardiac magnetic resonance (CMR) or cardiac computed tomography (CT), which are based on post-acquisition 3D reconstruction from multiple tomographic images and displaying only 3D rendered snapshots.

Data regarding clinical applications of 3DE are burgeoning and gradually capturing an established place in the noninvasive clinical assessment of anatomy and function of cardiac structures. Recently, joint European Association of Echocardiography and American Society of Echocardiography recommendations have been published, aiming to provide clinicians with a systematic approach to 3D image acquisition and analysis. Finally, the recent update of the recommendations for the chamber quantification using echocardiography recommended 3DE for the assessment of the left and right ventricular size and function. However, despite all these evidences 3DE has not yet been adopted for the clinical routine in most echocardiography laboratories. This chapter tries too identify the bareers that have hampered the diffusion of 3DE in the clinical arena and to offer some practical advices on how to implement 3DE in the clinical practice.

Keywords

Three-dimensional echocardiography · Two-dimensional echocardiography · Feasibility · Clinical value · Costs Cost/effectiveness · Workflow · Echocardiography laboratory · Routine clinical practice · Data management Reporting · Data set acquisition · Post-processing

Introduction

The heart has a complex anatomy and it is in constant motion. Conventional two-dimensional (2D) echocardiography can only provide partial information (Fig. 4.1) about the spatial and temporal relationships of cardiac structures during the cardiac cycle (Fig. 4.2, Video 4.8). Furthermore, conventional 2D echocardiography requires a difficult mental process by the operator to reconstruct a stereoscopic image of the heart based on the interpretation of multiple tomographic slices (Fig. 4.3). Sometimes, the mental exercise of reconstruction may be inadequate to obtain a precise diagnosis even for an experienced observer, especially when dealing with complex congenital abnormalities of the heart or unexpected anatomical findings. Finally, it can be difficult to con-

Electronic Supplementary Material The online version of this chapter (https://doi.org/10.1007/978-3-030-14032-8_4) contains supplementary material, which is available to authorized users.

D. Muraru · L. P. Badano (✉)
University of Milano-Bicocca, and Istituto Auxologico Italiano, IRCCS, San Luca Hospital, Milano, Italy
e-mail: denisa.muraru@unimib.it; luigi.badano@unimib.it

L. P. Badano et al. (eds.), *Textbook of Three-Dimensional Echocardiography*, https://doi.org/10.1007/978-3-030-14032-8_4

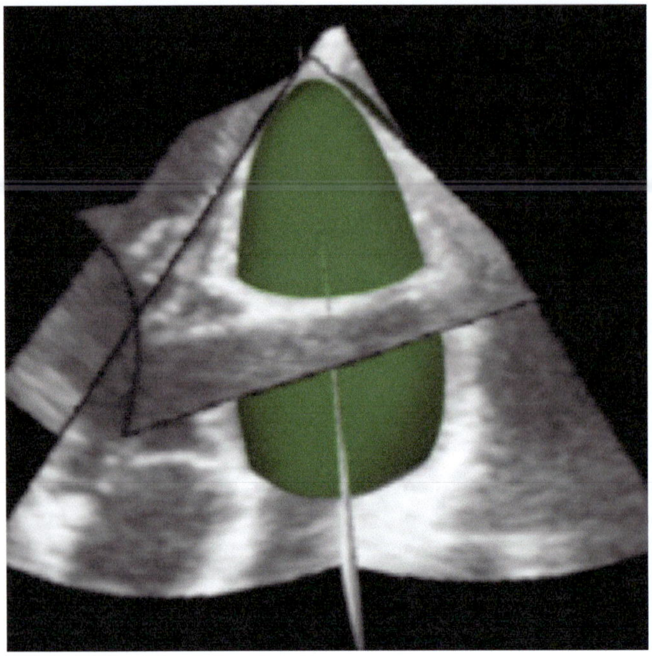

Fig. 4.1 Two-dimensional echocardiography is a tomographic imaging modality that provides information about the morphology and function of the different cardiac structures by obtaining a number of thin slices of the heart. The image shows a series of echocardiographic longitudinal and transversal views of the left ventricle and the 3D beutel of the cavity in green to demonstrate that what the echocardiographer actually visualizes it is just a very small amount of the endocardial surface and myocardial mass (less than 10%). Two-dimensional echocardiography is based on the assumption that what we see in the thin slices is the same that happens in the large endocardial surface and muscle mass which lies in between on two adjacent slices. This assumption has been proven not to be true in many cardiac conditions (i.e. ischemic heart disease)

vey or demonstrate a meaningful representation of cardiac pathology to those not fully conversant with 2D echocardiographic views and appearances.

Over the last decade, three-dimensional (3D) echocardiography has transitioned from a research tool to an imaging technique useful in everyday clinical practice for both diagnostic and procedure monitoring purposes, thus expanding the diagnostic capabilities of cardiac ultrasound [1–5]. 3D echocardiography may allow a more readily appreciated, intuitive, objective and quantitative evaluation of cardiac anatomy and physiology that would reduce the subjectivity in image interpretation.

At present there is enough scientific evidence to endorse the use of 3D echocardiography as the echocardiographic technique of choice to: (1) measure cardiac chamber volumes without the need for geometrical modelling [6]; (2) visualization of detailed in vivo anatomy of cardiac valves and congenital abnormalities [5, 7]; (3) monitor and assess effectiveness of surgical or percutaneous transcatheter interventions [8, 9]. However, despite these documented advantages, the technique is still quite far to be used in the clinical routine of most of echocardiograpy laboratories.

In this chapter, we will try to identify and discuss the main reasons that have limited the penetration of 3D echocardiography among clinical echocardiographers and to provide hints for an effective implementation of the technique in the clinical routine of echocardiography laboratories.

Identifying the Barriers Against the Routine Use of 3D Echocardiography in Clinical Practice

Apart the obvious skepticism that surrounds any new technology when it appears in the clinical arena, there are objective facts that may explain the resistance of echocardiographers to embrace 3D echocardiography (Table 4.1).

Underappreciation of the Added Clinical Value of 3D vs. Conventional 2D Echocardiography

This is the first, and probably the most important, reason for the relative underuse of 3D echocardiography in the clinical routine. With 3D echocardiography, a paradigm shift occurred in echocardiography (Fig. 4.4). We have moved from a technique based on geometrical assumptions (i.e. the left ventricular outflow tract is rounded; all left ventricles can be assimilated to rotational ellipsoids; the regurgitant orifices are always rounded; etc.) and calculations (use of relatively simple area, linear and velocity measurements to obtain volumes, pressure gradients and valve orifice areas) to a technique that allows the echocardiographer to actually see (and show!) the anatomy and measure the size and the function of cardiac structures (chambers, valves and defects) without any geometrical assumption about their shape. In addition, and differently from the anatomist and the cardiac surgeon (who can only examine the still heart), the echocardiographer can see the functional anatomy of the cardiac structures in the beating heart.

Not only 3D echocardiography allows a more accurate and reproducible measurement of the volumes of cardiac chambers such as left ventricle, left and the right atria compared to 2D echocardiography, but allows also to reliably measure volumes and ejection fraction of the right ventricle [11, 12]. The latter were impossible to obtain with 2D echocardiography and we know that they improve the prognostic stratification of patients with various cardiac conditions [13, 14] and also facilitates the communication with other health professionals. Conventional echocardiography parameters used to describe right ventricular function such as TAPSE (tricuspid annular plane systolic excursion), FAC (fractional area shortening), RIMP (right ventricular index of myocardial performance), FWLS (free wall longitudinal strain) may sound strange to colleagues who are not fully conversant in echocardiography, but terms like volumes and ejection fraction are readily understood by every healthcare professional.

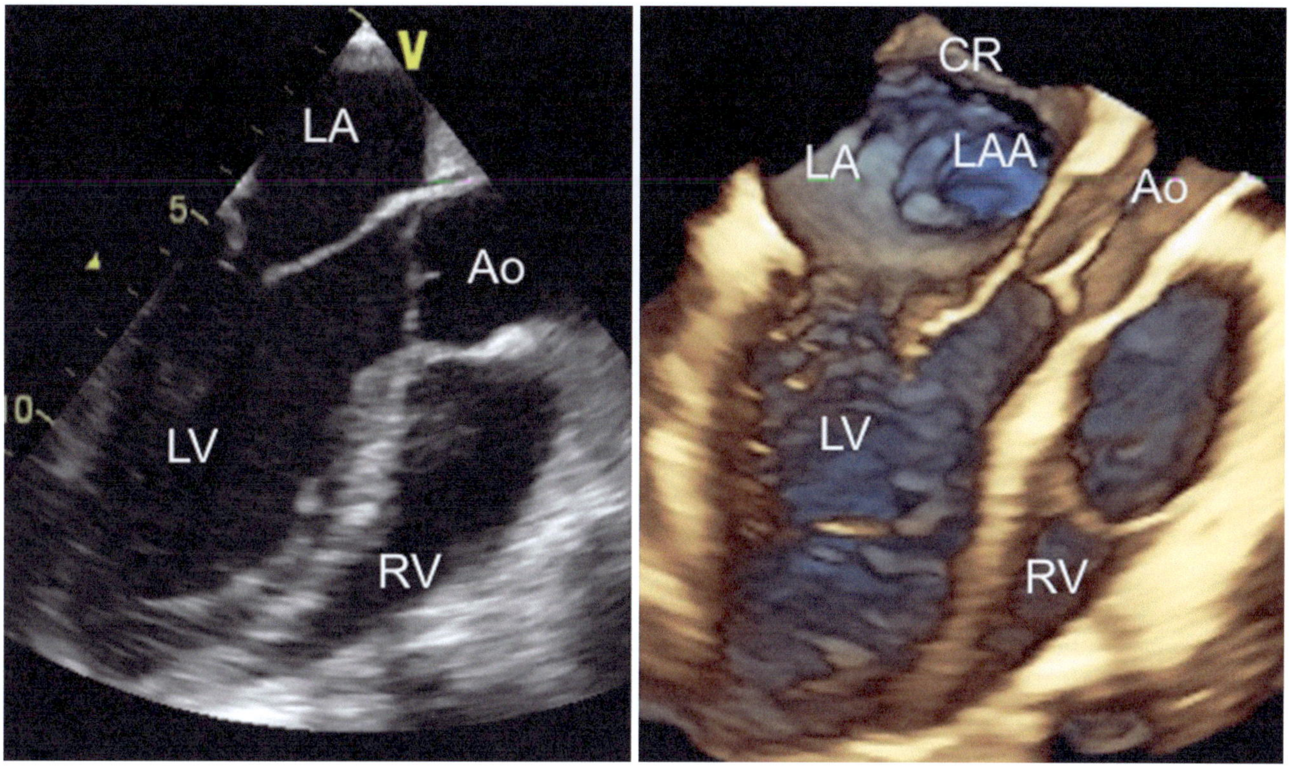

Fig. 4.2 Standard parasternal long-axis view obtained with 2D transesophageal echocardiography (*left panel*) and the same view obtained cropping a full volume data set of the left ventricle obtained with 3D echocardiography (*right panel*). Note the depth perception and visualization of structures (such as the left atrial appendage, LAA and the coumadin ridge, CR) which are not visible with 2D imaging. *Ao* aorta, *LA* left atrium, *LV* left ventricle, *RV* right ventricle

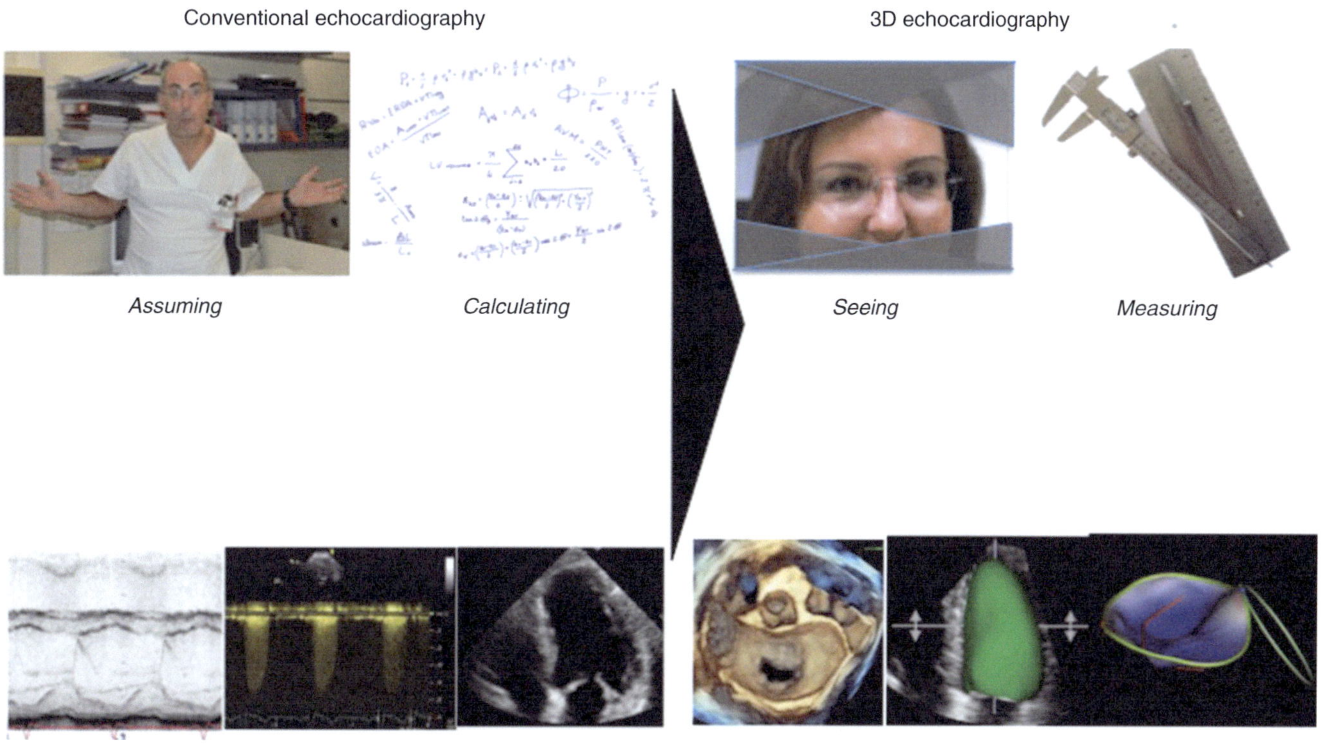

Fig. 4.3 Paradigm shift that has occurred in echocardiography after the introduction of 3D echocardiography in the clinical routine

Assessment of the heart valves with conventional echocardiography requires mental integration of data obtained from several 2D views obtained from different approaches (Fig. 4.3) and making geometrical assumptions about the shape of structures and orifices [7, 15]. Moreover, structures like the tricuspid valve are only seen partially (no more than two leaflets in each view) using 2D echocardiography (see also Chap. 18) [16, 17]. In any case, 2D echocardiography views provide only limited visualization of cardiac valve structures and visualize them from a single side (e.g. ventricular side using either transthoracic or transesophageal approach) which is the opposite of the view that the surgeon has when he/she opens the left/right atrium or the aorta. Conversely, 3D echocardiography (independent on the transthoracic or the transesophageal approach) allows the visualization of the whole valve from both sides in an anatomically sound spatial orientation (Fig. 4.5) allowing also the so called "*surgical view*" (as the valves appear to the surgeon when they open the atria or the aortic root). Finally, also the tricuspid valve can be seen *en face* in more than 90% of patients to allow a comprehensive assessment of its morphology and function (Fig. 4.6) [18, 19]. Not only valves can be properly imaged to visualize their morphology but dedicated software packages are available for the quantitative assessment of their geometry and to size their components (Fig. 4.7) [20–23].

Finally, septal defect can be imaged en face to allow anatomically sound measurements of their actual size without geometrical assumptions about their shape.

Table 4.1 Main reasons which have limited the expansion of 3D echocardiography in clinical practice

Underappreciation of the added clinical value of 3D vs. conventional 2D echocardiography
Need of specific education and training, skepticism about any new technique
Feasibility of 3D echocardiography and current technology limitations
Limited temporal and spatial resolution
Limited acquisition volume
Workflow related issues
Time constrain to perform echo studies
Limited number of 3D scanners in the laboratory
Data management
Complex 3D data set post-processing and interpretation of data
No DICOM tool to manage 3D data sets
Costs
Costs of 3D echocardiography systems
Lack of reimbursement

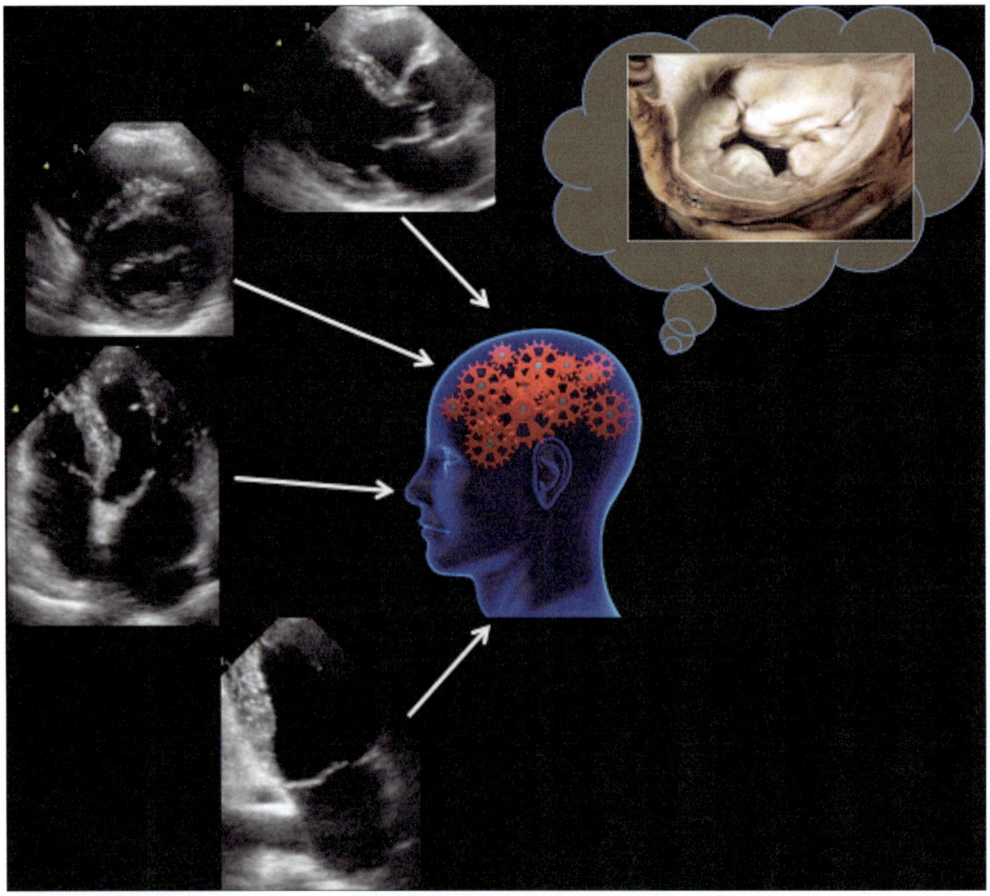

Fig. 4.4 Process of mental reconstruction of the anatomy of the mitral valve by integrating data coming from several tomographic views of the same valve obtained from different approaches. The accuracy of the reconstruction depends critically on the experience of the echocardiographers (e.g. how many diseased valves he/she have seen in the anatomical theater and/or in the operating room) [10]. Reprinted by permission from Springer Nature, Muraru D, Badano LP. Physical and Technical Aspects and Overview of 3D-Echocardiography. In: Manual of Echocardiography, Casas Rojo E, Fernandez-Golfin C, Zamorano J. (eds). Springer, Cham, 2017, pages 1–44

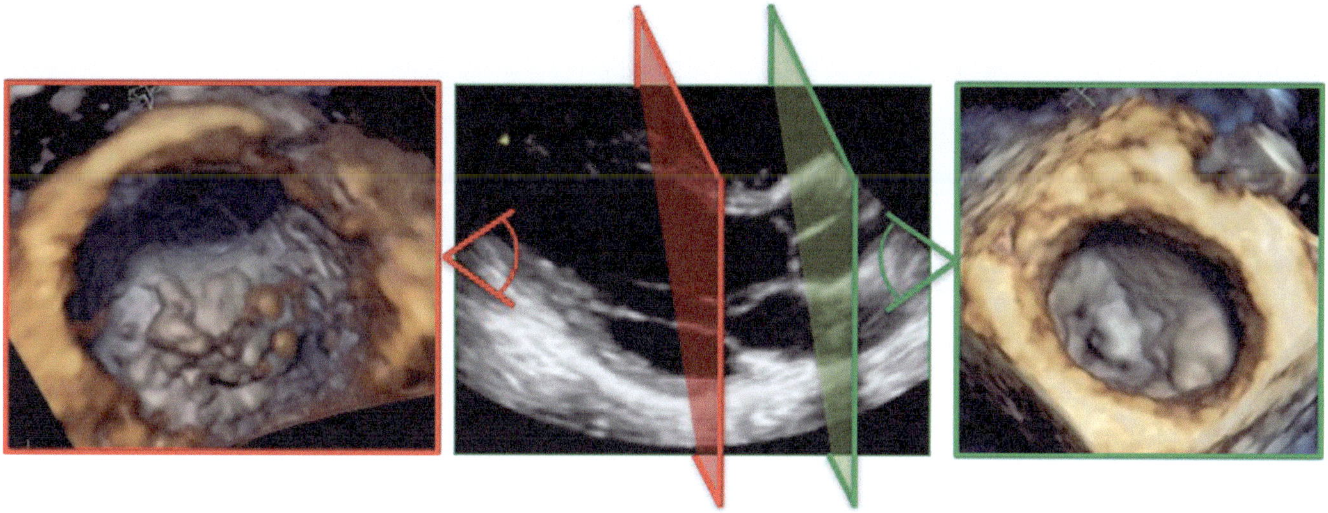

Fig. 4.5 Three-dimensional echocardiography visualization of the mitral valve from the ventricular (left panel) and atrial (right panel) perspectives. The position of the cut planes is shown in the central 2D longitudinal view plane as panels of the same color of the 3D echocardiography image frames

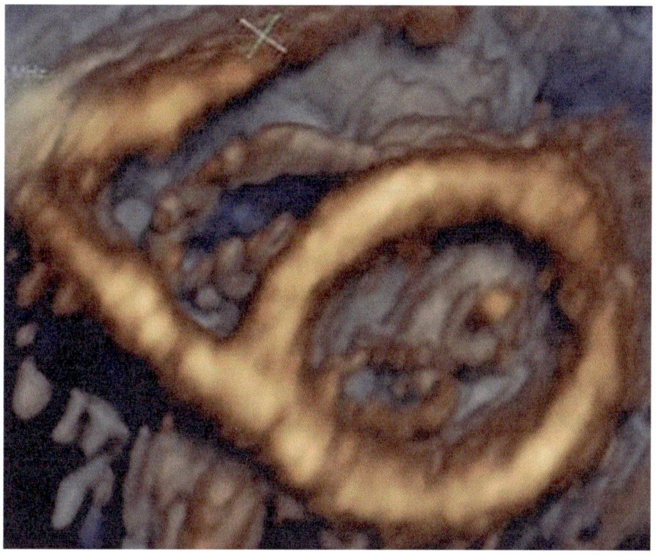

Fig. 4.6 Volume rendering of the mitral and tricuspid valves from the ventricular perspective. Transthoracic acquisition from the apical approach

Need of Specific Education and Training

3D echocardiography may sound easy but it is not. For effective application of the technique, echocardiographers need specific education and training. They have to learn how to acquire volumetric data sets without artifacts (Table 4.2, **accompanying figures and videos in Table**) [24], and navigate within the data set to visualize the desired cardiac structure [2]. New functions like cropping, slicing, translating, rotating and thresholding are available to manipulate the data sets in order to visualize the cardiac structure of interest. Various ways to display the information are available (see also Chap. 2). To learn how to acquire a good quality 3D data set, and properly post-process it, requires an investment in time and efforts. However, it is also true that learning to use 3D echocardiography is not that difficult and, if properly trained, an expert echocardiographer can easily learn how to acquire and postprocess 3D echocardiography data sets in a week (http://didattica.dctv.unipd.it/ecobad3d.php).

There are a few suggestions to acquire adequate 3D echocardiography data sets: (1) use a cut-out echocardiography bed to properly position the patient and the probe on his/her chest; (2) start with 2DE to localize the cardiac structure of interest and orient the probe in order to have the cardiac structure of interest in the centre of the scanning sector (where spatial resolution is the highest), then switch to live 3DE or zoom mode; (3) optimize the quality of 2D image—"*suboptimal 2DE images produce suboptimal 3DE data sets*" (do not worry if the 2D view is foreshortened or not properly oriented according to conventional 2D views, look at the best definition of endocardium and cardiac structures); (4) Check that the cardiac structure of interest is comprehensively included into the data set by using the multislice display; (5) select the highest resolution option that accommodates the cardiac structure of interest (i.e. the highest number of cardiac cycles, the smallest volume size and the lowest image depth).

Multibeat full-volume refers to the acquisition of volumes of information over several consecutive cardiac cycles (generally ranging from two to seven heart beats) that are combined to produce a single volumetric data set (see Chap. 2). This acquisition mode compensates for the poor temporal resolution of real-time (live) large volumes and it is very useful when large volumes need to be acquired with an adequate temporal resolution (i.e. acquisition of right or left ventricular data sets

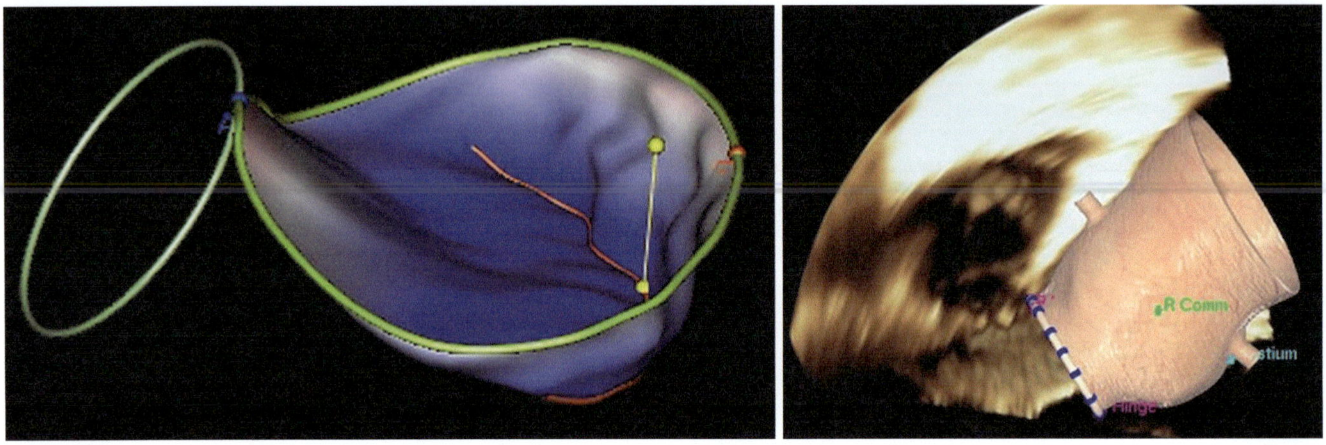

Fig. 4.7 Surface rendering display of the mitral valve apparatus (*left panel*) and the aortic root (*right panel*) used for quantitative assessment of these structures

Table 4.2 Most frequent artifacts (white arrows) occurring with three-dimensional echocardiography and practical ways to deal with them

Artifact	Image	Causes	How to deal with it
Stitching artifact	Image 4.1 (Stitching), Video 4.1 (Stitching)	1. Irregular arrhythmia (yellow circle) 2. Uncooperative patient unable to held his/her breath during acquisition 3. Probe movements during acquisition 4. Bed/patient movements during acquisition 5. Prominent P wave that the system mistakes for the R wave in some cardiac cycles to trigger the subvolume acquisition (red and green circles)	1. Limit the number of beats to acquire to the minimum to reach the target volume rate, then wait for a series of sinus beats (if frequent ectopic beats) or a series of regular R-R (if atrial fibrillation). Otherwise, acquire single beat by reducing the data set volume and depth to the minimum; 2. Try to motivate the patient and reduce the number of cardiac cycles to acquire to the minimum; 3. Seat comfortably and hold the probe steadily; 4. Ask nurses, fellows or students not to bend on the examination bed during acquisition; 5. Change ECG lead in order to find one with different voltages of P and R waves
Drop-outs	Image 4.2 (Drop out left and right), Videos 4.2a and 4.2b (Drop out left and right)	1. Thin cardiac structures (e.g. interatrial septum—*right panel*; normal aortic valve cusps) 2. Shadowing from hyperreflective structure (e.g. fibrosis—*left panel*, calcification etc.) 3. Low gain setting during acquisition	1. Try to acquire from an acoustic window in which the cardiac structure is perpendicular to the direction of the ultrasound beams; 2. Change the acquisition window/probe orientation in order to avoid the shadowing; 3. Acquire again with the proper gain settings 4. Check with saline contrast and/or color Doppler, as appropriate, if it is a true hole or a drop out artifact
Over gain	Image 4.3 (Overgain), Video 4.3 (Overgain)	Wrong machine settings	• Reduce overall gain (background depth should be perceived) • Time Gain Compensation slides in a straight line slightly over 50% • Reduce compression/dynamic range in mid range
Under gain	Image 4.4 (Under gain), Video 4.4 (Under gain)	Wrong machine settings	• Increase overall gain (background depth should be perceived) • Time Gain Compensation slides in a straight line slightly over 50% • Compression/dynamic range in mid range
Poor resolution	Image 4.5 (Poor resolution)	Suboptimal acoustic window/volume size/depth selection	• Reduce volume size to the minimum to encompass the cardiac structure of interest • Reduce depth at minimum to include the structure of interest • Use an acoustic window in which the cardiac structure of interest is oriented perpendicular to the direction of the acoustic beam (e.g. apical approach for aortic or atrio-ventricular valves, subcostal approach for interatrial septum; parasternal approach for interventricular septum)
Reverberations	Image 4.6 (Reverberations), Video 4.5 (Reverberations)	Persistence of sound in an enclosed space after its generation that may give the wrong impression of a stuck occluder in a bileaflet mechanical valve	Look at the data set after rotating in order not to have strong reflectors (e.g. mechanical valve occluders) between the transducer and the structure to evaluate. Use longitudinal cut planes in addition to transversal ones
Near field clutter	Image 4.7 (Near field clutter), Video 4.6 (Near field clutter)	Produced by the high-amplitude-oscillations of the piezoelectric crystals of the transducers	Slice the data set and look at the wall motion in order to exclude the presence of apical thrombi
Stationary	Image 4.8 (Stationary), Video 4.7 (Stationary)	Produced by reverberations from structures outside the heart (e.g. ribs)	The mass is not moving with the heart. This is particularly in sliced images

for quantitation purposes). This acquisition mode provides images that are not truly real-time, since the images are not available until the last recorded cardiac cycle is acquired. Some technical details are needed to acquire multibeat 3D data sets that are adequate for postprocessing and image rendering. The ECG trace should be optimized in order to display a distinct R wave voltage used by the system to trigger the acquisition. Since the most frequent artifact of multibeat 3D echocardiography data sets is the stitching artifact due to arrhythmias and patient and/or respiratory motion, the number of acquisition beats should be adjusted according to patient's ability to cooperate and clinical status, taking into account that the larger number of beats are acquired, the higher will be the temporal resolution and the wider the volume obtained. If the patient is unable to hold his/her respiration during multibeat acquisition or if there are significant rhythm disturbances (irregular atrial fibrillation or frequent ectopic beats) one should reduce the number of beats to be acquired or try to use the single beat full-volume acquisition (if available). Then, the volume size should be optimized in order to acquire the smaller volume able to encompass the cardiac structure of interest in order to improve spatial resolution (i.e. the number of scan lines per volume) while maintaining adequate temporal resolution since the two are inversely related.

Finally, appropriate gain and compression should be set before acquisition, since there are limits on how much gain and/or compression can be added or removed by postprocessing once a 3DE data set is acquired. In addition, low gain settings can artificially eliminate certain structures, while high gain settings can mask structures (both leading to significant misdiagnosis). As a general rule, both gain and compression should be set in the mid-range and the time-gain compensation should be used to overcompensate for the brightness of the image to allow the maximum flexibility during postprocessing.

3D color Doppler is an important acquisition mode in 3D echocardiography since both anterograde or regurgitant jets may be quite variable in shape, size and extension, and therefore they may be better assessed with a 3D visualization.

Before starting to acquire a 3D data set, one need to pay attention to the image resolution issue and the orientation of the cardiac structure of interest in relation to the ultrasound beam direction. The resolution of images varies according to the dimension employed. For current 3D transducers it is around 0.5–1 mm in the axial (y) dimension, around 1.5–2.0 mm in the lateral (x) dimension, and around 2.5–3 mm in the elevation (z) dimension. As a result, we will obtain the best images (less degree of spreading, i.e. distortion) when using the axial dimension and the worst (greatest degree of spreading) when we use the elevation dimension. These concepts have an immediate practical application in the choice of the best approach to image a particular cardiac structure. If the goal is to obtain an *en-face* view of the mitral valve from the left atrium or an *en-face* view of the aortic valve (the so called "*surgical views*"), the best results are expected to be obtained by using the parasternal short axis approach, because structures are imaged using the axial and lateral dimensions (Fig. 4.8, Videos 4.9a and 4.9b). Conversely, the worst result is expected to be obtained using the apical approach which uses the lateral and elevation dimensions. However, it is also true that both aortic and mitral valve leaflet are oriented parallel to the ultrasound beam when closed. Therefore, a limited number of scan lines will hit the valve leaflets in closure position leading to frequent drop-out artifacts (particularly, in case of normal, thin, valve leaflets). Conversely, both valves are perpendicular to the scan lines when imaged from the apical approach producing better image quality. As a result, the

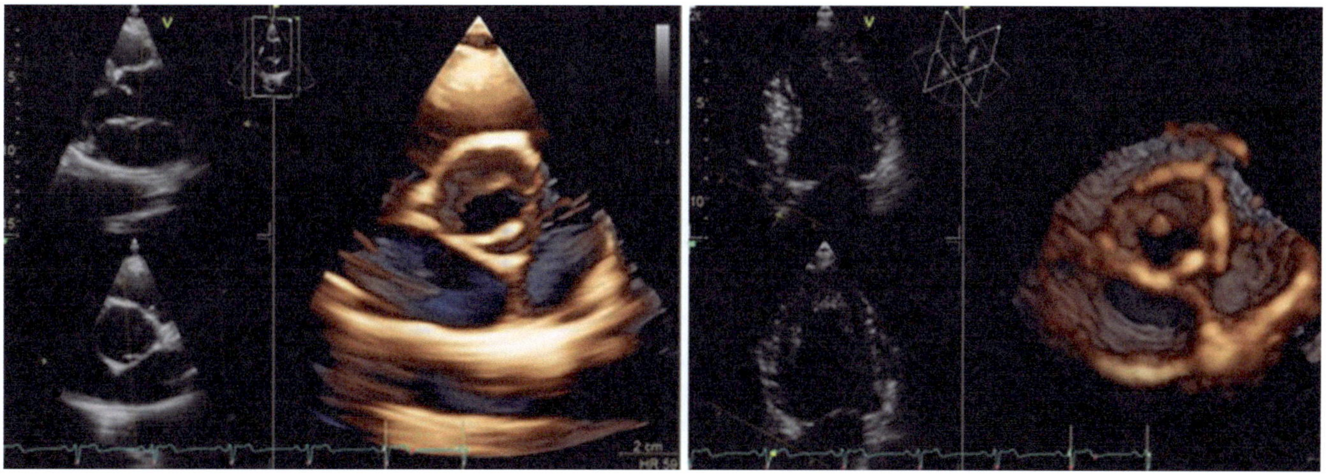

Fig. 4.8 Volume rendering of a bicuspid aortic valve by cropping data sets obtained from either the parasternal (***left panel***) (Video 4.9a left) and the apical (***right panel***) (Video 4.9b right) approach. The image obtained from the parasternal approach has better quality (more spatial resolution and less blurring) than the apical one

echocardiographer should try both approaches, trying to image the valve with an oblique orientation to the probe when acquired from the parasternal approach, and select the approach which provides the best results.

The inverse relationship between frame rate, volume size and spatial resolution has been described in Chap. 2. The practical implications for the echocardiographer are straightforward: (1) acquisitions with high temporal and spatial resolution can be obtained only at the expense of reducing the size of the acquired volume (e.g. zoom mode acquisitions); (2) large volumes can maintain adequate temporal resolution only if scan line density is reduced (reduced spatial resolution); (3) conversely in order to maintain adequate spatial resolution of large volumes, the temporal resolution (i.e. the volume rate) should be reduced. Accordingly acquisitions should be adapted to the specific clinical question to be answered: (1) to assess valve anatomy, the zoom mode acquisition (small volume size, high temporal and spatial resolution) is the preferred acquisition mode; (2) to assess spatial relationships among different cardiac structures, large volumes with relatively low volume rate (in order to preserve spatial resolution) should be used; (3) whereas to assess heart chamber size and function you need large volumes with temporal resolution >18 vps [25], and spatial resolution can be reduced as required.

Viewing a volume rendered 3D data set of the heart is analogous to standing outside a museum and being unable to see in without opening the door and entering the room or taking some or part of the walls away (Fig. 4.9). Once cropped away a part of the data set, one is able to enter inside the heart but necessarily, the image that is presented to the observer for interpretation is only part of all the information contained within the 3D volume (Fig. 4.10). To understand this concept, imagine yourself standing in the middle of a room: at any given point in time, you can only see the part of the room that is in front of you. To add information from what is behind, you need to rotate or change your position in space in relation to the rest of the room. In other words, despite the fact that the 3D structure of the room and its contents are available to be visualized, only part of it can be visualized at any given point in time from any given position.

Since the volume rendered 3D data set of the heart can be opened to display intracardiac structures by choosing a cutting plane and the image beyond this plane visualized as if the heart is cut by a surgeon, the word "view" (referred to heart's orientation to the body axis) will be no longer used, being replaced by the word "anatomical planes" or simply "planes" (referring to the heart itself) to describe orientation of the images [26]. The most frequently used planes in dissection are: (1) *the sagittal plane*, a vertical plane which divides the heart into right and left portions (Fig. 4.11); (2) the *transverse plane*, a vertical plane which divides the heart into anterior and posterior portions (Fig. 4.12); and (3) the *transverse plane*, an oblique, coronal plane which runs parallel to the ground and divides the heart into superior and inferior portions (Fig. 4.13). The use of anatomic planes to display the cardiac structures allows a parallelism between anatomic specimens and 3D echocardiography images and facilitates the communication with surgeons and anatomists.

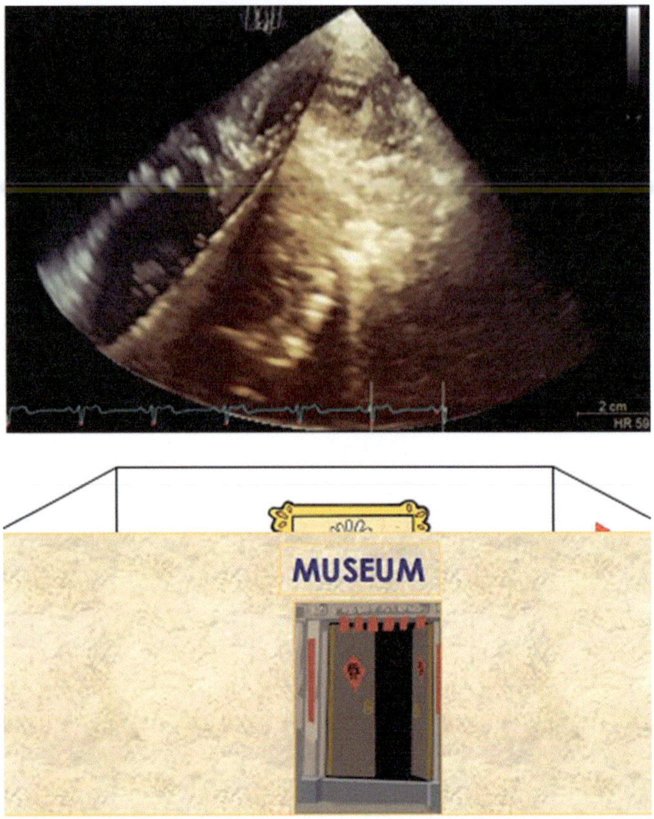

Fig. 4.9 Uncropped full-volume 3D data set acquired from the apical approach. Despite the fact that all cardiac structures are included into the pyramid of data, they cannot be viewed. This is similar to the impossibility to see the paintings and statues collected in a museum standing outside the main entrance, or to see the cardiac structures without opening the cardiac chambers

The action of entering the museum/heart to visualize the cardiac structures is called *cropping*. Cropping the volumetric data set means to partially remove volumetric data in order to enter the data set and visualize the cardiac structure of interest. Usually there are three cropping modalities: the single arbitrary cropping plane, the cropping box, and the dart tool (Fig. 4.14).

In order to display a specific cardiac structure, after having cropped the 3D data set, the echocardiographer should *rotate* the cropped volume to reorient the data set until the desired structure is properly oriented and visualized (Chap. 2, Fig. 2.10). To visualize different cardiac structures within the data set (or the same structure from different perspectives, Fig. 4.5) you need to change your position and point of view. This action is called *navigating*.

After having removed the undesired volumetric data, rotated the data set and properly positioned the point of view, the adequate display of cardiac structures requires some

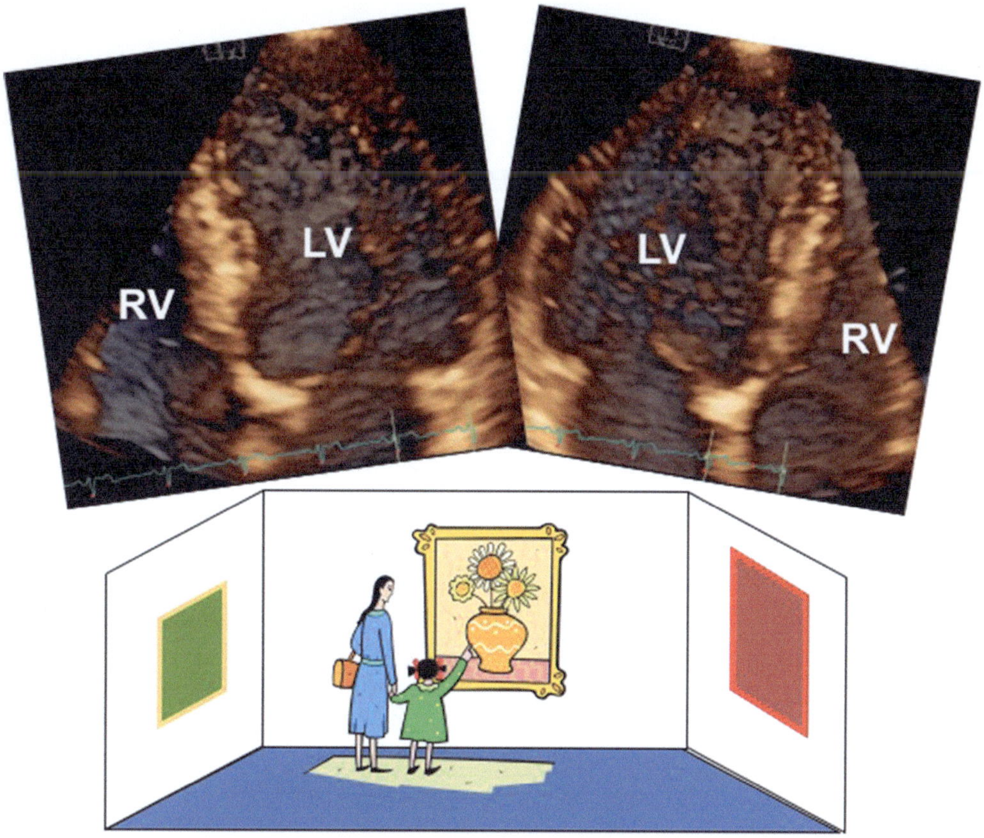

Fig. 4.10 The full volume data set has been cropped using an oblique/coronal plane to show the two halves of an equivalent four-chamber view (see also Fig. 4.13). Once entered into the museum/opened the heart, part of the content is visualized. What you actually see depends on where you are positioned and the direction you are looking at (see text)

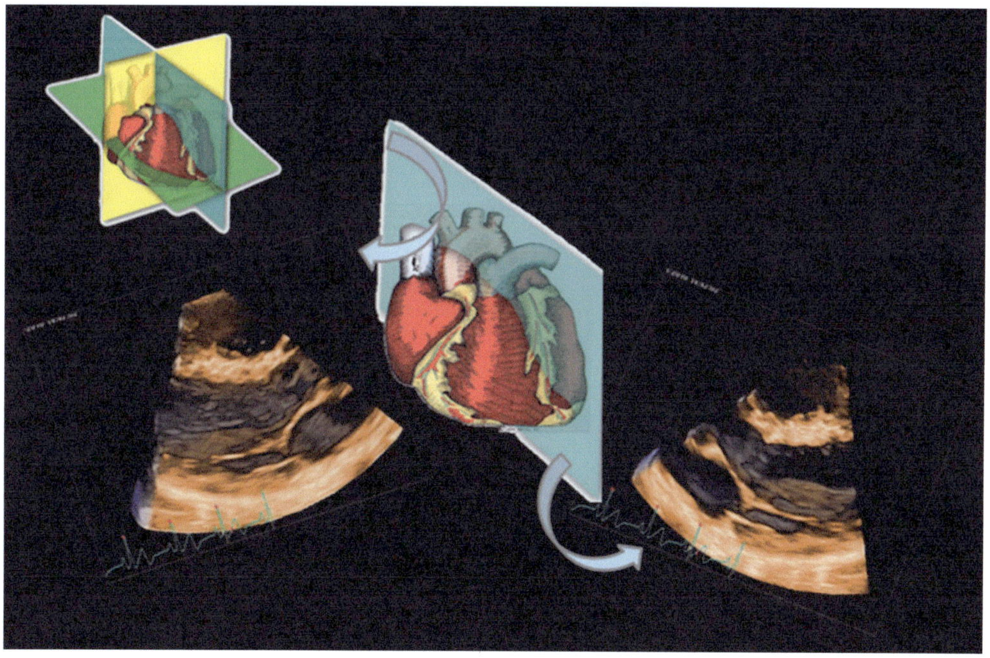

Fig. 4.11 The 3D data set of the heart can be dissected using anatomically sound section planes: a sagittal plane (long axis or longitudinal) is a vertical plane that divides an organ into right and left portions

thresholding. Thresholding allows the echocardiographer to determine how much of the volumetric data is part of the cardiac structure of interest, deemed noise or part of the cavity (Fig. 4.15, Videos 4.10a, 4.10b, and 4.10c). This is mainly controlled using the gain settings.

Once the cardiac structure of interest has been localized within the volumetric dataset, one can choose among different ways to display it on a 2D monitor. There are three broad classes of techniques for displaying 3D images: volume rendering, surface rendering, and 2D tomographic slices. The different display techniques have been discussed in Chap. 2 and the choice among them is generally determined by the clinical application and it is under user's control.

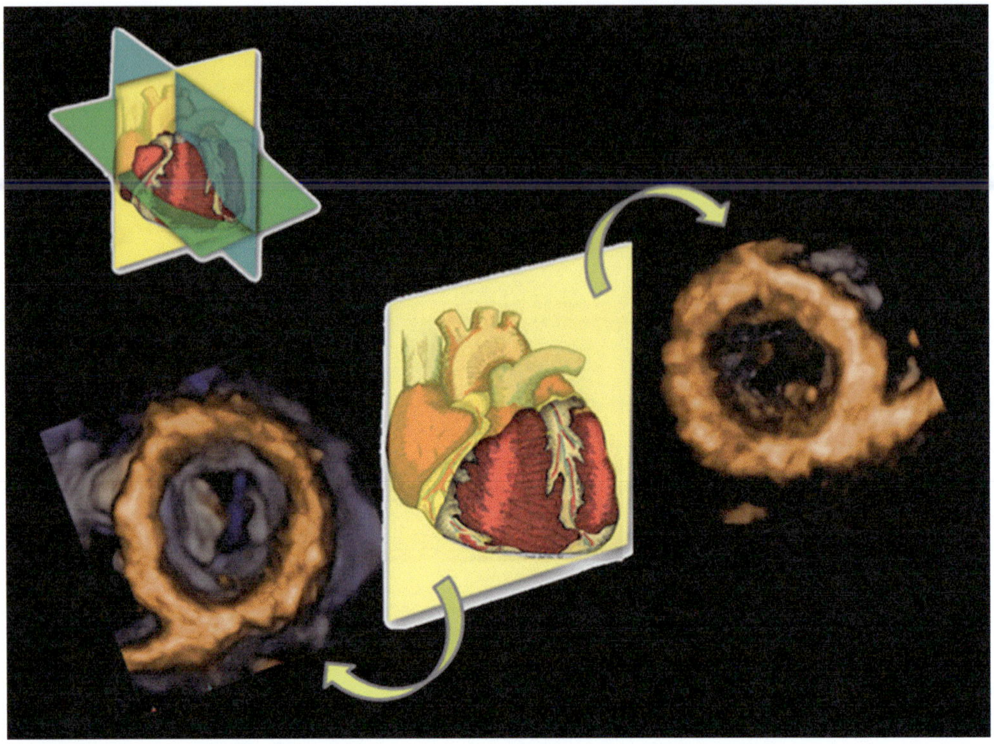

Fig. 4.12 The transverse section plane (frontal) is a vertical plane that divides an organ into anterior and posterior portions

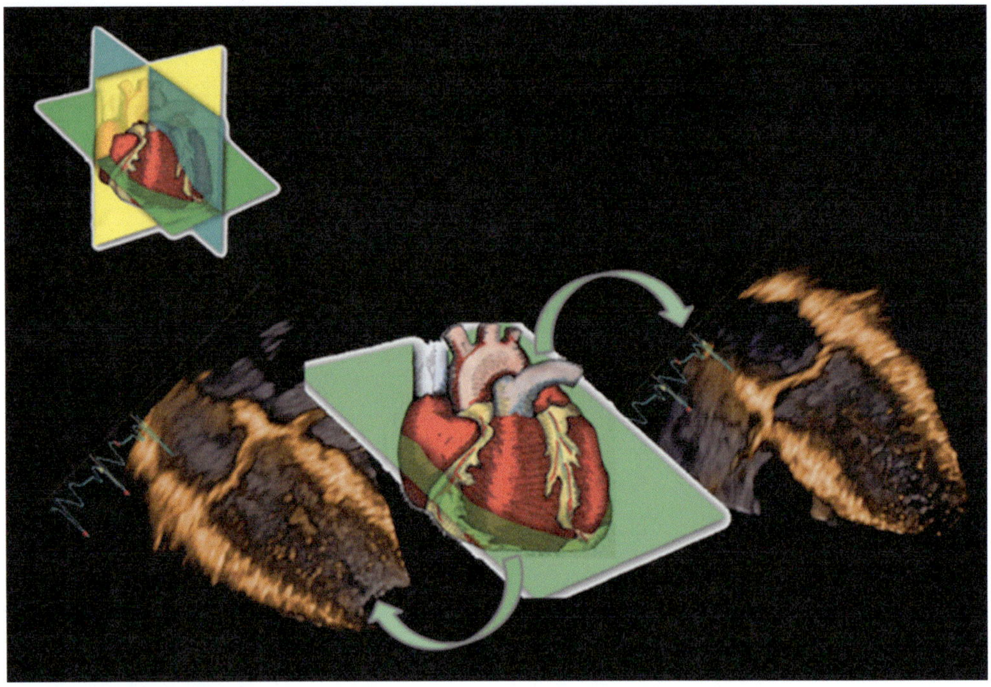

Fig. 4.13 A four-chamber view is the result of cutting the heart using an oblique, coronal section plane which runs parallel to the ground and divides the organ into superior and inferior portions

Feasibility of 3D Echocardiography and Current Technology Limitations

With current technology, feasibility of transthoracic and transesophageal 3D echocardiography are around 80%–85% and 90%–95%, respectively. Feasibility of 3D echocardiography is significantly lower than 2D echocardiography either from transthoracic or transesophageal approach. As a rule of thumb, when 2D images are of fair or poor quality, 3D data set can only be worse. In addition, 3D data sets have lower spatial and temporal resolution than 2D images and, since volume rendered 3D images tissue colorization is function of the position of the voxel in space, any tissue characterization is more difficult examining 3D than 2D images. However, in

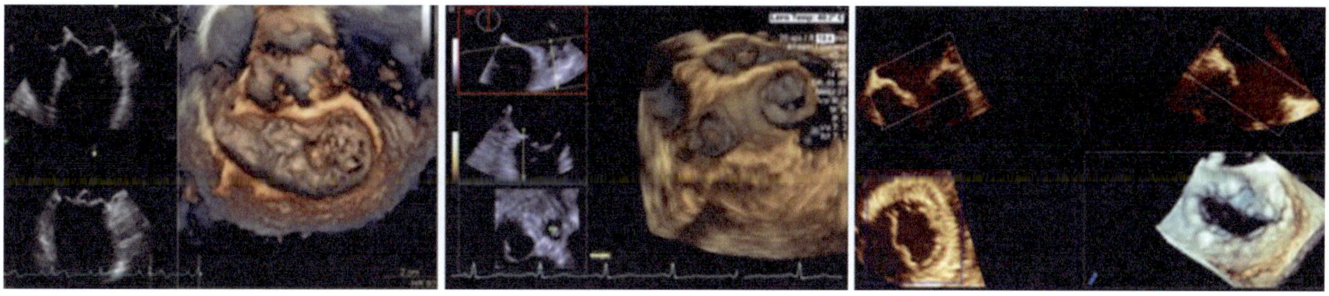

Fig. 4.14 Tools used to crop the 3D echocardiography data set. The position and orientation of the single arbitrary cropping plane (*left panel*) are shown as a yellow dotted line on the 2D images on the left, and the direction of visualization is shown by the yellow arrow. The dart by which the operator has to simply draw an arrow on one of the 2D slices on the left, from the selected point of view directed towards the structure of interest (*central panel*). The length of the arrow will define the thickness of the parallel cropping volume. The cropping box that allows to select a volume of interest of desired size and thickness within the 3D data set (*right panel*)

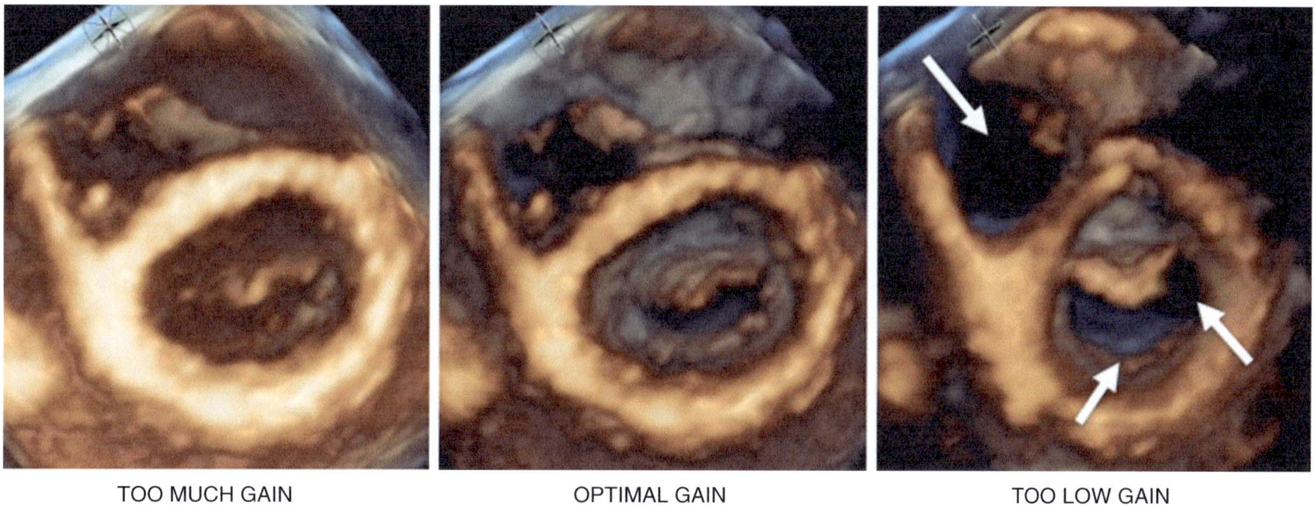

Fig. 4.15 Effects of gain optimization (thresholding) on the volume rendering of the mitral valve seen from the ventricular perspective in a 3D echocardiography data set acquired from transthoracic approach. The data set is usually acquired with a little of overgain in order to avoid drop-out artifacts (***left panel***, Video 4.10a Too much gain). Accurate thresholding allows to optimize the visualization of the mitral valve by removing the noise and choosing the proper depth color map (***central panel***, Video 4.10b Optimal). Too much gain reduction may create drop-out effects (***right panel, arrows***, Video 4.10c Too low gain)

patient in whom the echocardiographer can obtain adequate quality data sets, the amount of morphological and quantitative information provided by 3D echocardiography cannot be compared with that obtained from conventional 2D echocardiography (see above). Moreover, transducers are rapidly becoming more efficient while providing better signal/noise ratio images and the computational power of computers is increasing exponentially. Therefore many of current 3D echocardiography technological limitations will be attenuated or will disappear very soon.

Impact of 3D Echocardiography on the Workflow of the Laboratories

The main issue raised by echocardiographers against the use of the new echocardiographic technologies is the lack of time to perform new acquisitions/measurements. However, this is a misperception since 3D echocardiography actually saves time. Using a single acquisition from the apical approach, you can obtain multiple 2D views (multislice display), accurate and reproducible measurements of left/right ventricular volumes, ejection fraction, stroke volume, output, mass and (some systems) all myocardial deformation components and torsional parameters. To obtain the same parameters with 2D echocardiography, multiple views have to be acquired from different approaches a considerable amount of time should be spent in manually tracing endocardium and some parameters (such as right ventricular volumes of left ventricular torsion cannot be measured). Similarly, a single acquisition is sufficient to obtain anatomically sound images of valve morphology from both sides (and the images can be shown to colleagues and patients). Conversely, multiple acquisition from different approaches and an uncertain mental reconstruction are needed to obtain the same information by 2D echocardiography. Finally, the whole tricuspid valve can rarely be seen by 2D echocardiography. Also during stress echocardiography, the use of either the multiplane [27] or the full-volume [28] acquisition shortens both acquisition and image analysis time.

On the other end, it is true that current 3D echocardiography probes do not allow a 2D image quality comparable to that obtained with conventional 2D transducers, therefore it forces the echocardiographers who want to obtain 3D data sets to switch from one transducer to another in order to complete the echo study. Moreover, the workflow of the laboratory will be significantly affected if only a limited number of echo systems in the laboratory have the 3D module and patients need to be moved from a scanning room to another to have the 3D acquisition. Both these limitation may increase the time spent for each 3D echocardiography study and affect the whole lab productivity. To overcome these limitations you can: (1) adapt your acquisition protocol; (2) identify the clinical conditions that may benefit most from the 3D acquisition and schedule those patients to be studied in the rooms where a 3D system is available.

Despite a complete 3D echocardiography acquisition protocol has been recommended for both transthoracic and trasnesophageal acquisition [2], this is neither feasible nor useful for clinical purposes. We usually obtain a complete 2D and Doppler study [29] and then, if needed, we add the 3D acquisition at the end of the study to address specific clinical questions (i.e. anatomy of the mitral valve in degenerative regurgitation, mitral valve area in mitral stenosis, left/right ventricular function, sizing LVOT in aortic stenosis or septal defects, visualizing the tricuspid valve, clarifying difficult anatomy, etc.), this workflow will allow a single probe change and time/effective use of 3D echocardiography. To limit the negative impact of having to change the room to complete the echo study with 3D acquisitions and facilitate secretary and sonographer work, we have set a specific procedure to identify which patient will benefit most of a 3D echocardiography study (Table 4.3).

Table 4.3 Main indications to a 3D echocardiographic study in order to address suitable patients to the scanning rooms equipped with 3D scanners (if a limited number of them are available in the laboratory) and to limit the negative impact of the need to change the scanning room to complete the study with 3D echocardiography acquisitions on the laboratory work-flow

Pts with left ventricular dysfunction candidates at device implantation or complex surgical procedures
Pts with heart failure, or right heart diseases that may affect right ventricular size and function
Pts. who are candidates to mitral valve surgery or interventional procedures
Pts. with mitral stenosis
Pts with bicuspid aortic valve who are candidates to surgery
Pts. with congenital heart disease
Pts with unclear anatomy at 2D
Pts with significant tricuspid valve regurgitation or suspected stenosis

In addition, all patients undergoing routine transesophageal echocardiography are studied with a 3D echocardiography probe.

Added Complexity in Data Management and Result Interpretation

Compared to the comfortable similarity among the ways the different echocardiographic systems display 2D echocardiography images and make the calculations to obtain quantitative parameters like left ventricular volumes (we have just to find the right button on the console!), with 3D echocardiography every company has developed its own algorithms to post-process the data sets and to measure geometry and function of cardiac structures. Moreover, there is no DICOM standard to display, post-process and perform quantitative analysis of 3D echocardiography data sets. All these may represent significant limitations in multi-vendor echocardiography laboratories in which the echocardiographers have to learn different workflows and use different algorithms for the same task (i.e. visualize the mitral valve or measure left ventricular ejection fraction). In addition, despite it has been shown that left ventricular volumes and ejection fraction measured with different systems are very similar [30], other parameters (i.e. 3D strain components) [31] are significantly different among different systems.

Then, volumes of cardiac chambers measured by 3D echocardiography are significantly larger than those calculated by 2D echocardiography [32–34], therefore they are not comparable when we perform a 3D echocardiography study during the follow-up of patients whose previous echocardiographic examinations have been obtained with 2D echocardiography. The referring physicians who receive the report in which volumes have been measured by 3D echocardiography may be induced to think that some remodeling of the cardiac chamber may have occurred, whereas only the way to measure chamber volumes has changed. The best way to report cardiac chamber volumes during the transition between 2D and 3D echocardiography remains to be established. Different strategies may be considered: (1) reporting both 2D and 3D volumes, but this may be confusing for the referring physician; (2) reporting only 3D volumes (more accurate and reproducible than 2D ones [6]) and writing a note that despite the fact they are different but the 2D ones were similar/different compared to previous examinations; (3) continuing to report 2D volumes in patients in long-term follow-up and use 3D volumes only in newcomers. There are pros and cons for any of these strategies.

Left ventricular ejection fraction may also be significantly different when obtained from 2D and 3D echocardiography volumes (Fig. 4.16). This happens particularly in patients with extensive wall motion abnormalities (biplane algorithms

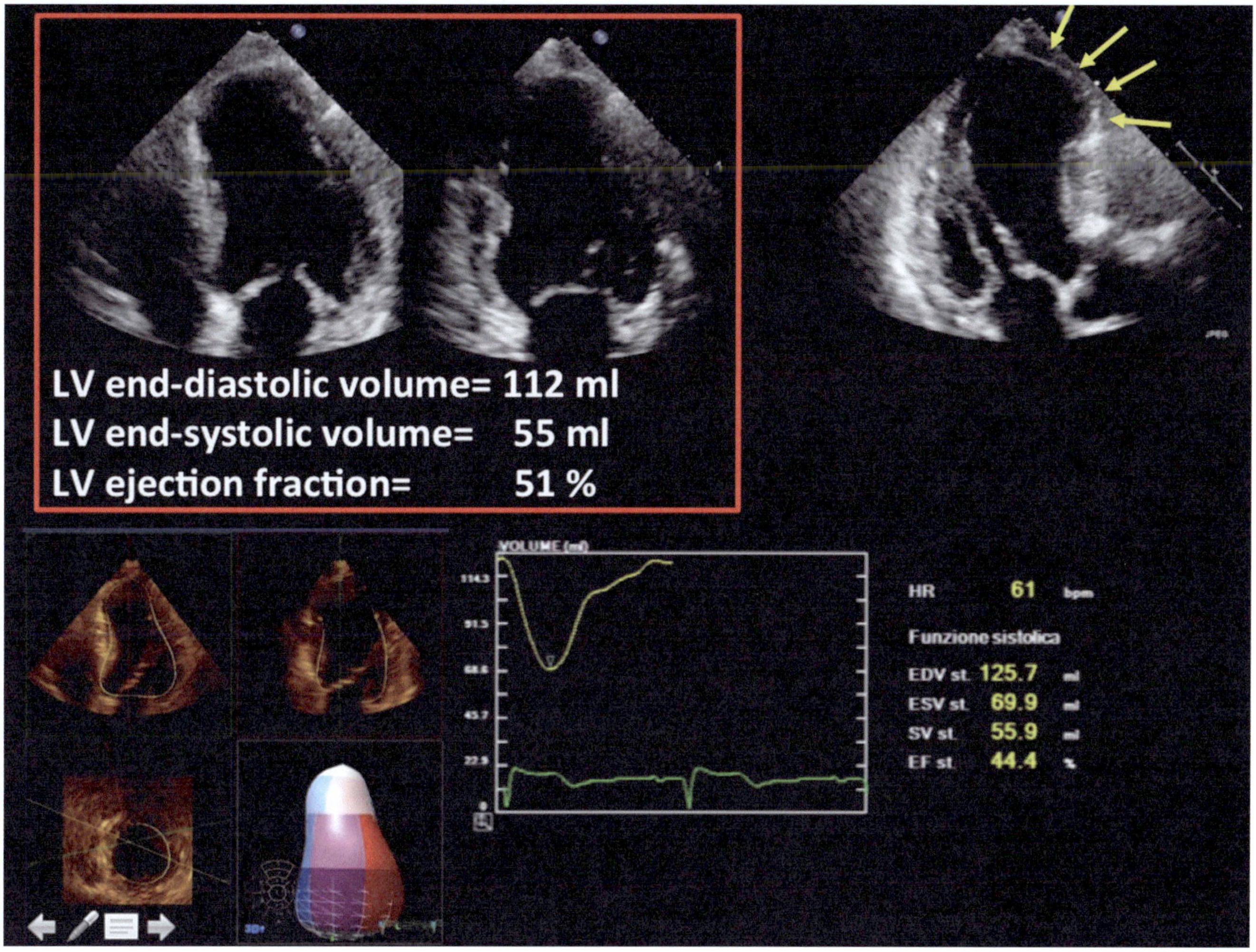

Fig. 4.16 Comparison of left ventricular volumes and ejection fraction calculations performed with 2D biplane discs' summation algorhythm and measured with 3D echocardiography in a patient with previous anterior myocardial infarction and extensive wall motion abnormalities. The use of the four- and two-chamber views by the 2D echocardiography algorithm (*red square*) does not take into account of the large aneurysm involving mainly the mid and apical part of the anterior septum (*yellow arrows*). As a result, 2D echocardiography underestimate left ventricular volumes and overestimate ejection fraction compared to 3D echocardiography (*lower panels*)

to calculate left ventricular volume take into account only wall motion abnormalities in left ventricular myocardial segments visualized in the four- and two chamber views, whereas 3D echocardiography takes into account all the 16 left ventricular myocardial segments. In patients with grossly distorted geometry (aneurysms, etc.), the discrepancy between left ventricular ejection fraction values maybe so large to change patient management [35] or to induce physicians to think about deterioration or improvement of left ventricular function while it is just the different way of measuring it. The best way to communicate the clinical significance of these changes remains to be defined. Moreover, all cut-off values of ejection fraction on which we base our decisions to indicate valve surgery, device implantation etc. derive from controlled randomized trials that used 2D echocardiography to obtain left ventricular ejection fraction values.

Finally, the reference values for cardiac chamber volumes measured with 3D and 2D are significantly different and cannot be used interchangeably [32–34]. Accordingly, echocardiography reports need to be prepared differently, accordingly with the echocardiography technique used, and clinicians need to remember different cut-off values to differentiate normal from enlarged volumes. It should be the task of scientific societies to provide indications on how to manage the transition between the 2D and the 3D era in the evolution of echocardiography.

Costs of the New Technology and Lack of Reimbursement

The problem of the higher costs of 3D echocardiography systems compared to conventional 2D machines should be viewed in perspective and not just as the cost of the probe and related software only. Technology cost should be balanced against the possibility to avoid preoperative transesophageal echocardiography to assess a sizable number of patients who are candidate to mitral valve surgery [36, 37]; better selection of heart failure patients candidates to ICD and/or CRT implants, or ACE-inhibitor treatment [35]; monitoring of interventional procedures without the use of ionizing energies or costly intravascular catheters [9, 38]. Moreover, also the costs of the additional tests driven by inaccurate 2D echocardiography diagnosis (due to limited visualization, need of mental reconstruction and geometrical assumptions about structure geometry) and by the larger variability in cardiac chamber volume and function calculations performed by 2D echocardiography in comparison with the 3D measurements [39], should be taken into account. All these savings, and the additional educational and communication opportunities offered by 3D display of cardiac anatomy (as well as 3D printing and holography, see also Chap. 2) well justify the cost/effectiveness of 3D technology.

Future Directions

3D echocardiography is the most recent among the various echocardiography techniques and the one with the largest room for future improvement.

The expected improvement in both temporal and spatial resolution will allow to acquire larger data sets which will include the whole heart and will change our way of pathophysiological thinking. Not anymore considering left/right ventricular or atrial function as the various cardiac structures work in isolation, but we will assess and understand the "cardiac function", being able to appreciate the interrelationships among cardiac structures (i.e. atrio-ventricular coupling, ventricular interdependence etc.) and assess their relative contribution to "cardiac function".

Highly performant fully automated software packages will allow accurate and reproducible quantitative analysis of the geometry and function of cardiac chambers [40] and valve structures [23, 41] independent on the expertise of the single echocardiographer, to provide clinicians, interventionists and cardiac surgeons reliable data to be used to address management, plan and monitoring interventions, and assess their outcome.

3D echocardiography data sets potentially allow morphometric quantitation of every cardiac structure. However, to obtain this goal we need dedicated software packages taking into account the morphological (the same software cannot be used to display and quantitate the aorta and the mitral valve) and the functional (e.g. the atria have a three phases function and not just diastole and systole like ventricles) peculiarities of the various cardiac structures. In particular, we lack software packages to assess the right heart structures. 3D echocardiography analysis of right ventricular shape [42, 43] and mechanics in various directions (i.e. longitudinal, circumferential and area strain) [44] is a promising area in future clinical practice. In pulmonary hypertension patients, a significant correlation was demonstrated between right ventricular ejection fraction and both 3D global longitudinal [45] and area strain with the latter being a strong independent predictor of mortality [46]. Finally, recently developed methodology for analysis of 3D echocardiography-derived global and regional right ventricular shape indices based on analysis of the right ventricular curvature demonstrated good results in patients with pulmonary arterial hypertension, showing that the curvature of the right ventricular inflow tract is a more robust predictor of death than right ventricular ejection fraction, volumes, or other regional curvature indices [42].

References

1. Surkova E, Muraru D, Aruta P, et al. Current clinical applications of three-dimensional echocardiography: when the technique makes the difference. Curr Cardiol Rep. 2016;18:109.
2. Lang RM, Badano LP, Tsang W, et al. EAE/ASE recommendations for image acquisition and display using three-dimensional echocardiography. Eur Heart J Cardiovasc Imaging. 2012;13:1–46.
3. Badano LP, Boccalini F, Muraru D, et al. Current clinical applications of transthoracic three-dimensional echocardiography. J Cardiovasc Ultrasound. 2012;20:1–22.
4. Morbach C, Lin BA, Sugeng L. Clinical application of three-dimensional echocardiography. Prog Cardiovasc Dis. 2014;57:19–31.
5. Simpson J, Lopez L, Acar P, et al. Three-dimensional echocardiography in congenital heart disease: an expert consensus document from the European Association of Cardiovascular Imaging and the American Society of Echocardiography. J Am Soc Echocardiogr. 2017;30:1–27.
6. Lang RM, Badano LP, Mor-Avi V, et al. Recommendations for cardiac chamber quantification by echocardiography in adults: an update from the American Society of Echocardiography and the European Association of Cardiovascular Imaging. Eur Heart J Cardiovasc Imaging. 2015;16:233–70.
7. Zoghbi WA, Adams D, Bonow RO, et al. Recommendations for noninvasive evaluation of native valvular regurgitation: a report from the American Society of Echocardiography Developed in Collaboration with the Society for Cardiovascular Magnetic Resonance. J Am Soc Echocardiogr. 2017;30(4):303–71.
8. Perk G, Lang RM, Garcia-Fernandez MA, et al. Use of real time three-dimensional transesophageal echocardiography in intracardiac catheter based interventions. J Am Soc Echocardiogr. 2009;22:865–82.
9. Zamorano JL, Badano LP, Bruce C, et al. EAE/ASE recommendations for the use of echocardiography in new transcatheter interventions for valvular heart disease. Eur Heart J. 2011;32:2189–214.

10. Muraru D, Badano LP. Physical and technical aspects and overview of 3D-echocardiography. In: Casas Rojo E, Fernandez-Golfin C, Zamorano J, editors. Manual of echocardiography. Cham: Springer; 2017. p. 1–44.
11. Muraru D, Spadotto V, Cecchetto A, et al. New speckle-tracking algorithm for right ventricular volume analysis from three-dimensional echocardiographic data sets: validation with cardiac magnetic resonance and comparison with the previous analysis tool. Eur Heart J Cardiovasc Imaging. 2016;17:1279–89.
12. Medvedofsky D, Addetia K, Patel AR, et al. Novel approach to three-dimensional echocardiographic quantification of right ventricular volumes and function from focused views. J Am Soc Echocardiogr. 2015;28:1222–31.
13. Surkova E, Muraru D, Iliceto S, Badano LP. The use of multimodality cardiovascular imaging to assess right ventricular size and function. Int J Cardiol. 2016;214:54–69.
14. Nagata Y, Wu VC, Kado Y, et al. Prognostic value of right ventricular ejection fraction assessed by transthoracic 3D echocardiography. Circ Cardiovasc Imaging. 2017;10(2). pii: e005384.
15. Baumgartner H, Hung J, Bermejo J, et al. Recommendations on the echocardiographic assessment of aortic valve stenosis: a focused update from the European Association of Cardiovascular Imaging and the American Society of Echocardiography. J Am Soc Echocardiogr. 2017;30:372–92.
16. Addetia K, Yamat M, Mediratta A, et al. Comprehensive two-dimensional interrogation of the tricuspid valve using knowledge derived from three-dimensional echocardiography. J Am Soc Echocardiogr. 2016;29:74–82.
17. Stankovic I, Daraban AM, Jasaityte R, Neskovic AN, Claus P, Voigt JU. Incremental value of the en face view of the tricuspid valve by two-dimensional and three-dimensional echocardiography for accurate identification of tricuspid valve leaflets. J Am Soc Echocardiogr. 2014;27:376–84.
18. Muraru D, Badano LP, Sarais C, Solda E, Iliceto S. Evaluation of tricuspid valve morphology and function by transthoracic three-dimensional echocardiography. Curr Cardiol Rep. 2011;13:242–9.
19. Muraru D, Surkova E, Badano LP. Revisit of functional tricuspid regurgitation; current trends in the diagnosis and management. Korean Circ J. 2016;46:443–55.
20. Mihaila S, Muraru D, Piasentini E, et al. Quantitative analysis of mitral annular geometry and function in healthy volunteers using transthoracic three-dimensional echocardiography. J Am Soc Echocardiogr. 2014;27:846–57.
21. Muraru D, Badano LP, Vannan M, Iliceto S. Assessment of aortic valve complex by three-dimensional echocardiography: a framework for its effective application in clinical practice. Eur Heart J Cardiovasc Imaging. 2012;13:541–55.
22. Muraru D, Cattarina M, Boccalini F, et al. Mitral valve anatomy and function: new insights from three-dimensional echocardiography. J Cardiovasc Med (Hagerstown). 2013;14:91–9.
23. Calleja A, Thavendiranathan P, Ionasec RI, et al. Automated quantitative 3-dimensional modeling of the aortic valve and root by 3-dimensional transesophageal echocardiography in normals, aortic regurgitation, and aortic stenosis: comparison to computed tomography in normals and clinical implications. Circ Cardiovasc Imaging. 2013;6:99–108.
24. Faletra FF, Ramamurthi A, Dequarti MC, Leo LA, Moccetti T, Pandian N. Artifacts in three-dimensional transesophageal echocardiography. J Am Soc Echocardiogr. 2014;27:453–62.
25. Yodwut C, Weinert L, Klas B, Lang RM, Mor-Avi V. Effects of frame rate on three-dimensional speckle-tracking-based measurements of myocardial deformation. J Am Soc Echocardiogr. 2012;25:978–85.
26. Nanda NC, Kisslo J, Lang R, et al. Examination protocol for three-dimensional echocardiography. Echocardiography. 2004;21:763–8.
27. Eroglu E, D'Hooge J, Herbots L, et al. Comparison of real-time tri-plane and conventional 2D dobutamine stress echocardiography for the assessment of coronary artery disease. Eur Heart J. 2006;27:1719–24.
28. Badano LP, Muraru D, Rigo F, et al. High volume-rate three-dimensional stress echocardiography to assess inducible myocardial ischemia: a feasibility study. J Am Soc Echocardiogr. 2010;23:628–35.
29. Evangelista A, Flachskampf F, Lancellotti P, et al. European Association of Echocardiography recommendations for standardization of performance, digital storage and reporting of echocardiographic studies. Eur J Echocardiogr. 2008;9:438–48.
30. Muraru D, Cecchetto A, Cucchini U, et al. Intervendor consistency and accuracy of left ventricular volume measurements using three-dimensional echocardiography. J Am Soc Echocardiogr. 2018;31(2):158–68.e1.
31. Badano LP, Cucchini U, Muraru D, Al Nono O, Sarais C, Iliceto S. Use of three-dimensional speckle tracking to assess left ventricular myocardial mechanics: inter-vendor consistency and reproducibility of strain measurements. Eur Heart J Cardiovasc Imaging. 2013;14:285–93.
32. Badano LP, Miglioranza MH, Mihaila S, et al. Left atrial volumes and function by three-dimensional echocardiography: reference values, accuracy, reproducibility, and comparison with two-dimensional echocardiographic measurements. Circ Cardiovasc Imaging. 2016;9:e004229.
33. Muraru D, Badano LP, Peluso D, et al. Comprehensive analysis of left ventricular geometry and function by three-dimensional echocardiography in healthy adults. J Am Soc Echocardiogr. 2013;26:618–28.
34. Peluso D, Badano LP, Muraru D, et al. Right atrial size and function assessed with three-dimensional and speckle-tracking echocardiography in 200 healthy volunteers. Eur Heart J Cardiovasc Imaging. 2013;14:1106–14.
35. Hare JL, Jenkins C, Nakatani S, Ogawa A, Yu CM, Marwick TH. Feasibility and clinical decision-making with 3D echocardiography in routine practice. Heart. 2008;94:440–5.
36. Pepi M, Tamborini G, Maltagliati A, et al. Head-to-head comparison of two- and three-dimensional transthoracic and transesophageal echocardiography in the localization of mitral valve prolapse. J Am Coll Cardiol. 2006;48:2524–30.
37. Gutierrez-Chico JL, Zamorano Gomez JL, Rodrigo-Lopez JL, et al. Accuracy of real-time 3-dimensional echocardiography in the assessment of mitral prolapse. Is transesophageal echocardiography still mandatory? Am Heart J. 2008;155:694–8.
38. Balzer J, van Hall S, Rassaf T, et al. Feasibility, safety, and efficacy of real-time three-dimensional transoesophageal echocardiography for guiding device closure of interatrial communications: initial clinical experience and impact on radiation exposure. Eur J Echocardiogr. 2010;11:1–8.
39. Thavendiranathan P, Liu S, Verhaert D, et al. Feasibility, accuracy, and reproducibility of real-time full-volume 3D transthoracic echocardiography to measure LV volumes and systolic function: a fully automated endocardial contouring algorithm in sinus rhythm and atrial fibrillation. JACC Cardiovasc Imaging. 2012;5:239–51.
40. Tsang W, Salgo IS, Medvedofsky D, et al. Transthoracic 3D echocardiographic left heart chamber quantification using an automated adaptive analytics algorithm. JACC Cardiovasc Imaging. 2016;9:769–82.
41. Calleja A, Poulin F, Woo A, et al. Quantitative modeling of the mitral valve by three-dimensional transesophageal echocardiography in patients undergoing mitral valve repair: correlation with intraoperative surgical technique. J Am Soc Echocardiogr. 2015;28:1083–92.
42. Addetia K, Maffessanti F, Yamat M, et al. Three-dimensional echocardiography-based analysis of right ventricular shape in

pulmonary arterial hypertension. Eur Heart J Cardiovasc Imaging. 2016;17:564–75.
43. Addetia K, Maffessanti F, Muraru D, et al. Morphologic analysis of the normal right ventricle using three-dimensional echocardiography-derived curvature indices. J Am Soc Echocardiogr. 2018;31(5):614–23.
44. Lakatos B, Toser Z, Tokodi M, et al. Quantification of the relative contribution of the different right ventricular wall motion components to right ventricular ejection fraction: the ReVISION method. Cardiovasc Ultrasound. 2017;15:8.
45. Ozawa K, Funabashi N, Takaoka H, et al. Utility of three-dimensional global longitudinal strain of the right ventricle using transthoracic echocardiography for right ventricular systolic function in pulmonary hypertension. Int J Cardiol. 2014;174:426–30.
46. Smith BC, Dobson G, Dawson D, Charalampopoulos A, Grapsa J, Nihoyannopoulos P. Three-dimensional speckle tracking of the right ventricle: toward optimal quantification of right ventricular dysfunction in pulmonary hypertension. J Am Coll Cardiol. 2014;64:41–51.

Routine Assessment of the Left Ventricle

5

Karima Addetia, Luigi P. Badano, and Roberto M. Lang

Abstract

Non invasive assessment of left ventricular (LV) geometry and function is critically important for clinical decision making and represents the most frequent indication for an echocardiographic examination. Suitability for device implantation in patients with LV dysfunction, discontinuation of potentially cardiotoxic chemotherapy in cancer patients, indications to cardiac surgery or to treatment initiation in asymptomatic patients are among the most critical decisions that rely on an accurate measurement of LV ejection fraction. LV volume calculations by two-dimensional echocardiography is highly operator dependent, uses only partial information contained in a few predefined cross sections of the LV to assess global myocardial function, and relies on geometrical assumptions that may not be necessarily valid in every patient. In particular, geometric assumptions about LV shape make the calculations of LV volumes and ejection fraction more inaccurate in patients in whom this information is more critical (i.e. patients in whom there are extensive wall motion abnormalities or the LV geometry is distorted because of aneurysms). With three-dimensional echocardiography, we can measure (not calculate anymore!) LV volumes with no assumption regarding LV geometry. This technique has been extensively validated against cardiac magnetic resonance and was demonstrated to be more time-saving, reproducible, repeatable and accurate than conventional two-dimensional echocardiography for LV volumes and ejection fraction measurements.

Keywords

Left ventricle · Volumes · Ejection fraction · Shape

Introduction

When an echocardiogram is ordered, it is the expectation of the referring physician that an assessment of left ventricular (LV) function will be reported. In clinical practice, two-dimensional echocardiography remains the most frequently used imaging modality for LV size and function assessment. LV size is assessed using LV end-diastolic and end-systolic dimensions measured from the parasternal long-axis views while LV function is quantified most frequently using the biplane method of discs on images obtained from transthoracic apical approach [1]. Measurements should always be confirmed with "eye ball" assessment. LV dimensions are clinically important in multiple clinical situations such as in the diagnosis of dilated cardiomyopathy where an LV end-diastolic dimension >53 mm in a woman and >59 mm in a man signifies LV dilatation [1]. The most recent valvular heart disease guidelines [2] advocate mitral valve surgery in patients with severe mitral regurgitation and LV end-systolic dimension ≥40 mm and aortic valve surgery in patients with asymptomatic severe aortic regurgitation and LV end-systolic dimension >50 mm or LV end-diastolic dimension >65 mm. Accurate assessment of LV ejection fraction impacts clinical decision-making in a number of diseases including coronary artery disease, cardiotoxicity due to a variety of chemotherapeutic agents and heart failure with reduced ejection fraction [3, 4].

All of the above examples underscore the importance of quantification of LV size and function on clinical decision-

Electronic Supplementary Material The online version of this chapter (https://doi.org/10.1007/978-3-030-14032-8_5) contains supplementary material, which is available to authorized users.

K. Addetia (✉) · R. M. Lang
Noninvasive Cardiac Imaging Laboratories, Department of Medicine/Section of Cardiology, University of Chicago Medical Center, Chicago, IL, USA
e-mail: kaddetia@medicine.bsd.uchicago.edu; rlang@medicine.bsd.uchicago.edu

L. P. Badano
University of Milano-Bicocca, and Istituto Auxologico Italiano, IRCCS, San Luca Hospital, Milano, Italy
e-mail: luigi.badano@unimib.it

L. P. Badano et al. (eds.), *Textbook of Three-Dimensional Echocardiography*, https://doi.org/10.1007/978-3-030-14032-8_5

making. Until recently most of this information has been obtained from two-dimensional echocardiography, a modality that has a number of limitations. We begin this chapter by describing some of the limitations of two-dimensional echocardiography and highlighting some of the advantages of three-dimensional echocardiography (3DE) in the assessment of the LV. We will finally discuss the basics of 3DE LV data acquisition and display, and review the methods for quantitative LV analysis and assessment of LV morphology. Towards the end of the chapter a variety of clinical cases will be discussed with the intent of introducing new concepts.

Limitations of Two-Dimensional Echocardiography

With regard to the assessment of LV size and function, two-dimensional echocardiography has two main limitations. Firstly, even when images are acquired with great care to maximize the long axis of the LV on apical views, foreshortening of the LV is frequently inevitable; secondly, geometrical models are used to transform two-dimensional echocardiography LV areas and linear measurements into volume measurements. This is true both when using the biplane Simpson method and the area-length method to quantify LV size and function and limits the accuracy of the calculations.

LV foreshortening occurs when the acquired two-dimensional plane does not pass through the true LV apex resulting in an oblique view of the LV cavity (Fig. 5.1). When this oblique view is used to calculate LV end-diastolic and end-systolic volumes, the results underestimate the actual LV volumes [5, 6]. Prior studies have shown that 50% of two-dimensional echocardiography views acquired by experienced sonographers are not optimally positioned with respect to displacement and angulation of the transducer and only 12% of apical four-chamber and two-chamber views acquired are truly orthogonal [7]. The need for two-dimensional echocardiography views to be orthogonal is important because use of the latter have been shown to result in less underestimation of LV volumes [8]. The impact of foreshortening was elegantly demonstrated in 19 patients [5] by measuring the LV long-axis dimension in apical four- and two-chamber views obtained from conventional two-dimensional echocardiography images and anatomically correct apical views selected offline from 3DE pyramidal data sets (Fig. 5.2). The LV long-axis measurement was longer in both apical views when evaluated using the 3DE technique suggesting that the majority of two-dimensional echocardiography apical views were foreshortened. In fact, in that study 3DE LV mass more closely correlated with mass measured with cardiovascular magnetic resonance (CMR) (r = 0.90) compared to LV mass measured using two-dimensional echocardiography (r = 0.70). In fact, two-dimensional echocardiography underestimated LV mass by 39% when compared to CMR and the reason cited for this underestimation was foreshortening of the LV on two-dimensional echocardiography images.

The accuracy of traditional two-dimensional echocardiography algorithms for LV volume quantification is further hampered by the reliance of two-dimensional echocardiography volumetric calculations on the assumptions made by fixed geometric models such as a prolate ellipsoid, which can be inaccurate especially in the presence of wall motion abnormalities or LV aneurysms [9, 10].

Quantification of LV Size and Function Using Three-Dimensional Echocardiography

When using 3DE, three approaches are commonly used for LV quantification (Fig. 5.3, Video 5.1):

1. The *3D-guided biplane technique* (Fig. 5.3, left panel): This approach is based on selecting, from a 3DE pyramidal dataset of the LV, anatomically correct, non-foreshortened two-dimensional echocardiography apical four- and two-chamber views. The biplane Simpson method of discs is then applied to calculate LV volumes from non-foreshortened apical views. Because this method still relies on geometric modeling to calculate LV volumes, it is likely to be inaccurate in distorted ventricles.
2. The *triplane technique* (Fig. 5.3, central panel): this approach is based on the multiplane technique that uses the 3DE matrix probe to acquire simultaneous two-dimensional echocardiography views in the same heart beat (see also Chap. 2). After manual orientation of the reference view (conventionally the four-chamber view), the two additional views (two-chamber and apical long-axis) are automatically selected at 60° and 120° from the four-chamber view. The echocardiographer can adjust the acquisition angles in order to optimize view orientations, but only during acquisition. The main advantages of this approach are: (1) the echocardiographers can immediately realize if any foreshortening has occurred during acquisition; (2) wall motion abnormalities occurring in the infero-lateral LV wall and anterior septum (the LV walls most frequently involved in patients with myocardial infarction) are accounted in LV ejection fraction computation; (3) it is more accurate than conventional biplane algorithms in assessing LV volumes and ejection fraction [11, 12]; (4) it is feasible in patients with irregular atrial fibrillation or other arrhythmias, too; (5) more user friendly approach (the echocardiographers traces the

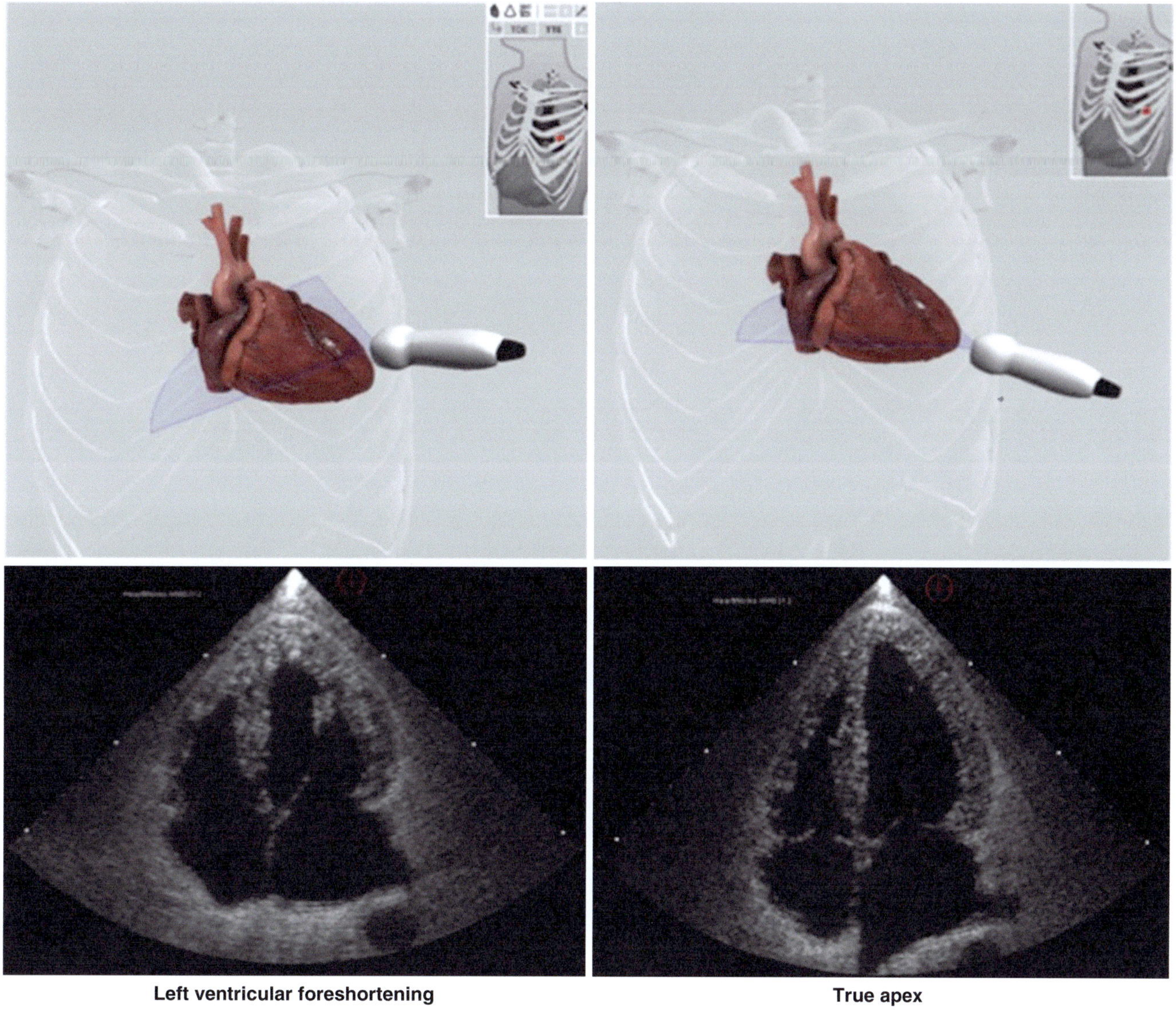

Fig. 5.1 Effects of the position and orientation of the probe on the apical four-chamber view of the left ventricle. When the ultrasound beam does not pass through the true apex of the left ventricle (*left upper panel*) the apical view results in an oblique (foreshortened) left ventricular cavity (*left lower panel*) which will lead to volume underestimation if selected for biplane Simpson or area-length analysis. Correct orientation of the apical view passing through the left ventricular apex (*right upper panel*) produces significantly longer left ventricular length (*right lower panel*)

endocardial border as he/she is used to do with conventional two-dimensional echocardiography) than with complex 3DE software packages. The issues with this technique are due to the fixed relationships that exists between the three views that does not allow avoidance of foreshortening of one or more of these views in some patients, the need of manual tracing of the endocardial border in three views, and the fact that this technique also relies on the same geometric assumptions about LV shape of the biplane discs' summation rule (even if they are mitigated by the addition of the third apical view).

3. *Direct volume quantification* (Fig. 5.3, right panel): This approach is based on semi-automated detection of LV endocardial surfaces throughout the cardiac cycle followed by measurement of LV volume contained within this surface. This approach [13–15] has the important advantage over the 3D-guided bi-plane and the triplane methods of not relying on geometric modeling. The calculated volume is obtained by directly counting voxels inside the endocardial surface. In addition, the endocardial surface can be automatically detected throughout the cardiac cycle, allowing precise identification of

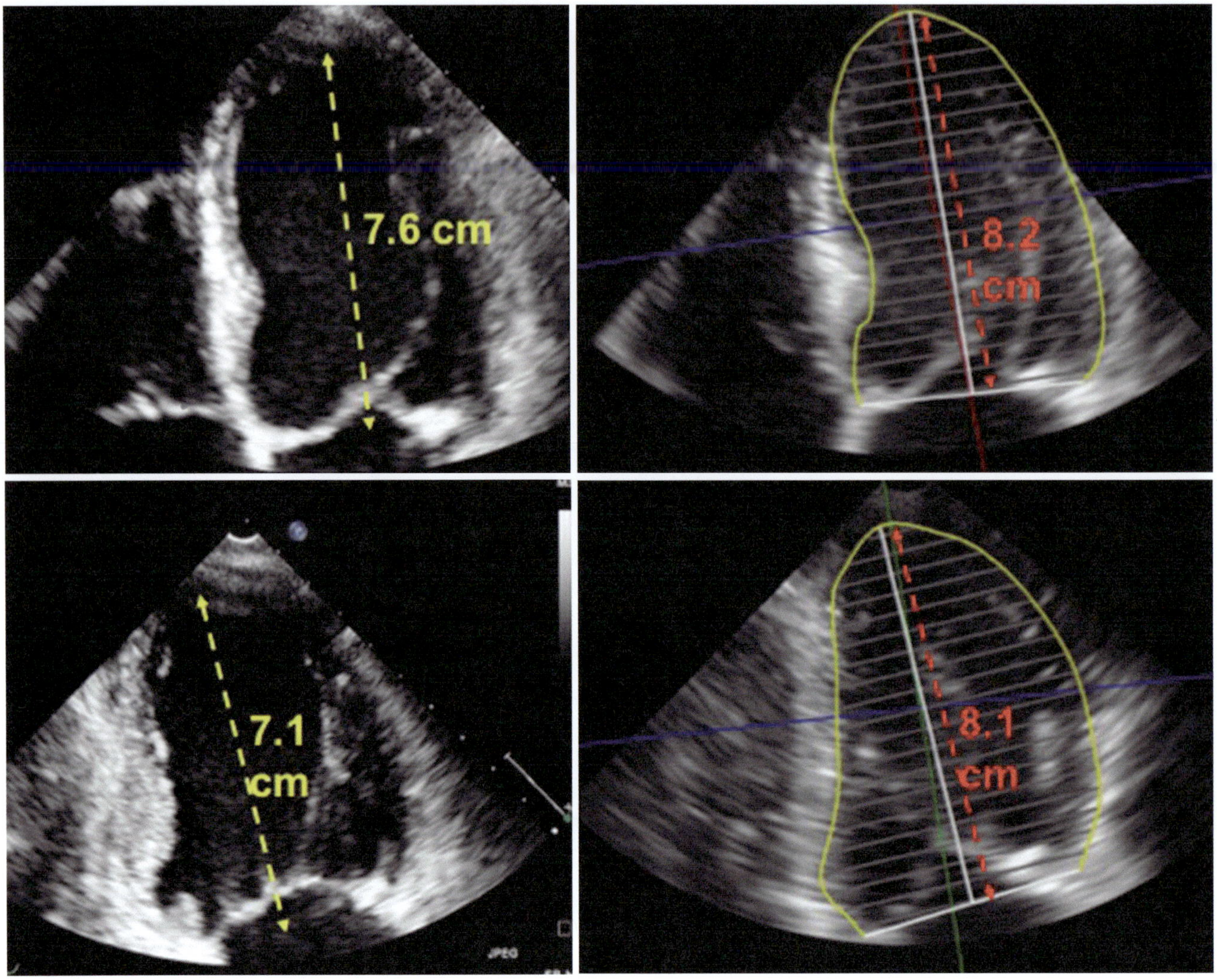

2DE

3DE

Fig. 5.2 Three-dimensional echocardiography (3DE) datasets allow the user to extract the anatomically correct apical views of the left ventricle (LV) for quantification of volumes and ejection fraction. This overcomes the errors associated with foreshortening of one or both the apical views. Left panels illustrate a slightly foreshortened four- and two-chamber apical views of the LV obtained from a two-dimensional echocardiography LV acquisition. Right panels depict the anatomically correct non-foreshortened LV views extracted from the pyramidal 3DE dataset. Note that the annulus to apex measurement is shorter in the foreshortened view than the non-foreshortened view and that in the non-foreshortened views the length of the LV is similar in both four- and two-chamber views

end-systolic frames in order to accurately measure end-systolic volumes from the correct frame.

Surface models are also useful for defining regions of the LV in position and time. This 3DE data can be used to assess LV synchrony, regional strain, curvature, and wall stress. However, at this time these extra steps are not performed in routine clinical practice. It is important to keep in mind that studies have shown that when endocardial borders are traced and borders manually adjusted on more than two cut planes the accuracy of volume quantification is improved [16, 17]. This is likely because fewer geometric assumptions are used. Transthoracic 3DE volumes are generally accurate even in very dilated and aneurysmal ventricles [18–20], provided that the sonographer takes care to include the entire ventricle within the acquisition volume [21].

It has been noted that while two-dimensional echocardiography methods of quantification are reasonably accurate for measurements in a group of subjects, confidence intervals are usually wide thereby limiting the ability of two-dimensional echocardiography to detect small changes in serial measurements in a single patient [10]. 3DE, however, as will be further discussed in the sections below, does not pose the same problem [22].

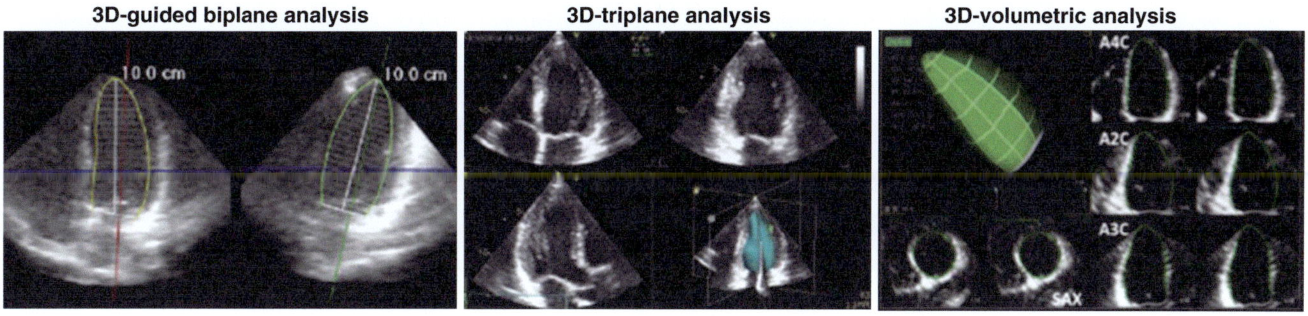

Fig. 5.3 Three approaches to measure left ventricular volumes using the matrix array probe: (*left panel*) three-dimensional-echocardiography (3DE)-guided biplane analysis based on selecting anatomically correct, non-foreshortened apical two- and four-chamber views from the 3DE dataset. These planes are then evaluated using the biplane Simpson's method of discs identical to that used with two-dimensional echocardiography; (*right panel and* Video 5.1). Triplane analysis which obtains three apical views which share the same apex by selectively activating three lines of piezoelectric elements at 0°, 60° and 120°. Volumes are obtained applying the Simpson's method of discs identical to that used with two-dimensional echocardiography; and (*central panel and* Video 5.1). Direct phase-by-phase volumetric analysis based on counting voxels contained inside the 3DE endocardial surface, which results in a volume measurement which is independent on assumptions about the shape of the LV

Three-Dimensional Acquisition and Display of the Left Ventricle

Originally, 3DE was based on the reconstruction from a sequential multi-plane acquisition, gated to the electrocardiogram and respiration (see also Chap. 1). This approach was time consuming, and prone to motion artifacts and was therefore replaced by volumetric imaging that enabled acquisition in real time of a pyramid of data using matrix array transducers. For measurement purposes, the LV is generally acquired as a full-volume dataset over 4–6 heartbeats (called a "multi-beat" acquisition) during a single breath-hold. In this process, dynamic sub-volumes are "stitched" together and scanned during consecutive cardiac cycles. While this breath-hold-based approach enables the acquisition of images with higher frame rates (higher temporal resolution) and higher spatial resolution, the disadvantage is that "stitch artifacts" (see Chap. 2) can occur as a result of changes in the position of the heart relative to the transducer. Single-beat acquisitions avoid stitch artifacts secondary to arrhythmias and respiratory motion but it results in datasets that have lower temporal and poorer spatial resolution. This impacts negatively on the ability of the operator to visualize structures when cropping into the dataset offline due to drop-out while simultaneously affecting the identification of the true end-systolic frame, which has a variable impact on the calculation of end-systolic volumes and consequently ejection fraction. However, a new generation of piezoelectric elements and probes has been developed that can acquire 3DE data set of the LV with enough temporal and spatial resolution to allow reliable measurement of LV volumes [23, 24].

3DE acquisition of the LV is generally performed from the apical approach on transthoracic echocardiography and from the mid-esophageal four-, two-, or three-chamber views on transesophageal echocardiography [25]. Depending on the shape of the LV and its position within the chest, a more off-axis transducer position may be appropriate for acquisition. The goal is simply to ensure the acquisition of the entire LV within the pyramidal dataset (Fig. 5.4). To guarantee optimal image quality, transducer frequency and overall gain should be adjusted appropriately. Sector width and depth should also be adjusted to ensure that the LV is captured devoid of adjacent structures that will reduce frame rate. Prior to 3DE acquisition the two-dimensional echocardiography image must be optimized. Multiplane visualization of the LV showing the azimuthal, the elevation and trasversal planes may help ensure that the entire LV is contained within the imaging sector (Fig. 5.5). Real-time imaging of the LV may also help optimize gain settings. Real-time imaging can also be used to visualize structural changes in the LV such as masses or thrombi and help with the location of wires of catheters used during interventional procedures. Gain settings should typically be higher than those used for two-dimensional echocardiography. Once the image is optimized a full-volume 3DE acquisition can be performed as above described. To optimize an LV dataset for volume and EF assessment a full-volume, 4–6 beat acquisition should be performed using a single breath-hold. If the patient is on mechanical ventilation, the latter can be briefly interrupted to allow acquisition of optimal data sets. In the operating room, data acquisitions should be avoided during the use of electrocautery as these can interfere with image quality and introduce artifacts. LV contrast opacification may be of value if the borders are sub-optimally visualized. Border clarity can be confirmed during full-volume acquisitions.

Of note there is no general agreement as to how the 3D LV dataset should be displayed. The suggestion from the 3D guidelines is to orient the LV so that the right-sided structures are on the left and the apex is up, similar to conventional apical four-chamber view [26]. However, the way the

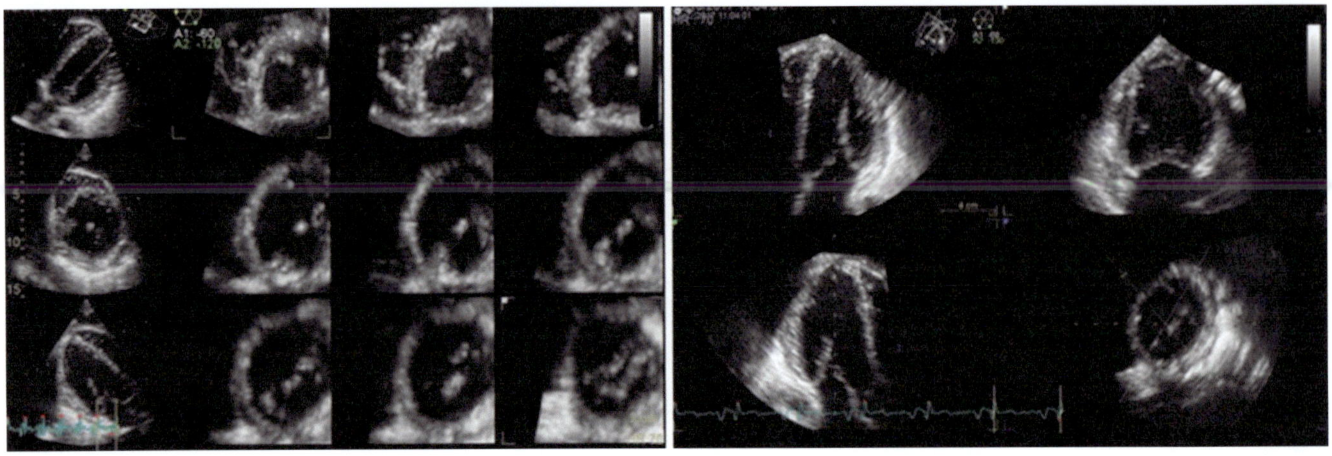

Fig. 5.4 Measurement of left ventricular (LV) volumes from a data set of the left ventricle obtained from the subcostal approach. With 3DE, the important points are that the cardiac structure of interest is included in the acquired data set and there is a clear visualization of the endocardial border. It does not matter the acquisition window or if the corresponding two-dimensional view is foreshortened. Then, during the postprocessing, the operator can rotate and translate the cut planes in order to obtain proper tomographic planes on which to perform measurements and border tracings. This allows to measure LV volumes in patients with poor or no apical acoustic window (e.g. chest deformities, reconstructive surgery after mastectomy etc.). Left panel: Multislice display of a 3DE data set acquired from subcostal approach. Note the orientation of the bottom and top dashed lines on the longitudinal views on the left to obtain proper transversal cut planes (short axes). Right panel: the 3DE data set has been re-aligned to obtain four- and two chamber, and apical long axes to measure LV volumes

3DE data set of the LV is displayed depends on the clinical question the clinicians wants to address: volume rendering display to show anatomy (Fig. 5.6, Videos 5.2a, 5.2b, and 5.2c); multislice display to show wall motion, masses or distribution of LV hypertrophy (Fig. 5.7, Videos 5.3a, 5.3b, 5.3c, and 5.3d); surface rendering display to show function (Fig. 5.8).

Quantitative Analysis of the LV: Volumes, and Ejection Fraction

Of the three methods described above for the quantification of LV volumes and ejection fraction (3DE-guided biplane, triplane and volumetric analysis) the favored method is the direct volume quantification because, as described above, this method avoids the need for geometric assumptions while minimizing the underestimation of LV volumes [27]. 3DE has shown improved reproducibility when compared with two-dimensional imaging [24, 28–30]. Intra-, inter-observer and test-re/test variability of LV volume measurements using the standard two-dimensional echocardiography biplane technique are higher than those obtained with 3DE-based measurements [22–24]. This translates into the need for smaller number of patients to test a hypothesis and thus into potential cost savings in clinical trials, which makes 3DE an attractive alternative to other costly imaging modalities. Perhaps even more important, however is the fact that the higher test/re-test reproducibility of 3DE assessment when compared with two-dimensional echocardiography makes 3DE the ideal technique for individual patient follow-up because smaller changes LV ejection fraction and/or volumes may be identified sooner [22, 24].

A methodology with good reproducibility is certainly desirable but even more so if it is accurate. Several studies have compared 3DE-derived volumes and ejection fractions with CMR finding excellent agreement, as reflected by correlation coefficients >0.85 as well as small biases and tight limits of agreement. However, several studies have reported that despite the high correlation with CMR, 3DE consistently underestimated LV volumes [29–34]. In order to determine out how much foreshortening contributes to this underestimation versus geometric modeling errors, the two-dimensional echocardiography biplane technique, 3DE-guided biplane technique and the volumetric approach were compared side-by-side against CMR in the same group of patients [28]. In this study, an incremental improvement in accuracy was noted, with the two-dimensional echocardiography technique being the least accurate. When the investigators looked specifically at the population of 20 patients in whom the two-dimensional echocardiography results were the least accurate, they noted that the inaccuracy of the two-dimensional echocardiography results was predominantly due to foreshortening of the LV on apical images. The most accurate method, of course was the volumetric or "deformable shell" method which accounts for foreshortening and, to some extent, geometrical modeling errors [28].

To further understand the factors contributing towards the underestimation of LV volumes by 3DE in comparison with CMR and to validate the new endocardial surface analysis technique for LV volumes quantification using CMR as the reference standard a multi-center study was

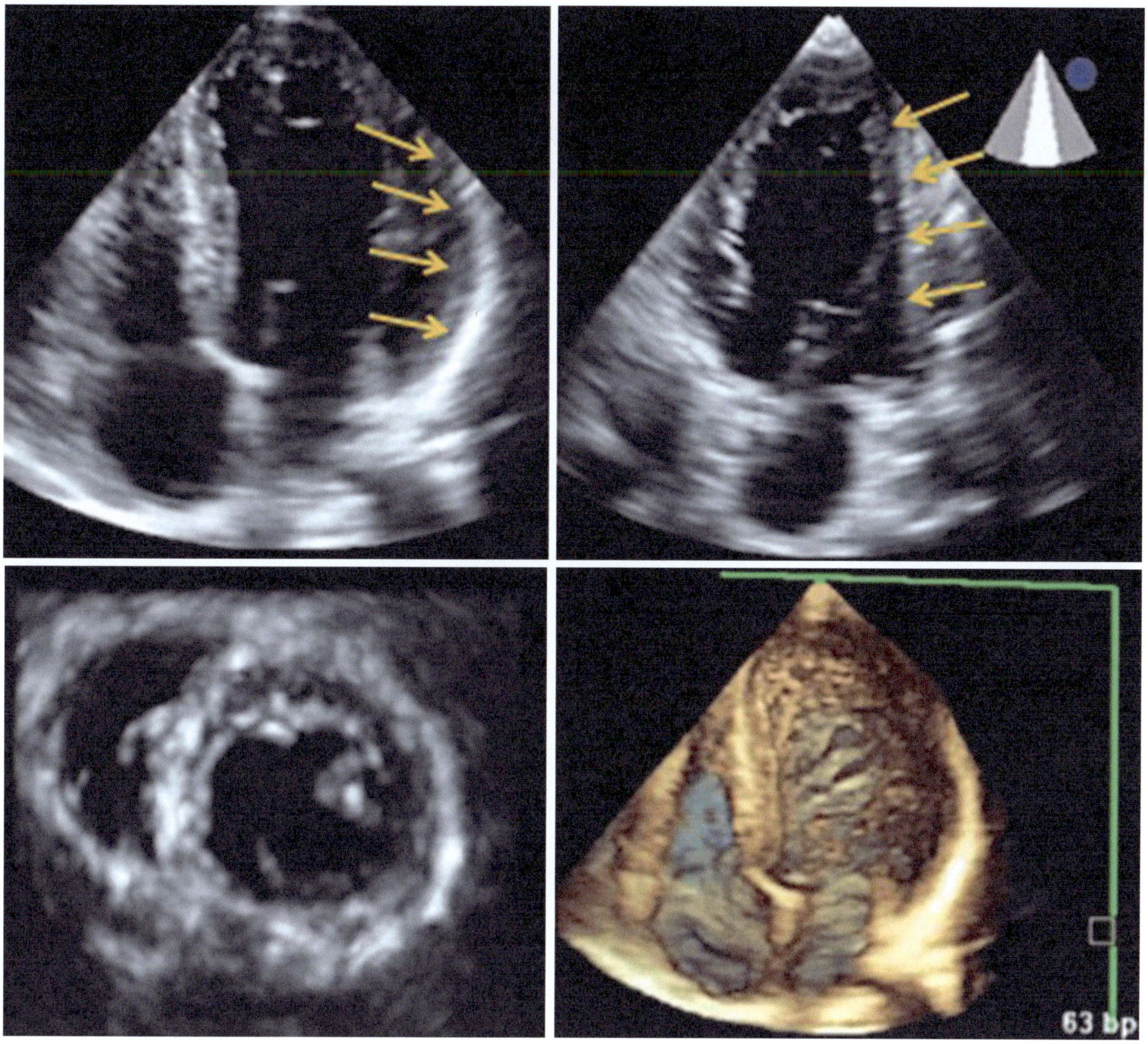

Fig. 5.5 Acquisition of a full-volume dataset of the left ventricle and left atrium. To ensure an optimal dataset, the whole extent of left ventricular myocardium should be seen both in orthogonal longitudinal planes (top row) and in the transverse plane (bottom left)

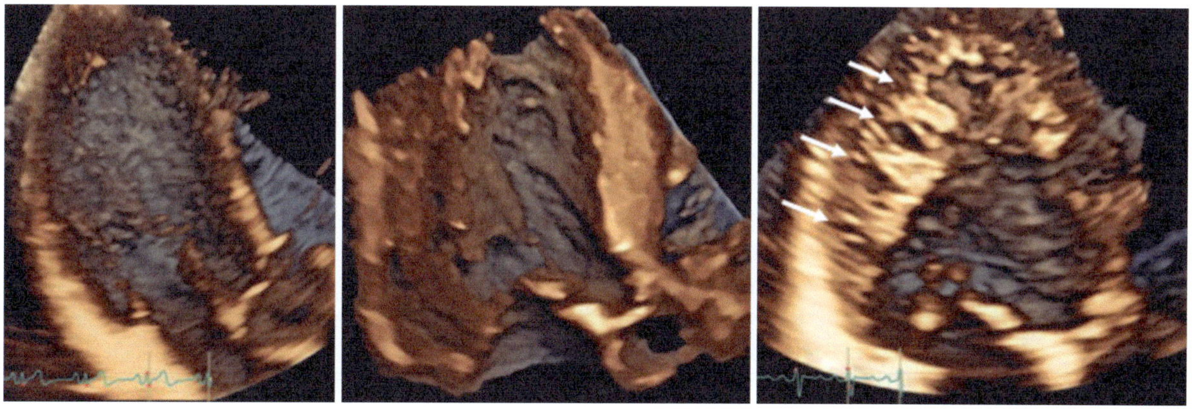

Fig. 5.6 Volume rendering display of the left ventricle to assess anatomy. *Left panel and* Video 5.2a ***left***: left ventricle obtained from a healthy subject. *Central panel and* Video 5.2b ***central***: left ventricle obtained from a patient with left ventricular hypertrophy. *Right panel and* Video 5.2c ***right***: left ventricle obtained from a patient with left ventricular no compaction (deep trabeculae shown with white arrows)

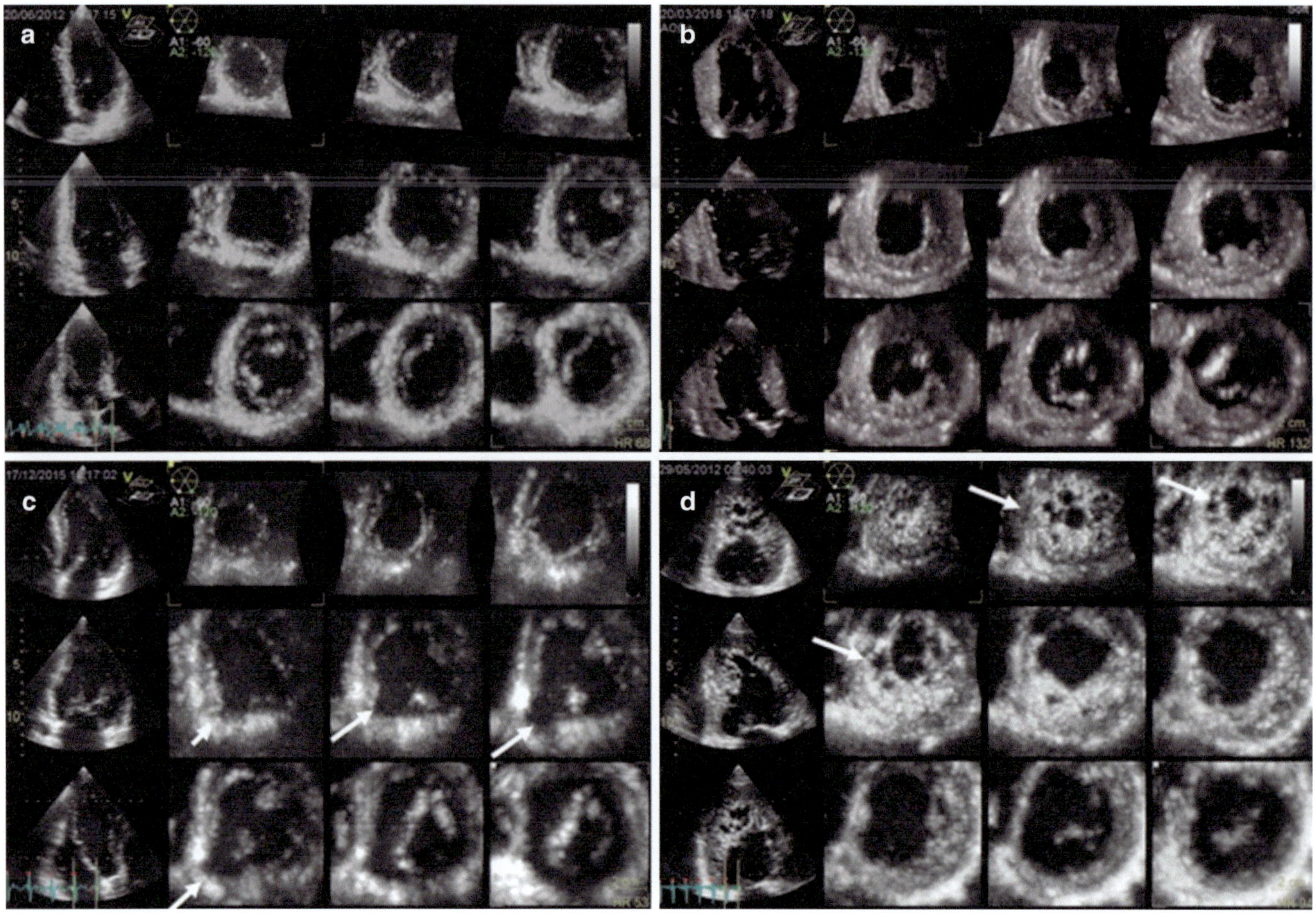

Fig. 5.7 Multislice display of the left ventricle in a healthy subject (panel A and Video 5.3a); in a patient with hypertenive heart disease (panel B and Video 5.3b); in a patient with ischemic heart diseases (panel C and Video 5.3c), the white arrows show an aneurysm of the inferior wall; and in a patient with left ventricular no compaction (panel D and Video 5.3d, the white arrows show the extension of the trabeculated area)

performed [27]. This study reported that 3DE-derived volumes correlated highly with CMR, in agreement with previous studies, but the underestimation was even larger than what was previously reported in single-center studies. After ruling out every possible source of error, endocardial border tracing, which, in human ventricles, is further complicated by the presence of endocardial trabeculae, was found to be the primary source of error leading to volume underestimation in humans. Due to reduced spatial resolution of current semiautomated endocardial border tracing algorithms, the automated endocardial border traced by the software package usually identifies the black and white interface on the screen which corresponds to the tip of trabeculae and not to the compacted part of the endocardium as it happens with CMR that has high spatial resolution. This error can be minimized by learning to correctly identify the true endocardial boundaries in 3DE images beyond what appears to be the blood-trabeculae interface (Fig. 5.9). It was shown that agreement between 3DE and CMR measurements improved when the trabeculae were excluded from the LV cavity on CMR [27]. Agreement between 3DE and CMR was also improved with increasing investigator experience noting that experienced investigators tend to place the LV endocardial borders as far outward as possible. Several more recent studies have demonstrated the added value of contrast enhancement in accurate delineation of LV endocardial boundaries, resulting in improved quantification of ventricular volumes [35, 36].

It must not be forgotten, however that CMR is not a perfect gold standard. There are errors and variations associated for example with the manner in which the basal slice is traced [37]. These errors can propagate and affect volume and ejection fraction assessment in CMR.

Despite the known limitations of CMR as a reference technique, all LV analysis algorithms used in commercially-available 3DE systems have been independently validated against CMR and close correlations between 3DE and CMR measurements have been reported, albeit with a small underestimation of LV volumes by 3DE as already discussed. Although this assumption has never been tested, it has been

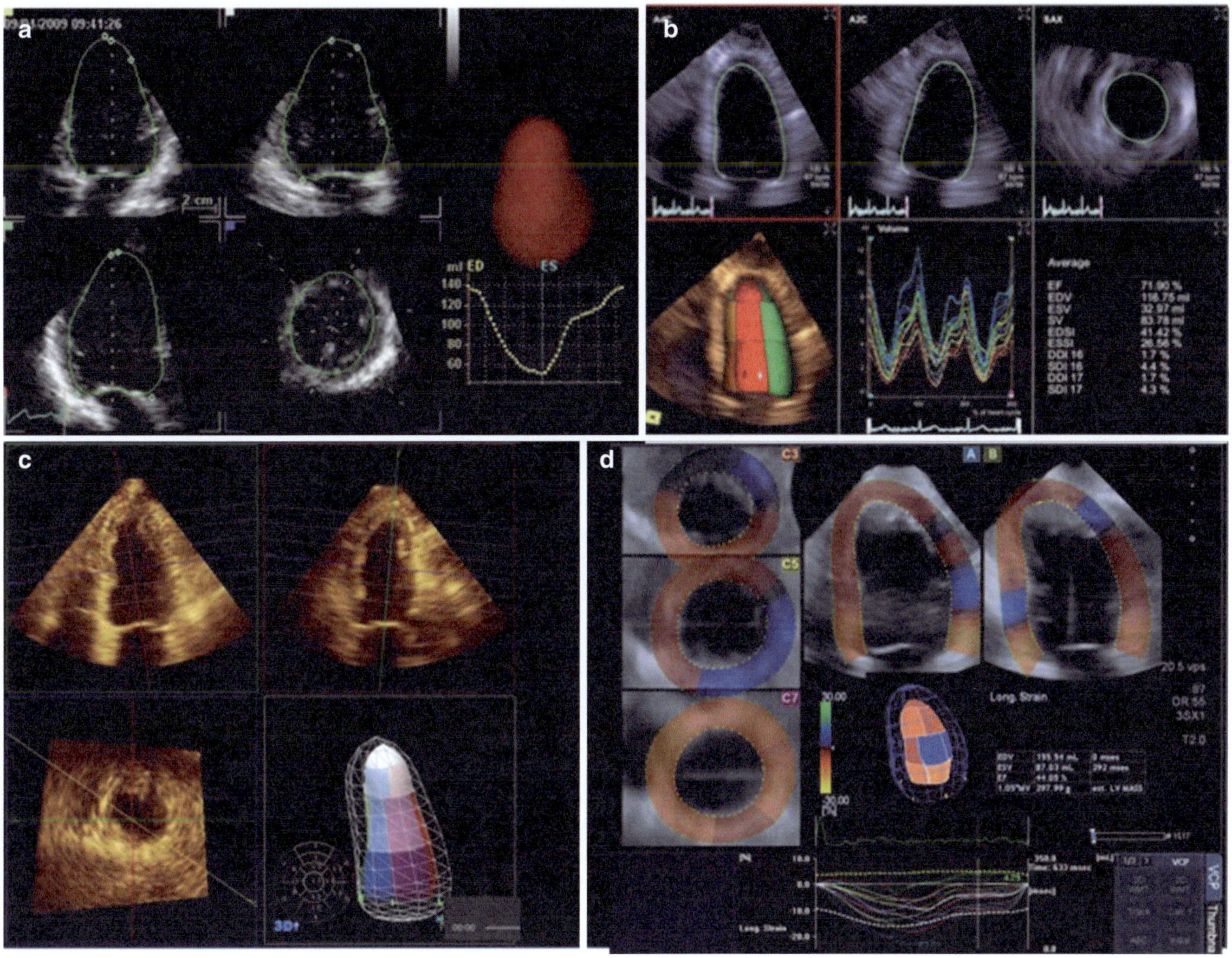

Fig. 5.8 Surface rendering display of the left ventricle to assess function using GE Vingmed (Horten, NO, ***panel A***), Siemens Healthineer (Mountainview, USA, ***panel B***), Philips Medical Systems (Andover, USA, ***panel C***) and Canon Medical Systems (Japan, ***panel D***) echocardiography systems. The use of both the wireframe (showing the end-diastolic volume, ***panels C and D***) and the solid surface (changes of volume over time) rendering allows a better appreciation of left ventricular function

assumed that all 3DE systems are equally accurate and provide consistent measurements of LV volumes and ejection fraction. However, a significant intervendor variability of LV 3D strain was reported by our group and by other investigators [38, 39], which casts some doubts over the actual consistency of LV measurements obtained with different 3DE systems. The assessment of intervendor consistency of LV volume measurements by 3DE has important scientific and clinical implications. From the scientific point of view, it would be important to know if the reference values of LV volumes and ejection fraction that have been obtained using one vendor-specific 3DE system (Table 5.1) can be applied to studies employing different 3DE systems. From the clinical point of view, physicians need to know how to adequately deal with patients that require serial follow-up echocardiographic examinations for LV size and function monitoring by 3DE (e.g. patients with asymptomatic severe valvular heart diseases, previous myocardial infarction or cardiac surgery, or undergoing chemotherapy, etc.). Can these patients be scanned by any 3DE system in the laboratory or is it mandatory to have them examined always with the same 3DE system in order to reliably assess changes in LV volumes and ejection fraction? A recent paper [40] reported consistent LV volume and ejection fraction values among three of the most popular software packages: 4D Auto LVQ (GE Vingmed, Horten, NO), 3DQ ADV (QLab 9.0, Philips Medical Systems, Andover, MA) and eSie LVA (Siemens, CA, USA) (Fig. 5.10).

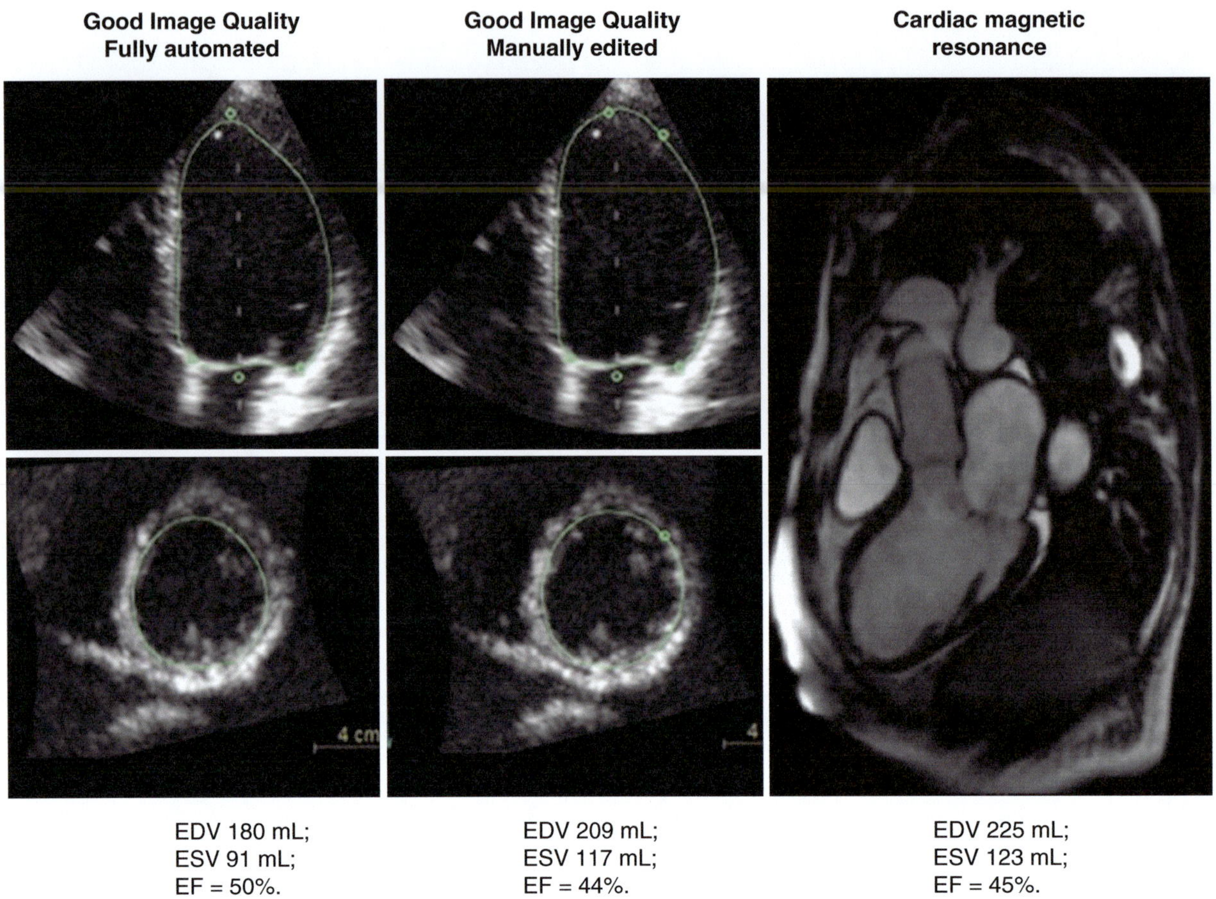

Fig. 5.9 Effect of manual editing of the automatically traced endocardial border on left ventricular volumes and ejection fraction. Despite the good quality of the data set, a fully automated quantitation of left ventricular volumes produces a significant underestimation of volumes and overestimation of ejection fraction (*left panel*) compared to proper manual editing in order to trace the compacted part of left ventricular wall (*central panel*). Left ventricular volumes and ejection fraction measured with cardiac magnetic resonance are reported for comparison (*right panel*)

Table 5.1 Reference values for left ventricular volumes and ejection fraction measured with three-dimensional echocardiography

	Aune E, et al. 2010 [41]	Fukuda S, et al. 2010 [43]	Chahal NS, et al. 2012 [42]	Muraru D, et al. 2013 [44]	Bernard A, et al. 2017 [46]
Study population	Scandinavian (n = 166)	Japanese (n = 410)	United Kingdom (n = 494) and Asian Indian (n = 484)	Italian (n = 226)	European (n = 440)
Echocardiography system	iE33	Sonos 7500, iE33, Vivid 7, Vivid E9, SC2000, Artida	iE33	Vivid E9	Vivid E9 and iE33
Upper limits of end-diastolic volume, (mL/m^2)					
Men	86	74	White = 67 Indian = 59	85	97
Women	74	64	White = 58 Indian = 55	78	82
Upper limits of end-systolic volume (mL/m^2)					
Men	41	29	White = 29 Indian = 26	34	42
Women	33	25	White = 24 Indian = 23	28	35
Lower limits of ejection fraction (%)					
Men	49	53	White = 49 Indian = 52	54	50
Women	49	55	White = 52 Indian = 52	57	51

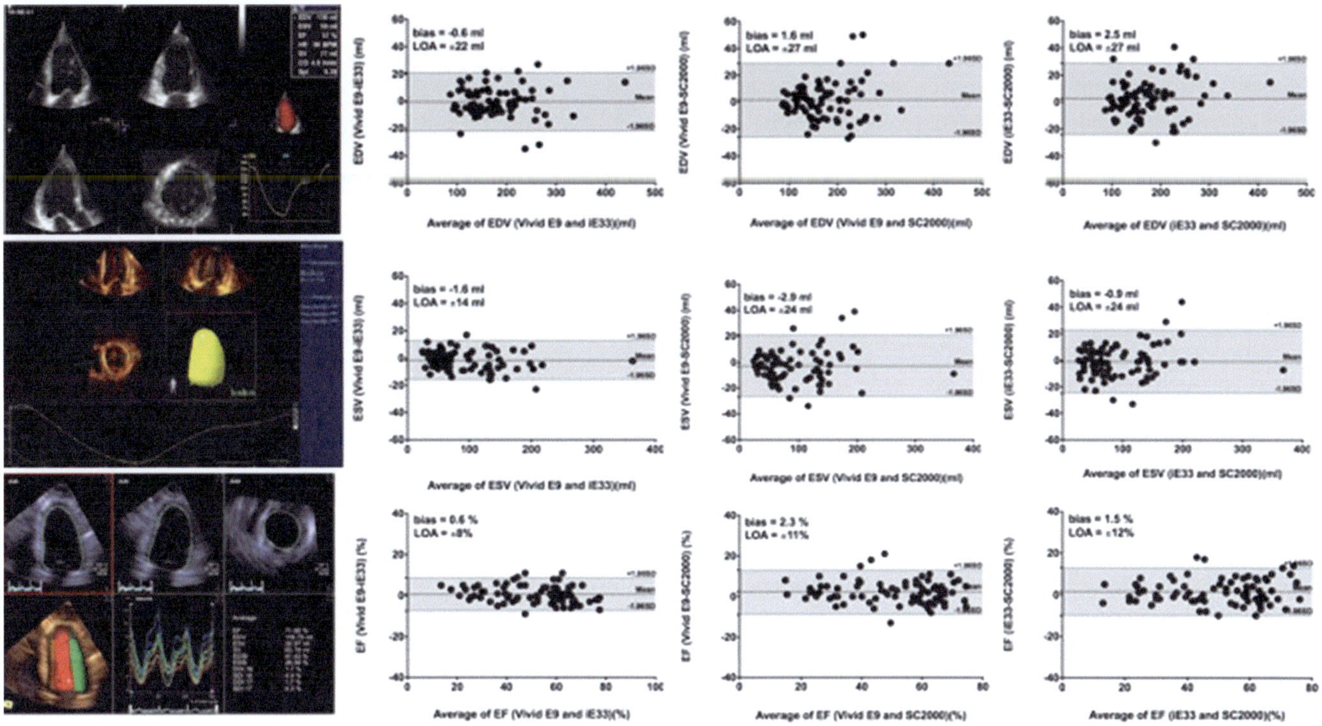

Fig. 5.10 The Bland-Altman plots show (from the left to the right) the results of the head-to-head comparison of end-diastolic and end-systolic volumes and ejection fraction in the same patients measured using (from the upper to the lower panel) GE Vingmed (Horten, NO), Siemens Healthineer (Mountainview, USA, panel B), Philips Medical Systems (Andover, USA, panel C) echocardiographic systems and software packages

Normative Values for Three-Dimensional Left Ventricular Volumes and Ejection Fraction

Beyond validation of new analysis software packages, the focus of 3DE research should be on the establishment of reference values and establishment of outcomes data for different 3DE volumes and ejection fraction cut-offs in different disease states. The identification of normal reference values is important for 3DE to assume a place in the clinical routine. The recent chamber quantification guidelines recommend 3DE quantification of LV volumes and ejection fraction when the expertise to do so exists in a particular echocardiographic laboratory. These guidelines also provide, for the first time, normative data for 3DE LV volumes (upper limits of the normal range for the end-diastolic volume was set a 79 mL/m^2 for men and 71 mL/m^2 for women; for the end-systolic volume it was 32 mL/m^2 for men and 28 mL/m^2 for women) and ejection fraction (lower limits of the normal range was set at 52% for men and 54% for women) [41–44]. Recently, another study called the Normal Reference Ranges for Echocardiography study (NORRE) reported normal reference ranges for the cardiac chambers in white Europeans aged 25–75 years using machines and software from two vendors [44]. A summary of the reference values for LV volumes and ejection fraction obtained with 3DE is shown in Table 5.1. The different studies enrolled quite different populations of healthy volunteers. Interestingly, the upper normal values (mean values +2 SDs) for 3DE end-diastolic and end-systolic volumes reported by Chahal NS et al. [42] for United Kingdom white subjects (e.g. 67 mL/m^2 and 29 mL/m^2 in males) were lower than the upper normal limits reported by two-dimensional echocardiography in current guidelines (75 mL/m^2 and 30 mL/m^2, respectively), contradicting all previous studies showing a larger underestimation of LV volumes measured by two-dimensional echocardiography than by 3DE. Finally, making a simple calculation from the data provided in the paper by Chahal NS et al. [42], it seems that the European subjects were all in a low flow state (stroke volume index 30 mL/m^2 in men, and 26 mL/m^2 in women). These data raised the issue of the accuracy of the measurements performed in this study, particularly when no reference modality or at least comparison with the simple stroke volume measurement with two-dimensional echocardiography and Doppler has been provided [45]. The only multicenter study was the NORRE study [46] which enrolled healthy subjects from 22 laboratories across Europe. Interestingly, this study reported the largest LV volumes among the published reports.

Ongoing efforts are being made by the American Society of Echocardiography that has designed the *World Alliance Societes of Echocardiography (WASE) normal values study* to establish reference ranges for all ethnic groups and populations.

Regional Wall Motion Analysis

The main problem with using two-dimensional echocardiography to assess LV wall motion is that two-dimensional echocardiography is a tomographic technique which obtains thin slices of the cardiac structures (Fig. 5.11). Independent of the number of long- and short-axes of the LV we can acquire in a conventional two-dimensional echocardiography study, less than 10% of the LV endocardial surface and myocardial mass are visualized. The assumption is that wall motion abnormalities respect the classic segmentation of the LV and occur uniformly in each segment. Therefore, what we see in the myocardium included in each thin slice is also what happens in the relatively wide blind area of myocardium between two two-dimensional echocardiography views. Unfortunately, this is not the case in most of the patients with ischemic heart disease and the location and extent of wall motion abnormalities is quite variable among patients with the same coronary artery disease (Fig. 5.12, Videos 5.4a and 5.4b). Conversely, 3DE allows the imaging of all walls in a single echocardiographic loop (Fig. 5.6). Foreshortening is less of a problem with 3DE than it is with two-dimensional echocardiography. For these reasons, 3DE is well suited to determine the location and extent of regional wall motion abnormalities. 3DE can also quantify wall motion using available tools (Fig. 5.13), resulting in a variety of parameters of regional systolic and diastolic function. Regional volumes derived from 3DE datasets are accurate when compared to a CMR reference (r values generally 0.8 and higher) [14, 47]. A study in patients with recent myocardial infarctions showed a reasonable correlation

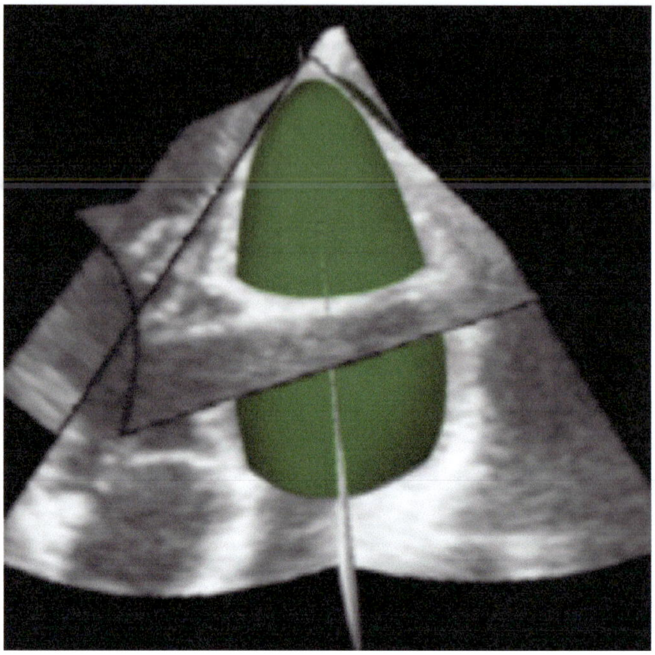

Fig. 5.11 Two-dimensional echocardiography is a tomographic imaging modality that provides information about the morphology and function of the different cardiac structures by obtaining a number of thin slices of the heart. The image shows a series of echocardiographic longitudinal and transversal views of the left ventricle and the 3DE beutel of the cavity in green to demonstrate that what the echocardiographer actually visualizes it is just a very small amount of the endocardial surface and myocardial mass (less than 10%). Two-dimensional echocardiography is based on the assumption that what we see in the thin slices is the same that happens in the large endocardial surface and muscle mass which lies in between on two adjacent slices. This assumption has been proven not to be true in many patients with ischemic heart disease

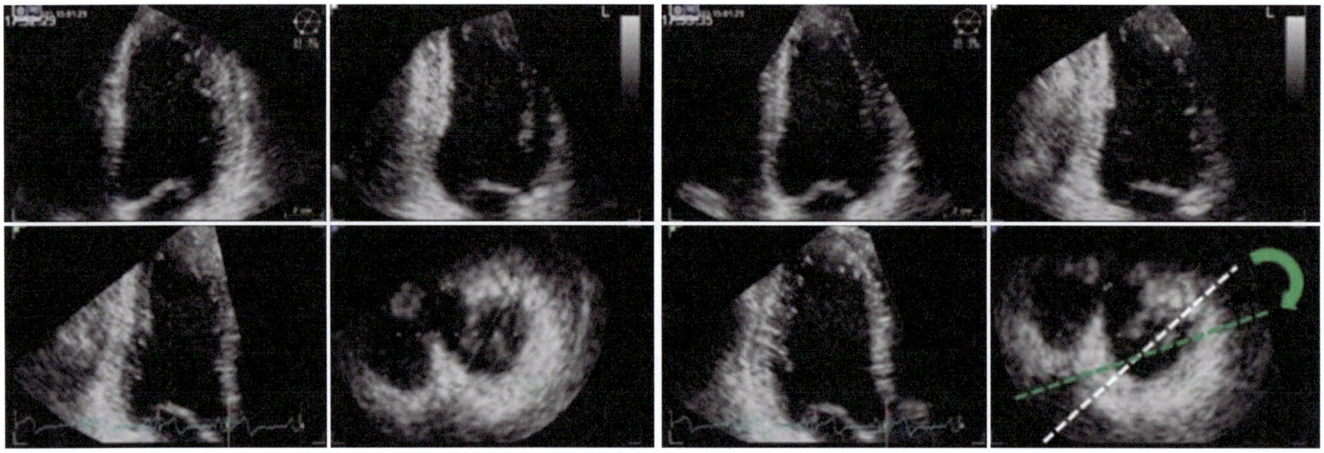

Fig. 5.12 Effects of 15° rotation of the cut planes (reproducing a 15° rotation of the two-dimensional probe) on left ventricular regional wall motion. The apical views shown in the *left panel and* Video 5.4a have been obtained from the same data set used to obtain the views shown in the *right panel and* Video 5.4b which are rotated 15° (green dashed line) compared to the original ones (white dashed line). Despite the views look similar, left ventricular regional wall motion is completely different. On the left, there are wall motion abnormalities at the apical segment of the inferior septum and in large part of the anterior septum. On the right, there is no wall motion abnormality of the inferior septum, the extent of wall motion abnormalities in the anterior septum are limited and there is a wall motion abnormality in the anterior wall. Clinical consequences of acquiring slightly rotated two-dimensional apical views during follow-up studies of the same patient or during different steps of a stress echo protocol can easily be imagined

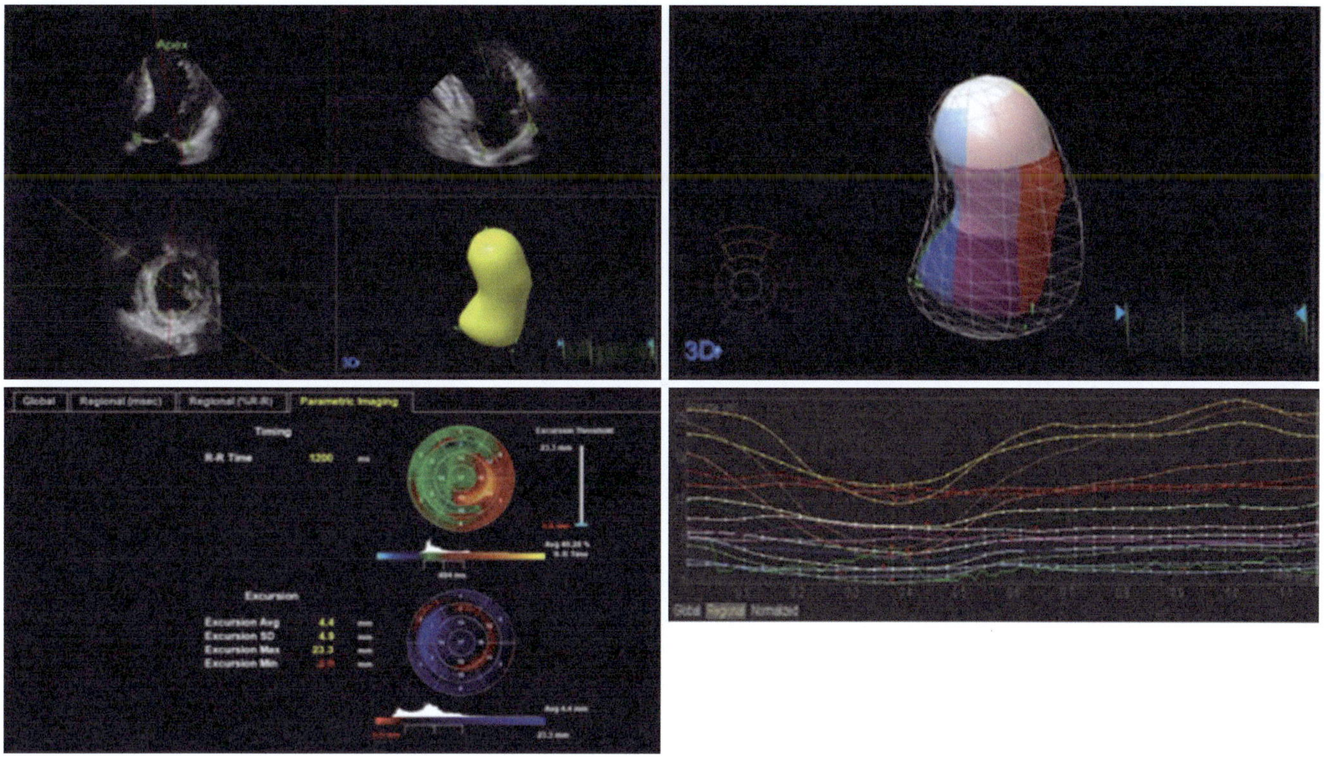

Fig. 5.13 Quantitative evaluation of regional wall motion using Q-Lab (Philips Medical Systems, Andover, USA). *Left upper panel*, semiautomated endocardial border tracing provides a map of left ventricular endocardial surface to obtain left ventricular beutel (in yellow). *Right upper panel*, the 17 myocardial segments are assimilated to pyramids with the base on the endocardium and the apex in the center of gravity of left ventricular cavity. Each segment is identified with a different color and a number. *Left lower panel*, myocardial segment function can be quantitated in terms of both time (the quickest contracting segments in green and the slowest in red, upper bull-eye) and endocardial excursion (in blue the larger excursion and in red the segments with less excursion, lower bell-eye). *Right lower panel*, the function of each pyramidal segment can also be quantitated in terms looking at the change of segmental volume over time during the cardiac cycle (each line color corresponds to the segmental colors on the left ventricular beutel). A sort of segmental ejection fraction can be calculated for each segment. Moreover, the standard deviation of the times from end-diastole to minimal segmental volume for the 16 myocardial segments (the apical cap is excluded) provides the systolic dyssynchrony index (SDI) which is an index of intraventricular dyssynchrony (see Chap. 6)

(r = 0.74) between wall motion score index by 3DE and the extent of delayed gadolinium enhancement by CMR [48]. Quantitative analysis from 3DE datasets could potentially become the manner in which LV wall motion will be evaluated in the future instead of the two-dimensional echocardiography experience-dependent visual interpretation.

Incremental Prognostic Value of Left Ventricular Geometry and Function Parameters Measured by Three-Dimensional Echocardiography

LV volumes and ejection fraction are powerful predictors of clinical events in a variety of cardiac conditions [49–53]. Since 3DE has been reported to provide more accurate (especially in ventricles which do not conform to a pre-defined geometric shape) and more reproducible (by avoiding the issues related to the measurement of LV volumes which change in shape over time and the effect of the different orientation of the tomographic views from one study to the next) measurements of LV volumes, these benefits should also translate into added prognostic value of 3DE LV geometry and function parameters when compared with those calculated using conventional two-dimensional echocardiography.

Stanton and coworkers [54] compared the power of two-dimensional and 3DE to predict all-cause mortality or cardiac hospitalization in 455 patients with high frequency of cardiovascular risk factors followed for 6.6 ± 3.4 years. There were 194 events (43%, including 75 deaths). In stepwise Cox regression analyses, the associations of cardiac hospitalization and mortality with clinical variables (age, chronic renal failure and heart failure) were augments by 3DE ejection fraction and end-systolic volume (incremental model X^2 value = 14.67; $p < 0.001$), more than by two-dimensional echocardiography parameters (incremental model X^2 value = 9.72; $p = 0.002$).

Yingchoncharoen and coworkers [55] compared the value of LV volumes and ejection fraction obtained by two- and 3DE to predict postoperative LV dysfunction (i.e. ejection

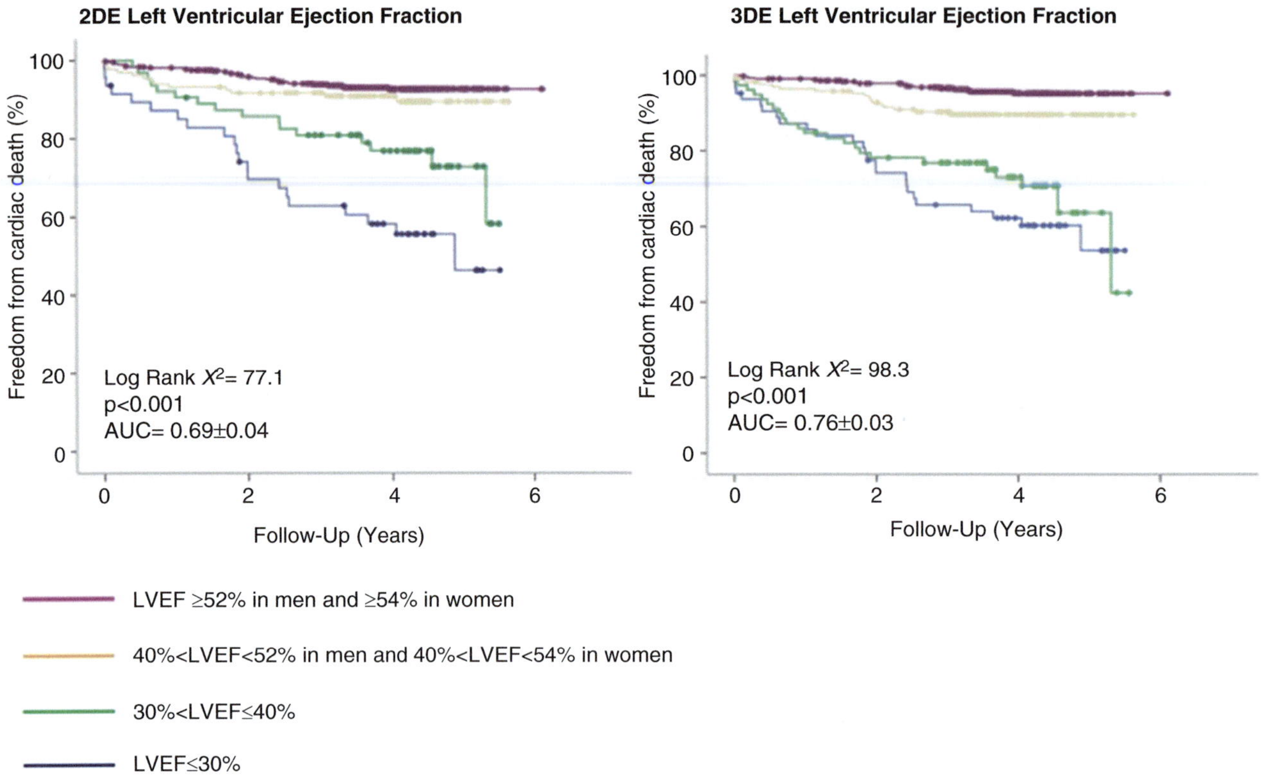

Fig. 5.14 Kaplan Meier curves two- (*left panel*) and three-dimensional (*right panel*) echocardiography left ventricular ejection fraction to predict cardiac death for the different ranges of left ventricular ejection fraction according to current guidelines [1]. *Abbreviations*: *2DE* two-dimensional echocardiography, *3DE* three-dimensional echocardiography, *AUC* area under the R.O.C. curve, *LVEF* left ventricular ejection fraction

fraction >45%) and occurrence of atrial fibrillation in 67 patients who underwent mitral valve surgery. They found that there was no association between two-dimensional end-systolic volumes and outcomes (hazard ratio = 1.02; p 0.18). Post-operative LV dysfunction or atrial fibrillation was associated with preoperative 3DE end-systolic volume index (hazard ratio = 1.06; confidence interval 1.04–1.16) independent of age and presence of coronary artery disease. 3DE LV end-systolic volume ≥40 mL/m^2 was the best cut-off value to predict postoperative outcome.

Medvedofsky and coworkers [56] compared the ability of parameters of LV geometry and function obtained with two-dimensional and 3DE to predict mortality in 416 inpatients followed for 5 ± 3 years. During this period 208 patients (50%) died. Among the various indexes of LV function, 3DE global longitudinal strain was the strongest predictor of cardiovascular mortality, superior to both two-dimensional and 3DE ejection fraction, and ejection fraction calculated with two-dimensional echocardiography was the weakest among the LV function indexes.

Genovese and coworkers [57] sought to identify the added prognostic value of using 3DE to measure LV ejection fraction over conventional two-dimensional echocardiography calculations in 724 unselected patients with various heart diseases who had complete two- and 3DE studies. During an average follow-up time of 3.7 ± 1.1 years, 80 cardiac deaths, 107 deaths due to other causes, and 243 composite endpoints (death and re-hospitalization for heart failure) occurred. 3DE showed a significantly higher predictive power to stratify cardiac death risk when compared with two-dimensional echocardiography (Fig. 5.14). At multivariable stepwise Cox regression analysis including baseline patient characteristics (demographics and cardiovascular risk factors), two- and 3DE LV ejection fraction, 3DE LV ejection fraction was selected as an independent predictor of both all-causes and cardiac death ($p < 0.001$ for both).

Future Directions

Despite the obvious benefits of using 3DE for quantification of LV size and function, widespread use of 3DE for this purpose is not the clinical routine in many laboratories. The reason for this is likely due to the time and training required to obtain accurate and reproducible 3DE measurements. An automated quantification technique could potentially circumvent some of these problems. A recent study introduced novel software which can quantify LV volumes and EF from 3DE transthoracic datasets with minimal input from the user [58]. The study showed that inter-observer reproducibility of LV

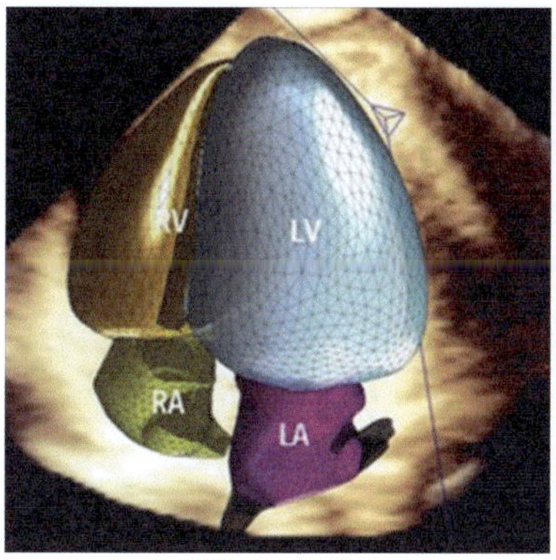

	Inter-observer variability		
	Automated 3D program with contour adjustment	3D Manual program	CMR
LV EDV	9 ± 4%	15 ± 12%	4 ± 6 %
LV ESV	10 ± 4%	18 ± 18%	8 ± 8 %
LV EF	9 ± 6%	21 ± 8%	8 ± 7 %

Fig. 5.15 Inter-observer variability using the HeartModel software package (Philips Medical Systems, *first column of the table*) the manual 3DE assessment program provided by QLab which uses the deformable shell method (ventral column) and cardiac magnetic resonance (left column). See text for details

volumes when using an automated algorithm was far superior than with a non-automated form of assessment (including two-dimensional echocardiography Simpsons and other commercially available 3DE software package) (Fig. 5.15). This finding is important because laboratories often have multiple readers and by reducing inter-reader variability, smaller changes in LV volumes and EF can be detected over time. This is important for follow-up of patients over time.

3DE is the ideal non-invasive, fast and inexpensive method for the quantification of LV volumes and EF. It eliminates the errors associated with foreshortening and geometric assumptions and approaches very closely the gold-standard CMR measurements. It facilitates the calculation of LV shape and the analysis of regional LV function and it diminishes inter- and intra-observer variability [59]. The major barrier to incorporation into the clinical routine is the fact that it is time-consuming and requires additional expertise (see also Chap. 4). With new 3DE analysis programs on the horizon [25, 58] which incorporate automated algorithms requiring little user interaction with the dataset the possibility of routine 3DE use in the clinical arena is a very real possibility in the very near future even if feasibility in the clinical routine is still suboptimal [60].

Clinical Cases

Clinical Case 5.1: The Problem with Foreshortening on Two-Dimensional Echocardiography

As discussed previously in this chapter, foreshortening is an important source of volume underestimation on two-dimensional echocardiography. In this case two-dimensional echocardiography images from two separate pairs of apical four- and two-chamber datasets were analyzed using biplane Simpson analysis for volumes and ejection fraction and compared to a 3DE dataset. All datasets were obtained in the same subject. The first pair of apical four- and two-chamber views analyzed included a foreshortened four-chamber view and a non-foreshortened two-chamber view (Data set 1). The second pair analyzed included non-foreshortened four- and two-chamber views (Data set 2). The third dataset analyzed was the 3DE dataset (Data set 3) (See Fig. 5.16). Not surprisingly biplane Simpson volumes obtained in Case 5.1 were smaller than those obtained in Case 5.2. Interestingly, the volumes and ejection fraction obtained from the 3DE dataset were comparable to those obtained from Case 5.2. This may be because in this particular subject, the LV was symmetrically-shaped. There were no wall motion abnormalities. The main source of error in volumes between two-dimensional echocardiography and 3DE were due to foreshortening.

Clinical Case 5.2: The Added Value of Using Three-Dimensional Echocardiography to Assess Left Ventricular Function in Patients with Extensive Wall Motion Abnormalities

Both biplane are-length and discs' summation algorithm, currently used to calculate LV volumes with two-dimensional echocardiography take into account only regional wall motion abnormalities visualized in the apical four- and two chamber views (12 out of 16 LV segments). These algorithms do not take into account of regional wall motion abnormalities occurring in the infero-lateral and/or anterior septal segments which are the more frequently affected segments in patients with myocardial infarction.

We present the case of a 52-year-old man sent to the echocardiography laboratory for pre-discharge evaluation of LV function after recanalized anterior-septal myocardial infarction. By applying the biplane discs' summation algorithm to conventional two-dimensional echocardiography apical four- and two-chamber views end-diastolic and end-systolic volumes were 112 mL and 51 mL, respectively

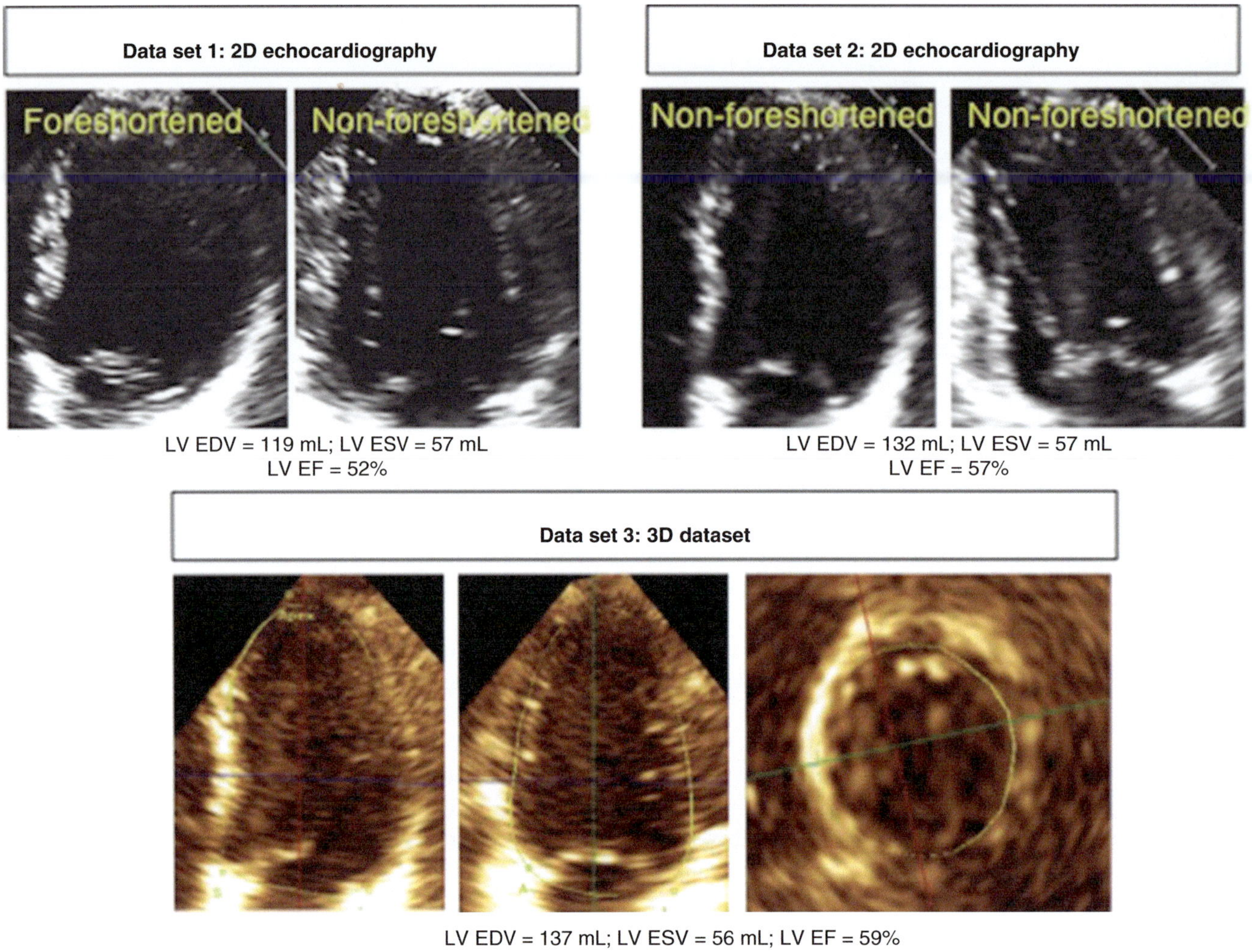

Fig. 5.16 All three data sets come from the same patient. The biplane Simpson's method of discs is used to calculate end-diastolic and end-systolic volumes and ejection fractions on the two-dimensional echocardiography datasets (Data sets 1 and 2) while the deformable shell method is used in the 3DE dataset (Data set 3). See text for details

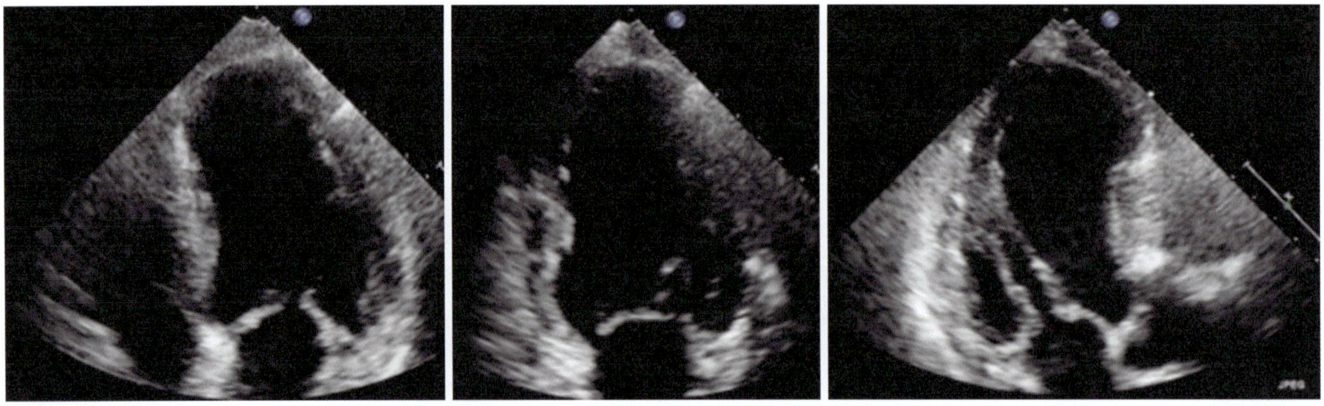

Fig. 5.17 Two-dimensional echocardiography imaging of a patient with recent anterior acute myocardial infarction. Apical four-chamber view (left panel and Video 5.5a **left**), two-chamber view (central panel and Video 5.5b **central**) and long-axis view (right panel and Video 5.5c **right**). See text for details

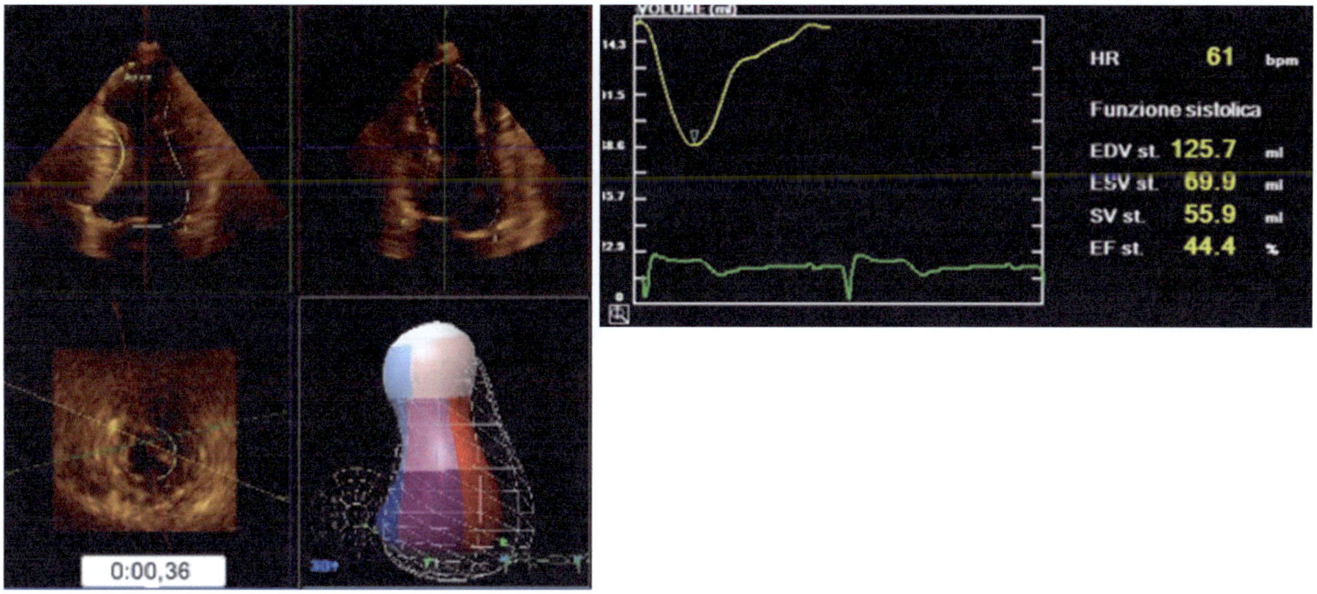

Fig. 5.18 Same patient as in Fig. 5.17. Measurement of left ventricular volumes and ejection fraction using a 3DE data set of the left ventricle. 3DE takes into account the contribution to left ventricular function of all the 16 myocardial segments (apical cap does not contribute to ejection fraction) (Video 5.6)

(Fig. 5.17, Videos 5.5a, 5.5b, and 5.5c). The calculated ejection fraction was 51%. However, the apical long-axis view showed an akinesis of mid anterior septum and a large apical aneurysm which were not taken into account by the discs' summation algorithm. By measuring LV EF by three-dimensional echocardiography which takes into account the functional contribution of all 16 myocardial segments, the LVEF drops to 44% (Fig. 5.18, Video 5.6).

References

1. Lang RM, Badano LP, Mor-Avi V, et al. Recommendations for cardiac chamber quantification by echocardiography in adults: an update from the American Society of Echocardiography and the European Association of Cardiovascular Imaging. J Am Soc Echocardiogr. 2015;28:1–39.e14.
2. Nishimura RA, Otto CM, Bonow RO, et al. 2014 AHA/ACC Guideline for the Management of Patients With Valvular Heart Disease: executive summary: a report of the American College of Cardiology/American Heart Association Task Force on Practice Guidelines. Circulation. 2014;129:2440–92.
3. Epstein AE, DiMarco JP, Ellenbogen KA, et al. 2012 ACCF/AHA/HRS focused update incorporated into the ACCF/AHA/HRS 2008 guidelines for device-based therapy of cardiac rhythm abnormalities: a report of the American College of Cardiology Foundation/American Heart Association Task Force on Practice Guidelines and the Heart Rhythm Society. J Am Coll Cardiol. 2013;61:e6–75.
4. Plana JC, Galderisi M, Barac A, et al. Expert consensus for multimodality imaging evaluation of adult patients during and after cancer therapy: a report from the American Society of Echocardiography and the European Association of Cardiovascular Imaging. J Am Soc Echocardiogr. 2014;27:911–39.
5. Mor-Avi V, Sugeng L, Weinert L, et al. Fast measurement of left ventricular mass with real-time three-dimensional echocardiography: comparison with magnetic resonance imaging. Circulation. 2004;110:1814–8.
6. Takeuchi M, Nishikage T, Mor-Avi V, et al. Measurement of left ventricular mass by real-time three-dimensional echocardiography: validation against magnetic resonance and comparison with two-dimensional and m-mode measurements. J Am Soc Echocardiogr. 2008;21:1001–5.
7. King DL, Harrison MR, King DL, et al. Ultrasound beam orientation during standard two-dimensional imaging: assessment by three-dimensional echocardiography. J Am Soc Echocardiogr. 1992;5:569–76.
8. Nosir YF, Vletter WB, Boersma E, et al. The apical long-axis rather than the two-chamber view should be used in combination with the four-chamber view for accurate assessment of left ventricular volumes and function. Eur Heart J. 1997;18:1175–85.
9. Chukwu EO, Barasch E, Mihalatos DG, et al. Relative importance of errors in left ventricular quantitation by two-dimensional echocardiography: insights from three-dimensional echocardiography and cardiac magnetic resonance imaging. J Am Soc Echocardiogr. 2008;21:990–7.
10. Chuang ML, Beaudin RA, Riley MF, et al. Three-dimensional echocardiographic measurement of left ventricular mass: comparison with magnetic resonance imaging and two-dimensional echocardiographic determinations in man. Int J Card Imaging. 2000;16:347–57.
11. Nucifora G, Badano LP, Dall'Armellina E, Gianfagna P, Allocca G, Fioretti PM. Fast data acquisition and analysis with real time triplane echocardiography for the assessment of left ventricular size and function: a validation study. Echocardiography. 2009;26:66–75.

12. Malm S, Frigstad S, Segberg E, Steen PA, Skjaerpe T. Real-time simultaneous triplane contrast echocardiography gives rapid, accurate and reproducible assessment of left ventricular volumes and ejection fraction: a comparison with magnetic resonance imaging. J Am Soc Echocardiogr. 2006;19:1494–501.
13. Caiani EG, Corsi C, Sugeng L, et al. Improved quantification of left ventricular mass based on endocardial and epicardial surface detection with real time three dimensional echocardiography. Heart. 2006;92:213–9.
14. Corsi C, Lang RM, Veronesi F, et al. Volumetric quantification of global and regional left ventricular function from real-time three-dimensional echocardiographic images. Circulation. 2005;112:1161–70.
15. Muraru D, Badano LP, Piccoli G, et al. Validation of a novel automated border-detection algorithm for rapid and accurate quantitation of left ventricular volumes based on three-dimensional echocardiography. Eur J Echocardiogr. 2010;11:359–68.
16. Marsan NA, Henneman MM, Chen J, et al. Real-time three-dimensional echocardiography as a novel approach to quantify left ventricular dyssynchrony: a comparison study with phase analysis of gated myocardial perfusion single photon emission computed tomography. J Am Soc Echocardiogr. 2008;21:801–7.
17. van Dijk J, Dijkmans PA, Gotte MJ, Spreeuwenberg MD, Visser CA, Kamp O. Evaluation of global left ventricular function and mechanical dyssynchrony in patients with an asymptomatic left bundle branch block: a real-time 3D echocardiography study. Eur J Echocardiogr. 2008;9:40–6.
18. Ahmed S, Nanda NC, Miller AP, et al. Usefulness of transesophageal three-dimensional echocardiography in the identification of individual segment/scallop prolapse of the mitral valve. Echocardiography. 2003;20:203–9.
19. Flachskampf FA, Chandra S, Gaddipatti A, et al. Analysis of shape and motion of the mitral annulus in subjects with and without cardiomyopathy by echocardiographic 3-dimensional reconstruction. J Am Soc Echocardiogr. 2000;13:277–87.
20. Matsumura Y, Saracino G, Sugioka K, et al. Determination of regurgitant orifice area with the use of a new three-dimensional flow convergence geometric assumption in functional mitral regurgitation. J Am Soc Echocardiogr. 2008;21:1251–6.
21. Little SH, Igo SR, Pirat B, et al. In vitro validation of real-time three-dimensional color Doppler echocardiography for direct measurement of proximal isovelocity surface area in mitral regurgitation. Am J Cardiol. 2007;99:1440–7.
22. Jenkins C, Bricknell K, Chan J, Hanekom L, Marwick TH. Comparison of two- and three-dimensional echocardiography with sequential magnetic resonance imaging for evaluating left ventricular volume and ejection fraction over time in patients with healed myocardial infarction. Am J Cardiol. 2007;99:300–6.
23. Tamborini G, Piazzese C, Lang RM, et al. Feasibility and accuracy of automated software for transthoracic three-dimensional left ventricular volume and function analysis: comparison with two-dimensional echocardiography, three-dimensional transthoracic manual method, and cardiac magnetic resonance imaging. J Am Soc Echocardiogr. 2017;30:1049–58.
24. Thavendiranathan P, Liu S, Verhaert D, et al. Feasibility, accuracy, and reproducibility of real-time full-volume 3D transthoracic echocardiography to measure LV volumes and systolic function: a fully automated endocardiac contouring algorithm in sinus rhythm and atrial fibrillation. JACC Cardiovasc Imaging. 2012;5:239–51.
25. Medvedofsky D, Mor-Avi V, Amzulescu M, et al. Three-dimensional echocardiographic quantification of the left heart chambers using an automated adaptive analytics algorithm: multicentre validation study. Eur Heart J Cardiovasc Imaging. 2018;19:47–58.
26. Lang RM, Badano LP, Tsang W, et al. EAE/ASE recommendations for image acquisition and display using three-dimensional echocardiography. Eur Heart J Cardiovasc Imaging. 2012;13:1–46.
27. Mor-Avi V, Jenkins C, Kuhl HP, et al. Real-time 3-dimensional echocardiographic quantification of left ventricular volumes: multicenter study for validation with magnetic resonance imaging and investigation of sources of error. JACC Cardiovasc Imaging. 2008;1:413–23.
28. Jacobs LD, Salgo IS, Goonewardena S, et al. Rapid online quantification of left ventricular volume from real-time three-dimensional echocardiographic data. Eur Heart J. 2006;27:460–8.
29. Jenkins C, Bricknell K, Hanekom L, Marwick TH. Reproducibility and accuracy of echocardiographic measurements of left ventricular parameters using real-time three-dimensional echocardiography. J Am Coll Cardiol. 2004;44:878–86.
30. Soliman OI, Geleijnse ML, Theuns DA, et al. Reverse of left ventricular volumetric and structural remodeling in heart failure patients treated with cardiac resynchronization therapy. Am J Cardiol. 2008;101:651–7.
31. Arai K, Hozumi T, Matsumura Y, et al. Accuracy of measurement of left ventricular volume and ejection fraction by new real-time three-dimensional echocardiography in patients with wall motion abnormalities secondary to myocardial infarction. Am J Cardiol. 2004;94:552–8.
32. Qin JX, Jones M, Shiota T, et al. Validation of real-time three-dimensional echocardiography for quantifying left ventricular volumes in the presence of a left ventricular aneurysm: in vitro and in vivo studies. J Am Coll Cardiol. 2000;36:900–7.
33. Shimada YJ, Shiota T. A meta-analysis and investigation for the source of bias of left venrticular volumes and function by three-dimensional echocardiography in comparison with magnetic resonance imaging. Am J Cardiol. 2011;107:126–38.
34. Dorosz JL, Lezotte DC, Weitzenkamp DA, et al. Performance of three-dimensional echocardiography in measuring left ventricular volumes and ejection fraction: a systematic review and meta-analysis. J Am Coll Cardiol. 2012;59:1799–808.
35. Jenkins C, Moir S, Chan J, et al. Left ventricular volume measurement with echocardiography: a comparison of left ventricular opacification, three-dimensional echocardiography, or both with magnetic resonance imaging. Eur Heart J. 2009;30:98–106.
36. van der Heide JA, Mannaerts HF, Yang L, et al. Contrast-enhanced versus non-enhanced three-dimensional echocardiography of left ventricular volumes. Neth Heart J. 2008;16:47–52.
37. Beerbaum P, Barth P, Kropf S, et al. Cardiac function by MRI in congenital heart disease: impact of consensus training on interinstitutional variance. J Magn Reson Imaging. 2009;30:956–66.
38. Badano LP, Cucchini U, Muraru D, et al. Use of three-dimensional speckle tracking to assess left ventricular myocardial mechanics: intervendor consistency and reproducibility of strain measurements. Eur Heart J Cardiovasc Imaging. 2013;14:285–93.
39. Gayat E, Ahmad H, Weiner L, Lang RM, Mor-Avi V. Reproducibility and inter-vendor variability of left ventricular deformation measurements by three-dimensional speckle-tracking echocardiography. J Am Soc Echocardiogr. 2011;24:878–85.
40. Muraru D, Cecchetto A, Cucchini U, et al. Intervendor consistency and accuracy of left ventricular volume measurements using three-dimensional echocardiography. J Am Soc Echocardiogr. 2018;31:158–68.
41. Aune E, Baekkevar M, Rodevand O, Otterstad JE. Reference values for left ventricular volumes with real-time 3-dimensional echocardiography. Scand Cardiovasc J. 2010;44:24–30.
42. Chahal NS, Lim TK, Jain P, et al. Population-based reference values for 3D echocardiographic LV volumes and ejection fraction. JACC Cardiovasc Imaging. 2012;5:1191–7.

43. Fukuda S, Watanabe H, Daimon M, et al. Normal values of real-time 3-dimensional echocardiographic parameters in a healthy Japanese population: the JAMP-3D Study. Circ J. 2012;76:1177–81.
44. Muraru D, Badano LP, Peluso D, et al. Comprehensive analysis of left ventricular geometry and function by three-dimensional echocardiography in healthy adults. J Am Soc Echocardiogr. 2013;26:618–28.
45. Badano LP. Defining normative values for 3D LV volumes: the devil is in the details. JACC Cardiovasc Imaging. 2013;6:530.
46. Bernard A, Addetia K, Dulgheru R, et al. 3D Echocardiographic reference ranges for normal left ventricular volumes and strain: results from the EACVI NORRE study. Eur Heart J Cardiovasc Imaging. 2017;18:475–83.
47. Nesser JH, Sugeng L, Corsi C, et al. Volumetric analysis of regional left ventricular function with real-time three-dimensional echocardiography: validation by magnetic resonance and clinical utility testing. Heart. 2007;93:572–8.
48. Thorstensen A, Dalen H, Hala P, et al. Three-dimensional echocardiography in the evaluation of global and regional function in patients with recent myocardial infarction: a comparison with magnetic resonance imaging. Echocardiography. 2013;30:682–92.
49. Pfeffer MA, Swedberg K, Granger BB, et al. Effects of candesartan on mortality and morbidity in patients with chronic heart failure: the CHARM-Overall programme. Lancet. 2003;362:759–66.
50. Packer M, Fowler MB, Roecker EB, et al. Effect of carvedilol on the morbidity of patients with severe chronic heart failure: results of the Carvedilol Prospective Randomized Cumulative Survival (COPERNICUS) study. Circulation. 2002;106:2194–87.
51. The SOLVD Investigators. Effect of enalapril on survival in patients with reduced left ventricular ejection fractions and congestive cardiac failure (for the SOLVD Investigators). N Engl J Med. 1991;325:293–302.
52. Dickstein K, Kjekshus J. OPTIMAAL trial steering committee of the OPTIMAAL study group. Effects of losartan and captopril on mortality and morbidity in high-risk patients after acute myocardial infarction: the OPTIMAAL randomised trial. Lancet. 2002;360:752–60.
53. St. John SM, Pfeffer MA, Plappert T, et al. Quantitative two-dimensional echocardiographic measurements are major predictors of adverse cardiovascular events after acute myocardial infarction. The protective effects of captopril. Circulation. 1994;89:68–75.
54. Stanton T, Jenkins C, Haluska BA, Marwick T. Association of outcome with left ventricular parameters measured by two-dimensional and three-dimensional echocardiography in patients at high cardiovascular risk. J Am Soc Echocardiogr. 2014;27:65–73.
55. Yingchoncharoen T, Negishi T, Stanton T, Marwick TH. Incremental value of three-dimensional echocardiogarphy in the evaluation of left ventricular size in mitral regurgitation: a follow-up study after mitral valve surgery. J Am Soc Echocardiogr. 2014;27:608–15.
56. Medvedofsky D, Maffessanti F, Weinert L, et al. 2D and 3D echocardiography-derived indices of left ventricular function and shape: relationship with mortality. JACC Cardiovasc Imaging. 2018;11(11):1569–79.
57. Genovese D, Ermacora D, Cavalli G, et al. Incremental prognostic value of left ventricular ejection fraction measured with three-dimensional echocardiography in a large cohort of patients with various heart diseases. Eur Heart J. 2017;38(Suppl 1). Abstract ehx501.P154.
58. Tsang W, Salgo IS, Medvedofsky D, et al. Transthoracic 3D echocardiographic left heart chamber quantification using an automated adaptive analytics algorithm. JACC Cardiovasc Imaging. 2016;9:769–82.
59. Addetia K, Bhave NM, Tabit CE, et al. Sample size and cost analysis for pulmonary arterial hypertension drug trials using various imaging modalities to assess right ventricular size and function end points. Circ Cardiovasc Imaging. 2014;7:115–24.
60. Mevedofsky D, Mor-Avi V, Byku I, et al. Three dimensional echocardiographic automated quantification of left heart chamber volumes using and adptive analytics algorithm: feasibility and impact of Image quality in non selected patients. J Am Soc Echocardiogr. 2017;30:879–85.

6 Advanced Assessment of the Left Ventricle

Masaaki Takeuchi, Karima Addetia, and Roberto M. Lang

Abstract

The left ventricle has a unique shape that changes unpredictably in pathological conditions, and a complex mechanics due to a peculiar architectural arrangement of myocardial fibers. Both left ventricular geometry and mechanics cannot be comprehensively analyzed by exploring it with a tomographic imaging technique such as two-dimensional echocardiography (2DE). The need of making assumptions about left ventricular shape and mechanics to calculate geometrical and functional parameters from simple linear dimensions and area measurements is a major limitation of 2DE. Three-dimensional echocardiography, by encompassing the whole left ventricle in the acquisition volume, provides actual measurements of volumes, shape and mass, independent on any assumption about geometry, and allows to follow the motion of myocardial speckles frame-to-frame to allow actual measurement of the various components of myocardial deformation and ventricular torsion.

Keywords

Left ventricular mass · Left ventricular shape
Left ventricular torsion · 3D strain · Speckle tracking

M. Takeuchi (✉)
Department of Laboratory and Transfusion Medicine, University of Occupational and Environmental Health Hospital, School of Medicine, Kitakyushu, Japan
e-mail: takeuchi@med.uoeh-u.ac.jp

K. Addetia · R. M. Lang
Noninvasive Cardiac Imaging Laboratories, Department of Medicine/Section of Cardiology, University of Chicago Medical Center, Chicago, IL, USA
e-mail: kaddetia@medicine.bsd.uchicago.edu; rlang@medicine.bsd.uchicago.edu

Left Ventricular Volumes and Ejection Fraction

As discussed in Chap. 5, the main reasons why conventional two-dimensional echocardiography significantly underestimates left ventricular (LV) volumes when compared against cardiac magnetic resonance (CMR) as a standard reference [1, 2] can be summarized in: (1) foreshortening of apical views; (2) algorithms for LV volume calculations based on geometrical assumptions about the left ventricular shape.

To overcome these issues, several 3DE software packages for the quantification of LV volumes have been developed (Fig. 6.1) and validated against CMR [1–8]. With 3DE, LV volumes continue to be underestimated when compared with CMR [9, 10], but importantly, this underestimation is half that reported for 2DE. The major reason for the discrepancy between LV volumes obtained using 3DE and CMR depends on the proper identification of endocardial border using 3DE. Currently, due to the suboptimal spatial resolution, the quality of the 2D images extracted from the 3DE datasets is often not adequate to provide clear delineation of the boundary between the compacted and non-compacted myocardial layers. Previous reports clearly demonstrate that small differences (1 mm) in border endocardial tracing may alter significantly LV volume measurements [11]. In addition, individual echocardiographers have their own preferences for endocardial border tracing, which result in a considerable degree of inter-observer variability for LV volume measurements. Fully automated LV endocardial border identification software packages from high volume rate 3D full volume datasets have recently been developed to circumvent these limitations [4, 12]. Just recently, another novel 3D fully automated analysis software appeared in the clinical arena [13, 14]. This software (HeartModel, Philips Medical Systems, Andover, USA) simultaneously detects the LV and left atrial endocardial surface using an adaptive analytic algorithm that consisted of knowledge-based identification of initial global shape and orientation followed by patient specific adaptation. After acquisi-

L. P. Badano et al. (eds.), *Textbook of Three-Dimensional Echocardiography*, https://doi.org/10.1007/978-3-030-14032-8_6

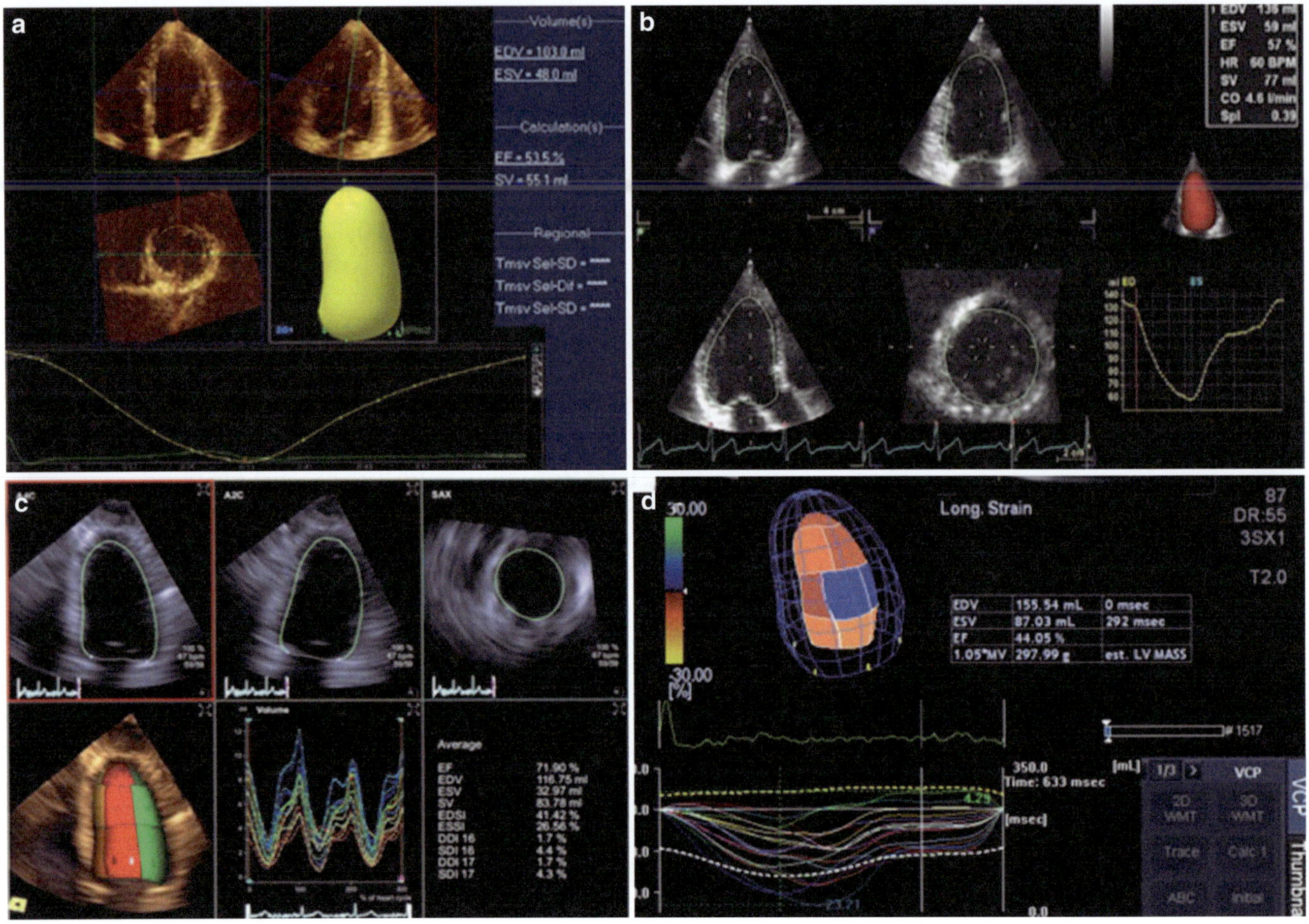

Fig. 6.1 Commercially available software packages to quantify left ventricular (LV) volumes and ejection fraction using three-dimensional data sets. (**a**) 3DQ Adv (Philips Medical Systems, Andover, MA). After initialization of anatomical landmark (both sides of the mitral annulus and apical endocardium), the software determines endocardial border in 3D space at end-diastole and end-systole. Sequential analysis throughout one cardiac cycle generates time domain LV volume curves, from which LV end-diastolic and end-systolic volumes and LV ejection fraction are obtained. (**b**) 4D AutoLVQ (GE Vingmed, Horten, NO) allows either manual (identification of both sides of the mitral annulus and LV apex in all three apical cut planes), semiautomated (identification of LV apex and the center of mitral annulus in just one apical cut plane) or fully automated (no intervention from the operator required) initialization to identify endocardial border. (**c**) eSie LVA (Siemens Healthineer, CA, USA) works only in single-beat acquisitions and provides a fully automated initialization of LV endocardium; (**d**) 3D Wall Motion Tracking (WMT, Toshiba Medical Systems Corporation, Tokyo, JP) works in multibeat acquisition and fully automated initialization of the LV endocardium

tion of a single-beat 3DE full volume dataset, the operator initiates the analytical software without the need for manual identification of any anatomical landmarks. The software then proceeds to automatically identify the end-diastolic and end-systolic frames, together with the LV end-diastolic and end-systolic volumes, LVEF and maximal left atrial volume (Fig. 6.2). While this novel software is supposed to be used without contour editing, intra- and inter-observer variabilities are 0%, and <5% with the use of minor editing. Test-retest variability is also low. Another advantage of this software is that it uses one beat acquisition of full volume datasets with reasonably high volume rates. Multi-beat full volume data acquisition is frequently associated with stitching artifacts, particularly when acquired in patients with irregular heart rates or who are unable to withhold respiration during data acquisition. One beat acquisition is less demanding for both sonographers and patients, expanding the applicability of this methodology to patients in whom multi-beat acquisition is not possible. Since the initial results of this software were promising [13, 14], further studies will be required to expand the clinical applicability of this methodology in different clinical settings [15].

Left Ventricular Mass

Except in the athletic heart, LV hypertrophy is a maladaptive response of LV remodeling, which may be associated with adverse outcomes [16]. The presence and/or severity of LV hypertrophy provides useful information regarding future prognosis [17]. Echocardiographic determination of LV mass corrected by body surface area or height (LV mass index) has

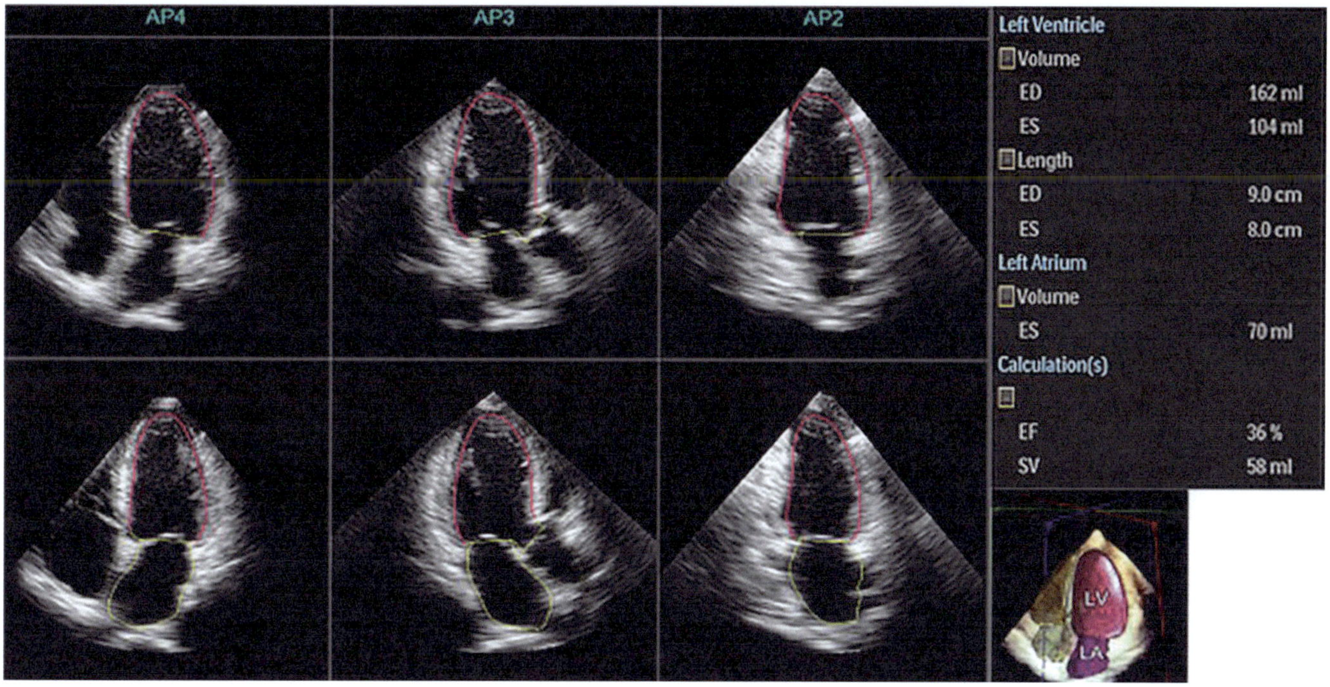

Fig. 6.2 Fully automated left chamber quantification software (HeartModel, Philips Medical Systems, Andover, USA). The user acquires one-beat 3D full volume dataset which encompass both the left ventricle and left atrium. Thereafter, the software automatically selects the end-diastolic and end-systolic frames, and determines the endocardial border of both the ventricle and the atria

Table 6.1 Reference normal values of left ventricular mass by echocardiography and cardiac magnetic resonance

	Male	Female
M-mode (g/m^2) [18]	49–115	43–95
2D echo [18]	50–102	44–88
3D echo Japanese [22]	40–88	34–78
3D echo Italian [24]	57–97	58–90
3D echo Japanese [23]	53–85	45–77
3D echo American [23]	52–88	46–74
CMR	45–83	35–70

CMR cardiac magnetic resonance

been traditionally acquired using M-mode and two-dimensional echocardiography, and their normal reference values have been well established [18] (Table 6.1). However, LV mass assessment by two-dimensional echocardiography suffers from the same limitations which affect the reproducibility and the accuracy of volumes and ejection fraction calculations. The currently recommended algorithm for LV mass calculation, the cubed formula (most commonly applied to linear dimensions of the LV obtained with two-dimensional echocardiography), has been validated against post-mortem pathology findings, however it relies on the geometric assumption that the LV is a prolated ellipsoid [19]. This assumption is inaccurate in both remodeled and non-symmetrically contracting ventricles. The other two algorithms based on two-dimensional echocardiography (the truncated ellipsoid and the area-length) also rely on geometric assumptions about the circular shape of the short-axis view, are affected by the foreshortening of the apical four-chamber view, and by the uncertain position of the transversal axis in the apical view, though they are more robust in distorted LV with wall motion abnormalities. Not surprisingly, the normal ranges obtained using these techniques are more widely distributed compared to values obtained using CMR (Table 6.1).

Theoretically, 3DE avoids these limitations and has multiple advantages for the measurement of LV mass. There are two methods for measuring LV mass using 3DE: the 3DE guided 2DE biplane method of disk and the 3DE border tracing method. With the latter, LV mass is calculated by subtracting the 3DE endocardial volume from the epicardial one to obtain the myocardial volume that is multiplied by the myocardial specific gravity (1.05 g/mL) to calculate the LV mass (Fig. 6.3).

Although both 3DE methods have been demonstrated to be accurate for LV mass measurements against CMR [20, 21], the former has still the limitation of geometric assumption, whereas the latter often requires laborious and time consuming manual editing of both endocardial and epicardial borders, which precludes its widespread clinical use. Thus, normal reference values for 3DE LV mass across a wide range of ages have not been provided in recent guidelines due to the paucity of studies reporting normal values [22–24]. Currently, 3DE quantification software for LV mass has becomes more user-friendly (Fig. 6.4). To date only three studies have provided normal ranges of LV mass using 3D echocardiography [24–26]. Interestingly, in these studies the

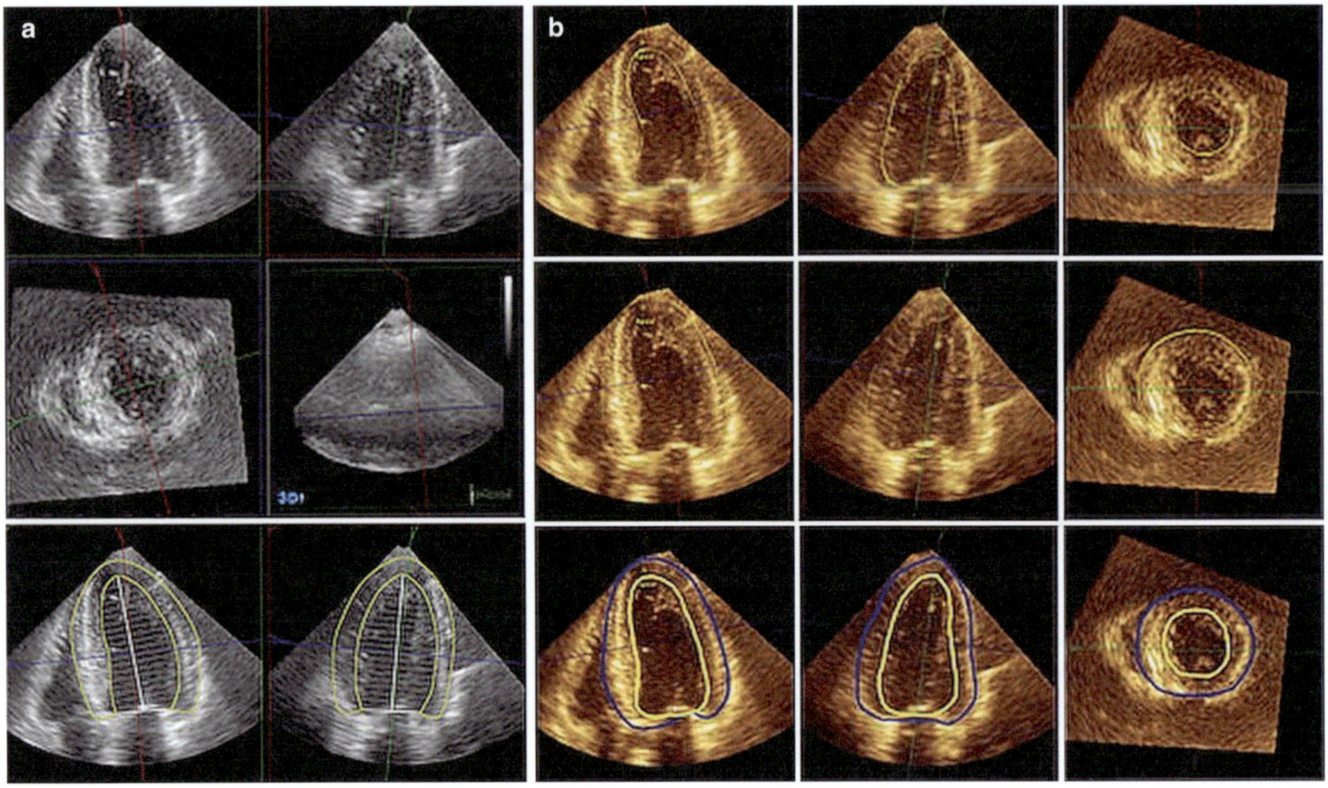

Fig. 6.3 Left ventricular mass measurements using three-dimensional echocardiography (3DE). (**a**) 3DE guided two-dimensional biplane method of disks' summation. After extracting two orthogonal two-dimensional left ventricular long axis views from the 3DE full volume datasets, the user traces the endocardial and epicardial border. The software measures endocardial and epicardial volumes using the biplane method of disks' summation. LV mass is measured by substracting the LV epicardial volume from the LV endocardial volume and multiplying this number by the specific muscle mass gravity (1.05). (**b**) Subtraction of 3D determined epicardial and endocardial volume method. LV epicardial border and endocardial border are manually determined in 3D space, and both epicardial and endocardial volume are obtained. LV mass is determined by substracting (LV epicardial volume − LV endocardial volume) × myocardial specific gravity (1.05)

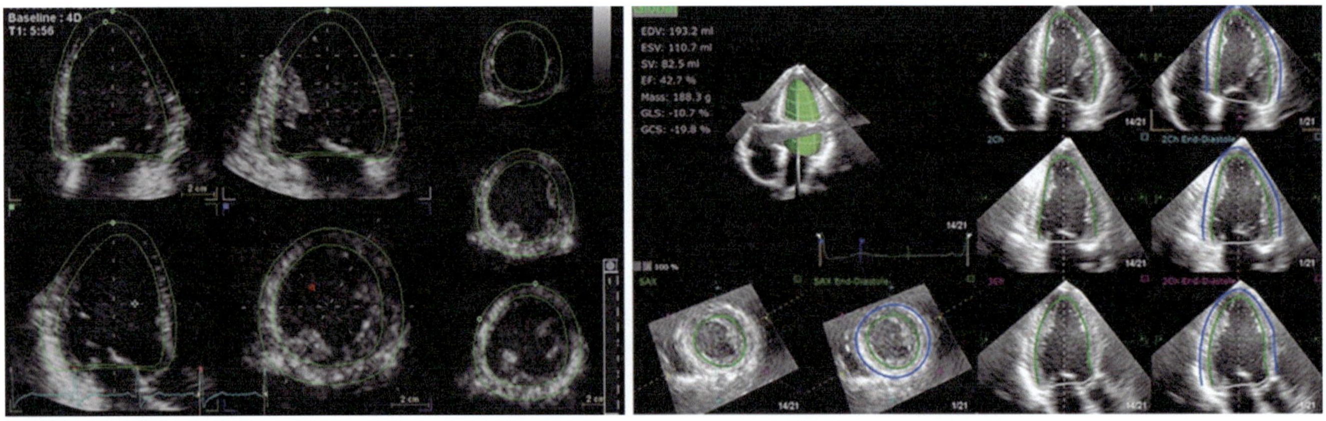

Fig. 6.4 Left ventricular mass measurements with novel software packages: *left panel*, 4D AutoLVQ (GE Vingmed, Horten, NO); *right panel*, 4D LV function (TomTec Imaging Systems, Unterschleissen, D). Apical four-chamber, two-chamber and long-axis views and a number of short-axis views at end-diastole are automatically extracted from the 3DE dataset. Non-foreshortened apical views are identified by initializing the LV apex and the center of the mitral annular plane at end-diastole, and then connecting both sides of the mitral annulus with the largest LV long-axis dimensions. Subsequently, the LV endocardial surface will be automatically identified (green line). Manual adjustments of the endocardial surface will be performed when necessary using both longitudinal and transversal views. Subsequently, the software packages delineate the epicardial surface in a similar way on the same frame. LV mass is calculated as: (LV epicardial volume − LV endocardial volume) × 1.05

normal ranges reported for 3DE are narrower than those from 2DE, and similar to CMR values. Despite the fact that 3DE has been recommended to measure LV mass by echocardiography, particularly in abnormally shaped ventricle or in individuals with asymmetric or localized hypertrophy [25], whether the use of 3DE cut-off values for LV mass index would provide more clinically useful prognostic information compared to traditional methods should be determined in the future studies.

Left Ventricular Shape

LV volume, ejection fraction and mass do not completely characterize the left ventricle. Another important determinant of LV performance is its shape. There are many ways to describe LV shape. Probably, the best known and simplest method is the sphericity index. On two-dimensional echocardiography, the sphericity index has been defined as the short to long-axis dimension ratio in the end-diastolic apical four-chamber view [26]. Unlike two-dimensional echocardiography, which is limited to flat tomographic planes, 3DE can yield volumes to more accurately quantify sphericity. With 3DE, LV shape is defined by how different the shape of the ventricle is from a sphere, with a perfect spherical ventricle having a value of 1.0. While the concept of 3DE sphericity had already been applied to the LV using data acquired form cardiac angiography [27], the use of 3DE to describe this parameter is fairly recent [28–30]. Mannaerts et al. [30] were the first to define the use of the 3DE derived sphericity index. This index was defined as the ratio between the actual LV volume and the volume of a sphere with a diameter equal to the length of the LV long axis (Fig. 6.5).

$$\text{Sphericity Index} = \text{LV EDV} / \left[4/3 \times \pi \times \left(L/2 \right)^3 \right]$$

where: EDV is the LV end-diastolic volume and L is the LV end-diastolic major long axis obtained from two-dimensional echocardiography or the longest distance between the center of the mitral annulus and the endocardial apex as extracted from the 3DE LV dataset.

LV sphericity, measured using 3DE, has been used to describe LV remodeling after myocardial infarction and pre- and post-mitral valve surgery [30, 31]. It has been demonstrated that patients with dilated cardiomyopathy who have more spherical ventricles have worse prognosis [32]. A recent study reported age-related changes in LV sphericity index [33]. Another study suggested that circumferential contractility is important in the preservation of LV shape by showing that circumferential LV strain rate deterioration correlates with LV remodeling [34].

The sphericity index, however, is a relatively crude index, as it is associated with global changes in LV shape and does not take into account regional differences. The latter have been shown to be clinically significant. For instance, regional shape changes at the apex often precede global LV dilation [35]. It has been shown that LV chambers that dilate globally after a myocardial infarction and have a high sphericity index

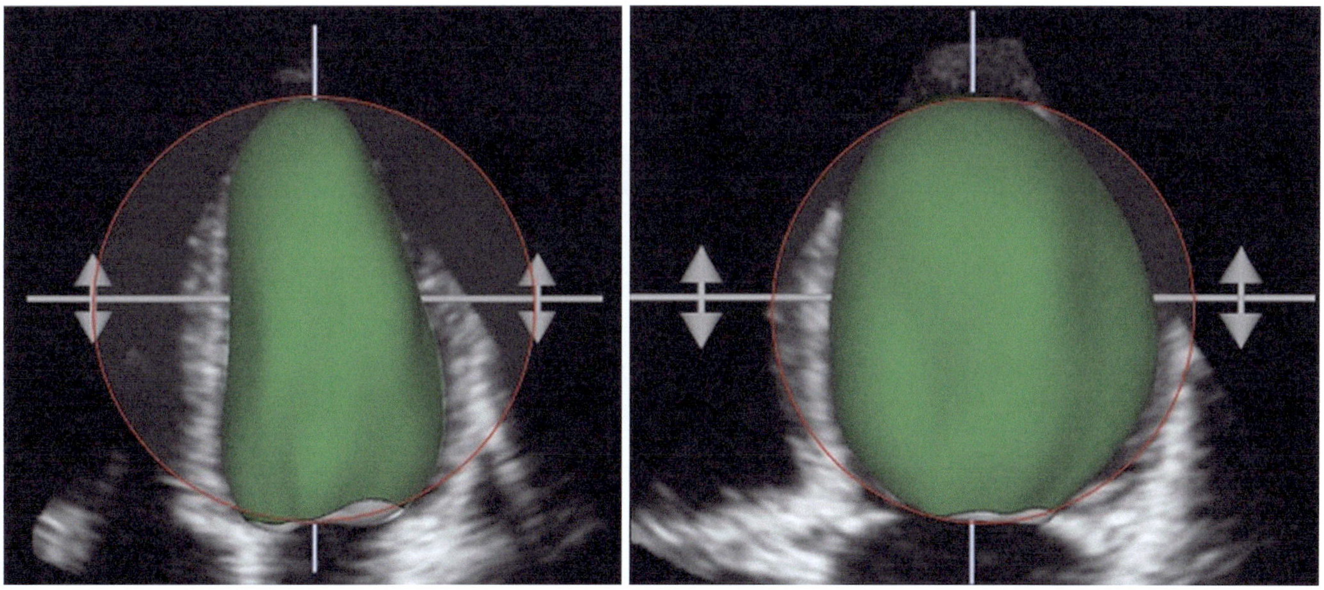

Normal heart

Dilated Cardiomyopathy

Fig. 6.5 The sphericity index indicates how close the left ventricular (LV) cavity approximates a sphere. Sphericity is computed as a ratio between actual LV volume and the volume of a sphere whose diameter is the LV long-axis length. The normal left ventricle on the left is elongated with a shape of a bullet. The left ventricle of a patient with dilated cardiomyopathy on the right is more rounded and closer to a spherical geometry tend to have more severe mitral regurgitation than LV chambers in which dilation is confined to the apex (a high apical conicity index without increased sphericity). This means that it is the dilation of the basal and mid segments that play the biggest role in functional ischemic mitral regurgitation.

Alternative approaches to characterize LV shape do exist. Curvature is one of these [36]. Curvature is defined as the amount by which a surface deviates from being flat. Numerically, it is the reciprocal of the radius of a circle that tangentially fits the curved surface of interest. A large radius represents a small curvature (flatter region) while a small radius represents a larger curvature (a more round or convex region) (Fig. 6.6). Normal values of LV ellipsoidal, spherical and conical indices and their change from diastole to systole have been reported [29]. The LV becomes more conical and less spherical at end-systole when compared to end-diastole. Regional curvature analysis of 3DE datasets of the LV has been used to describe regional LV remodeling. Patients with dilated cardiomyopathy had significantly smaller curvature values, indicating rounder global LV shape throughout the cardiac cycle [36]. Regional analysis also identified a loss of septal and apical curvatures in these patients. Systolic apical mean curvature correlated highly with LV ejection fraction (r = 0.89).

Left Ventricular Myocardial Mechanics

2DE strain acquired with speckle tracking analysis has rapidly become the most useful clinical research tool to quantify cardiac chamber mechanics [37]. Among the different 2DE strain and strain rate parameters, global longitudinal strain is the most robust and useful for identifying latent LV dysfunction in patients receiving potentially cardiotoxic drugs and for predicting prognosis in different clinical scenarios [38]. However, global 2DE strain values are traditionally derived from the three standard apical views which only include a little amount of LV myocardium (Fig. 6.7). Moreover, during systole, the basal LV myocardium moves toward the apex while rotating clockwise whereas the apical myocardium rotates counterclockwise. Thus, due to this complex myocardial motion speckles may move in and out from a fixed and thin cross-sectional 2DE view resulting in the potential for

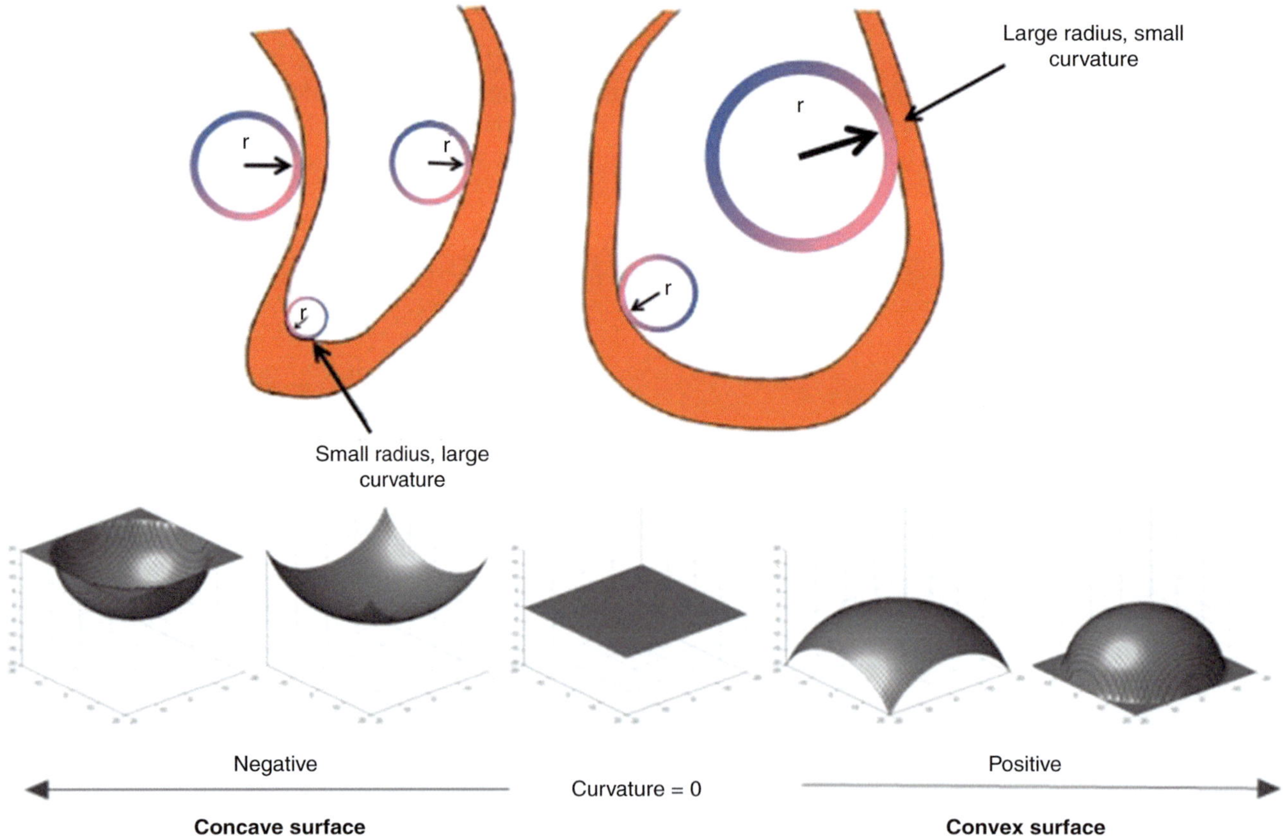

Fig. 6.6 Curvature is numerically quantified as the reciprocal of the radius of a circle that tangentially fits the curved surface of interest (see various circles positioned against the walls shown). A large radius represents a small curvature (flatter region) while a small radius represents a larger curvature (a more convex region). A concave surface is describes with a negative curvature. A flat surface has zero curvature and a convex surface has a positive curvature

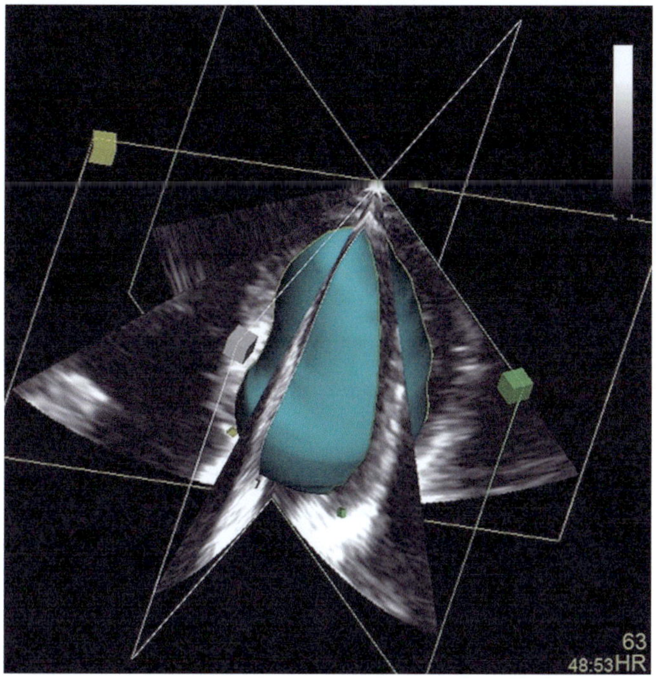

Fig. 6.7 The relationship between the amount of left ventricular (LV) myocardium encompassed by the three two-dimensional views used to measure global LV longitudinal strain by 2D speckle tracking and the large amount of myocardium (blue surface of the beutel) which is not evaluated by 2D speckle tracking echocardiography

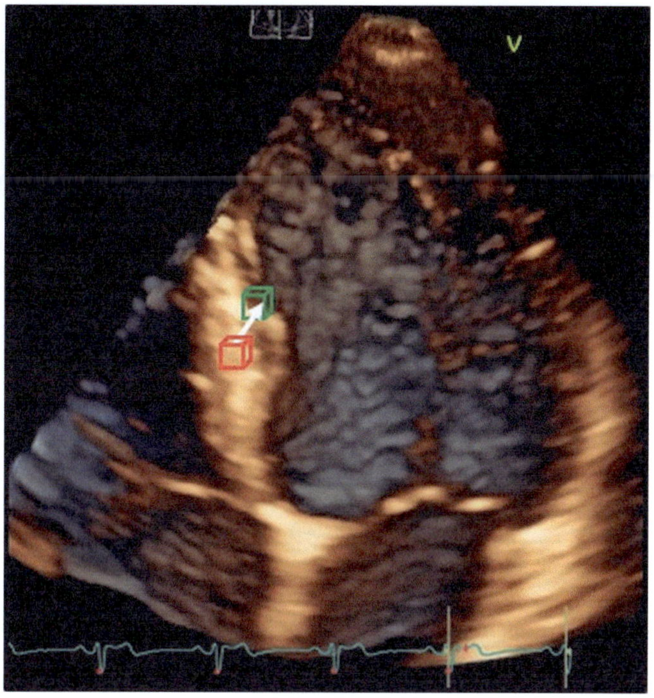

Fig. 6.8 The principle of "block-matching" used for three-dimensional speckle tracking. A specific 3D patterns of natural acoustic markers are tracked from end-diastole (red cube) to end-systole (green cube)

measurement errors [39, 40]. Although more complex, current computer technology has enabled 3DE speckle tracking analysis which has the potential to eliminate some of the aforementioned limitations of 2DE speckle tracking technique [41, 42].

2DE speckle tracking technique is based on the presence of distinctive patterns of gray scale values within the ultrasound images of myocardial tissue due to constructive and destructive interference of reflections from the individual myocardial scatterers (reflections occurring at transition between different tissue densities). These natural acustic markers are commonly referred to as "speckles". The speckles included within a spatial unit (kernel) are arranged in distinct patterns which are unique for each kernel within the ultrasound image [43], serving as a unique target that can be tracked frame-by-frame during the cardiac cycle by the 2DE speckle tracking algorithm [39, 44]. 2DE speckle tracking technique relies on the assumption that speckles are moving linearly within the scan plane of the 2DE image in consecutive frames of the same cardiac cycle. However, due to the different spatial orientation of myocardial fibers in the various layers of LV wall, LV mechanics is more complex and myocardial deformation involves a combination of apex-to-base shortening and thickening with simultaneous clockwise rotation of base and counterclockwise rotation of the apex [45, 46]. Accordingly, speckles have a complex motion in the 3D space, and thus are subject to through-plane motion from the 2DE scan planes during the cardiac cycle. Recent developments of ultrasound transducer technology have allowed the possibility of 3DE imaging of the LV with relatively high spatial and temporal resolution, thus allowing 3DE strain measurements which have the potential to eliminate some of the aforementioned limitations of 2DE speckle tracking technique.

The post-processing of the 3DE data set to measure the different myocardial strain components starts with the automatic generation of a region of interest (ROI) from an endocardial and an epicardial border traces, followed by the automated segmentation of the LV into a 17-segment model. Each ROI contains cubes with specific 3D patterns of natural acoustic markers that are matched and searched through the cardiac cycle by the 3DE speckle tracking algorithm, a process called "block matching" (Fig. 6.8). The 3DE speckle tracking algorithm calculates the quality of each match, identifies any outliers and removes them before performing the weighted spatial averaging of the results. The results are mapped to an average myocardial mesh, so that the shape of the mesh model of the LV can be updated for all frames. Finally, quantitative results of LV deformation are derived from this mesh model (Fig. 6.9). Since the blocks are tracked in a 3D volume, they can be followed in any direction thus avoiding the out-of-plane motion of the speckles. Furthermore, 3DE speckle tracking is a time saving

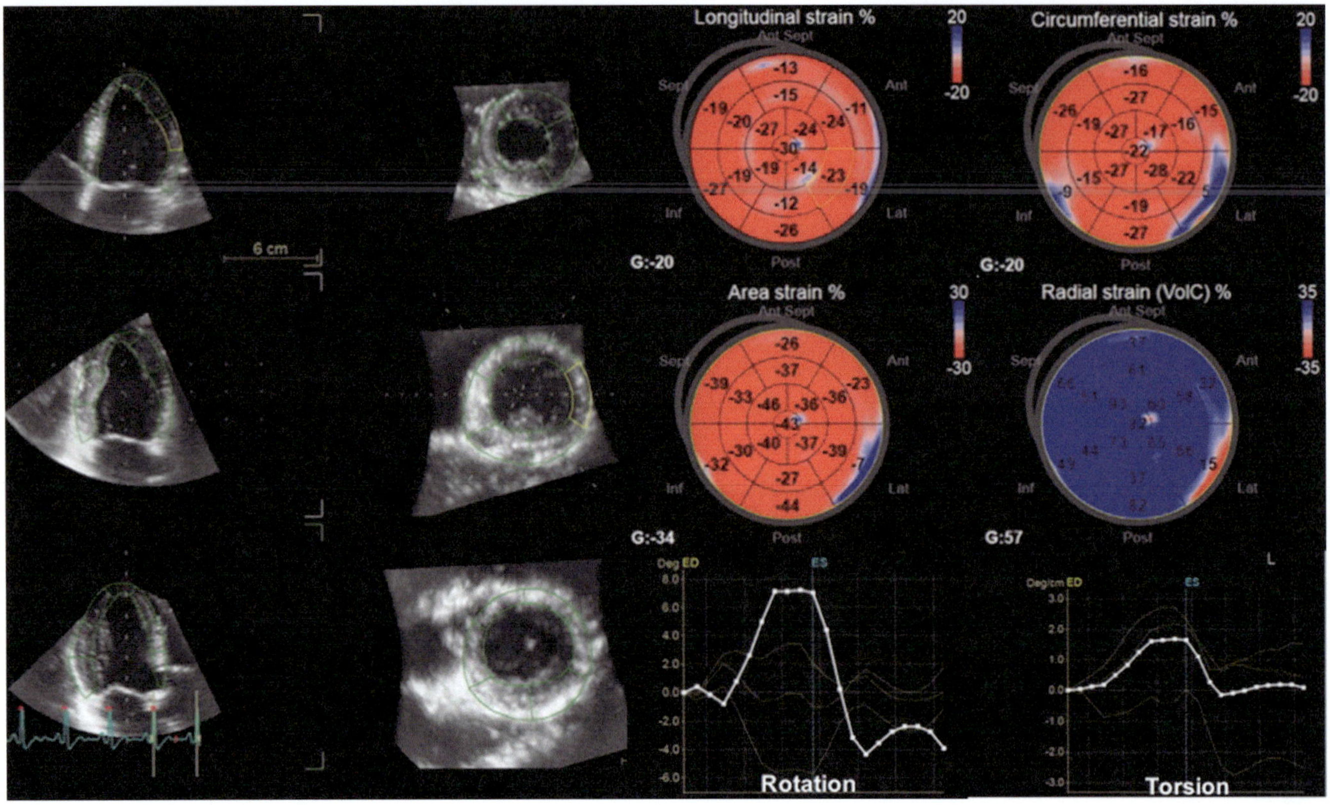

Fig. 6.9 Analysis of left ventricular mechanics with three-dimensional echocardiography speckle tracking technique. A region of interest encompassing left ventricular myocardium is delineated using a series of longitudinal and transversal cut planes obtained from a full volume data set of the left ventricle with a temporal resolution of about 30–40 vps (left panel, green borders). Then the software uses the block matching procedure to measure longitudinal, circumferential, area, and radial strain plus twist and torsion

technique, as it allows the measurement of all myocardial deformation components of the LV from a single volumetric data set of the left ventricle (Fig. 6.9) and avoids errors caused by heart rate variability that may occur when multiple acquisitions from different acoustic windows are needed as with two-dimensional echocardiography speckle tracking [47, 48]. Table 6.2 summarizes the main differences between two- and 3DE speckle-tracking.

Anatomy of Left Ventricular Wall and 3D Mechanic of Myocardial Deformation

Knowledge of the anatomical structure of the LV myocardial wall is key to understand and interpret 3D mechanics of myocardial deformation in clinical practice. LV myocardial fibers are oriented in a right-handed helix in the subendocardial layer of LV wall and a left-handed helix in the subepicardial layer, with circumferential fibers lying between the two. This complex anatomical structure of the myocardium in the LV wall explains the different patterns of myocardial deformation. According to a simplified model of myocardial mechanics, during systole the LV reduces the longitudinal and circumferential dimensions and twists along its long axis, while its wall thickens (radial dimension). Strain is a measure of the deformation that occurs in a myocardial segment at any time during the cardiac cycle in relation to its original dimensions and it is expressed as a percentage. Thus, a negative strain is the expression of the decrease in that dimension (i.e., shortening or thinning) and positive strain describes the increase in that dimension (e.g., lengthening or thickening) compared to its initial length (Fig. 6.9). Strain-rate is a measure of the velocity at which myocardial deformation occurs and it is expressed in seconds^{-1}. In addition, LV mechanics is also characterized by twist. Since mechanical activation occurs first in the subendocardium (right-handed helix), during isovolumic contraction, the base and the apex of the LV rotate in an anticlockwise direction. During the ejection phase, the apex rotates anti-clockwise whereas the base has a clockwise rotation due to the activation of the subepicardial left-handed helix [45, 46]. During isovolumic relaxation, the cardiac apex untwists by a clockwise rotation, generating active intraventricular suction forces that promote LV rapid filling [49]. Rotation refers to the change of the angle measured on a transverse LV plane and is expressed in degrees. Positive values represent anticlockwise rotation (as viewed from the apex), while negative values are used for clockwise rotation. Twist refers to the

Table 6.2 Comparison between the characteristics of two-dimensional and three-dimensional echocardiography speckle-tracking analysis

Characteristic	2DE strain	3DE strain
Acquisition	Three apical and three parasternal short-axis views	Single apical full volume of the left ventricle
Rhythm	Regular (2D views acquired in sequence)	Regular (multi-beat full-volume acquisition)
Temporal resolution	50–80 fps	30–40 vps
Feasibility in sinus rhythm	>90%	75–80%
Reliance on image quality	Very important	Critical
Myocardial deformation components	Longitudinal strain Circumferential strain Radial strain Ventricular twist Mechanical dispersion	Longitudinal strain Circumferential strain Radial strain Area strain Ventricular twist Ventricular torsion
Bull-eye map	Static (regional peak strain values)	Both static and dynamic
Global strain computation	Peak strain values	Either peak values or instantaneous strain values
Radial strain	Measured	Calculated by the law of volume conservation
Out-of-plane motion of speckles	Yes	No
Definition of end-systole	Timing of aortic valve closure	Timing of minimal left ventricular volume
Drift compensation	Yes	No

absolute difference of rotation between base and apex, and torsion is the ratio between LV twist and the length of the LV to allow comparability of LV twist among ventricles of different sizes.

Using 2DE speckle tracking analysis, all these parameters describing the mechanics of the left ventricle can be quantified (with the exception of LV torsion, because we do not know the actual distance between the apical and basal short axis views). However, to assess myocardial deformation by 2DE, the operator needs to acquire multiple views of the LV from different acoustic windows, at different times, with no precise anatomical landmarks for ensuring their proper position and orientation. Therefore, the use of 3DE strain is desirable. Since all of them can be obtained from a single data set, 3DE can avoid all these potential sources of error in a more time-efficient manner.

Normal Values of Three-Dimensional Left Ventricular Strain

Since strain values obtained with 2DE and 3DE speckle tracking analysis are different even when acquired in the same subjects [40], normal reference values for 3DE strain should be established before using this methodology clinically. Already, several studies have determined normal values of 3DE strain in a large number of healthy subjects over a wide range of ages. Kaku et al. [50] performed 3D speckle tracking analysis using vendor-independent software (4D LV function, TomTec Imaging Systems, Unterschleissen, Germany) in 313 healthy subjects. The mean values for global longitudinal, circumferential and radial strain were −20 ± 3%, −29 ± 5% and 88 ± 24%, respectively. A significant age-dependency, characterized by a reduction of strain value at the higher decades of life, was observed in global longitudinal strain. Muraru et al. [51] performed 3DE speckle tracking analysis using both vendor-specific software (4D AutoLVQ, GE Vingmed, Horten, Norway) and vendor-independent software (4D LV function, TomTec Imaging Systems, Unterschleissen, Germany) in 265 healthy subjects. The median values for global longitudinal, circumferential and radial strain with vendor-specific software were −19%, −18% and 52%, respectively. Corresponding value using vendor-independent software were −20%, −28% and 42%, respectively. Significant differences in all global strain values were noted between vendor-specific and vendor-independent software. Interestingly, when strain values obtained with vendor-independent software were compared between Kaku's study and Muraru's study, similar values for global longitudinal and circumferential strain were obtained. The large discrepancies between global radial strains are probably related to the inter-study differences in endocardial border tracing. Muraru also reported age-dependency of global longitudinal strain. These initial results clearly show that 3DE global longitudinal and circumferential strain are robust and reproducible parameters to quantify LV mechanics. However, the same software should be used in cross-sectional and longitudinal studies of the same patient, because the values are not interchangeable between vendor-specific software and vendor-independent software [52, 53].

Feasibility of Three-Dimensional Speckle-Tracking Echocardiography

The accuracy of 3DE speckle tracking largely depends on the quality of the LV data set, with sufficient temporal resolution (volume rate), which requires a sufficient amount of dedicated training and skill. These basic technical requirements may dramatically limit the feasibility of 3DE speckle tracking in the clinical routine [41]. Currently, the feasibility of 3DE speckle tracking in everyday practice is lower than the feasibility of 2DE speckle tracking. After excluding patients with irregular rhythm and unable to breathhold, the reported feasibility of 3DE speckle tracking in different studies ranges from 63 to 83% [47, 54], being lower than that for 2DE speckle tracking (80–97%) [55, 56]. Recently, we reported a feasibility of 3DE global longitudinal strain of 90% in a large cohort of healthy subjects [51], which was lower than the feasibility of 2DE global longitudinal strain (95%). As reported in other studies [57–59], LV basal segments are the most difficult to track by the 3DE speckle tracking software, because of their active excursion and their position in the far field, which adversely affects the spatial resolution of speckles.

Clinical Advantage of Three-Dimensional over Two-Dimensional Left Ventricular Strain

Only a few studies have reported the advantages of 3DE over 2DE strain measurement in the clinical setting.

Intraventricular Dyssynchrony

3DE speckle tracking provides comprehensive information of regional myocardial contraction patterns and has the potential for accurate LV dyssynchrony assessment and determination for optimal pacemaker lead position in patients requiring cardiac resynchronization therapy. Tanaka et al. [60] reported that time-domain color-coded 3DE radial strain of the left ventricle provided precise patterns of mechanical activation that were useful for the determination of optimal LV lead position in patients scheduled to undergo biventricular pacing (Fig. 6.10). The same group of authors demonstrated that 3DE speckle tracking analysis is also useful to compare mechanical activation patterns in patients with chronic right ventricular pacing and those with left bundle branch block [61]. Publications have also demonstrated that 3DE speckle tracking echocardiography clearly detects the improvement of both global strain values and LV mechanical dispersion from right ventricular pacing to biventricular pacing in patients with congestive heart failure [62]. All of these studies suggest that 3DE speckle tracking analysis is more useful than 2DE speckle tracking analysis to assess LV dyssynchrony in patients with optimal echocardiography image quality.

Prognostic Value

One of major advantages of 2DE strain, especially global longitudinal strain is that it provides useful prognostic information in various cardiovascular disease states. Myocardial contractile reserve is closely coupled to the severity of LV dysfunction and subsequent prognosis. Matsumoto et al. [63] performed two- and 3DE speckle tracking analysis at rest and during 20 mcg/kg/min of dobutamine infusion in patients with dilated cardiomyopathy, investigating which strain parameter was the best predictor of future events. They reported that an absolute increase in 3DE global circumferential strain change $\leq$2.7% from rest to dobutamine infusion is a best predictor for future adverse outcomes compared to 2DE global circumferential strain at rest or an increase in 2DE global circumferential strain from rest to dobutamine infusion. Multivariable analysis revealed that an increase in 3DE global circumferential strain was the only independent predictor of cardiovascular events. Thus, objective assessment of myocardial contractile reserve using 3DE global circumferential strain during dobutamine stress echocardiography appears to be the best method for predicting future adverse outcome in dilated cardiomyopathy.

There is growing interest in the identification of patients with asymptomatic severe aortic stenosis who are at high risk of developing symptoms and/or sudden cardiac death. In this regard, 2DE global longitudinal strain has demonstrated incremental prognostic value in patients with aortic stenosis [64, 65]. In a recent study involving 104 asymptomatic severe aortic stenosis patients with preserved LVEF, both 2DE and 3DE global longitudinal strain had significant predictive power for predicting future adverse cardiovascular events [66]. However, after correcting for other parameters, 3DE global longitudinal strain remained the only independent predictor of future adverse outcome using a multivariate analysis. Further studies are required to determine whether 3DE global longitudinal strain is superior to other emerging predictors, such as biomarkers or interstitial fibrosis assessed by CMR.

Three-Dimensional Echocardiography Evaluation of Myocardial Perfusion

It has been recognized for quite some time that assessment of perfusion by 2DE is limited by the specific planes used for assessment and these planes depend on the acquisition made at the time of the echocardiographic study. 3DE technology allows volumetric imaging and as such it offers an opportunity for improved perfusion assessment without the need for re-positioning of the probe to acquire multiple views. Previous studies have shown good agreement between location and extent of perfusion defects on contrast-enhanced 3DE and tissue staining in animal studies undergoing experimental coronary occlusion [67, 68]. Perfusion defects in contrast-enhanced 3DE datasets can be visualized as dark areas. Figure 6.11 shows a contrast-enhanced 3DE dataset obtained in a patient with left anterior descending coronary artery stenosis. The images were obtained after a stress agent (in this case adenosine). The apical myocardial wall is black illustrating the lack of contrast enhancement and the presence of a perfusion defect.

Quantitative analysis of regional myocardial contrast is not clinically performed but it has been done in experimental mod-

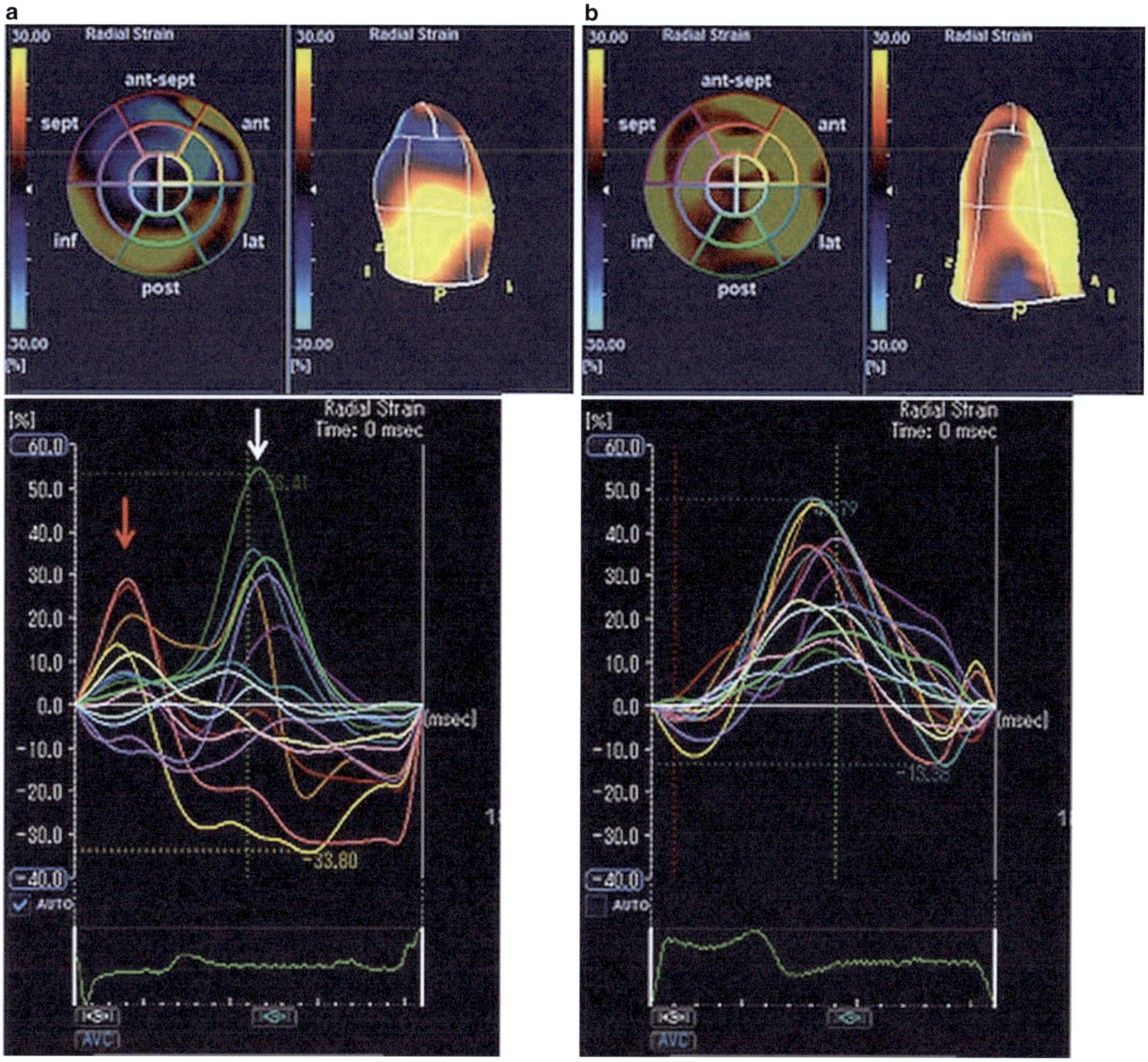

Fig. 6.10 Assessment of left ventricular dyssynchrony by 3D speckle tracking in a 64 year old patient with non-ischemic dilated cardiomyopathy and a QRS duration of 158 ms. (**a**) Before CRT therapy: Upper panels show the parametric map of left ventricular (LV) myocardial thickening (radial strain) with 16-segment model (left) and plastic bag model (right). Yellow color denotes myocardial thickening (positive radial strain), and blue color denotes myocardial thinning (negative radial strain). Both maps show 3D display of LV dyssynchrony (myocardial thickening of inferoposterolateral wall and thinning of interventricular septum). Lower panel shows radial strain curve in each of the 16 LV segments. There are two peaks. The earlier peak is characterized by wall thickening of the interventricular septum at early systole, whereas the late peak is characterized by wall thickening of the inferoposterolateral wall after aortic valve closure (AVC; vertical green dotted line). LV end-diastolic and end-systolic volume and ejection fraction were 203 mL, 131 mL and 29%, respectively. (**b**) After CRT therapy. Compared to (**a**), myocardial thickening was more homogeneous. Segmental strain curves also show that the time to peak strain is reached before AVC in the majority of segments, reflecting less dyssynchronous contraction. This is associated with reversed LV remodeling: end-diastolic and end-systolic volumes decreased (153 mL and 84 mL; respectively) and ejection fraction improved (45%). Courtesy of Dr. Hidekazu Tanaka, Kobe University Graduate School of Medicine, Japan

els. During the process, 3DE myocardial regions of interest are defined by segmenting the 3DE shell contained between the endo- and epicardial surfaces. Myocardial contrast enhancement curves can then be obtained from these 3DE segments by measuring beat-by-beat contrast intensity during a transition from no contrast to fully enhanced myocardium.

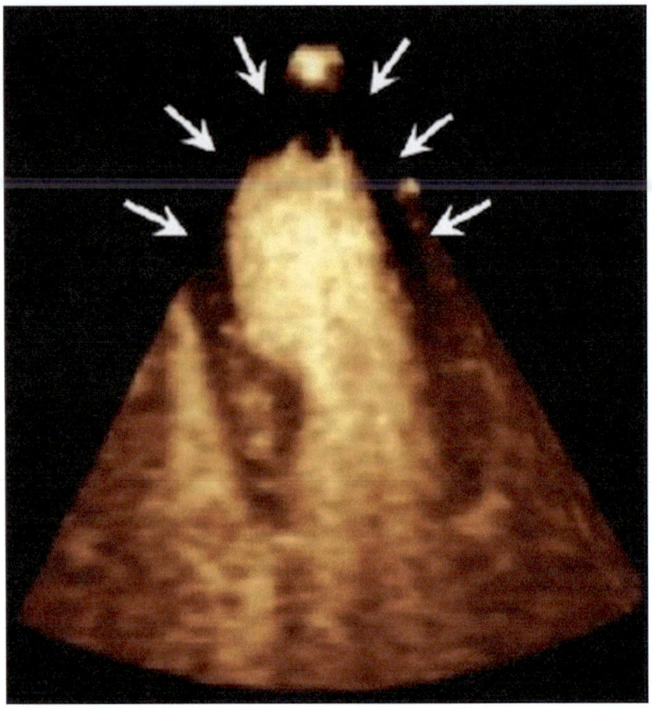

Fig. 6.11 Contrast-enhanced three-dimensional echocardiography dataset obtained in a patient with critical stenosis of the left anterior descendent coronary branch. The apex shows lack of contrast enhancement indicating a perfusion defect

Conclusions: Future Directions

Although the relationship between 3DE image quality and volume rate is a trade-off, the best situation for 3DE is one-beat acquisition with high volume rates and high temporal and spatial resolution imaging. Acquisition of good image quality 3D datasets requires expertise. However, the emerging role of fully automated analytical software is critical, because it allows on-line measurement of LV mechanical parameters on cart, but also eliminates inter-observer variability resulting in high reproducibility. 3DE determination of LV function has becoming increasingly important and relevant in daily clinical practice.

References

1. Jenkins C, Bricknell K, Chan J, Hanekom L, Marwick TH. Comparison of two- and three-dimensional echocardiography with sequential magnetic resonance imaging for evaluating left ventricular volume and ejection fraction over time in patients with healed myocardial infarction. Am J Cardiol. 2007;99:300–6.
2. Jenkins C, Bricknell K, Hanekom L, Marwick TH. Reproducibility and accuracy of echocardiographic measurements of left ventricular parameters using real-time three-dimensional echocardiography. J Am Coll Cardiol. 2004;44:878–86.
3. Muraru D, Badano LP, Piccoli G, et al. Validation of a novel automated border-detection algorithm for rapid and accurate quantitation of left ventricular volumes based on three-dimensional echocardiography. Eur J Echocardiogr. 2010;11:359–68.
4. Thavendiranathan P, Liu S, Verhaert D, et al. Feasibility, accuracy, and reproducibility of real-time full-volume 3D transthoracic echocardiography to measure LV volumes and systolic function: a fully automated endocardial contouring algorithm in sinus rhythm and atrial fibrillation. JACC Cardiovasc Imaging. 2012;5:239–51.
5. Chang S-A, Lee S-C, Kim E-Y, et al. Feasibility of single-beat full-volume capture real-time three-dimensional echocardiography and auto-contouring algorithm for quantification of left vnetricular volume: validation with cardiac magnetic resonance imaging. J Am Soc Echocardiogr. 2011;24:853–9.
6. Shibayama K, Watanabe H, Iguchi N, et al. Evaluation of automated measurement of left ventricular volume by novel real-time 3-dimensional echocardiographic system: validation with cardiac magnetic resonance imaging and 2-dimensional echocardiography. J Cardiol. 2013;61:281–8.
7. Nesser HJ, Mor-Avi V, Gorissen W, et al. Quantification of left ventricular volumes using three-dimensional speckle tracking: comparison with MRI. Eur Heart J. 2009;30:156–73.
8. Jacobs LD, Salgo IS, Goonewardena S, et al. Rapid online quantification of left ventricular volume from real-time three-dimensional echocardiographic data. Eur Heart J. 2006;27:460–8.
9. Shimada YJ, Shiota T. A meta-analysis and investigation for the source of bias of left ventricular volumes and function by three-dimensional echocardiography in comparison with magnetic resonance imaging. Am J Cardiol. 2011;107:126–38.
10. Dorosz JL, Lezotte DC, Weitzenkamp DA, Allen LA, Salcedo EE. Performance of 3-dimensional echocardiography in measuring left ventricular volumes and ejection fraction: a systematic review and meta-analysis. J Am Coll Cardiol. 2012;15(59):1799–808.
11. Mor-Avi V, Jenkins C, Kühl HP, et al. Real-time 3-dimensional echocardiographic quantification of left ventricular volumes: multicenter study for validation with magnetic resonance imaging and investigation of sources of error. J Am Coll Cardiol Img. 2008;1:413–23.
12. Macron L, Lim P, Bensaid A, et al. Single-beat versus miltibeat real-time 3D echocardiography for assessing left ventricular volumes and ejection fraction: a comparison study with cardiac magnetic resonance. Circ Cardiovasc Imaging. 2010;3:450–5.
13. Tsang W, Salgo IS, Medovedofsky D, et al. Real-time automated transthoracic three-dimensional echocardiographic left heart chamber quantification using an adaptive analytics algorithm. J Am Coll Cardiol Img. 2016;9:769–82.
14. Medvedofsky D, Mor-Avi V, Amzulescu M, et al. Three-dimensional echocardiographic quantification of the left heart chambers using an automated adaptive analytics algorithm: multicentre validation study. Eur Heart J Cardiovasc Imaging. 2018;19:47–58.
15. Mevedofsky D, Mor-Avi V, Byku I, et al. Three dimensional echocardiographic automated quantification of left heart chamber volumes using and adptive analytics algorithm: feasibility and impact of image quality in non selected patients. J Am Soc Echocardiogr. 2017;30:879–85.
16. Bluemke DA, Kronmal RA, Lima JAC, et al. The relationship of left ventricular mass and geometry to incident cardiovascular events: the mesa (multi-ethnic study of atherosclerosis) study. J Am Coll Cardiol. 2008;52:2148–55.
17. Armstrong AC, Gidding S, Gjesdal O, Wu C, Bluemke DA, Lima JAC. LV mass assessed by echocardiography and CMR, cardiovascular outcomes, and medical practice. J Am Coll Cardiol Img. 2012;5:837–48.
18. Lang RM, Badano LP, Mor-Avi V, et al. Recommendations for cardiac chamber quantification by echocardiography in adults: an update from the American Society of Echocardiography and the European Association of Cardiovascular Imaging. J Am Soc Echocardiogr. 2015;28:1–39.e14.

19. Devereaux RB, Alonso DR, Lutas EM, et al. Echocardiographic assessment of left ventricular hypertrophy: comparison to necropsy findings. Am J Cardiol. 1986;57:450–8.
20. Mor-Avi V, Sugeng L, Weinert L, et al. Fast measurement of left ventricular mass with real-time three-dimensional echocardiography: comparison with magnetic resonance imaging. Circulation. 2004;110:1814–8.
21. Takeuchi M, Nishikage T, Mor-Avi V, et al. Measurement of left ventricular mass by real-time three-dimensional echocardiography: validation against magnetic resonance and comparison with two-dimensional and m-mode measurements. J Am Soc Echocardiogr. 2008;21:1001–5.
22. Fukuda S, Watanabe H, Daimon M, et al. Normal values of real-time 3-dimensional echocardiographic parameters in a healthy Japanese population—the JAMP-3d study. Circ J. 2012;76:1177–81.
23. Mizukoshi K, Takeuchi M, Yasufumi N, et al. Normal values of left ventricular mass index assessed by transthoracic three-dimensional echocardiography. J Am Soc Echocardiogr. 2016;29:51–61.
24. Muraru D, Badano LP, Peluso D, et al. Comprehensive analysis of left ventricular geometry and function by three-dimensional echocardiography in healthy adults. J Am Soc Echocardiogr. 2013;26:618–28.
25. Marwick TH, Gillebert TC, Aurigemma G, et al. Recommendations on the use of echocardiography in adult hypertension: a report from the Eropean Association of Cardiovascular Imaging (EACVI) and the American Society of Echocardiography. J Am Soc Echocardiogr. 2015;28:727–54.
26. Chan SY, Mancini GB, O'Brien DW, Armstrong PW. Novel methodology for echocardiographic quantification of cardiac shape. Can J Cardiol. 1997;13:153–9.
27. Mitchell GF, Lamas GA, Vaughan DE, Pfeffer MA. Left ventricular remodeling in the year after first anterior myocardial infarction: a quantitative analysis of contractile segment lengths and ventricular shape. J Am Coll Cardiol. 1992;19:1136–44.
28. Maffessanti F, Lang RM, Corsi C, Mor-Avi V, Caiani EG. Feasibility of left ventricular shape analysis from transthoracic real-time 3-D echocardiographic images. Ultrasound Med Biol. 2009;35:1953–62.
29. Maffessanti F, Sugeng L, Takeuchi M, et al. Feasibility of regional and global left ventricular shape analysis from real-time 3d echocardiography. In: Conference proceedings: Annual International Conference of the IEEE Engineering in Medicine and Biology Society IEEE Engineering in Medicine and Biology Society Annual Conference; 2009. p. 3641–4.
30. Mannaerts HF, van der Heide JA, Kamp O, Stoel MG, Twisk J, Visser CA. Early identification of left ventricular remodelling after myocardial infarction, assessed by transthoracic 3D echocardiography. Eur Heart J. 2004;25:680–7.
31. Maffessanti F, Caiani EG, Tamborini G, et al. Serial changes in left ventricular shape following early mitral valve repair. Am J Cardiol. 2010;106:836–42.
32. Opie LH, Commerford PJ, Gersh BJ, Pfeffer MA. Controversies in ventricular remodelling. Lancet. 2006;367:356–67.
33. Kaku K, Takeuchi M, Otani K, et al. Age- and gender-dependency of left ventricular geometry assessed with real-time three-dimensional transthoracic echocardiography. J Am Soc Echocardiogr. 2011;24:541–7.
34. Hung CL, Verma A, Uno H, Shin SH, Bourgoun M, Hassanein AH, et al. Longitudinal and circumferential strain rate, left ventricular remodeling, and prognosis after myocardial infarction. J Am Coll Cardiol. 2010;56(22):1812–22.
35. Di Donato M, Dabic P, Castelvecchio S, et al. Left ventricular geometry in normal and post-anterior myocardial infarction patients: sphericity index and 'new' conicity index comparisons. Eur J Cardiothorac Surg. 2006;29(Suppl 1):S225–30.
36. Salgo IS, Tsang W, Ackerman W, et al. Geometric assessment of regional left ventricular remodeling by three-dimensional echocardiographic shape analysis correlates with left ventricular function. J Am Soc Echocardiogr. 2012;25:80–8.
37. Mor-Avi V, Lang RM, Badano LP, et al. Current and evolving echocardiographic techniques for the quantitative evaluation of cardiac mechanics: ASE/EAE consensus statement on methodology and indications endorsed by the Japanese Society of Echocardiography. J Am Soc Echocardiogr. 2011;24:277–313.
38. Plana JC, Galderisi M, Barac A, et al. Expert consensus for multimodality imaging evaluation of adult patients during and after cancer therapy: a report from the American Society of Echocardiography and the European Association of Cardiovascular Imaging. Eur Heart J Cardiovasc Imaging. 2014;15:1063–93.
39. Geyer H, Caracciolo G, Abe H, et al. Assessment of myocardial mechanics using speckle tracking echocardiography: fundamentals and clinical applications. J Am Soc Echocardiogr. 2010;23:351–69.
40. Wu VC-C, Takeuchi M, Otani K, et al. Effect of through-plane and twisting motion on left ventricular strain calculation: direct comparison between two-dimensional and three-dimensional speckle-tracking echocardiography. J Am Soc Echocardiogr. 2013;26:1274–81.e1274.
41. Jasaityte R, Heyde B, D'hooge J. Current state of three-dimensional myocardial strain estimation using echocardiography. J Am Soc Echocardiogr. 2013;26:15–28.
42. Muraru D, Niero A, Rodriguez-Zanella H, Cherata D, Badano L. Three-dimensional speckle-tracking echocardiography: benefits and limitations of integrating myocardial mechanics with three-dimensional imaging. Cardiovasc Diagn Ther. 2018;8:101–17.
43. Mondillo S, Galderisi M, Mele D, et al. Speckle-tracking echocardiography: a new technique for assessing myocardial function. J Ultrasound Med. 2011;30:71–83.
44. Blessberger H, Binder T. NON-invasive imaging: two dimensional speckle tracking echocardiography: basic principles. Heart. 2010;96:716–22.
45. Buckberg G, Hoffman JI, Mahajan A, et al. Cardiac mechanics revisited: the relationship of cardiac architecture to ventricular function. Circulation. 2008;118:2571–87.
46. Sengupta PP, Krishnamoorthy VK, Korinek J, et al. Left ventricular form and function revisited: applied translational science to cardiovascular ultrasound imaging. J Am Soc Echocardiogr. 2007;20:539–51.
47. Reant P, Barbot L, Touche C, et al. Evaluation of global left ventricular systolic function using three-dimensional echocardiography speckle-tracking strain parameters. J Am Soc Echocardiogr. 2012;25:68–79.
48. Pérez de Isla L, Balcones DV, Fernández-Golfín C, et al. Three-dimensional-wall motion tracking: a new and faster tool for myocardial strain assessment: comparison with two-dimensional-wall motion tracking. J Am Soc Echocardiogr. 2009;22:325–30.
49. Burns AT, La Gerche A, Prior DL, et al. Left ventricular untwisting is an important determinant of early diastolic function. JACC Cardiovasc Imaging. 2009;2:709–16.
50. Kaku K, Takeuchi M, Tsang W, et al. Age-related normal range of left ventricular strain and torsion using three-dimensional speckle-tracking echocardiography. J Am Soc Echocardiogr. 2014;7:55–64.
51. Muraru D, Cucchini U, Mihăilă S, et al. Left ventricular myocardial strain by three-dimensional speckle-tracking echocardiography in healthy subjects: reference values and analysis of their physiologic and technical determinants. J Am Soc Echocardiogr. 2014;27:858–71.
52. Gayat E, Ahmad H, Weinert L, Lang RM, Mor-Avi V. Reproducibility and inter-vendor variability of left ventricular deformation measurements by three-dimensional speckle-tracking echocardiography. J Am Soc Echocardiogr. 2011;24:878–85.

53. Badano LP, Cucchini U, Muraru D, Al Nono O, Sarais C, Iliceto S. Use of three-dimensional speckle tracking to assess left ventricular myocardial mechanics: inter-vendor consistency and reproducibility of strain measurements. Eur Heart J Cardiovasc Imaging. 2013;14:285–93.
54. Hayat D, Kloeckner M, Nahum J, et al. Comparison of real-time three-dimensional speckle tracking to magnetic resonance imaging in patients with coronary heart disease. Am J Cardiol. 2012;109:180–6.
55. Marwick TH, Leano RL, Brown J, et al. Myocardial strain measurement with 2-dimensional speckle-tracking echocardiography: definition of normal range. JACC Cardiovasc Imaging. 2009;2:80–4.
56. Leitman M, Lysyansky P, Sidenko S, et al. Two-dimensional strain-a novel software for real-time quantitative echocardiographic assessment of myocardial function. J Am Soc Echocardiogr. 2004;17:1021–9.
57. Elen A, Choi HF, Loeckx D, et al. Three-dimensional cardiac strain estimation using spatio-temporal elastic registration of ultrasound images: a feasibility study. IEEE Trans Med Imaging. 2008;27:1580–91.
58. Negishi K, Negishi T, Agler DA, et al. Role of temporal resolution in selection of the appropriate strain technique for evaluation of subclinical myocardial dysfunction. Echocardiography. 2012;29:334–9.
59. Jasaityte R, Heyde B, Ferferieva V, et al. Comparison of a new methodology for the assessment of 3D myocardial strain from volumetric ultrasound with 2D speckle tracking. Int J Cardiovasc Imaging. 2012;28:1049–60.
60. Tanaka H, Hara H, Saba S, Gorcsan J. Usefulness of three-dimensional speckle tracking strain to quantify dyssynchrony and the site of latest mechanical activation. Am J Cardiol. 2010;105:235–42.
61. Tanaka H, Hara H, Adelstein EC, Schwartzman D, Saba S, Gorcsan J. Comparative mechanical activation mapping of RV pacing to LBBB by 2D and 3D speckle tracking and association with response to resynchronization therapy. J Am Coll Cardiol Img. 2010;3:461–71.
62. Thebault C, Donal E, Bernard A, et al. Real-time three-dimensional speckle tracking echocardiography: a novel technique to quantify global left ventricular mechanical dyssynchrony. Eur J Echocardiogr. 2011;12:26–32.
63. Matsumoto K, Tanaka H, Kaneko A, et al. Contractile reserve assessed by three-dimensional global circumferential strain as a predictor of cardiovascular events in patients with idiopathic dilated cardiomyopathy. J Am Soc Echocardiogr. 2012;25:1299–308.
64. Kearney LG, Lu K, Ord M, et al. Global longitudinal strain is a strong independent predictor of all-cause mortality in patients with aortic stenosis. Eur Heart J. 2012;13:827–33.
65. Yingchoncharoen T, Gibby C, Rodriguez LL, Grimm RA, Marwick TH. Association of myocardial deformation with outcome in asymptomatic aortic stenosis with normal ejection fraction. Circ Cardiovasc Imaging. 2012;5:719–25.
66. Nagata Y, Takeuchi M, Wu VC-C, et al. Prognostic value of LV deformation parameters using 2D and 3D speckle-tracking echocardiography in asymptomatic patients with severe aortic stenosis and preserved LV ejection fraction. J Am Coll Cardiol Img. 2015;8:235–45.
67. Bae RY, Belohlavek M, Tanabe K, Greenleaf JF, Seward JB. Rapid three-dimensional myocardial contrast echocardiography: volumetric quantitation of nonperfused myocardium after intravenous contrast administration. Echocardiography. 1999;16:357–65.
68. Yao J, De Castro S, Delabays A, Masani N, Udelson JE, Pandian NG. Bulls-eye display and quantitation of myocardial perfusion defects using three-dimensional contrast echocardiography. Echocardiography. 2001;18:581–8.

The Normal Mitral Valve

7

Sorina Mihaila Baldea, Dragos Vinereanu, and Roberto M. Lang

Abstract

Accurate characterization of the normal anatomy and function of the mitral valve apparatus is key to understand the pathophysiology of mitral valve diseases. Echocardiography is the first-line imaging technique used for the assessment of the mitral valve morphology and function. During the last five decades, echocardiography has evolved from M-mode to two-dimensional, and then three-dimensional imaging, introducing a new era in the cardiovascular imaging. The use of newly matrix array transthoracic and transesophageal transducers bestowed unique possibilities to assess the mitral valve apparatus in all three or four-dimensions (including time), without the need of offline reconstruction. Heart imagers were able to obtain for the first time "en face" visualization of the mitral valve from the atrial perspective, as only the surgeons were previously able to see it, and to describe in detail the complex anatomy of the valvular and subvalvular apparatus.

This chapter summarizes the current status of the acquisition and display of the mitral valve using three-dimensional transthoracic and transesophageal echocardiography and describes the normal anatomy of the mitral valve apparatus components.

Electronic Supplementary Material The online version of this chapter (https://doi.org/10.1007/978-3-030-14032-8_7) contains supplementary material, which is available to authorized users.

S. M. Baldea (✉) · D. Vinereanu
The University of Medicine and Pharmacy "Carol Davila", Bucharest, Romania

Department of Cardiology, Emergency University Hospital Bucharest, Bucharest, Romania

R. M. Lang
Noninvasive Cardiac Imaging Laboratories, Department of Medicine/Section of Cardiology, University of Chicago Medical Center, Chicago, IL, USA
e-mail: rlang@bsd.uchicago.edu, rlang@medicine.bsd.uchicago.edu

Keywords

Normal mitral valve · Three-dimensional echocardiography · Transesophageal · Transthoracic Data set Acquisitions and display · Mitral annulus Chordae · Papillary muscles

Introduction

Echocardiography is the most useful imaging technique for the non-invasive assessment of heart valves. Routine use of two-dimensional and Doppler echocardiography has greatly enhanced our understanding of valve morphology and function. However, two-dimensional echocardiography is a tomographic imaging technique that essentially provides single cut-planes of the heart [1], thereby being limited in the assessment of complex valve structures. With two-dimensional echocardiography, mental reconstruction from several tomographic views is required to imagine the stereoscopic morphology of the heart valves (see Fig. 4.2, Chap. 4). The accuracy of such a mental reconstruction depends critically on the experience of the operator, how many times he/she has seen the actual mitral valve either in the anatomical theatre or in the operating room. Different echocardiographers with different experience may imagine the heart valves in different ways.

Recent advances in three-dimensional echocardiography (3DE) have allowed the introduction of this technology in the routine clinical practice [2]. The advent of real-time 3DE using the new matrix array transesophageal and transthoracic transducers has resulted in improved temporal and spatial resolution of data sets with the possibility of performing a qualitative and quantitative analysis of valve morphology and function from a single volume acquisition [3]. The unique benefit of 3DE is the realistic "en face" view of the mitral valve (MV), which can be viewed from the same perspective (atrial or "surgical" view) of the cardiac surgeon

L. P. Badano et al. (eds.), *Textbook of Three-Dimensional Echocardiography*, https://doi.org/10.1007/978-3-030-14032-8_7

operating when he/she opens the left atrium, with the added value of seeing it in the beating heart allowing the echocardiographers to display the functional anatomy of the MV that cannot be appreciated in the still heart in the operating room. This visualization enables a better assessment of MV morphology and valve disease mechanisms, particularly in patients with degenerative mitral regurgitation [1]. Therefore, 3DE plays an increasingly role in the management of patients with MV disease, both for the diagnosis and follow-up, and also for guiding therapeutic procedures.

The Normal Mitral Valve by Three-Dimensional Echocardiography

The MV is a complex and dynamic three-dimensional apparatus that allows normal left ventricular (LV) filling and left atrial emptying during LV diastole, and ensures a unidirectional heart pump function, by sealing the left atrium from the LV chamber during the LV systole.

The main components of the MV apparatus are the annulus, the leaflets, the chordae tendineae, and the papillary muscles (Fig. 7.1). The integrated and coordinate interplay between all these components is mandatory to ensure normal MV function avoiding both stenosis and regurgitation.

3DE is well suited for the assessment of the three-dimensional geometry and dynamics of MV apparatus. Transesophageal and transthoracic 3DE have been successfully used to describe MV morphology in different pathological settings [4–6], to quantify MV disease severity [7, 8], and to guide MV interventions [9–11].

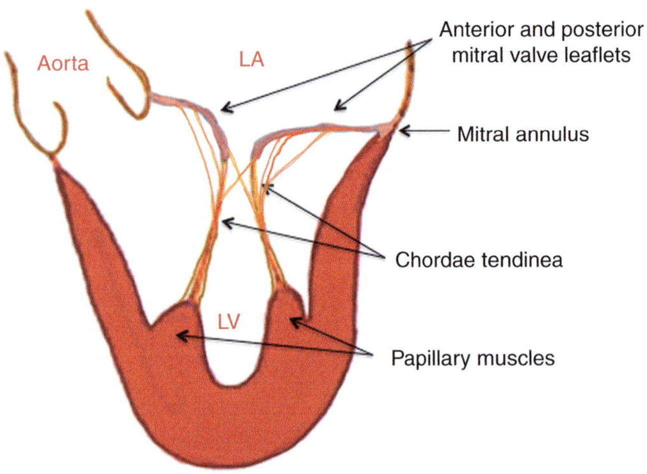

Fig. 7.1 Mitral valve apparatus components. Anterior and posterior mitral valve leaflets; mitral annulus, a fibrous ring at the juncture between the mitral leaflets, the left ventricle (LV) and the left atrium (LA); the chordae tendineae, attached to the valve and to the papillary muscles, sustaining the mitral valve leaflets when closed; the papillary muscles, which are inserted on the left ventricular (LV) wall and continue with the chordae tendineae

Acquisition of the Mitral Valve Apparatus Using Three-Dimensional Echocardiography

Several types of acquisition modalities have been used for the assessment of the MV apparatus using either transesophageal or transthoracic 3DE [12]. The availability of new transthoracic matrix-array transducers has allowed real-time volumetric imaging of the MV from the transthoracic approach [13], resulting in optimal visualization of both the MV leaflets, commissures, and MV orifice [14]. Dataset acquisitions for MV using transthoracic 3DE can be obtained either from the parasternal or the apical approach [12].

Transesophageal 3DE has a higher feasibility for the analysis of MV morphology when compared to the transthoracic approach [15]. Since the left atrium and the MV are the closest cardiac structures to the esophagus, transesophageal 3DE acquisition of the MV can be easily obtained from the mid-esophageal level. Improved temporal and spatial resolution of the volumetric acquisitions yields high quality data sets on which detailed morphological assessment of the mitral leaflets and annulus can be performed [16]. Transthoracic 3DE can also be a rapid, non-invasive and relatively feasible approach for assessing MV morphology [17]. Overall, the posterior mitral valve leaflet is best visualized from the parasternal window, while the anterior leaflet can be well seen from both apical and parasternal windows [18].

Multiplane Mode

The multiplane mode allows the visualization of the MV in two or more simultaneous tomographic planes recorded with either transthoracic or transesophageal 3DE. The reference plane is usually at 0° in the mid-esophageal four-chamber view of the LV, focusing on the MV, whereas the secondary pane is (by default) at 90° rotation from the reference plane (Fig. 7.2A). The operator may adjust the extent of the rotation of the secondary plane during acquisition as needed to optimize the view (see also Chap. 2). Tri-plane mode is also possible, with three different cut-planes of the MV acquired simultaneously at 0°, 60° and 120° by default. The two-dimensional cut-planes can also have color flow superimposed, in order to establish the relationship between the flow and the structural valve lesion (Fig. 7.2B).

Real-Time or Live 3DE

This modality is a volumetric acquisition that acquires beat by beat (single-beat acquisition), to ensure enough spatial and temporal resolution the pyramidal volume of acquisition is reduced by the operator. Data sets acquired in real-time usually have a suboptimal spatial and temporal resolution (depending

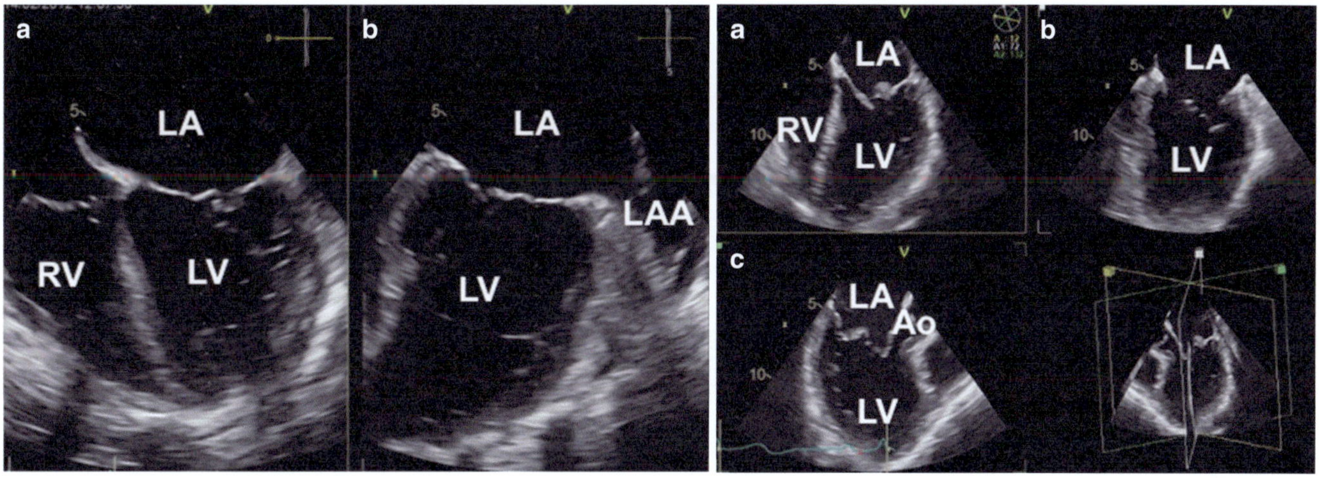

Fig. 7.2 Multiplane acquisition of the mitral valve. Biplane acquisition (*Left panel*). Two two-dimensional views of the mitral valve can be acquired from the same heart beat. The reference view is usually the four-chamber view (0° rotation, quad A) and the secondary view is at 90° (quad B), by default. However, both the reference view and the extent of the rotation at which to acquire the secondary view can be changed by the operator during acquisition only (see also Chap. 2). Triplane acquisition (*Right panel*), allowing three simultaneous views of the mitral valve at 0° (quad A), 60° (quad B) and 120° (quad C), respectively. *Ao* aorta, *LA* left atrium, *LAA* left atrial appendage, *LV* left ventricle, *RV* right ventricle

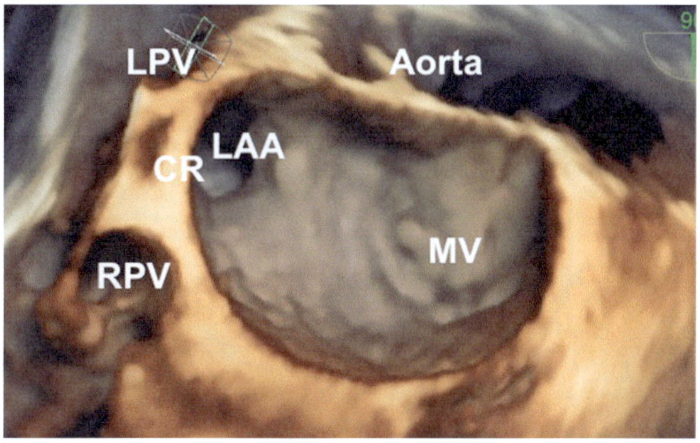

Fig. 7.3 Real time 3DE full-volume of the mitral valve and left atrial structures obtained using transesophageal echocardiography. This acquisition requires a single cardiac cycle for the acquisition of a pyramidal full-volume large enough to show the mitral valve (MV) from the atrial perspective and its anatomical relationships with the left atrial appendage (LAA), left (LPV), right pulmonary veins (RPV) and Coumadin ridge (CR). Despite the low temporal resolution (Video 7.1) of 5 vps, the quality of the data set allows precise assessment of the anatomy of the left atrial structures

on the size of the acquired volume). However, this modality allows the acquisition of 3DE data sets also in patients who cannot cooperate with breath holding and in those with irregular heart rhythm. The good quality of these images frequently allows the assessment of MV anatomy and the accurate diagnosis of complex MV pathologies (Fig. 7.3, Video 7.1).

3DE Zoom Mode

This acquisition modality permits a focused-wide sector view of the MV apparatus, including the MA, the chordae tendinea and the heads of papillary muscles (Fig. 7.4). Of note, by enlarging the region of interest, the temporal resolution of the image will decrease. However, this modality allows a complete visualization of the MV, which can be encompassed within the dataset (Fig. 7.5, Videos 7.2a and 7.2b).

Full-Volume Multibeat Acquisition

The full-volume mode has the largest acquisition sector possible (up to 90° × 90°), which is ideal for imaging all the components of the MV apparatus from a single dataset. Multislice display of the MV can be used to ensure that all mitral leaflets and annulus are contained within the pyramidal data set. Full-volume multi-beat acquisition is an ECG gated acquisition modality, which reconstructs the full-volume of the MV apparatus from four or six-triggered sub-volumes (Fig. 7.6, Videos 7.3a and 7.3b). The full-volume acquisition of the MV apparatus using the highest line density and maximum number of cardiac cycles should always be attempted when the rhythm is regular and the patient cooperates. The possibility of post-processing the full-volume data set using gain-adjustments and cropping it enables detailed en-face visualization of the MV leaflets, from both the left atrium and the LV perspective. The resultant images of the MV are similar to the ones acquired with the *zoom mode*, but with better image quality. Longitudinal cut-planes of the data set can be used to analyze the subvalvular MV apparatus, including chordae tendinea and the papillary muscles (Fig. 7.6, **right panel**). It has the advantage of providing optimal spatial and temporal resolution, which permits detailed diagnosis of complex MV pathologies [12]. However, this acquisition modality cannot be used

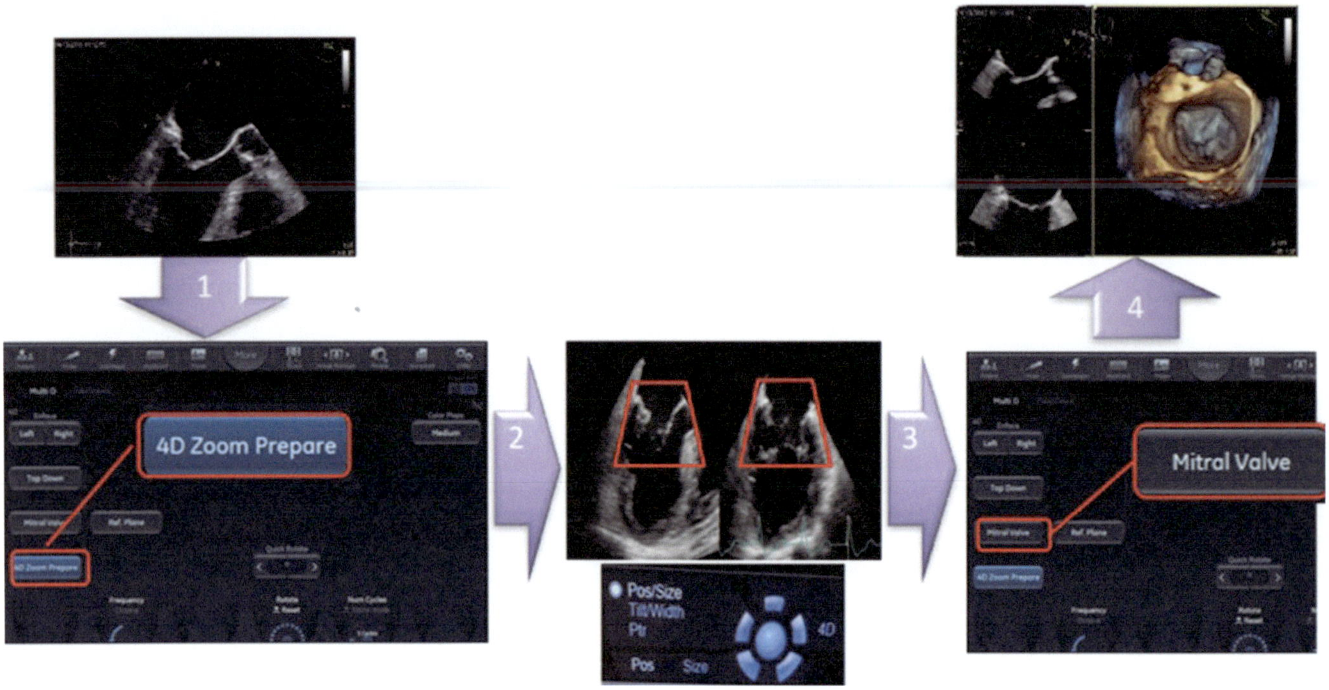

Fig. 7.4 Workflow to acquire the mitral valve apparatus using the zoom mode. Step 1. Obtain a proper two-dimensional view optimized for endocardial border visualization and encompassing the entire cardiac structure you want to visualize (e.g. mitral valve). Step 2. Position a region of interest (ROI, red trapezoids) of adequate size to include all cardiac structures of interest taking care that the structure of interests are included in the ROI bot in the azimuthal and elevation planes; Step 3. Acquire the 3DE data set using single- or multibeat acquisition; Step 4. Crop it as it is needed to show the structure of interest from the needed perspective (in the example, the mitral valve from the atrial perspective). The example shows the workflow used in Vivid E95 system (GE Vingmed, Horten, NO). However, the procedure is the same in any system. What changes are the buttons/knobs to control

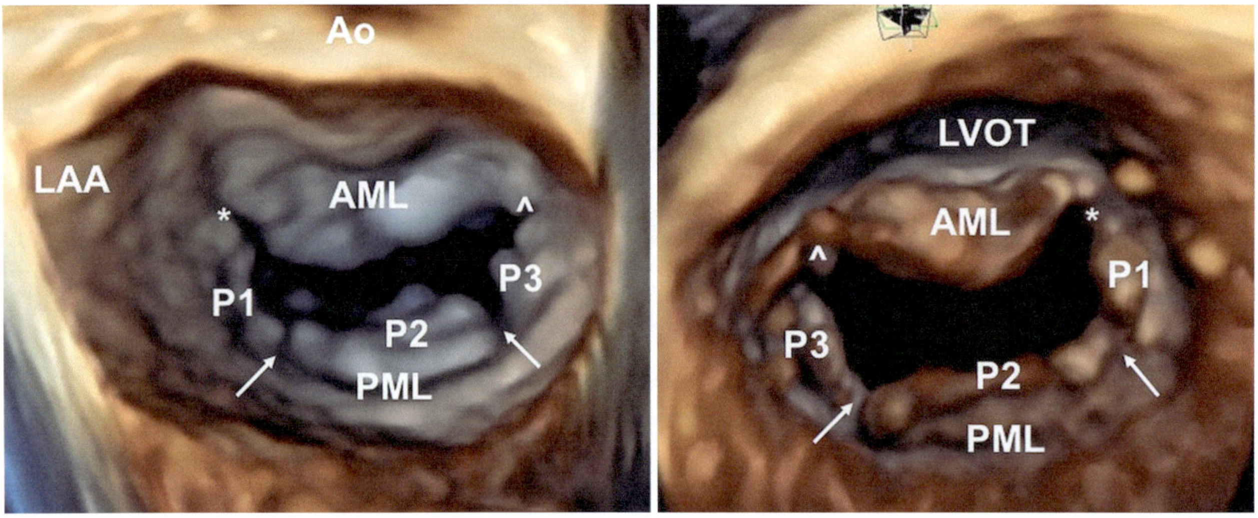

Fig. 7.5 Zoom mode acquisition of the mitral valve with transesophageal 3DE. *Left panel*, the mitral valve visualized from the left atrial perspective (so called "*surgical view*", see text) (Video 7.2a left). The anterior mitral leaflet (AML) is next to the aortic valve (Ao), positioned at 12 o'clock, while the posterior mitral leaflet (PML) is opposite to the aortic valve. The anterior-lateral (*) and posterior-medial (^) commissures are clearly seen. White arrows indicate the position of indentations (or pseudocleft) that subdivides the PML in three scallops (P1, P2, P3) which are listed starting from the left atrial appendage (LAA). *Right panel,* The mitral valve is visualized from the left ventricular perspective (Video 7.2b right). At 12 o'clock there is the left ventricular outflow tract (LVOT)

in patients with irregular rhythm or labored breathing, because of the occurrence of stitching artefacts. Color flow Doppler can also be acquired in this format to allow the visualization of mitral regurgitation jets (Fig. 7.7). It is recommended to also obtain a real-time 3DE data set at increased depth and focus from the mid-esophageal five-chamber view, to be able to visualize the sub-valvular apparatus and its relationship with the respective LV walls. Finally, a real-time or

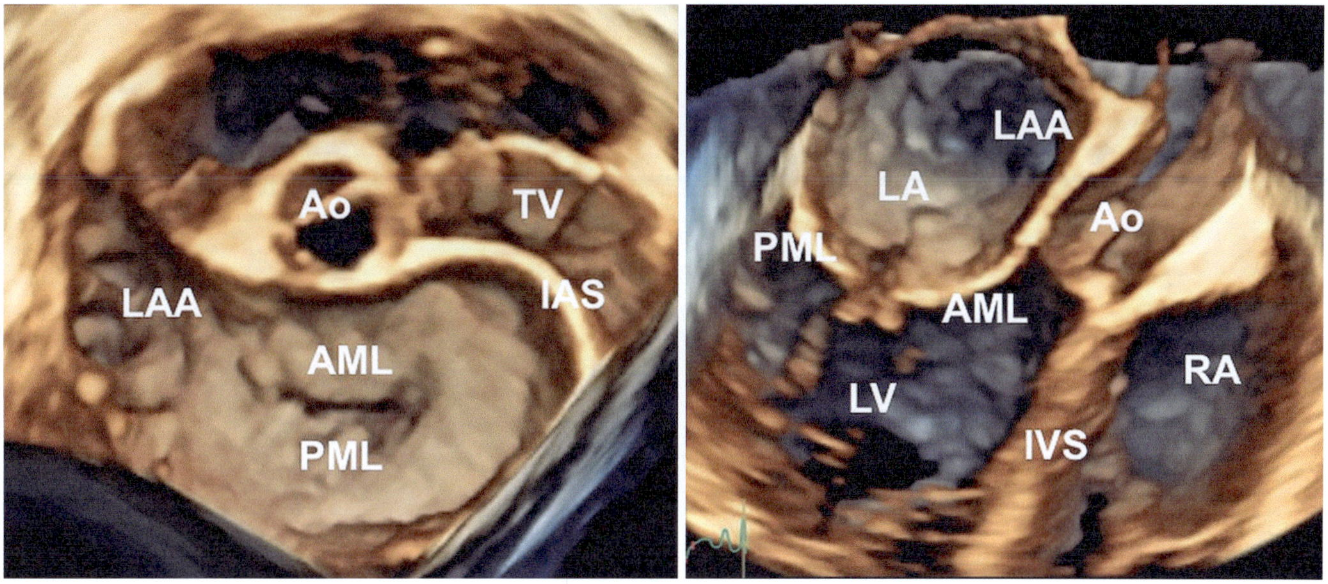

Fig. 7.6 Multi-beat ECG-gated acquisition allows to obtain a larger data set with adequate spatial and temporal resolution. The data set can be cropped in different ways to study the anatomical relationships of the mitral valve with adjacent cardiac structures. *Left panel*, transversal cut plane at the base of the heart (Video 7.3a Left). *Right panel*, Longitudinal cut plane at the center of aortic valve (Video 7.3b Right). *AML* anterior mitral leaflet, *Ao* aorta, *IAS* interatrial septum, *IVS* interventricular septum, *LA* left atrium, *LAA* left atrial appendage, *LV* left ventricle, *PML* posterior mitral leaflet, *RA* right atrium, *TV* tricuspid valve

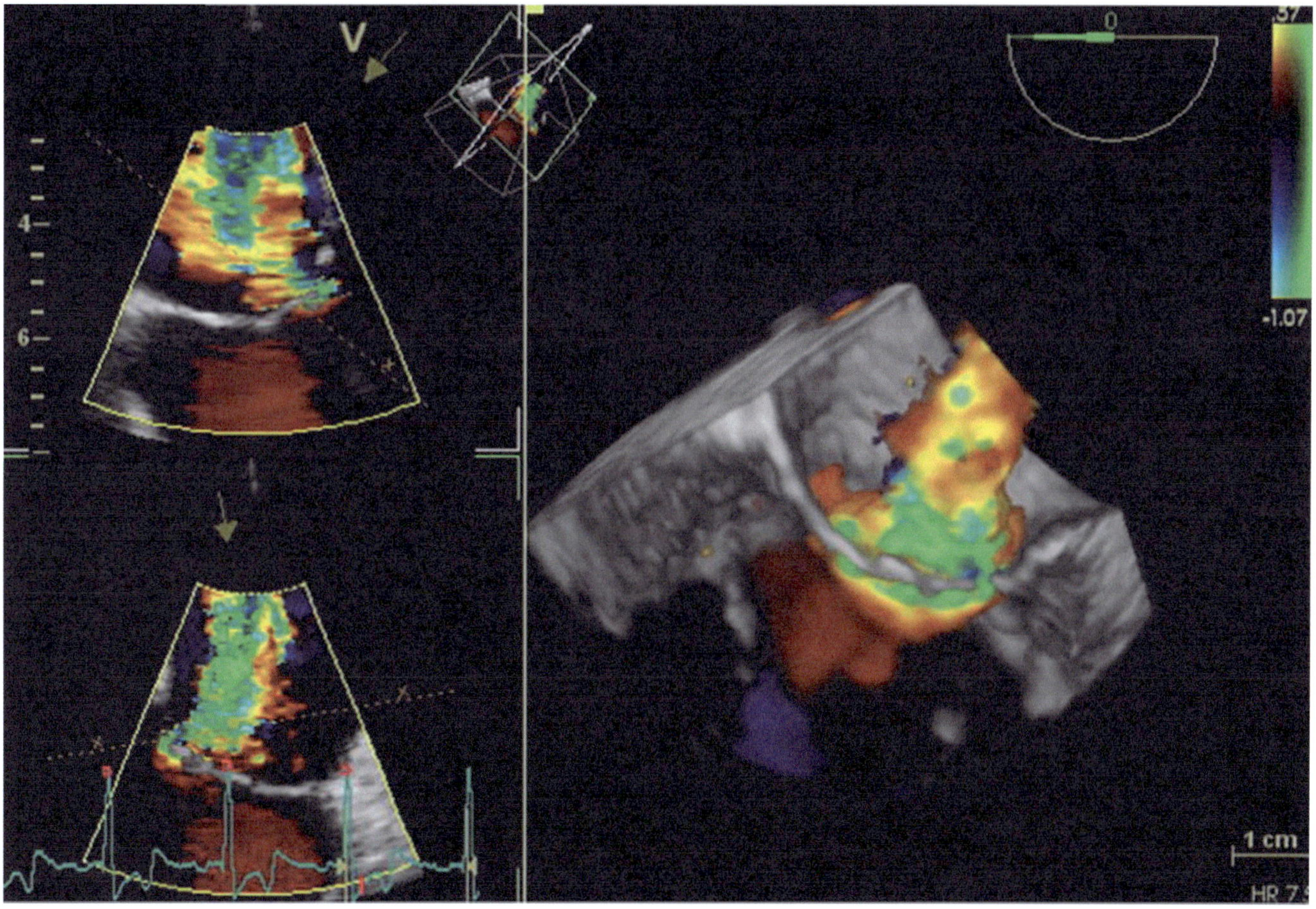

Fig. 7.7 Full-volume 3DE color acquisition of the mitral valve, showing a regurgitant jet into the left atrium Baseline color flow velocity has been shifted to see the flow-convergence of the jet

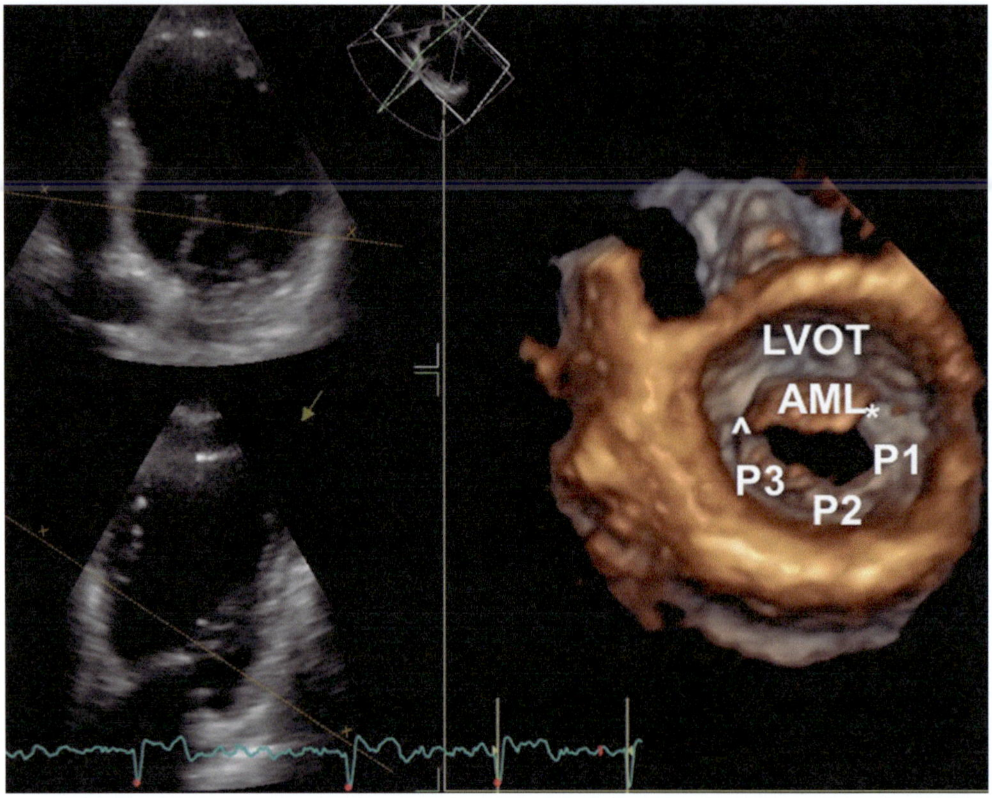

Fig. 7.8 Full-volume, multibeat 3DE transthoracic acquisition to visualize the mitral valve from the ventricular perspective (Video 7.4). *LVOT* left ventricular outflow tract, *AML* anterior mitral leaflet, *P1, P2, P3* scallops of posterior mitral leaflet

multibeat acquisition of the MV apparatus should be obtained from the transgastric approach, using the two-chamber view, to analyze the chordae and the papillary muscles [18].

Because of its high temporal and spatial resolution this acquisition methodology is also recommended to be used with the transthoracic approach (Fig. 7.8, Video 7.4), to visualize and quantitate the components of the MV apparatus.

Display and Analysis of the Acquired Datasets of Mitral Valve Apparatus

The Multiplane Display

3DE examination of the MV apparatus begins with a preliminary visualization using the multi-plane modality, in order to identify pathological segments, and thoroughly analyze the sub-valvular apparatus in the longitudinal axis (Fig. 7.2). The addition of color flow allows a matching of the structural lesion with the regurgitant jet (Fig. 7.9, Video 7.5).

Volumetric Display

The MV can be displayed *en face*, either from the left atrial (Fig. 7.5 **Left panel**) or from the LV perspective (Fig. 7.5 **Right panel**).

Abnormalities of papillary muscle and chordal attachments to the LV and MV surfaces can be also assessed using different oblique cut-planes of the data set (Fig. 7.6 **Right panel**).

From the volumetric data set several anatomically oriented cut planes can be obtained to explore in details the functional anatomy of selected regions of the MV apparatus or to perform quantitative analyses (e.g. distances, areas) (Fig. 7.10).

The Normal Anatomy of the Mitral Valve Apparatus and Particularities of the 3DE Acquisition and Display

Mitral Valve Leaflets

The MV has two leaflets that have different shapes and circumference length [19]. The anterior MV leaflet has a larger surface and a round free edge. It is attached to about one third of the MA circumference. The anterior MV leaflet connects with the aortic valve through a fibrous curtain, which is localized at the base of the anterior MV leaflet (*the aortic-mitral curtain*) [20]. The height of the posterior MV leaflet is less than the anterior leaflet, however, both leaflets have similar surface area because the posterior leaflet has a larger annular attachment (two-thirds of the MA circumference)

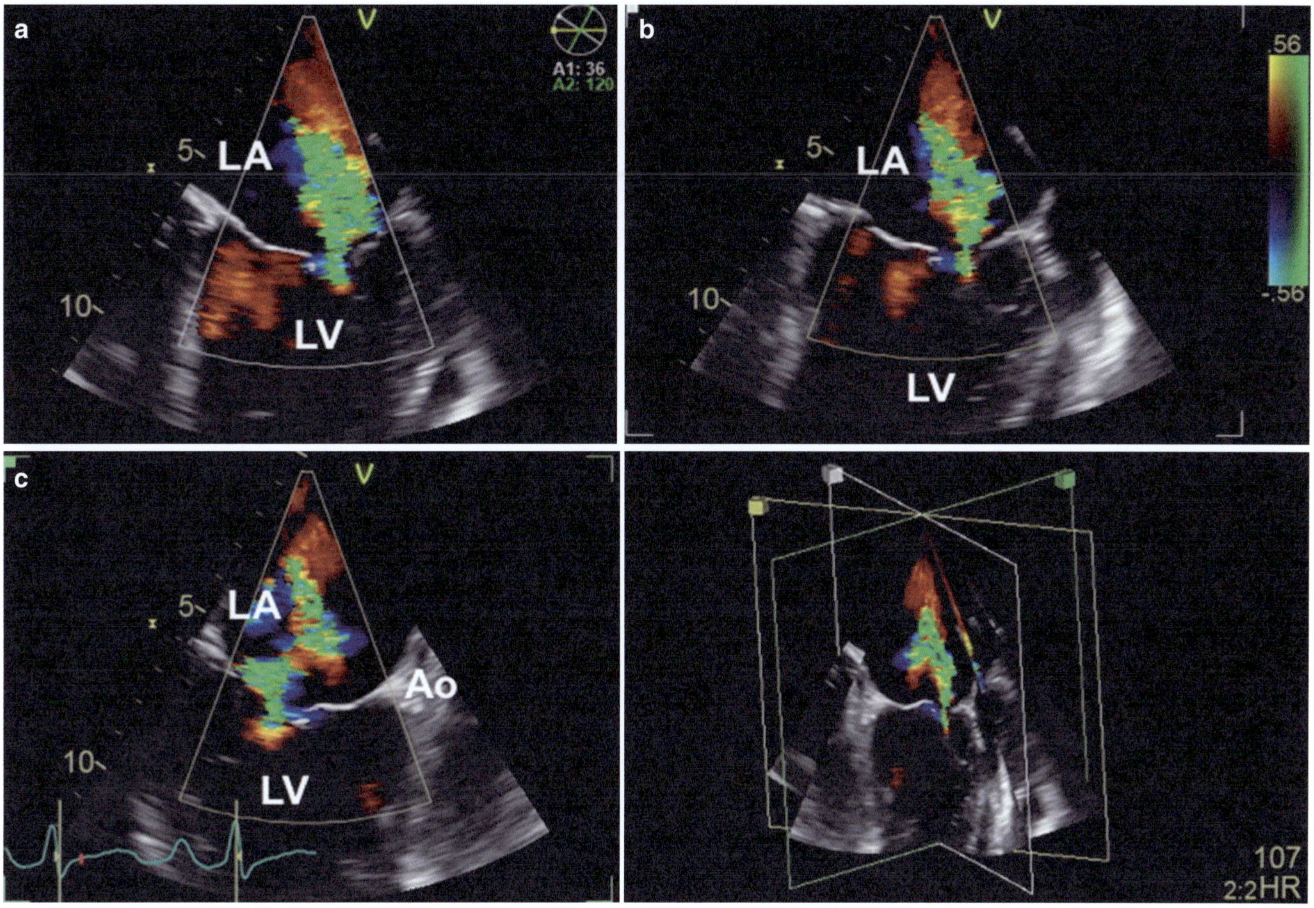

Fig. 7.9 Triplane acquisition (**a**, four-chamber view; **b**, two-chamber view; and **c**, apical long-axis view) of the regurgitant jet of a mitral valve from a single cardiac beat to visualize both the direction and extension of the jet in the left atrium (LA), and to measure the vena contracta size (Video 7.5). *Ao* aorta, *LV* left ventricle

[21]. When the leaflets are closed, the MV resembles a smile, when visualized from the atrial perspective. The anterior and the posterior leaflets are separated by two commissures, designated as anterior-lateral and posterior-medial commissures (Fig. 7.5). The posterior leaflet is divided in P1, P2 and P3 scallops by deep indentations or clefts [22–24]. Usually, the anterior leaflet does not show any cleft, but the leaflet is subdivided in A1, A2 and A3 regions that oppose the scallops of the posterior leaflets (Fig. 7.5).

The subdivision of MV leaflets in scallops is used in clinical practice to describe the location of prolapsed or flailed segments or different leaflets lesions [12].

Data sets of the MV can be easily post-processed using gain adjustments, cropping and translating tools, leading to a clear visualization of the MV from either the atrial or the ventricular perspective (Fig. 7.5). The classic display of the MV from the atrial perspective is obtained by rotating the data set in order to place the MV leaflets in the center of the image, and the left atrial appendage to the left, with the aortic valve at 12 o'clock (Fig. 7.5 **left panel**). The anterior MV leaflet is connected to the left and non-coronary cusps of the aortic valve via the *mitral-aortic curtain*. The aortic cusp opposite to the anterior MV leaflet is the right coronary cusp. The prolapsing segments of the MV leaflets are best visualized from the left atrial perspective ("*surgical view*").

The ventricular perspective of the MV offers a detailed visualization of the anterior and the posterior MV leaflets of the commissures and of the LV outflow tract (Fig. 7.5 **Right panel**). The ventricular perspective of the MV is best suited for assessing MV clefts that predominantly affect the anterior leaflet [17] and for quantifying MV stenosis [25].

Beyond the enface view of the MV, 3DE allows any cut-plane to be obtained from a full-volume data set of the MV in order to analyze any structure of interest (Fig. 7.10). The MV leaflets height measured by 3DE correlate with the ones measured by multislice-computed tomography [14, 26].

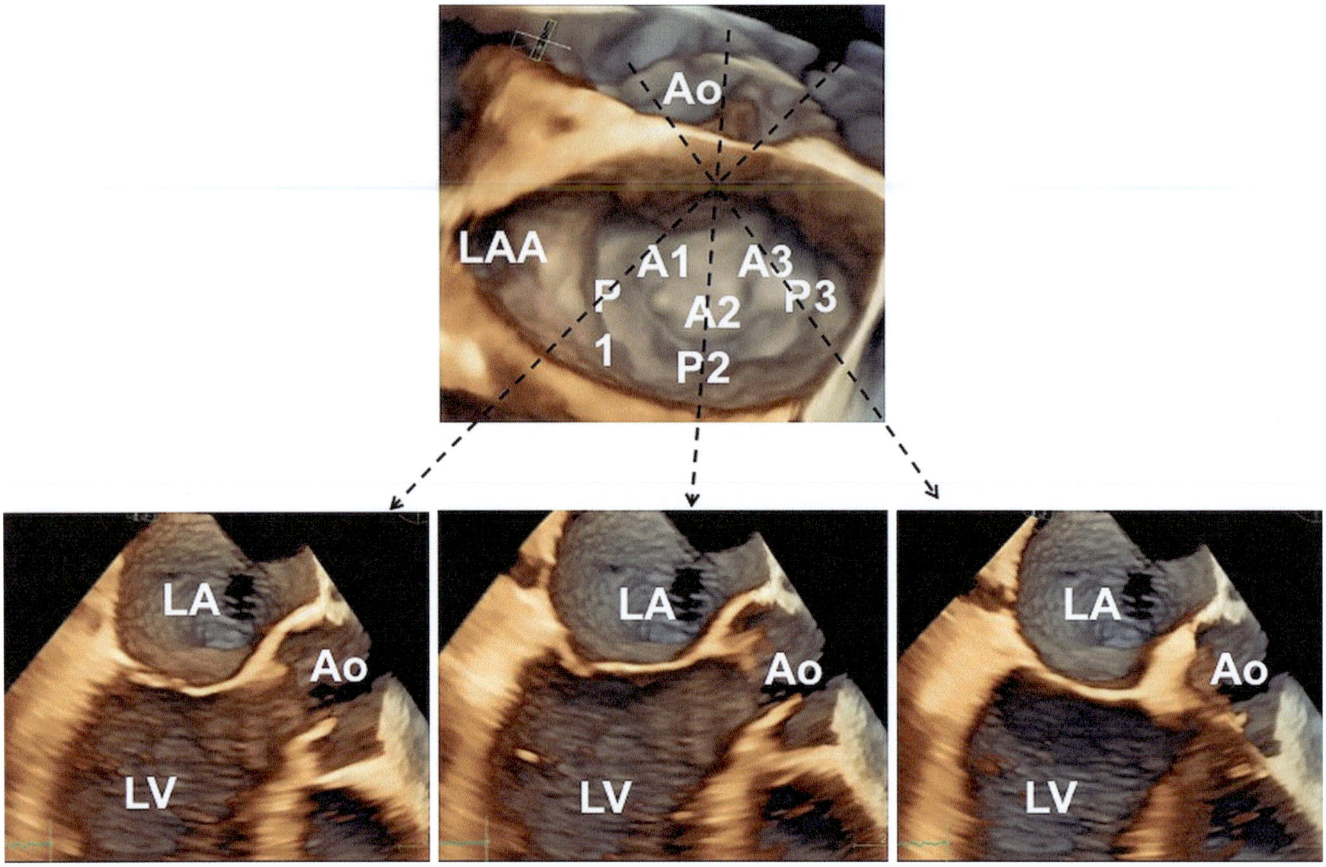

Fig. 7.10 Anatomically oriented cut planes obtained from a full volume data set of the mitral valve to examine the functional anatomy of the mitral valve scallops. Three longitudinal cut-planes (black dashed lines) have been obtained at the level of A1–P1, A2–P2, and A3–P3. *A1, A2, A3* scallops of anterior mitral leaflet, *Ao* aorta, *LA* left atrium, *LAA* left atrial appendage, *LV* left ventricle, *P1, P2, P3* scallops of posterior mitral leaflet

Mitral Annulus

The MA is a fibrous hinge-line structure that marks the junction between the left atrium, the LV and the mitral leaflets [19]. In normal individuals, the MA is an anatomically ill-defined structure, with a D-shape as seen from above, in a single horizontal cut-plane (Fig. 7.11). However, the MA has a complex three-dimensional shape, resembling to a saddle (Fig. 7.12) [27, 28], which has an important role in reducing the stress on the leaflets [29]. The MA is conventionally divided into the anterior and posterior portions, located higher than the lateral and medial commissural parts (also called "the valleys") [30]. The *anterior annulus* spans between the left and the right fibrous trigons and is anatomically coupled to the aortic annulus via the *aortic-mitral curtain* [21]. The *posterior annulus* is a discontinuous fibrous structure occasionally interrupted by fat, which makes it more susceptible to dilation [19, 31]. Even though the MA is a fibrous structure without intrinsic contraction, it has a very dynamic behavior during the cardiac cycle due to the adjacent muscular fibers of the left atrium and LV walls. The MA displays complex three-dimensional changes in size and shape during the entire cardiac cycle, which have been categorized in three main types: (1) the *translation function*, when the MA moves to and away from the LV apex; (2) the *contraction function*, due to the contraction of the adjacent fibers, which reduces the MA area; (3) the *folding function*, due to the reduction of the anterior-posterior size across its axis [30].

Due to its connection with the LV and left atrium free walls, the dynamics of the posterior annulus is more accentuated than the anterior annulus, which is fixed trough the *mitral-aortic curtain* to the aortic valve [32]. The contraction of the MA along its anterior-posterior axis leads to an increase in MA height during LV systole with a secondary accentuation of the saddle shape, which is an important factor resulting in MV leaflet coaptation [33, 34]. Due to its conformational changes, the MA decreases its area during early systole, in the so-called "contraction function" [35].

During the cardiac cycle, the MA also changes its relation with the surrounding structures. In normal individuals, the angle between the aorta and the MA plane steepens during LV contraction [14], allowing an easier emptying of the LV.

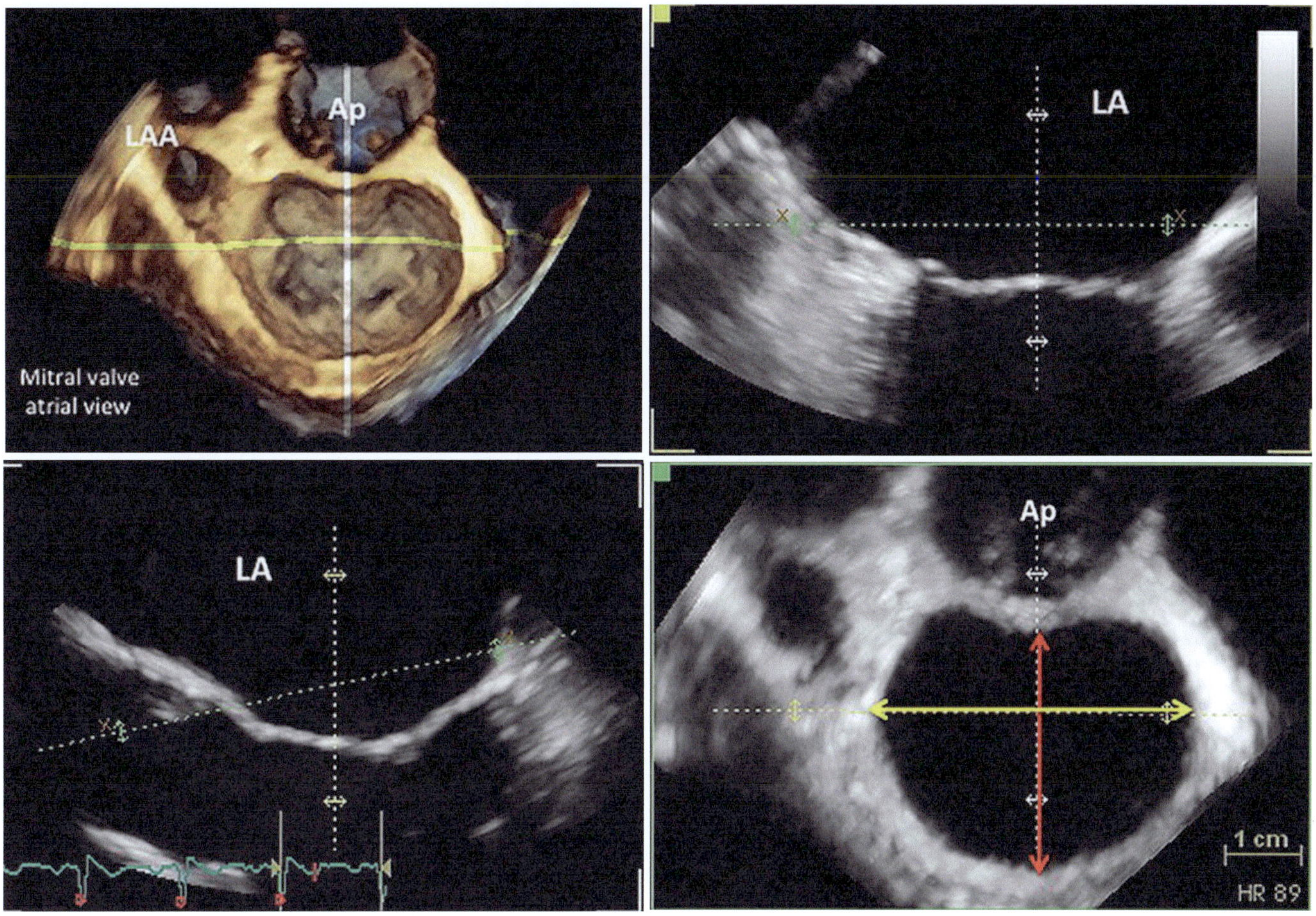

Fig. 7.11 Flexi slice at the level of the mitral valve annulus. The mitral valve is seen from the left atrial perspective, with the "D shape" of the mitral annulus. Cut-planes can be oriented in order to measure the true antero-posterior (in red) and anterolateral-posteromedial (in yellow) diameters of the mitral annulus. *Ao* aorta, *LA* left atrium, *LAA* left atrial appendage

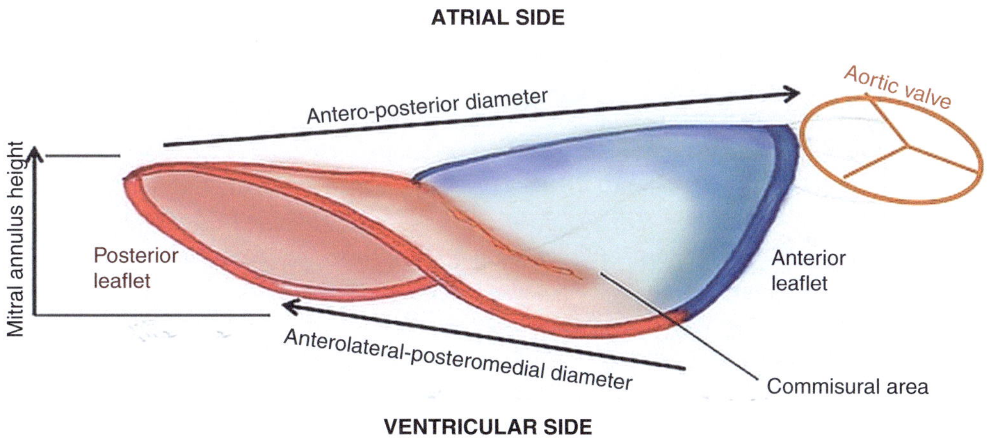

Fig. 7.12 Mitral annulus three-dimensional shape. The mitral annulus has a saddle shape, with two higher anterior and posterior horns, and two lower commissural valleys. The anterior-posterior diameter is the shortest diameter of the mitral annulus [28]

Assessment of MA dimensions is important to be able to determine appropriate annuloplasty ring or mitral prosthesis size, and two-dimensional echocardiography has been a pivotal method used for this purpose [36]. However, two-dimensional echocardiography allows only measurements of the MA diameters obtained from tomographic views, being unable to provide data about the complex 3D geometry of the MA. The only measurement recommended by current guidelines [36] is the anterior-posterior diameter of the MA obtained in the long axis-view of the LV, which uses the aorta as an anatomical landmark. However, in many cases the anterior-posterior diameter obtained with two-dimensional

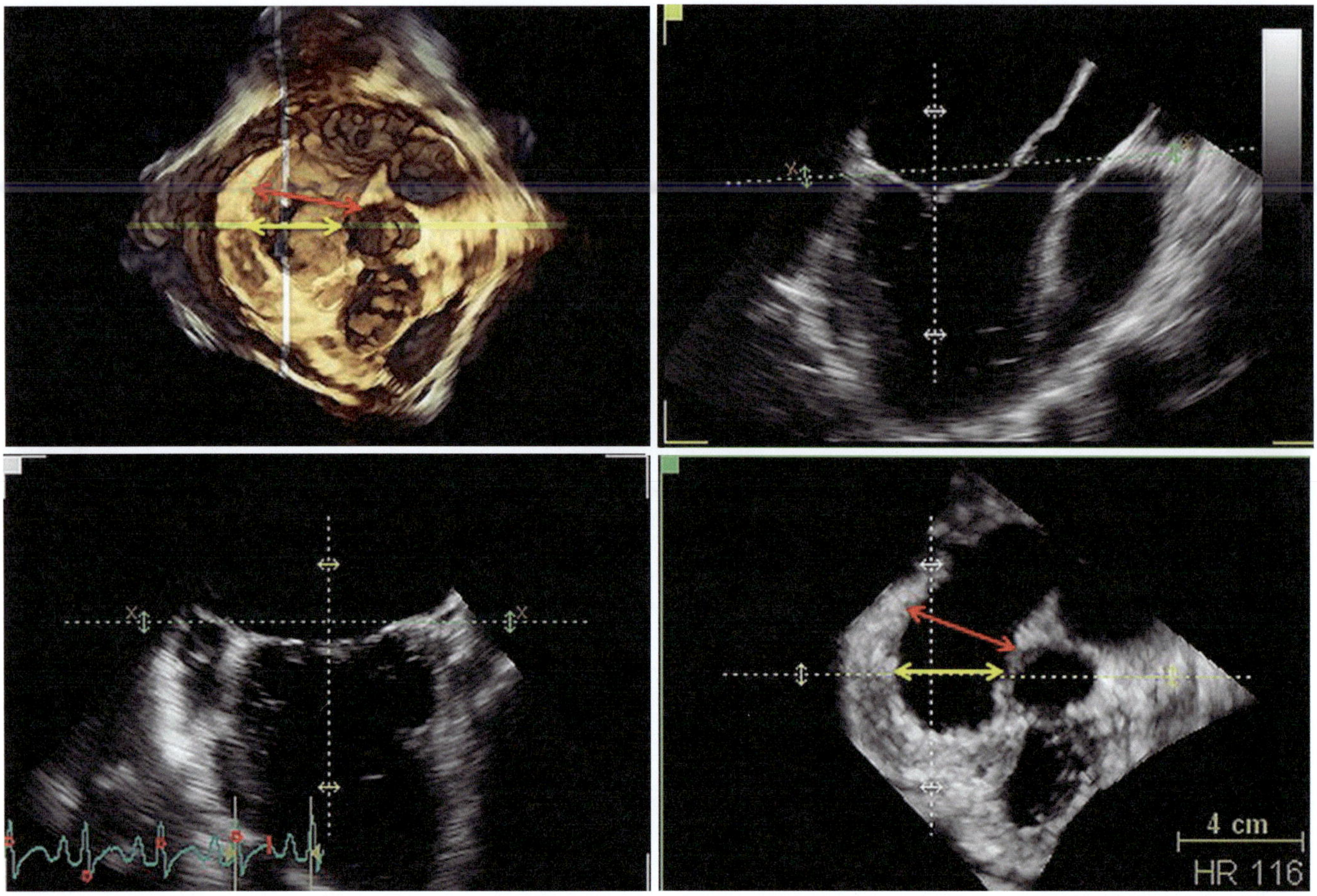

Fig. 7.13 Assessment of the anterior-posterior (AP) diameter of the mitral annulus. Long axis view of the ventricle, through the aortic valve, does not always provide the true anterior-posterior diameter of the mitral annulus. Using a cut-plane at the base of the heart obtained from a 3DE full-volume, the real shape of the mitral annulus and its diameters can be assessed. Red arrows—true AP diameter of the mitral annulus. Yellow arrows—apparent AP diameter, from a section through the aorta of the left ventricle and mitral valve

echocardiography may not be the true shortest diameter of the MA. If the longitudinal cut plane on which to measure the anterior posterior diameter of the MA is obtained from a 3D full-volume of the MV, it can be noticed that this diameter is not necessarily the shortest diameter of the MA (Fig. 7.13).

At present, 3DE offers the possibility of analyzing the MA in infinite cut-planes obtained from a single data set of the MV. A recent, important advance of the 3DE technology was the development of dedicated software packages to allow 3D surface rendering of the MV and quantitative analysis of the mitral apparatus geometry from a single 3D dataset of the MV (Fig. 7.14). Due to the initially low quality of the datasets obtained with transthoracic 3DE, the software packages were dedicated only for transesophageal 3D datasets [5, 15, 24, 37]. With the introduction of the most recent matrix array transducers, MV datasets obtained with transthoracic 3DE can be now analyzed with a feasibility of 73% in unselected patients, and with similar reproducibility to that of those obtained using the transesophageal approach [14]. These software packages allowed the completion of extensive research aimed at improving the characterization of the mechanisms leading to mitral regurgitation [4–6, 38–41].

Dedicated MV software performs a static analysis in the mid-systolic frame, by semi-automatically measuring different parameters describing MA geometry, such as the antero-posterior and anterolateral-posteromedial diameters of the MA, MA area and circumference, MA sphericity, MA height, non-planarity, MV tenting height, area and volume [14] (Fig. 7.15). The angle between the aorta and the MA plane analyzes the relationship of the MA with the surrounding structures, which is especially important after aortic valve replacement [42, 43]. All parameters of MA geometry can be also automatically tracked during the cardiac cycle, in order to perform a dynamic analysis of the MA geometry (Fig. 7.16).

In order to perform an in-depth analysis of the mechanisms of MV regurgitation, it is mandatory to have a thorough understanding of the normal size and shape of the MA.

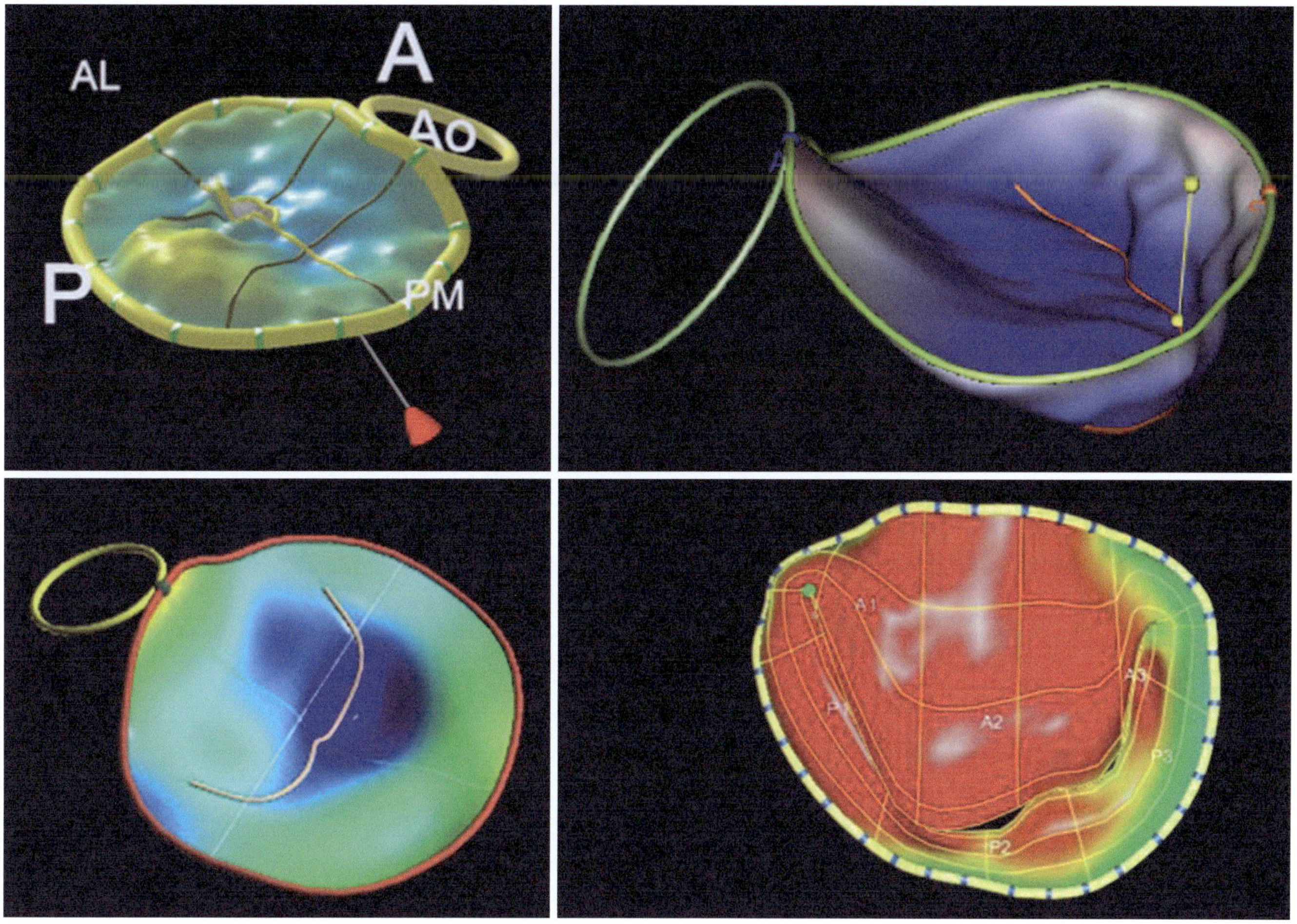

Fig. 7.14 Surface rendering of the mitral valve using different software packages for quantitative analysis of mitral annulus and leaflet geometry. *Upper left panel*, Mitral Valve Navigator (MVN; Philips Medical Systems, Andover, USA). *Upper right panel*, 4D MV-Assessment (TomTec Imaging Systems GMBH, Unterschleissheim, DE). *Lower left panel*, 4D Auto MVQ (Automatic Mitral Valve Quantitation, GE Vingmed, Horten NO). *Lower, right panel*, Syngo MVA (Mitral Valve Assessment, Siemens Healthineer, Mountainview, USA)

3D studies in normal individuals showed that MA decreases its area before the onset of LV systole, starting with left atrial contraction [35]. The MA area reaches its smallest size early during LV systole [14, 43]. Due to its contraction that occurs mainly along the anterior-posterior direction, the sphericity of the MA is minimal, the MA height and non-planarity are the highest during the LV systole [14, 44]. The MA enlarges its area towards end-systole [14] and diastole [28, 35], when it has a flatter shape. The MA area assessed by 3DE is similar to the one assessed with cardiac magnetic resonance and computerized tomography in normal subjects [14, 26, 44], and larger than the one measured by two-dimensional echocardiography studies [34, 45].

Conversely, in patients with degenerative MV disease, the MA is enlarged and more spherical, with decreased height [4, 5, 46] but preserved displacement [46]. In patients with functional mitral regurgitation, the MA is enlarged and more spherical [39], with decreased non-planarity and increased tenting volume of the MV leaflets [6, 47, 48]. The MA also has decreased "contraction" and "displacement" during LV systole in patients with functional mitral regurgitation [6].

Therefore, the use of MV dedicated software packages improves our understanding MV mechanics. It helps assess the suitability of MV repair and provides valuable information for annuloplasty ring design [12].

Chordae Tendineae

The chordae tendineae are string-like structures that attach the free edge of the MV leaflets to the postero-inferior LV wall or to both the papillary muscles [19]. Unlike the tricuspid valve, the MV does not have chordal attachments to the septum. This feature helps differentiate the MV from the TV in a transversal cut plane of the ventricles. According to their insertion into the mitral leaflets, chordae tendineae have been

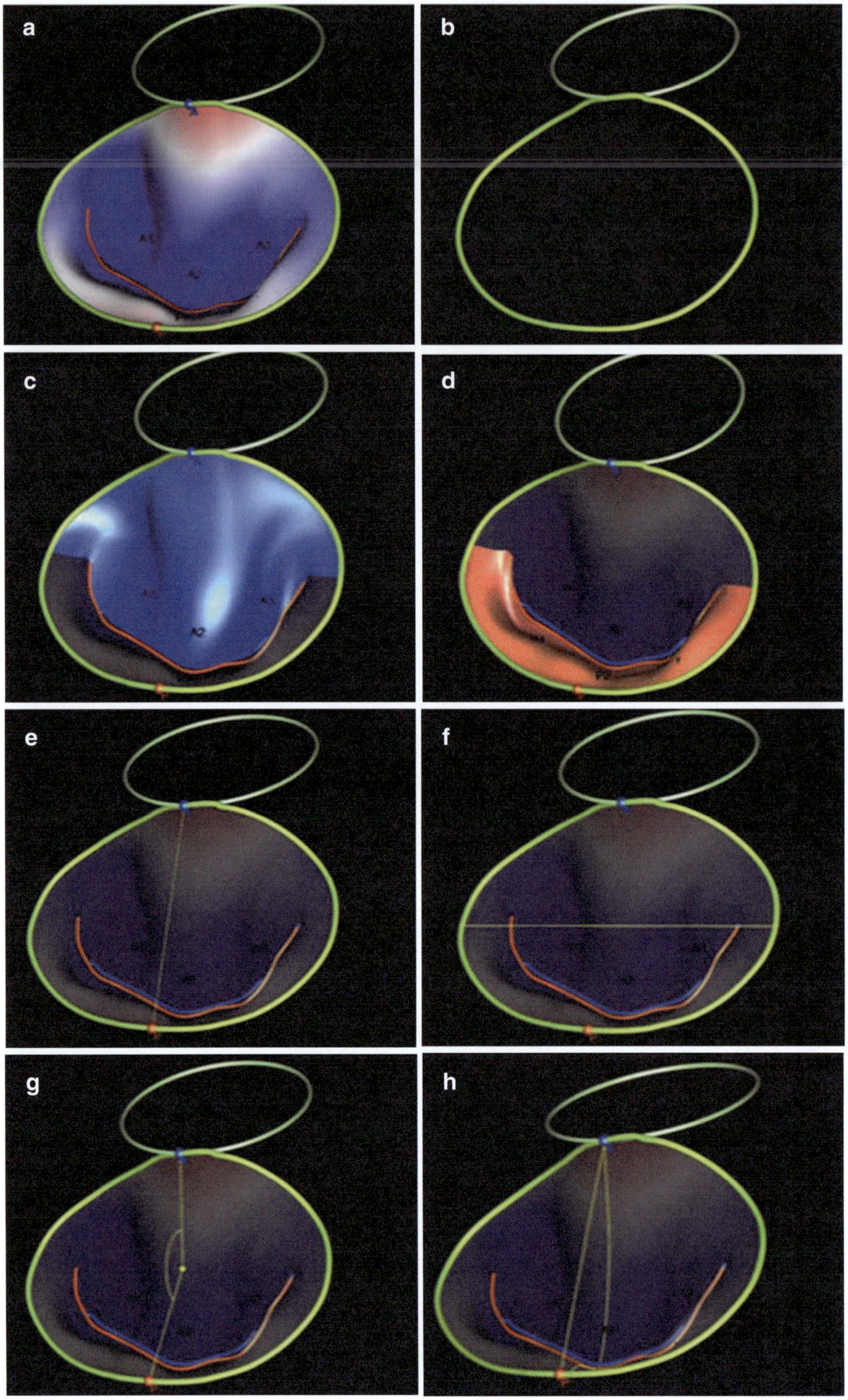

Fig. 7.15 Quantitative analysis of mitral annulus and leaflet geometry using three-dimensional transthoracic echocardiography and dedicated software package in a normal subject. Several parameters are measured in the mid-systolic frame to characterize the mitral valve geometry: (**a**) Mitral annulus area; (**b**) Mitral annulus circumference; (**c**) Anterior mitral leaflet area; (**d**) Posterior mitral leaflet area; (**e**) Mitral annulus antero-posterior diameter; (**f**) Mitral annulus anterior-lateral to posterior-medial diameter; (**g**) Mitral annulus non-planarity angle. (**h**) Mitral valve tenting area and volume

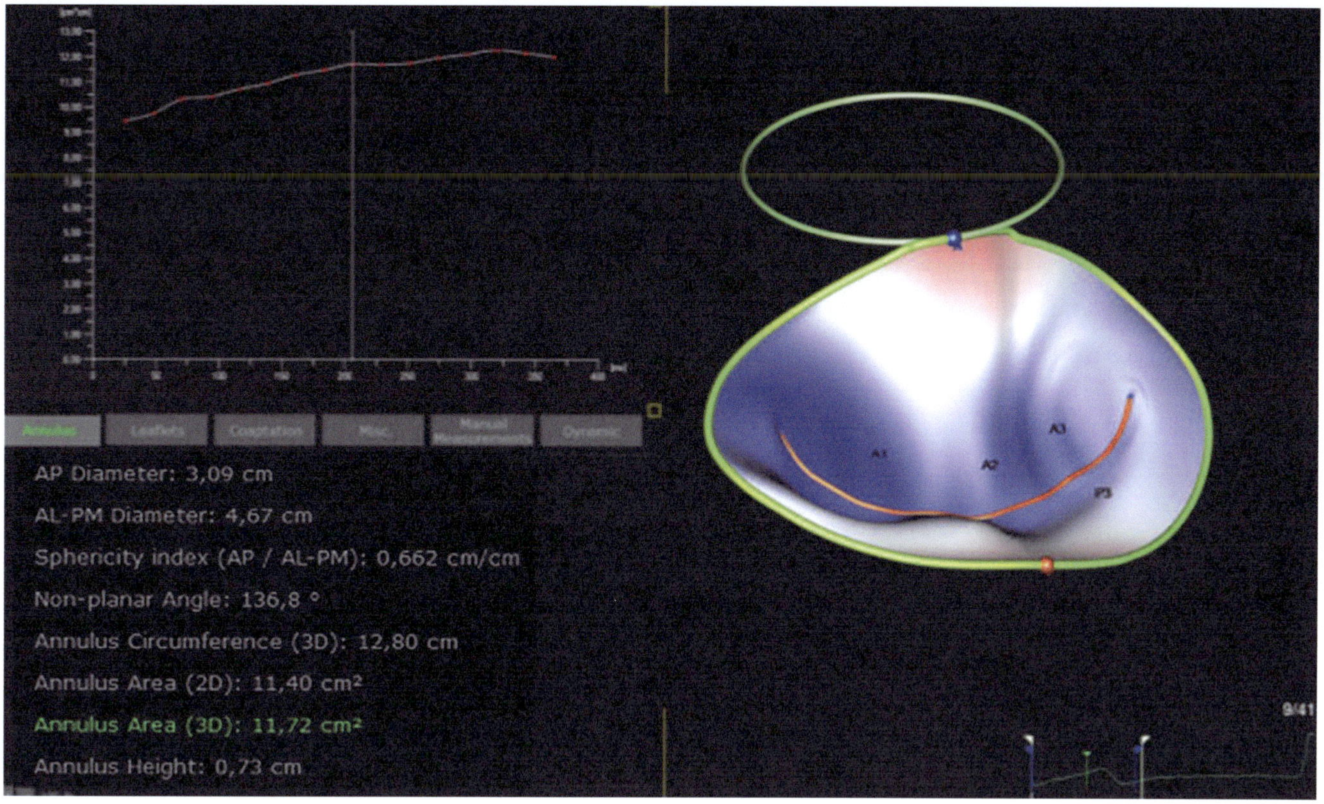

Fig. 7.16 Dynamic analysis of the mitral annulus area. The software package tracks the mitral annulus frame-by frame throughout the cardiac systole, providing information about frame-by-frame changes in size and geometry

classified into: (1) primary chordae, thin and delicate structures, inserted onto the free edge of the leaflets; (2) secondary chordae, which are thicker and insert on the body of the mitral leaflet, on its ventricular surface; and (3) tertiary chordae, which arise directly from the LV wall and insert at the base of the posterior leaflet [19].

A full volume data set of the MV apparatus is recommended to ensure the visualization of the MV chordae, both from the mid-esophageal four- or two-chamber view (Fig. 7.17 **left panel**) and from the trans-gastric approach, a longitudinal two-chamber view of the LV (Fig. 7.17 **Right panel**).

Multiplanar reconstruction of the 3DE data set to obtain both transversal and longitudinal cut planes allow visualization of the chordae insertions on the free margins (primary chordae), body (secondary chordae), and base (tertiary chordae) of the MV leaflets and measurement of their length [18] (Fig. 7.18). Conversely, chordae rupture with flail or prolapse can be best visualized from the left atrial perspective and/or by selected longitudinal cut planes [12].

Papillary Muscles

The papillary muscles are normally inserted on the apical and middle third regions of the LV walls [19]. There are usually two papillary muscles, located on the antero-lateral and the postero-medial surfaces of the LV walls, projected to the correspondent medial and lateral commissures of the mitral valve. They are continuing with chordae that sustain both the MV leaflets and ensure the correct MV leaflet coaptation during LV contraction. The anterior-lateral papillary muscle usually has a single head and dual blood supply from the circumflex branch and left anterior descending artery. The posterior-medial papillary muscle usually has two heads and its blood supply comes from the posterior left descending artery (the right or circumflex artery, depending on coronary dominance) [49, 50]. The location of the papillary muscles is very important to maintain an appropriate geometry of the MV during LV systole and to avoid prolapse of the leaflets or part of them [51–53]. Any change in LV geometry (LV remodeling due to ischemia or dilated cardiomyopathies)

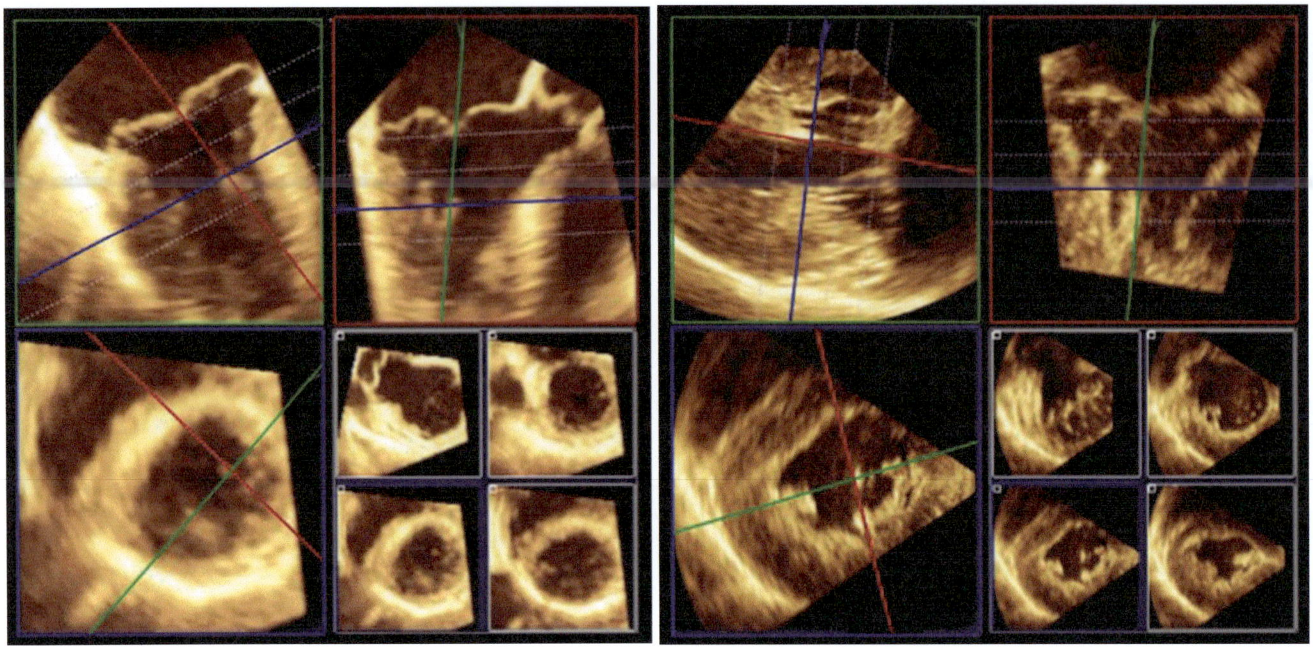

Fig. 7.17 Multiplane slicing of full volume 3DE data sets acquired from mid-esophageal (*left panel*) and transgastric approach (*right panel*) to study papillary muscles and chordae tendineae. *Left panel*, the two longitudinal planes (green and red upper quadrants) show the morphology of the anterior-lateral papillary muscle which is crossed by the green and the red planes in the transversal slice (blue panel). *Right panel*, transgastric approach allows better image quality that permits clear identification of chordae tendineae

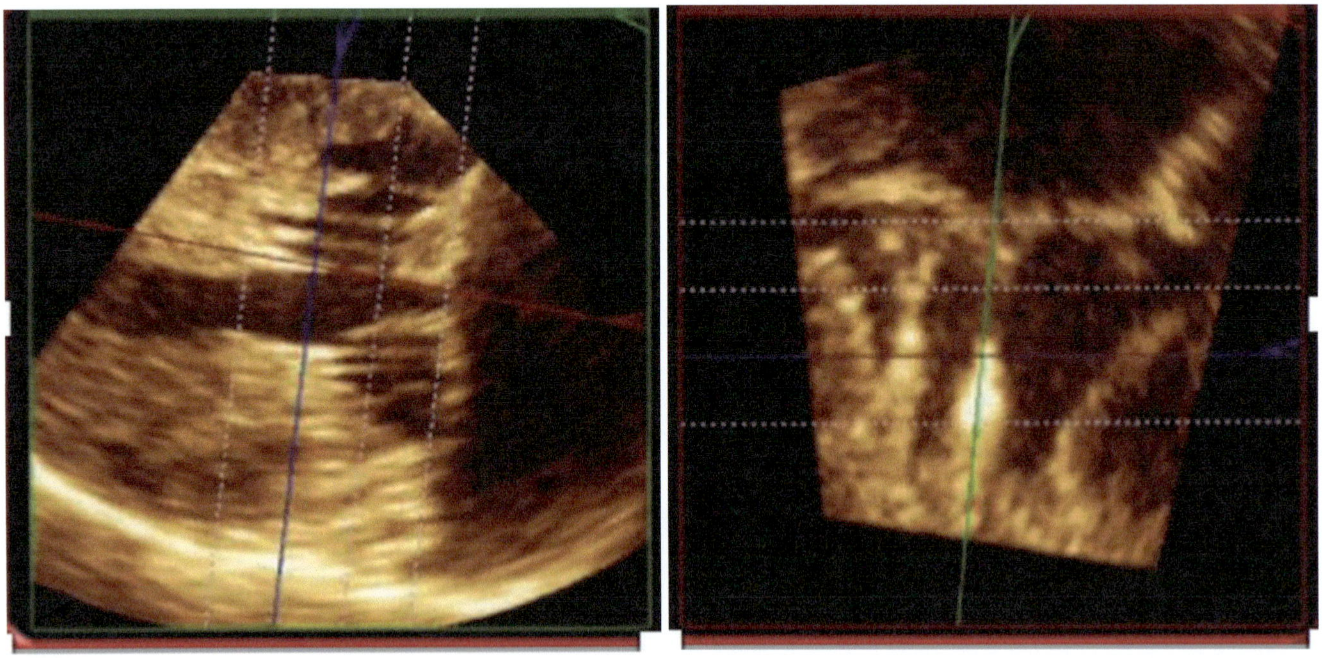

Fig. 7.18 Proper slicing of a 3DE full volume data set acquired from transgastric approach allows clear identification of chordae tendineae of different orders and to measure their length (upper panels), as well as localization and measurement of papillary muscle size

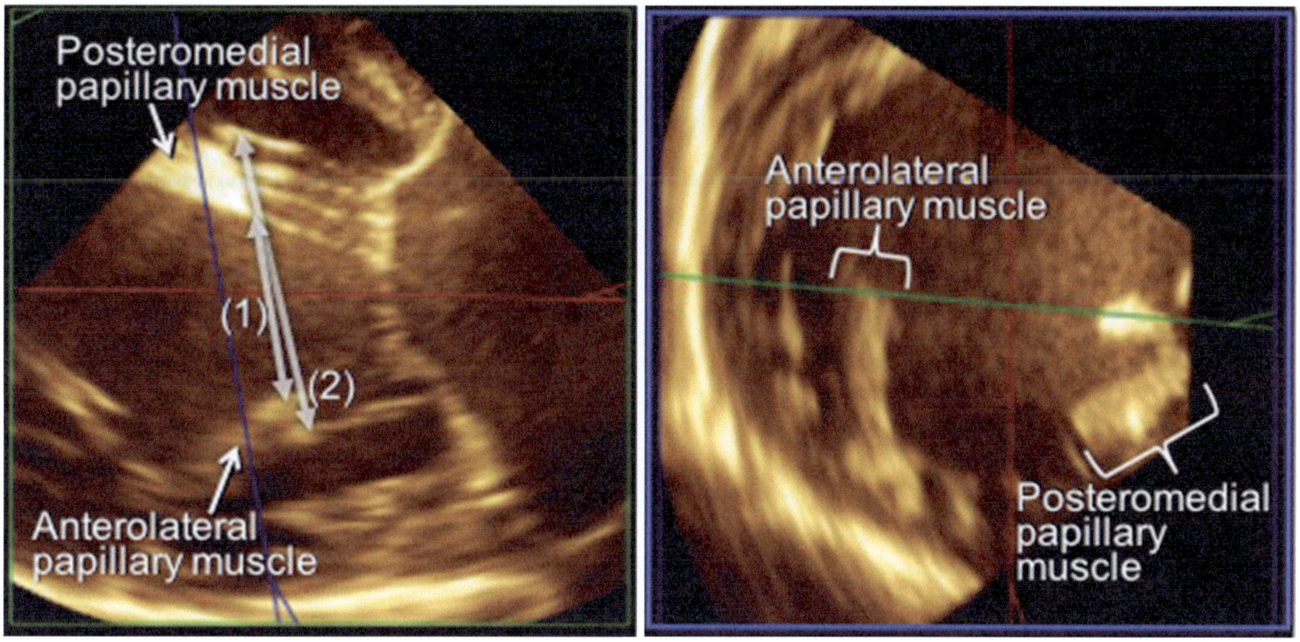

Fig. 7.18 (continued)

leads to a distortion of the papillary muscle orientation, with tethering of the chordae [54–56] and secondary MV leaflets tenting, causing functional MR [57–59].

To allow the quantitative assessment of papillary muscle position/displacement, 3DE data sets should encompass MV, aorta and enough LV to include at least the head of both papillary muscles (Fig. 7.19, Video 7.6). When the transthoracic approach is inadequate to provide optimal image quality, transesophageal 3DE can be performed to assess the MV apparatus from several unique views to obtain additional information [58] (Figs. 7.17 and 7.18).

Longitudinal displacement of papillary muscles can be measured taking MA center, MA plane and LV long axis as reference points (Figs. 7.20 and 7.21), whereas the, transversal displacement of papillary muscles can be assessed using MA center and aortic valve as reference points. Finally, papillary muscle positions can be defined by measuring the angles (α° e β°) formed between the anterior- lateral and the posterior- medial papillary muscles, with MA center and the aortic valve (Fig. 7.22) [60–64].

3DE is still evolving and its clinical applications are still subject of extensive research. Therefore, this technology should complement current two-dimensional echocardiographic techniques, in order to enhance our understanding of the topography of the lesions and their relationship with the

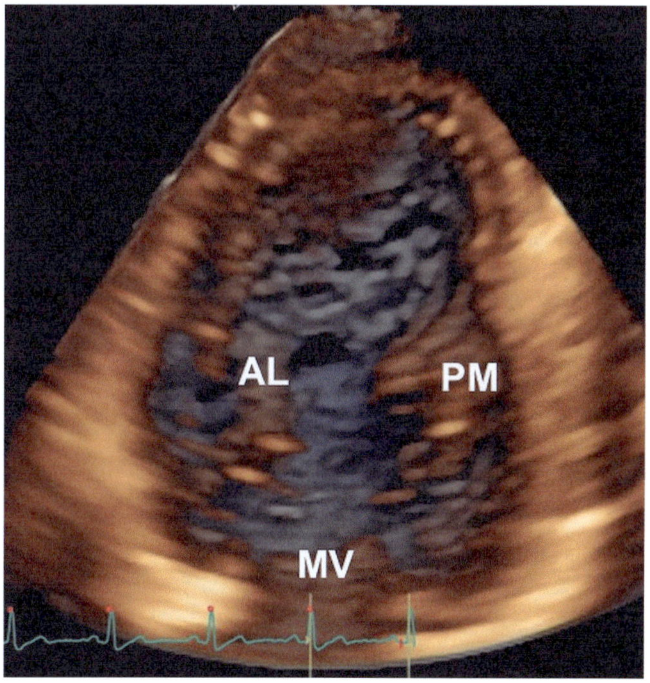

Fig. 7.19 Full volume 3DE data set of the left ventricle obtained with transthoracic echocardiography and cropped in a longitudinal axis to visualize both papillary muscles (Video 7.6). *AL* anterior-lateral papillary muscle, *PM* posterior-medial papillary muscle (with double head); *MV* mitral valve

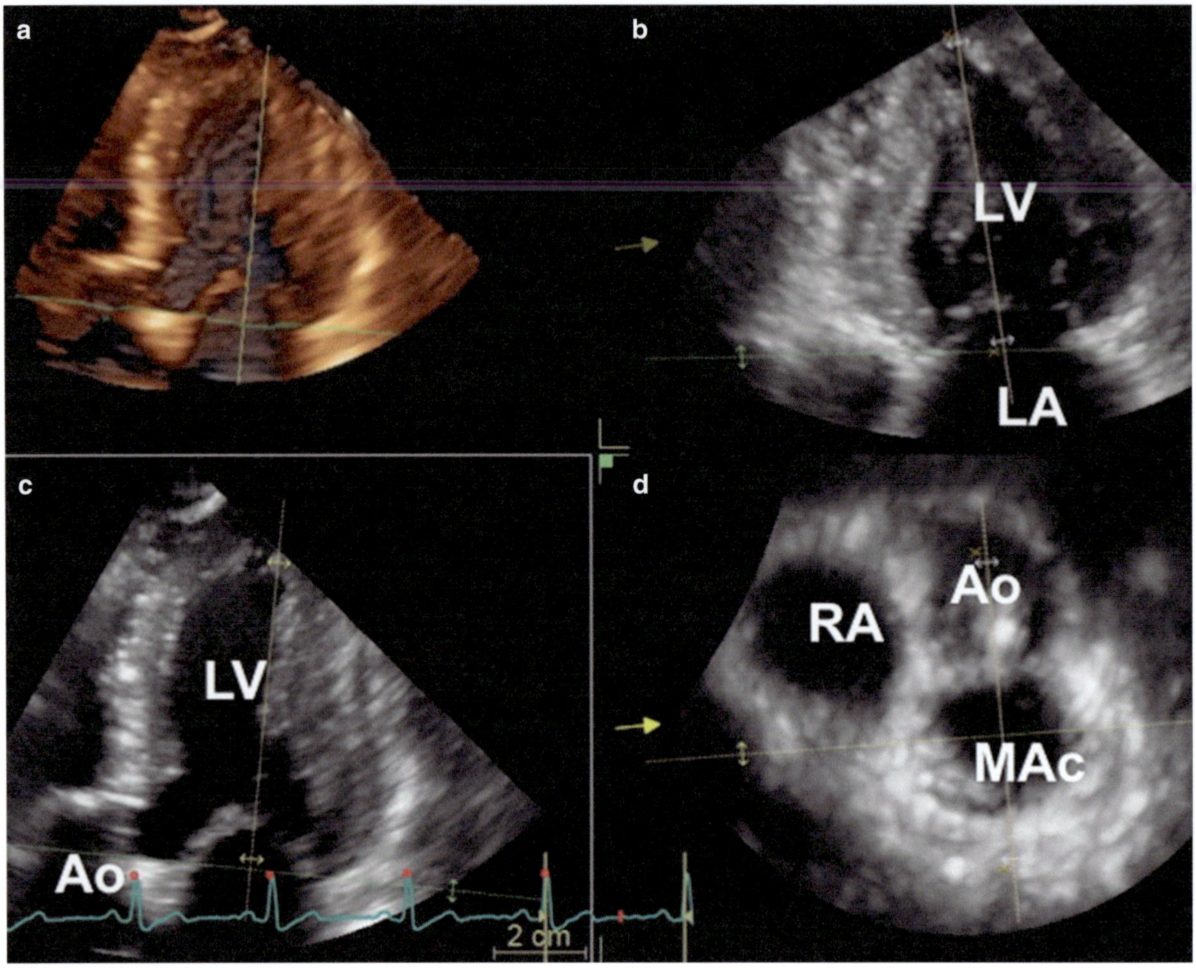

Fig. 7.20 Slicing of a transthoracic 3DE full volume data set to identify the center of the mitral annulus (MAc) as the crossing point between the anatomically oriented long axis (white line, *panel C*) and bi-commissural (yellow line, *panel B*) cut planes at the level of the mitral annulus identified by the green line

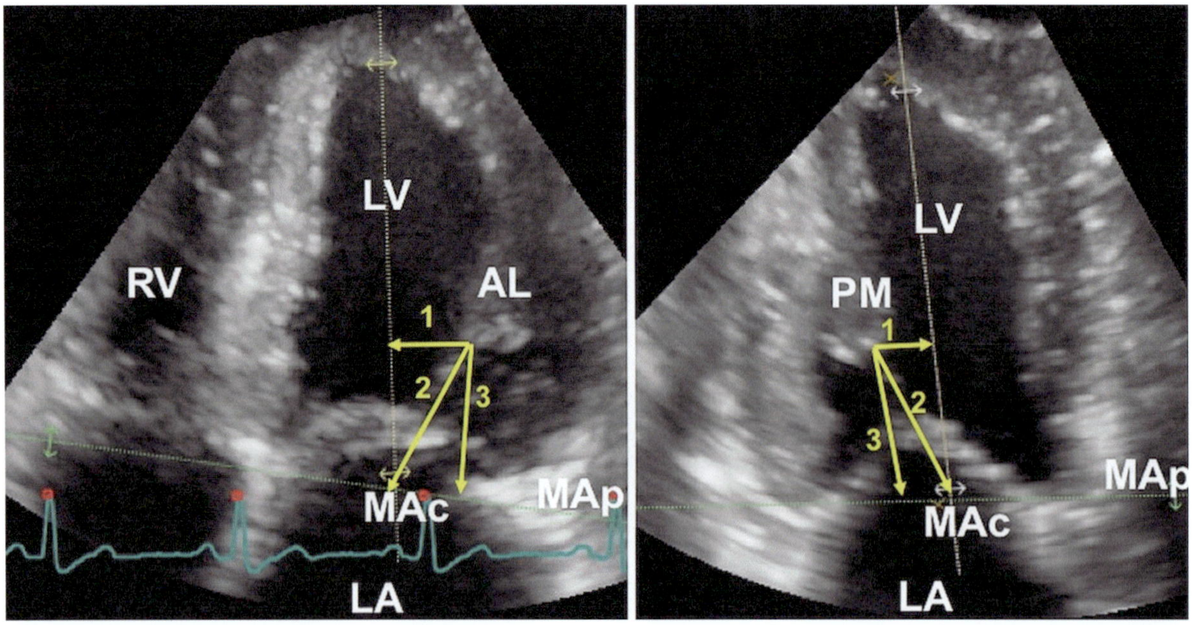

Fig. 7.21 Quantitative assessment of the transversal displacement of the anterior-lateral (AL) and posterior-lateral (PL) papillary muscles. The distances of the head of the papillary muscle from the longitudinal axis (yellow arrow #1) of the left ventricle (LV), from the center of the mitral annulus (MAc, yellow arrow #2) and the mitral annulus plane (MAp, yellow arrow #3) are measured. *LA* left atrium, *RV* right ventricle

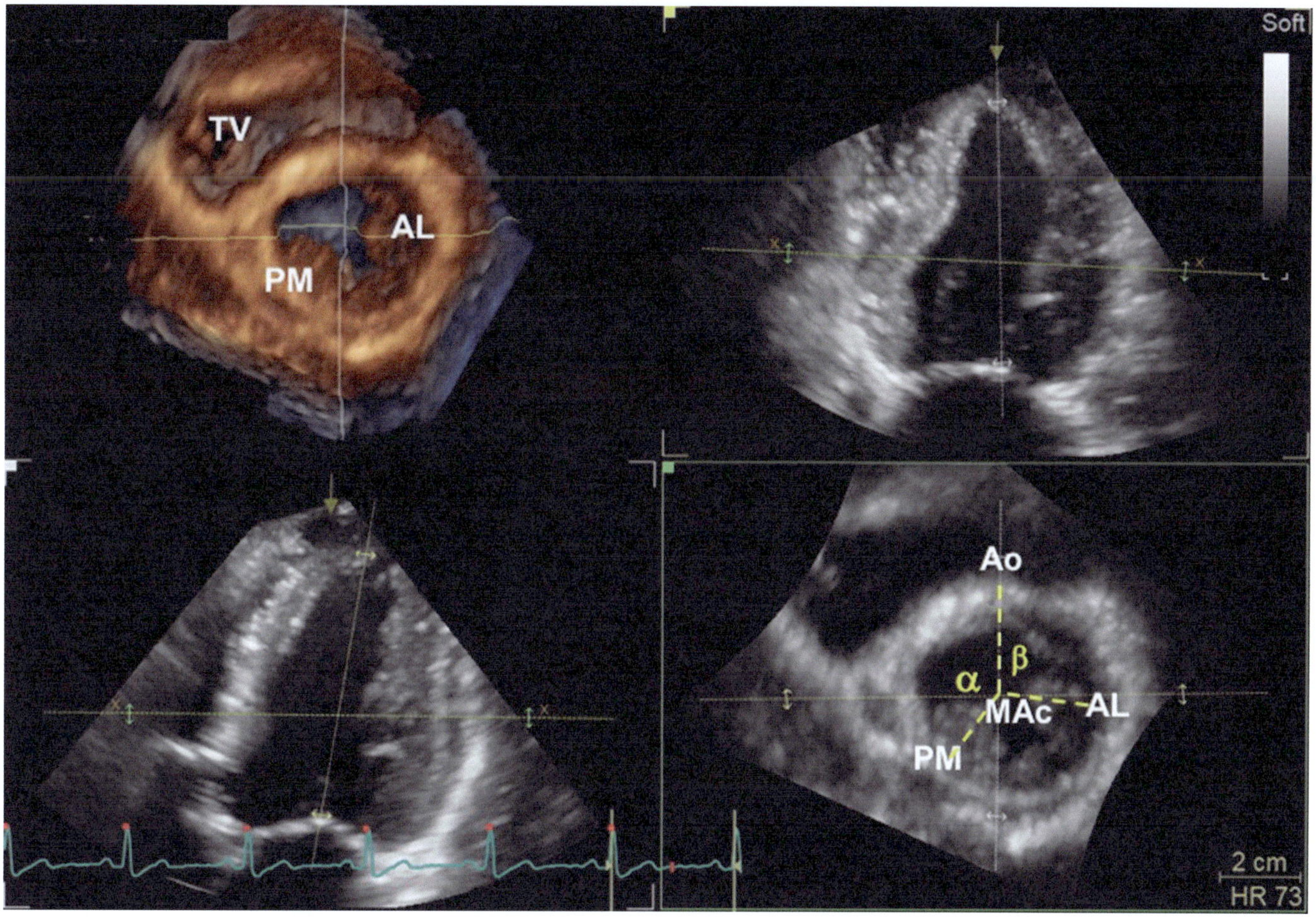

Fig. 7.22 Spatial orientation of the anterior-lateral (AL) and posterior-lateral (PL) papillary muscles is also defined by measuring the angles (α° and β°) formed between PL and AL, respectively, with the center of the mitral annulus (MAc) and the aortic valve

surrounding cardiac structures. The assessment of the MV is one of the most promising clinical applications of 3DE. The unique benefits of analyzing the mitral valve in infinite planes from a single 3D volume data set while having "en face" views of the valve helps to establish a closer connection of the heart-imager with the surgeon, to better plan MV procedures.

References

1. Badano LP, Boccalini F, Muraru D, et al. Current clinical applications of transthoracic three-dimensional echocardiography. J Cardiovasc Ultrasound. 2012;20:1–22.
2. Lang RM, Mor-Avi V, Sugeng L, Nieman PS, Sahn DJ. Three-dimensional echocardiography: the benefits of the additional dimension. J Am Coll Cardiol. 2006;48:2053–69.
3. Lang RM, Tsang W, Weinert L, Mor-Avi V, Chandra S. Valvular heart disease. The value of 3-dimensional echocardiography. J Am Coll Cardiol. 2011;58:1933–44.
4. Caiani EG, Fusini L, Veronesi F, et al. Quantification of mitral annulus dynamic morphology in patients with mitral valve prolapse undergoing repair and annuloplasty during a 6-month follow-up. Eur J Echocardiogr. 2011;12:375–83.
5. Grewal J, Suri R, Mankad S, et al. Mitral annular dynamics in myxomatous valve disease: new insights with real-time 3-dimensional echocardiography. Circulation. 2010;121:1423–31.
6. Topilsky Y, Vaturi O, Watanabe N, et al. Real-time 3-dimensional dynamics of functional mitral regurgitation: a prospective quantitative and mechanistic study. J Am Heart Assoc. 2013;2:e000039.
7. Thavendiranathan P, Phelan D, Thomas JD, Flamm SD, Marwick TH. Quantitative assessment of mitral regurgitation: validation of new methods. J Am Coll Cardiol. 2012;60:1470–83.
8. Thavendiranathan P, Phelan D, Collier P, Thomas JD, Flamm SD, Marwick TH. Quantitative assessment of mitral regurgitation: how best to do it. JACC Cardiovasc Imaging. 2012;5:1161–75.
9. Cavalcante JL, Rodriguez LL, Kapadia S, Tuzcu EM, Stewart WJ. Role of echocardiography in percutaneous mitral valve interventions. JACC Cardiovasc Imaging. 2012;5:733–46.
10. Altiok E, Becker M, Hamada S, et al. Real-time 3D TEE allows optimized guidance of percutaneous edge-to-edge repair of the mitral valve. JACC Cardiovasc Imaging. 2010;3:1196–8.
11. Wunderlich NC, Siegel RJ. Peri-interventional echo assessment for the MitraClip procedure. Eur Heart J Cardiovasc Imaging. 2013;14:935–49.
12. Lang RM, Badano LP, Tsang W, et al. EAE/ASE recommendations for image acquisition and display using three-dimensional echocardiography. Eur Heart J Cardiovasc Imaging. 2012;13:1–46.
13. Mor-Avi V, Sugeng L, Lang RM. Real-time 3-dimensional echocardiography: an integral component of the routine echocardiographic examination in adult patients? Circulation. 2009;119:314–29.
14. Mihaila S, Muraru D, Piasentini E, et al. Quantitative analysis of mitral annular geometry and function in healthy volunteers using transthoracic three-dimensional echocardiography. J Am Soc Echocardiogr. 2014;27:846–57.
15. Pepi M, Tamborini G, Maltagliati A, et al. Head-to-head comparison of two- and three-dimensional transthoracic and transesopha-

geal echocardiography in the localization of mitral valve prolapse. J Am Coll Cardiol. 2006;48:2524–30.
16. Sugeng L, Coon P, Weinert L, et al. Use of real-time 3-dimensional transthoracic echocardiography in the evaluation of mitral valve disease. J Am Soc Echocardiogr. 2006;19:413–21.
17. Miglioranza MH, Muraru D, Mihaila S, Haertel JC, Iliceto S, Badano LP. Isolated anterior mitral valve leaflet cleft: 3D transthoracic echocardiography-guided surgical strategy. Arq Bras Cardiol. 2015;104:e49–52.
18. Obase K, Jeevanandam V, Saito K, et al. Visualization and measurement of mitral valve chordae tendineae using three-dimensional transesophageal echocardiography from the transgastric approach. J Am Soc Echocardiogr. 2015;28:449–54.
19. Ho SY. Anatomy of the mitral valve. Heart. 2002;88(Suppl 4):iv5–10.
20. Levine RA, Durst R. Mitral valve prolapse: a deeper look. JACC Cardiovasc Imaging. 2008;1:304–6.
21. Silbiger JJ, Bazaz R. Contemporary insights into the functional anatomy of the mitral valve. Am Heart J. 2009;158:887–95.
22. Mantovani F, Clavel MA, Vatury O, et al. Cleft-like indentations in myxomatous mitral valves by three-dimensional echocardiographic imaging. Heart. 2015;101:1111–7.
23. Quill JL, Hill AJ, Laske TG, Alfieri O, Iaizzo PA. Mitral leaflet anatomy revisited. J Thorac Cardiovasc Surg. 2009;137:1077–81.
24. Grewal J, Mankad S, Freeman WK, Click RL, Suri RM, Abel MD, et al. Real-time three-dimensional transesophageal echocardiography in the intraoperative assessment of mitral valve disease. J Am Soc Echocardiogr. 2009;22(1):34–41.
25. Zamorano J, Cordeiro P, Sugeng L, et al. Real-time three-dimensional echocardiography for rheumatic mitral stenosis evaluation: an accurate and novel approach. J Am Coll Cardiol. 2004;43:2091–6.
26. Beaudoin J, Thai WE, Wai B, Handschumacher MD, Levine RA, Truong QA. Assessment of mitral valve adaptation with gated cardiac computed tomography: validation with three-dimensional echocardiography and mechanistic insight to functional mitral regurgitation. Circ Cardiovasc Imaging. 2013;6(5):784–9.
27. Levine RA, Handschumacher MD, Sanfilippo AJ, et al. Three-dimensional echocardiographic reconstruction of the mitral valve, with implications for the diagnosis of mitral valve prolapse. Circulation. 1989;80:589–98.
28. Kaplan SR, Bashein G, Sheehan FH, et al. Three-dimensional echocardiographic assessment of annular shape changes in the normal and regurgitant mitral valve. Am Heart J. 2000;139:378–87.
29. Salgo IS, Gorman JH 3rd, Gorman RC, et al. Effect of annular shape on leaflet curvature in reducing mitral leaflet stress. Circulation. 2002;106:711–7.
30. Silbiger JJ. Anatomy, mechanics, and pathophysiology of the mitral annulus. Am Heart J. 2012;164:163–76.
31. Angelini A, Ho SY, Anderson RH, Davies MJ, Becker AE. A histological study of the atrioventricular junction in hearts with normal and prolapsed leaflets of the mitral valve. Br Heart J. 1988;59:712–6.
32. Pai RG, Varadarajan P, Tanimoto M. Effect of atrial fibrillation on the dynamics of mitral annular area. J Heart Valve Dis. 2003;12(1):31–7.
33. Ormiston JA, Shah PM, Tei C, Wong M. Size and motion of the mitral valve annulus in man. I. A two-dimensional echocardiographic method and findings in normal subjects. Circulation. 1981;64:113–20.
34. Ormiston JA, Shah PM, Tei C, Wong M. Size and motion of the mitral valve annulus in man. II. Abnormalities in mitral valve prolapse. Circulation. 1982;65:713–9.
35. Mihaila S, Muraru D, Miglioranza MH, et al. Normal mitral annulus dynamics and its relationships with left ventricular and left atrial function. Int J Cardiovasc Imaging. 2015;31:279–90.
36. Baumgartner H, Falk V, Bax JJ, et al. 2017 ESC/EACTS Guidelines for the management of valvular heart disease. Eur Heart J. 2017;38:2739–91.
37. Veronesi F, Caiani EG, Sugeng L, et al. Effect of mitral valve repair on mitral-aortic coupling: a real-time three-dimensional transesophageal echocardiography study. J Am Soc Echocardiogr. 2012;25:524–31.
38. Kwan J, Shiota T, Agler DA, et al. Geometric differences of the mitral apparatus between ischemic and dilated cardiomyopathy with significant mitral regurgitation: real-time three-dimensional echocardiography study. Circulation. 2003;107:1135–40.
39. Kwan J, Qin JX, Popovic ZB, Agler DA, Thomas JD, Shiota T. Geometric changes of mitral annulus assessed by real-time 3-dimensional echocardiography: becoming enlarged and less nonplanar in the anteroposterior direction during systole in proportion to global left ventricular systolic function. J Am Soc Echocardiogr. 2004;17:1179–84.
40. Veronesi F, Corsi C, Sugeng L, et al. Quantification of mitral apparatus dynamics in functional and ischemic mitral regurgitation using real-time 3-dimensional echocardiography. J Am Soc Echocardiogr. 2008;21:347–54.
41. Tsang W, Veronesi F, Sugeng L, et al. Mitral valve dynamics in severe aortic stenosis before and after aortic valve replacement. J Am Soc Echocardiogr. 2013;26:606–14.
42. Tsang W, Meineri M, Hahn RT, et al. A three-dimensional echocardiographic study on aortic-mitral coupling in transcatheter aortic valve replacement. Eur Heart J Cardiovasc Imaging. 2013;14:950–6.
43. Kwan J, Jeon MJ, Kim DH, Park KS, Lee WH. Does the mitral annulus shrink or enlarge during systole? A real-time 3D echocardiography study. J Korean Med Sci. 2009;24:203–8.
44. Anwar AM, Soliman OI, Nemes A, et al. Assessment of mitral annulus size and function by real-time 3-dimensional echocardiography in cardiomyopathy: comparison with magnetic resonance imaging. J Am Soc Echocardiogr. 2007;20:941–8.
45. Anwar AM, Soliman OI, ten Cate FJ, et al. True mitral annulus diameter is underestimated by two-dimensional echocardiography as evidenced by real-time three-dimensional echocardiography and magnetic resonance imaging. Int J Cardiovasc Imaging. 2007;23:541–7.
46. Mihaila S, Muraru D, Miglioranza MH, et al. Relationship between mitral annulus function and mitral regurgitation severity and left atrial remodelling in patients with primary mitral regurgitation. Eur Heart J Cardiovasc Imaging. 2016;17:918–29.
47. Watanabe N, Ogasawara Y, Yamaura Y, Kawamoto T, Akasaka T, Yoshida K. Geometric deformity of the mitral annulus in patients with ischemic mitral regurgitation: a real-time three-dimensional echocardiographic study. J Heart Valve Dis. 2005;14(4):447–52.
48. Watanabe N, Ogasawara Y, Yamaura Y, et al. Mitral annulus flattens in ischemic mitral regurgitation: geometric differences between inferior and anterior myocardial infarction: a real-time 3-dimensional echocardiographic study. Circulation. 2005;112(9 Suppl):I458–62.
49. Chiechi MA, Lees WM, Thompson R. Functional anatomy of the normal mitral valve. J Thorac Surg. 1956;32:378–98.
50. Rusted IE, Scheifley CH, Edwards JE. Studies of the mitral valve. I. Anatomic features of the normal mitral valve and associated structures. Circulation. 1952;6:825–31.
51. Cochran RP, Kunzelman KS. Effect of papillary muscle position on mitral valve function: relationship to homografts. Ann Thorac Surg. 1998;66(6 Suppl):S155–61.
52. Nielsen SL, Nygaard H, Fontaine AA, et al. Papillary muscle misalignment causes multiple mitral regurgitant jets: an ambiguous mechanism for functional mitral regurgitation. J Heart Valve Dis. 1999;8:551–64.
53. Levine RA, Vlahakes GJ, Lefebvre X, et al. Papillary muscle displacement causes systolic anterior motion of the mitral valve.

Experimental validation and insights into the mechanism of subaortic obstruction. Circulation. 1995;91:1189–95.
54. Boltwood CM, Tei C, Wong M, Shah PM. Quantitative echocardiography of the mitral complex in dilated cardiomyopathy: the mechanism of functional mitral regurgitation. Circulation. 1983;68(3):498–508.
55. Chaput M, Handschumacher MD, Tournoux F, et al. Mitral leaflet adaptation to ventricular remodeling: occurrence and adequacy in patients with functional mitral regurgitation. Circulation. 2008;118:845–52.
56. He S, Fontaine AA, Schwammenthal E, Yoganathan AP, Levine RA. Integrated mechanism for functional mitral regurgitation: leaflet restriction versus coapting force: in vitro studies. Circulation. 1997;96:1826–34.
57. Lee AP, Acker M, Kubo SH, et al. Mechanisms of recurrent functional mitral regurgitation after mitral valve repair in nonischemic dilated cardiomyopathy: importance of distal anterior leaflet tethering. Circulation. 2009;119:2606–14.
58. Nagasaki M, Nishimura S, Ohtaki E, et al. The echocardiographic determinants of functional mitral regurgitation differ in ischemic and non-ischemic cardiomyopathy. Int J Cardiol. 2006;108:171–6.
59. Otsuji Y, Handschumacher MD, Schwammenthal E, et al. Insights from three-dimensional echocardiography into the mechanism of functional mitral regurgitation: direct in vivo demonstration of altered leaflet tethering geometry. Circulation. 1997;96:1999–2008.
60. Sakai T, Okita Y, Ueda Y, et al. Distance between mitral annulus and papillary muscles: anatomic study in normal human hearts. J Thorac Cardiovasc Surg. 1999;118:636–41.
61. Theriault-Lauzier P, Mylotte D, Dorfmeister M, et al. Quantitative multi-slice computed tomography assessment of the mitral valve complex for transcatheter mitral valve interventions part 1: systematic measurement methodology and inter-observer variability. EuroIntervention. 2016;12:e1011–20.
62. Hsuan CF, Yu HY, Tseng WK, et al. Quantitation of the mitral tetrahedron in patients with ischemic heart diseases using real-time three-dimensional echocardiography to evaluate the geometric determinants of ischemic mitral regurgitation. Clin Cardiol. 2013;36:286–92.
63. Veronesi F, Corsi C, Sugeng L, et al. Quantification of mitral apparatus dynamics in functional and ischemic mitral regurgitation using real-time 3-dimensional echocardiography. J Am Soc Echocardiogr. 2008;21:347–54.
64. Otsuji Y, Kumanohoso T, Yoshifuku S, et al. Isolated annular dilation does not usually cause important functional mitral regurgitation. Comparison between patients with lone atrial fibrillation and those with idiopathic or ischemic cardiomyoapthy. J Am Coll Cardiol. 2002;39:1651–6.

Mitral Valve Congenital Abnormalities and Stenosis

8

Hani Mahmoud-Elsayed

Abstract

Three-dimensional echocardiography (3DE) has tremendously improved our ability to diagnose and assess the severity of mitral valve congenital abnormalities such as congenital mitral cleft, congenital double orifice mitral valve and parachute mitral valve.

Rheumatic mitral valve stenosis is still a high-prevalent heart valve disease in many countries and degenerative, calcific, mitral stenosis is an emerging heart valve disease in the elderly. 3DE has become the reference imaging modality to assess the mitral valve stenosis qualitatively in terms of leaflet visualization, quantitation of the reduced diastolic opening, commissural calcification, leaflet mobility/pliability and assessment of the subvalvular apparatus. Moreover, 3DE provides accurate quantitative analysis of mitral stenosis severity and of mitral valve scoring system in order to assess the suitability for percutaneous mitral balloon valvuloplasty.

Finally, transesophageal 3DE is used to guide and assess the results of percutaneous mitral balloon valvuloplasty in the catheterization laboratory.

Keywords

Congenital mitral valve abnormalities · Cleft mitral valve
Double orifice mitral valve · Parachute mitral valve
Rheumatic mitral stenosis · Commissural fusion
Commissural calcification · Degenerative calcific mitral stenosis · Percutaneous mitral balloon valvuloplasty
Septal puncture · RATLe-90 maneuver

Electronic Supplementary Material The online version of this chapter (https://doi.org/10.1007/978-3-030-14032-8_8) contains supplementary material, which is available to authorized users.

H. Mahmoud-Elsayed (✉)
CardioVascular Imaging/Cardiology Department, Queen Elizabeth Hospital, University Hospitals Birmingham NHS Foundation Trust, Birmingham, UK
e-mail: Hani.elsayed@uhb.nhs.uk

Mitral Valve Congenital Malformations

Congenital abnormalities of the mitral valve (MV) represent a wide range of lesions that can be associated with other congenital heart abnormalities [1]. Congenital abnormalities of the MV have been detected in almost 0.5% of 13,400 patients [2].

Preoperative assessment of the anatomical problem is crucial for successful MV repair. As suboptimal repair was shown to be a strong predictor for redo surgeries [3].

The ability of three-dimensional echocardiography (3DE) to provide wide angle *en face* views of the MV from either the left atrium or the left ventricular perspective makes it superior to two-dimensional echocardiography in terms of accurate delineation of the anatomy and the spatial orientation of the different parts of the MV apparatus, which has a significant impact on the understanding of the underlying pathology and on the planning of repair procedures.

There are some anatomical variations that can be encountered during daily practice that may or may not affect the MV function. One of the most common anatomical variations are the cleft-like indentations defined as a visible tissue defect seen during systole, occupying the interscallop region of the posterior leaflet (not plicatures of leaflets' free edge at other location) and extending at least half depth of the adjacent mitral scallop height [4] (Fig. 8.1, Video 8.1). Normal indentations that delineates the scallops of the posterior mitral leaflet are usually not deep, but deep cleft-like indentations can be associated with mitral regurgitation [5] and failure of mitral repair [6].

Another, very rare, malformation of the MV is the presence of accessory MV tissue. This malformation is characterized by a mobile mass attached to the body of the anterior MV leaflet, floating in the left ventricular outflow tract with variable degree of obstruction (Fig. 8.2, Videos 8.2a and 8.2b). This malformation is more frequent on the MV, but it may involve both atrio-ventricular valves and/or be associated with other congenital malformations [7]. The mobile

L. P. Badano et al. (eds.), *Textbook of Three-Dimensional Echocardiography*, https://doi.org/10.1007/978-3-030-14032-8_8

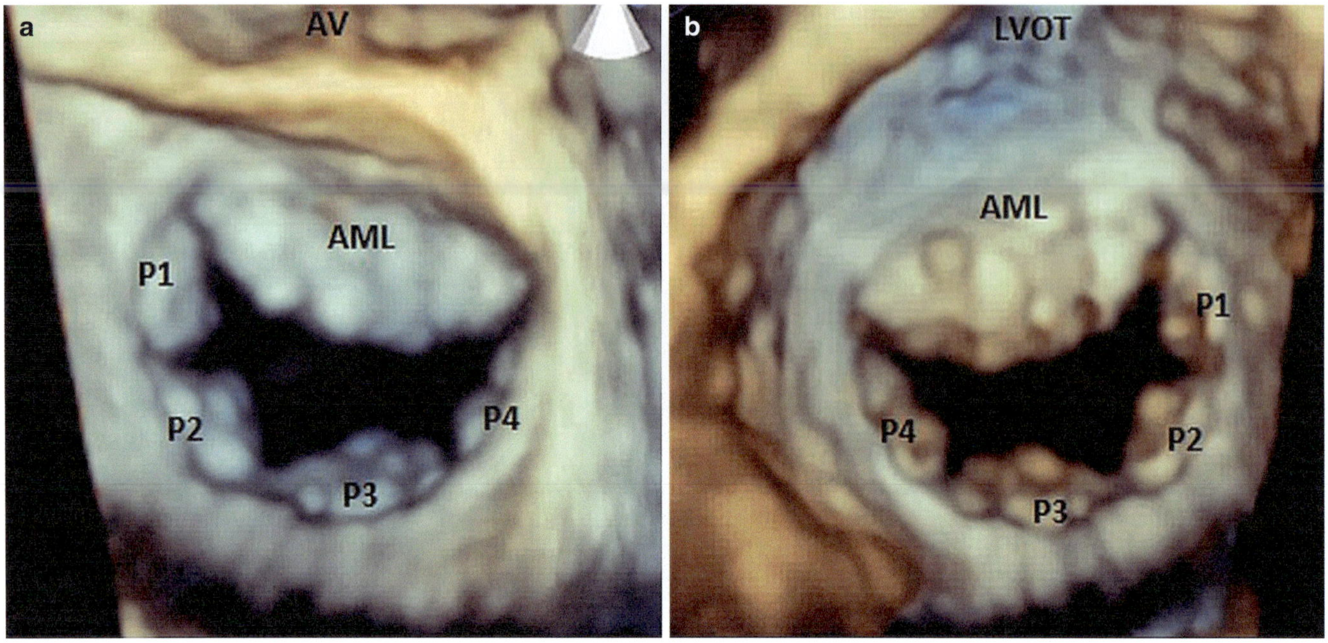

Fig. 8.1 Transesophageal 3DE zoom acquisition of the mitral valve which was cropped to show the mitral valve from both the left atrial (**a**) and the left ventricular (**b**) perspectives. The posterior mitral leaflet is divided into four distinct scallops (P1, P2, P3 and P4) by three cleft-like indentations (Video 8.1). *AV* aortic valve, *AML* anterior mitral leaflet, *LVOT* left ventricular outflow tract

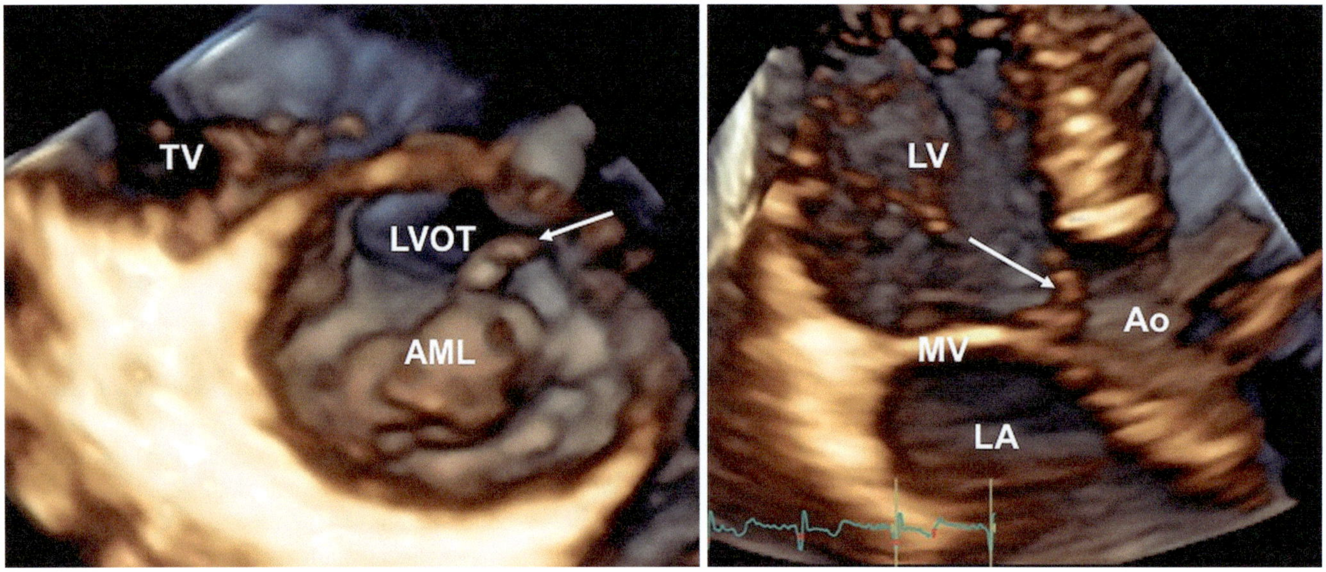

Fig. 8.2 Transthoracic 3DE showing the classic features of accessory mitral valve tissue. *Left panel*, transversal cut plane showing the mitral valve from the ventricular perspective and the accessory mitral valve tissue (white arrow) attached to the body of anterior mitral valve leaflet (Video 8.2a Left). *Right panel*, longitudinal cut plane from the same data set showing the motion of the accessory mitral valve tissue in the left ventricular outflow tract (Video 8.2b Right). *AML* anterior mitral valve leaflet, *Ao* aortic valve, *LA* left atrium, *LV* left ventricle, *LVOT* left ventricular outflow tract, *MV* mitral valve, *TV* tricuspid valve

type (pedunculated or leaflet like) is more frequent than the fixed type, and the presence of chordae tendineae is frequent with variable site of attachment [8].

Other well-known congenital abnormalities of the MV include: MV cleft, double orifice MV, congenital mitral stenosis, parachute MV, and supra-valvular ring.

Mitral Valve Cleft

The definition of MV cleft is the division of one of the leaflets (usually the anterior one) of the MV [9]. MV cleft can occur in isolation or in association with other congenital abnormalities. Although cleft can affect any segment of the

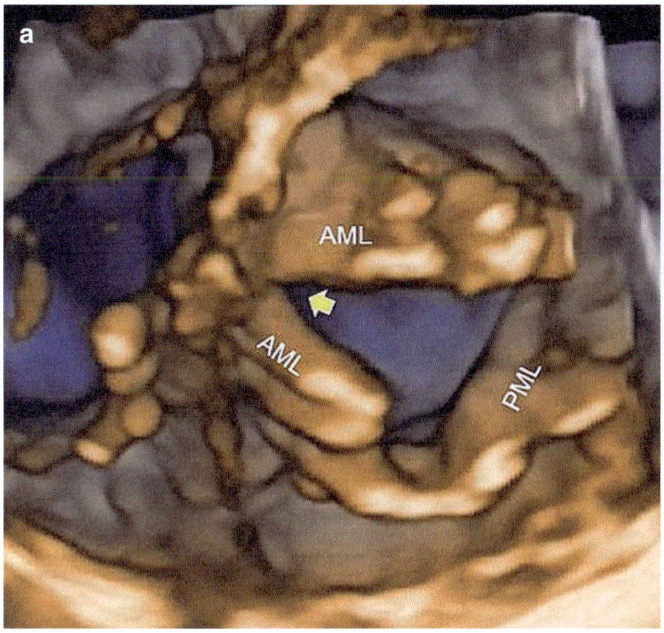

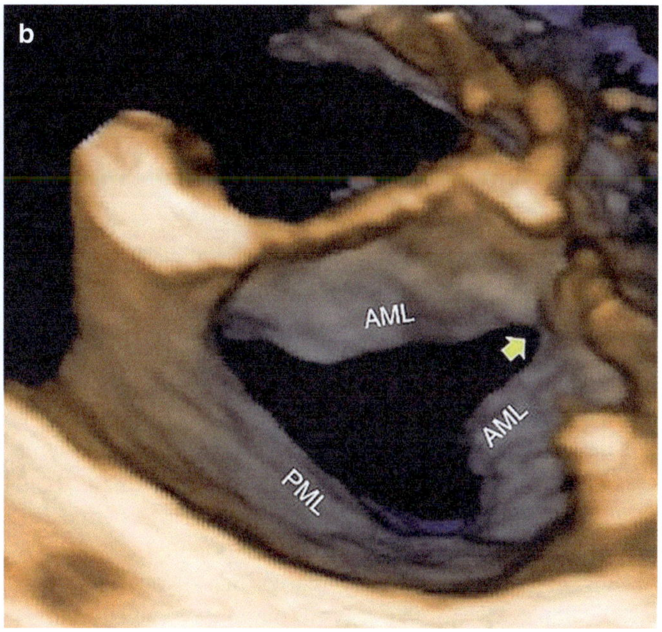

Fig. 8.3 Cleft of the anterior leaflet of the mitral valve. Transthoracic 3DE visualization of the mitral valve from the left ventricular (**a**, Video 8.3a Left) and left atrial (**b**, Video 8.3b Right) perspectives showing a cleft (yellow arrow) of the anterior mitral leaflet (AML) in a patient with ostium primum atrial septal defect. The cleft reaches the annulus splitting the AML into two parts while the posterior mitral leaflet (PML) is intact

MV leaflet, the most common locations are the middle segments (i.e. A2 or P2).

In patients with isolated cleft of the anterior mitral leaflet, the usual site of the cleft is towards left ventricular outflow tract, at 11 o'clock [3, 10]. Whereas, in patients with atrio-ventricular canal defects there is a counterclockwise rotation of the papillary muscles determining a different position of the cleft which is located towards the interventricular septum [1] (Fig. 8.3, Videos 8.3a and 8.3b). Less often, isolated cleft may be seen in the posterior leaflet of the mitral valve [11] (Fig. 8.4, Video 8.4). Although it may occur at any segment of the posterior leaflet, the predominant localization of the cleft is within scallop P2 [12]. Cleft of the posterior mitral leaflet has been reported to be associated with counterclockwise malrotation of the papillary muscles that may, again, lead one to suspect a common embryological origin with atrio-ventricular septal defect [13].

3DE is very helpful in establishing the diagnosis and delineating the exact anatomy and spatial orientation of the cleft through the anatomically oriented *en face* views for the MV where it appears as a slit-like defect in the leaflet extending from the annulus till the leaflet margin and causing full splitting of the affected leaflet.

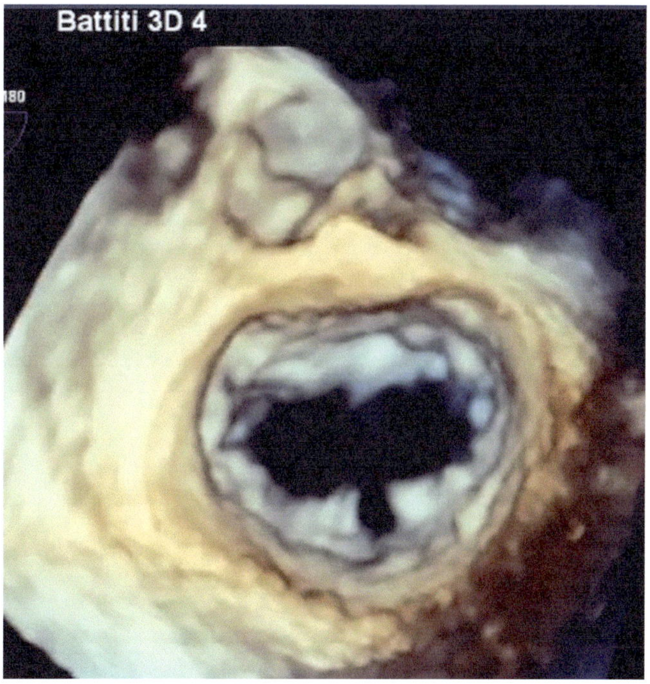

Fig. 8.4 Cleft of the posterior leaflet of the mitral valve. Transesophageal 3DE visualization of the mitral valve from the atrial perspective showing a cleft which splits the posterior leaflet in two parts (Video 8.4)

It was also shown that 3D echocardiography was an accurate tool to assess the severity of the associated mitral regurgitation [14].

Double Orifice Mitral Valve

Double orifice MV is a rare congenital anomaly that in most of the cases has been associated with other forms of congenital heart disease, but rarely found in an isolated form [15, 16]. Double orifice MV is defined as a single fibrous annulus with two orifices opening into the left ventricle [1] (Fig. 8.5, Videos 8.5a and 8.5b).

Double orifice MV is classified into three different types: the "incomplete bridge type", characterized by a small strand of tissue connecting the anterior and posterior leaflets at the leaflet edge level; the "complete bridge type", a fibrous bridge divides the atrioventricular orifice completely from the leaflet edge all the way through the valve annulus (Fig. 8.5); finally, the 'hole type' (eccentric), a secondary orifice with subvalvular apparatus occurs in the lateral commissure of the mitral valve [17].

3DE was proven to be sensitive and accurate in identifying double orifice MV, even in the newborn [18]. Through the anatomically oriented enface view of the MV from the left atrial and the left ventricular perspectives we can appreciate the double orifice pattern very easily (Fig. 8.5).

Congenital double orifice MV has to be differentiated from the iatrogenic causes of double orifice MV such as surgical Alfieri's stitch or trans-catheter MitraClip.

Mitral Ring

Mitral ring (supravalvar mitral ring or supramitral ring) is one of the components described by Shone et al. in Shone's syndrome (association of coarctation of the aorta, subaortic stenosis, parachute MV and supramitral ring) [19]. Exceptionally isolated, this lesion is more often associated with various other anomalies of the heart such as ventricular septal defects and left-sided obstructive lesions. Two types of mitral rings are described: the supramitral ring is a fibrous membrane originating just above the mitral annulus, beneath the orifice of the left atrial appendage within the muscular atrial vestibule, not adhering to the leaflets and associated with a normal subvalvular apparatus; and the intramitral ring is a thin membrane located within the funnel created by the leaflets of the mitral valve, closely adherent to the valve leaflets, always combined with abnormal subvalvular apparatus.

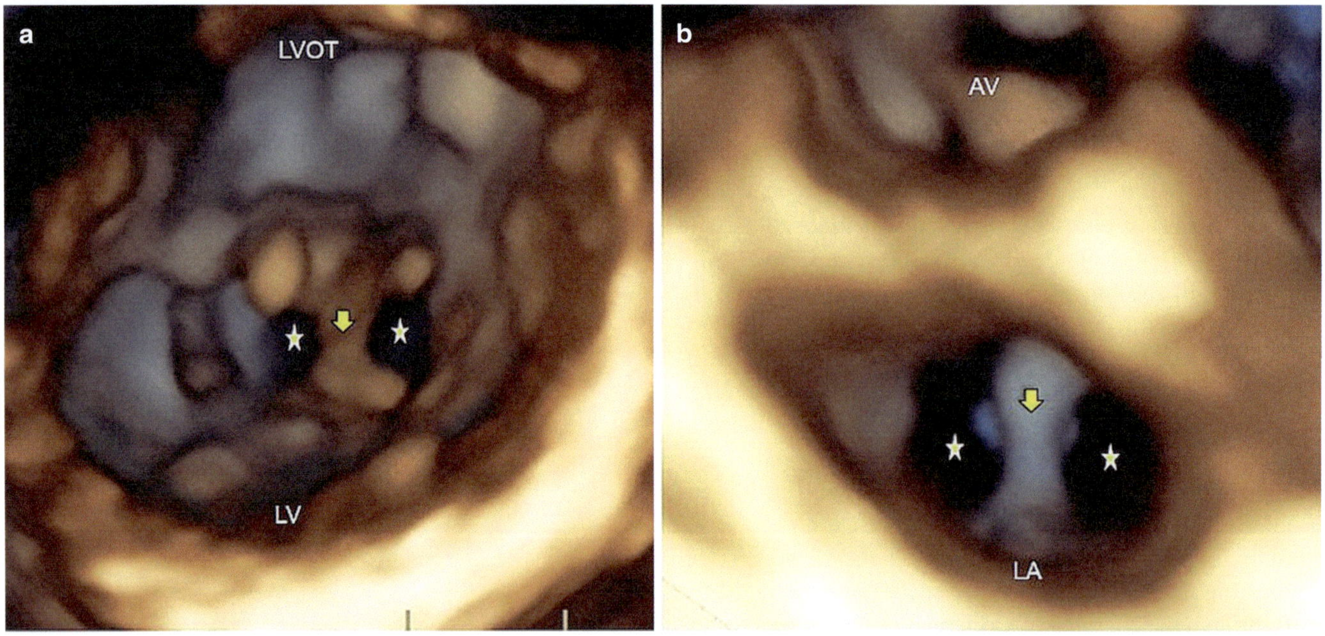

Fig. 8.5 Double orifice mitral valve. Transthoracic 3DE visualization of the MV from both ventricular (**a** and Video 8.5a left) and atrial (**b** and Video 8.5b right) perspectives clearly showed the double orifices (white stars) with a central bridge of abnormal tissue (yellow arrow) connecting the anterior with the posterior leaflet. The two orifices were asymmetric, being the medial orifice slightly larger than the lateral one. Valve leaflets were thin and normally sized. There were two papillary muscles that showed normal morphology and position. *AV* aortic valve, *LA* left atrium, *LV* left ventricle, *LVOT* left ventricular outflow tract

Arcade or Hammock Valve

Anomalous mitral arcade is a congenital abnormalities of the MV in which there is a direct connection of the papillary muscles to the MV leaflets, either directly or through the interposition of unusually short chordae.

Parachute Mitral Valve

True parachute MV is characterized by unilateral attachment of the chordae tendineae to a single (or fused) papillary muscle. This single papillary muscle is usually centrally placed and receives all chordae from both mitral valve leaflets [1] (Fig. 8.6, Videos 8.6a and 8.6b).

The dominant papillary muscle, classically posteromedial [20], is of normal size, whereas the other is elongated and displaced higher in the ventricle with its tip reaching to the annulus. The chordae tendineae are usually short and thickened, thus restricting the motion of the leaflets causing variable degrees of MV stenosis and, uncommonly, regurgitation.

Parachute MV is commonly seen in association with other obstructive lesions affecting the left heart such as Shone's syndrome [19].

The pathognomonic 2D "pear" shape of the mitral valve can be seen in the apical four-chamber view, with the left atrium forming the larger base of the pear and the mitral leaflets the apex [21].

This pathognomonic pattern can also be appreciated using 3DE (Fig. 8.6a). The spatial orientation of the chordae tendineae along the MV orifice and their attachment to a single papillary muscle can be easily detected with a single 3DE acquisition.

Mitral Stenosis

Introduction

Rheumatic fever remains the major cause of MV stenosis, particularly in developing countries [22, 23].

Rheumatic inflammation of the endocardium predisposes to multiple gross changes in the mitral valve, including leaflet thickening, that starts at the tips of the leaflets then progresses towards the bases, leaflet calcification, commissural fusion with reduction of the diastolic mitral valve opening, cordal thickening, fusion and shortening causing a funnel-shaped mitral valve apparatus [24]. Sometimes one of the earliest gross changes of the mitral valve is the disappearance of the indentations of the posterior leaflet hiding the demarcation of the three scallops [25] (Fig. 8.7).

3DE assessment of the MV apparatus should be incorporated into the routine trans-thoracic and/or trans-esophageal evaluation because it provides more physiological as well as morphological information [26]. By providing a unique "en face" view for the MV from both atrial and ventricular perspectives, as well as longitudinal cut planes, 3DE allows accurate morphologic analysis

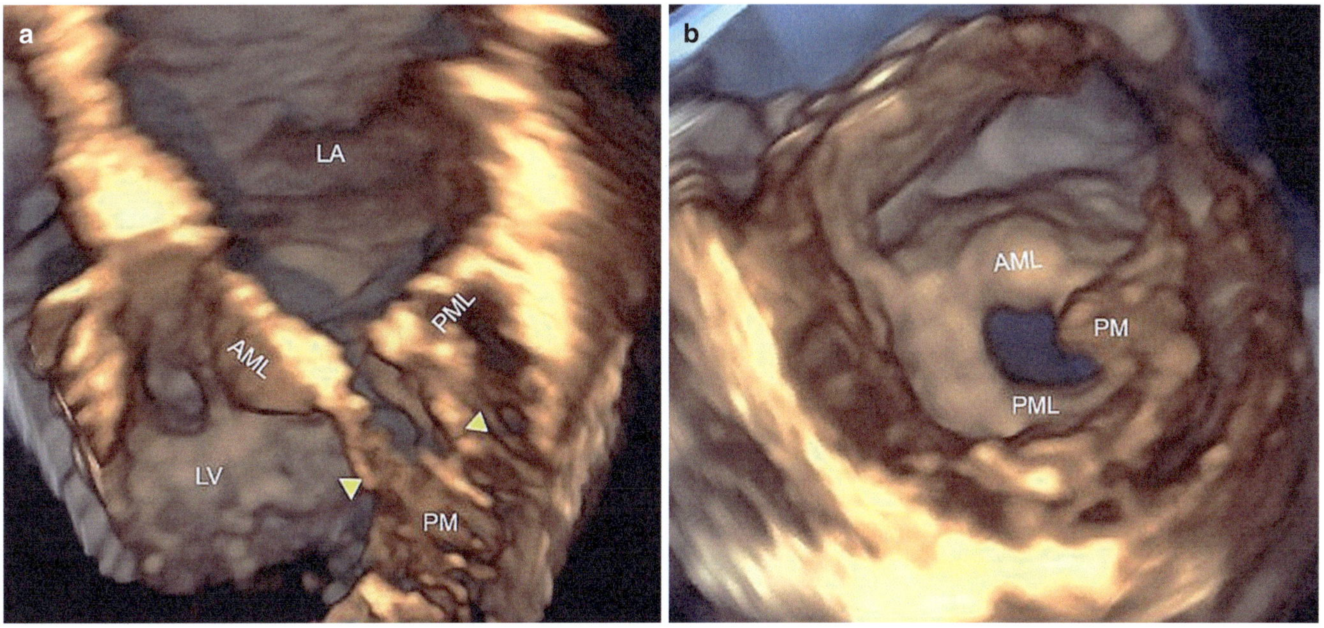

Fig. 8.6 Parachute mitral valve. Transthoracic 3DE visualization of a parachute mitral valve. A longitudinal cut plane (**a** Video 8.6a left) shows a fused papillary muscle (PM). All chordae tendineae are short and thickened and are inserted into this single papillary muscle. En face view of the mitral valve from the ventricular perspective (**b** Video 8.6b right) showing thickened valve leaflets with reduced diastolic excursion

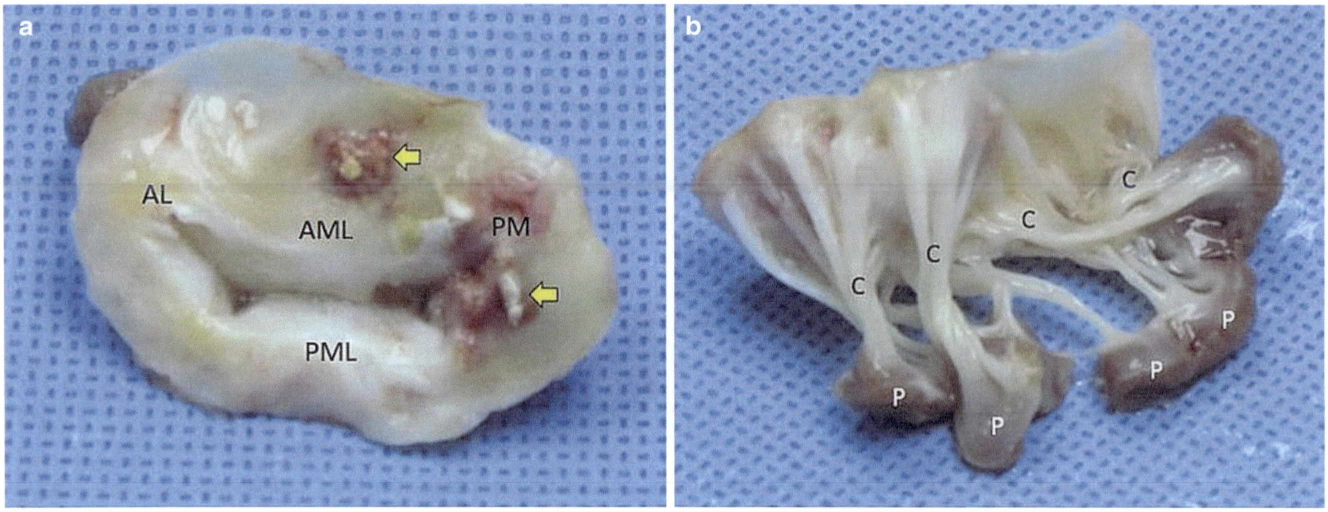

Fig. 8.7 Mitral stenosis. (**a**) Mitral valve after surgical valve replacement, from the left atrial perspective showing the anterior mitral leaflet (AML), posterior mitral leaflet (PML), anterolateral (AL) and posteromedial (PM) commissures. Calcifications (arrows) can be detected at the middle of the AML and around the PM commissure. (**b**) From the LV perspective, thickened and fused chordae (C) and their attachment into the papillary muscles (P). Courtesy of Dr. Marcel P. Harder, Consultant Cardiac Surgeon, Prince Sultan Cardiac Center, Al-Hassa, KSA

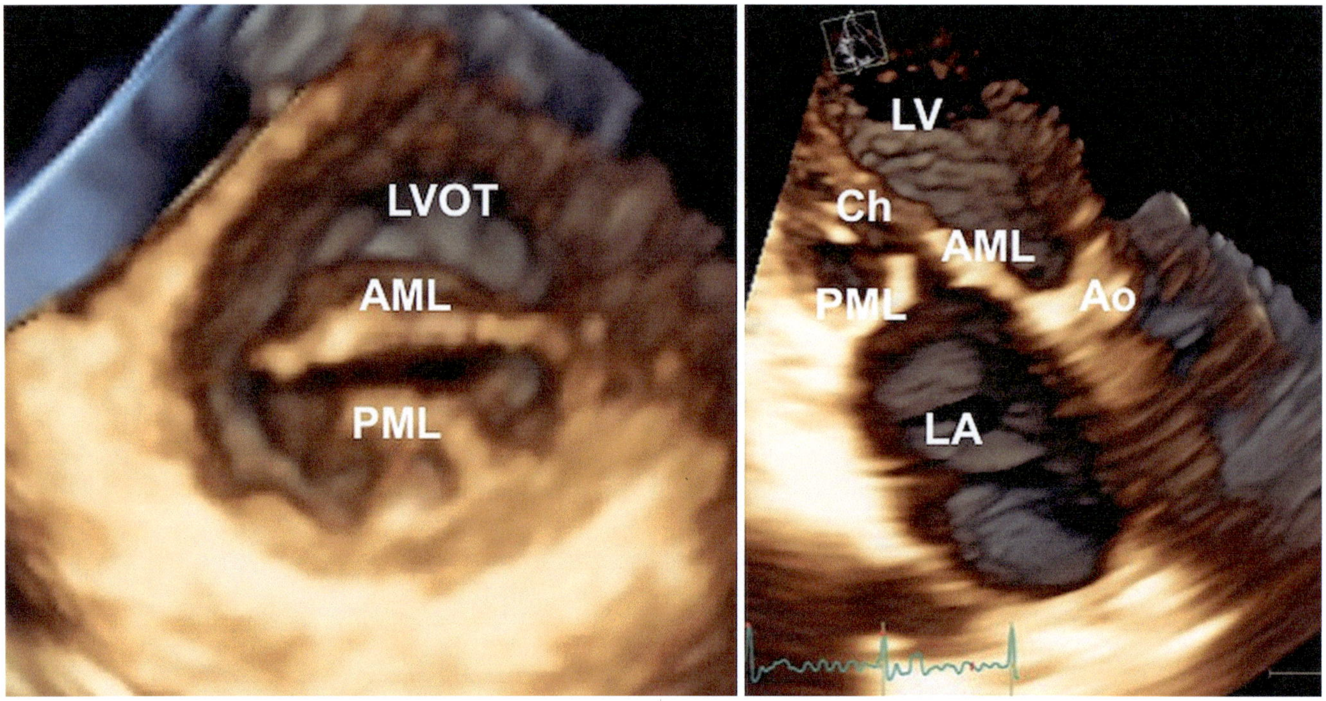

Fig. 8.8 Transthoracic 3DE visualization of a mitral stenosis. *Left panel*, the stenotic mitral valve orifice as it appears from the left ventricular perspective. The doming of the anterior mitral leaflet is visualized (Video 8.7a Left). *Right panel,* the various lesions of the MV apparatus occurring in rheumatic mitral stenosis (reduced excursion of thickened leaflets, shortened and thickened chordae tendineae; enlarged left atrium) can be detected using a longitudinal cut plane (Video 8.7b Right). *AML* anterior mitral leaflet, *Ao* aorta, *Ch* chordae tendineae, *LA* left atrium, *LV* left ventricle, *LVOT* left ventricular outflow tract, *PML* posterior mitral leaflet

of the entire MV apparatus and measurement of residual orifice area [27] (Fig. 8.8, Videos 8.7a and 8.7b).

Hemodynamic severity of mitral valve stenosis is best determined by MV area planimetry [28, 29].

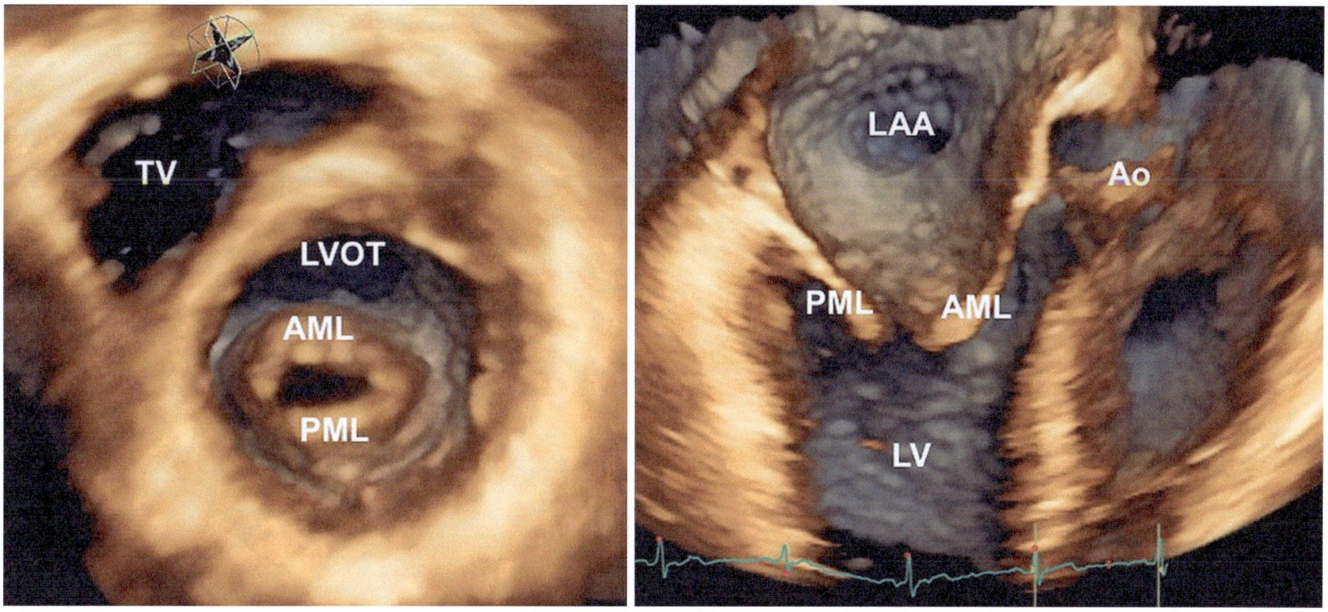

Fig. 8.9 Transesophageal 3DE visualization of a mitral stenosis. *Left panel*, the stenotic mitral valve orifice as it appears from the left ventricular perspective. There is extensive fusion of the commissures (Video 8.8a Left). *Right panel,* Longitudinal cut plane showing the thickened leaflets and the anatomical relationships with the surrounding cardiac structures (Video 8.8b Right). *LAA* left atrial appendage, *TV* tricuspid valve, *AML* anterior mitral leaflet, *Ao* aorta, *Ch* chordae tendineae, *LA* left atrium, *LV* left ventricle, *LVOT* left ventricular outflow tract, *PML* posterior mitral leaflet

Image Acquisition

MV is the classic valve for 3DE due to its relative slower motion and thicker leaflets compared to the other cardiac valves. 3DE data set for the mitral valve can be acquired using any mode of acquisition after optimizing the volume size in order to include the whole MV. Transesophageal 3DE zoom mode provides data sets of the MV with high temporal and spatial resolution. Transthoracic (Fig. 8.8) or transesophageal (Fig. 8.9, Videos 8.8a and 8.8b) full-volume, multiple-beat acquisition is usually needed if imaging of the entire MV apparatus [26].

Qualitative Assessment

The superiority of 3DE over conventional two-dimensional echocardiography for the qualitative morphologic description of the MV has been reported by many studies [27, 30–32]. By rotating and cropping the 3DE data set in various transversal and longitudinal cut planes better assessment of the leaflet mobility and pliability and of mitral commissures, in terms of extent of their fusion and presence of calcification can be obtained.

Leaflet Visualization

The whole extension of mitral leaflet length is difficult to be evaluated through a single two-dimensional echocardiography and different views are needed. By 3DE, it is possible to visualize and evaluate the whole leaflet extension in a single data set (Figs. 8.8 and 8.9). Despite the identification of thicknened leaflet scallop is possible and reproducible, it should be taken into account that the reduced spatial resolution of 3DE, compared to two-dimensional echocardiography, displays more thickened leaflets than what they actually are [33] (Fig. 8.10, Videos 8.9a and 8.9b).

Reduced Diastolic Opening (Funnel Shaped Valve)

The 3DE *en face* view for the MV from the ventricular perspective offers a unique opportunity to qualitatively assess the shape of the real MV orifice that is often not symmetrically oval or circular (Figs. 8.8 and 8.9).

Commissural Fusion

Commissural fusion can be assessed from the LV en-face view of the mitral valve using either transthoracic or transesophageal 3DE. Right-to-left tilting of that volume can show expose the antero-lateral commissure, while left-to-right tilting can expose the postero-medial commissure. See (Fig. 8.11, Video 8.10).

According to Carpentier's classification, commissural fusion can be classified as; grade I: partial fusion of the commissures (Fig. 8.12, Video 8.11); grade II: complete fusion with visible demarcation between the two leaflets (Fig. 8.9); grade III: complete fusion of one or both commissures

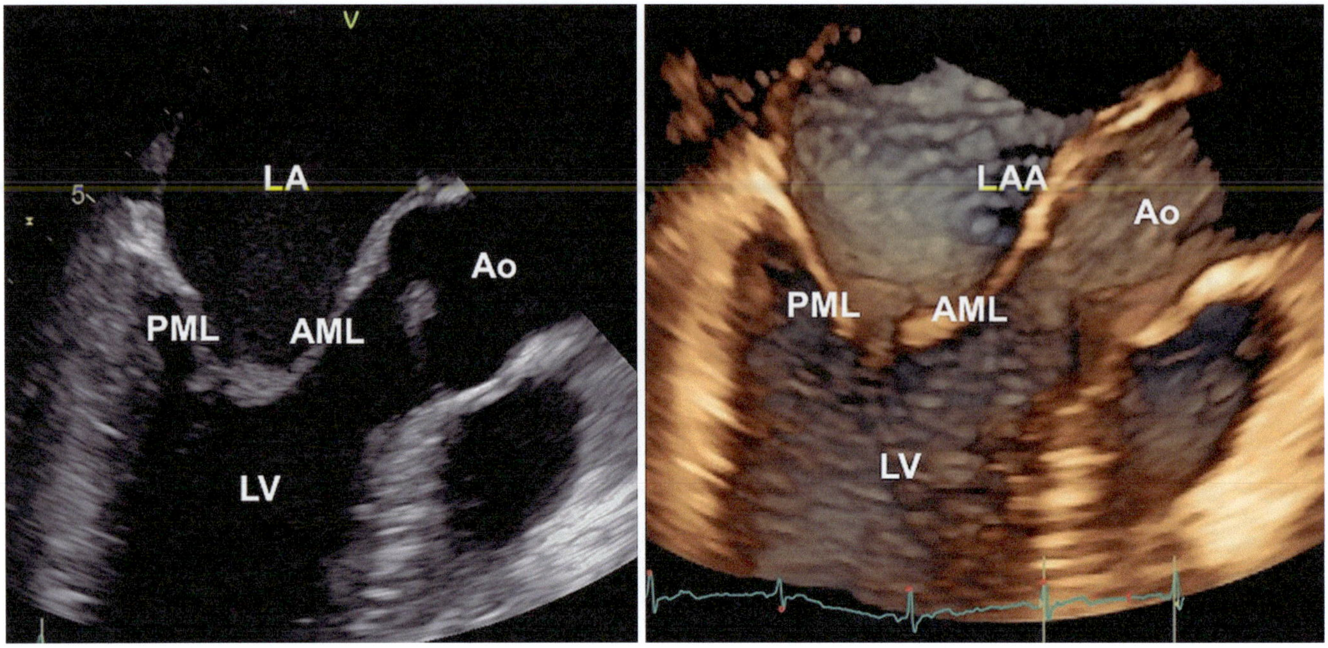

Fig. 8.10 Comparison of leaflet thickness as they are visualized with conventional two-dimensional echocardiography (***Left panel***, Video 8.9a left) and 3DE (***Right panel***, Video 8.9b right). The reduced spatial resolution of 3DE visualize thicker leaflets than conventional two-dimensional echocardiography. *AML* anterior mitral leaflet, *Ao* aorta, *Ch* chordae tendineae, *LA* left atrium, *LV* left ventricle, *LVOT* left ventricular outflow tract, *PML* posterior mitral leaflet

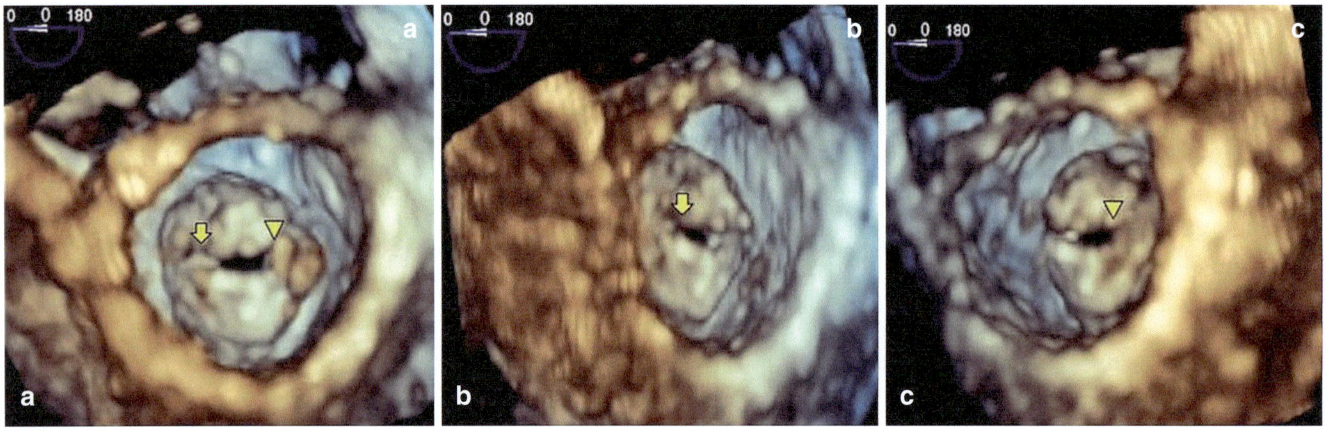

Fig. 8.11 Transesophageal 3DE showing a stenotic rheumatic mitral valve in an *en face* view from ventricular perspective (**a**). A left-to-right rotation of the data set allows the visualization the posteromedial commissure (arrow, **b**). A right-to-left rotation of the data set exposes the anterolateral commissure (arrow head, **c**) (Video 8.10)

without visible demarcation between leaflets (Fig. 8.13, Video 8.12).

It is not uncommon to find asymmetrical commissural fusion of MV (Fig. 8.11) which can be easily appreciated by 3DE [25].

Commissural Calcification

The assessment of leaflet calcification as well as its distribution along the mitral valve orifice, particularly at the commissures is of great importance to predict both the suitability and outcome of percutaneous mitral balloon valvuloplasty [33]. 3DE can be used to assess the extent and distribution of calcification in each scallop utilizing a single 3D data set [34].

Since the shades of color in 3DE code the distance of a structure from the probe rather than histological characteristics of the tissue, one of the limitations of 3DE is the inability to accurately differentiate between calcium and normal tissue if both are at the same distance from the probe, as both will appear with the same color. However, because calcifications usually protrude into the left atrial cavity and they are relatively less mobile than normal tissue, they can be

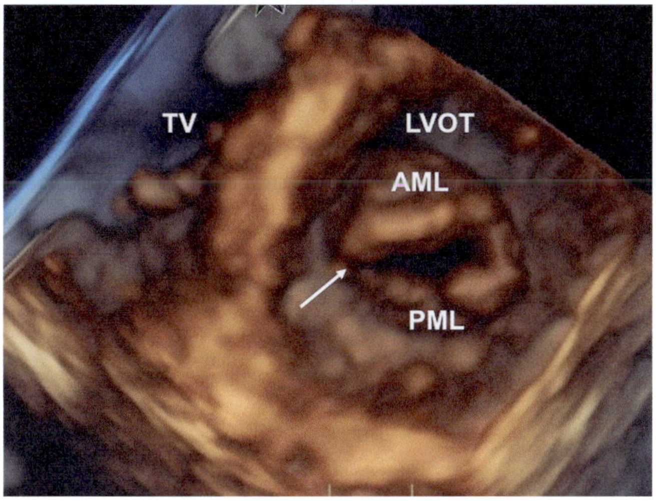

Fig. 8.12 Transesophageal 3DE showing a stenotic rheumatic mitral valve in an *en face* view from ventricular perspective (Video 8.11). The commissures are partially fused with the medial commissure (white arrow) being less involved than the lateral one. *AML* anterior mitral leaflet, *LV* left ventricle, *LVOT* left ventricular outflow tract, *PML* posterior mitral leaflet, *TV* tricuspid valve

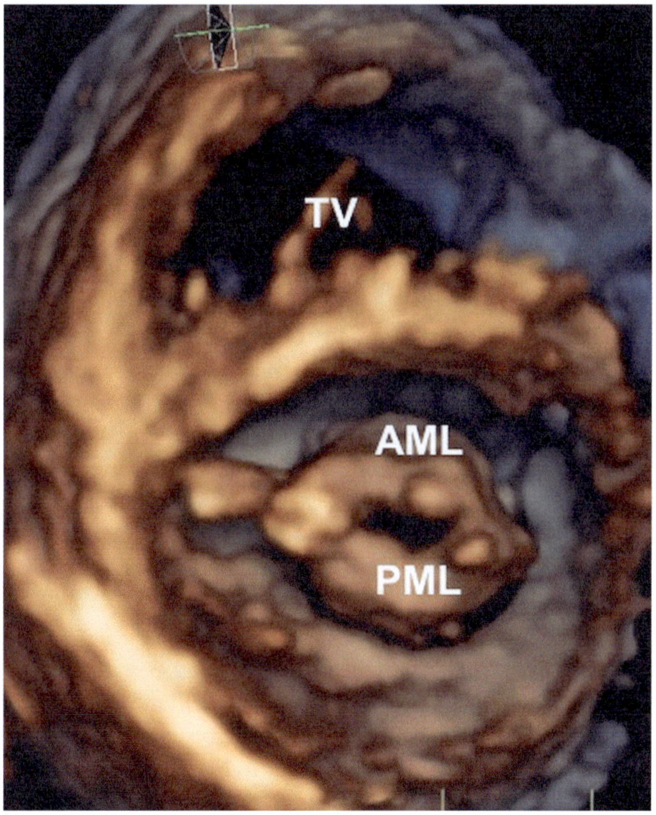

Fig. 8.13 Transesophageal 3DE showing a stenotic rheumatic mitral valve in an *en face* view from ventricular perspective. The commissures are completely fused (Video 8.12). *AML* anterior mitral leaflet, *PML* posterior mitral leaflet, *TV* tricuspid valve

identified and their location and distribution in relation to the commissures can be appreciated [25] (Fig. 8.14).

Leaflet Mobility and Pliability

Leaflet mobility can be well assessed and even scored by 3DE, and it was shown to be a good predictor of successful percutaneous mitral balloon valvuloplasty [33].

Diastolic doming of the anterior mitral leaflet is a very common finding in rheumatic mitral valve stenosis. It is due to restricted motion of the leaflet tips due to commissural fusion. If the body of the leaflet is still more-or-less healthy and mobile it domes into the left ventricular cavity towards the septum (Fig. 8.8). But if the leaflets become fibrosed or calcified this doming decreases (Fig. 8.12). Thus, doming is a sign of leaflet pliability. 3DE does not add too much over two-dimensional echocardiography in the assessment of pliability except if the doming was not symmetrical along the leaflet length.

Sub-valvular Apparatus

Two-dimensional echocardiography was shown to underestimate the subvalvular affection [35], while 3DE was used to assess and score the affection of the subvalvular apparatus with a good reproducibility [33] (Fig. 8.15, Video 8.13).

Quantitative Assessment

Residual Orifice Area Measurement

In patients with mitral stenosis, MV area can be calculated by plenty of methods e.g. the invasive Gorlin formula, pressure half time, the continuity equation, proximal isovelocity surface area method, and the planimetry using either two- or 3D imaging.

The invasively calculated Gorlin formula [36] has been considered the gold standard method for measuring residual orifice area.

Planimetry of the MV orifice was shown to be one the best methods to measure the residual orifice area as it is not affected by the hemodynamics [37]. However, the use of two-dimensional echocardiography to planimeter MV orifice area is limited to the availability of the parasternal window, is based on the assumption that the valve opens parallel to the long axis of the left ventricle and it is heavily operator dependent. It needs a skilled echocardiographer to make sure that the imaging plane is cutting exactly the narrowest MV orifice in diastole otherwise under and/or overestimation of the residual orifice area may occur.

There are many advantages in using 3DE to planimeter the mitral valve area: (1) it is independent on the approach (any acoustic window can be used, the only condition is that

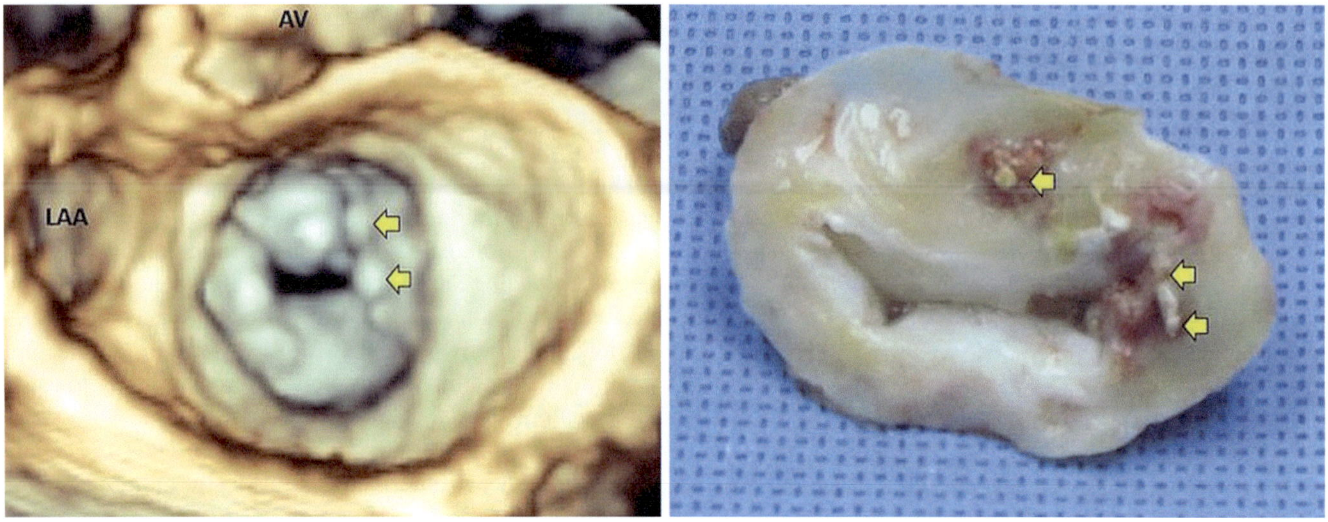

Fig. 8.14 Transesophageal 3DE showing the *en face* anatomically oriented view of the mitral valve from the atrial perspective with calcification spots (arrows) well seen near the posterior-medial commissure (*left panel*). Anatomical specimen of the mitral valve showing calcification spots (arrows) on the middle of the anterior mitral leaflet and around the posteromedial commissure (*right panel*). Courtesy of Dr. Marcel P. Harder, Consultant Cardiac Surgeon, Prince Sultan Cardiac Center, Al-Hassa, KSA

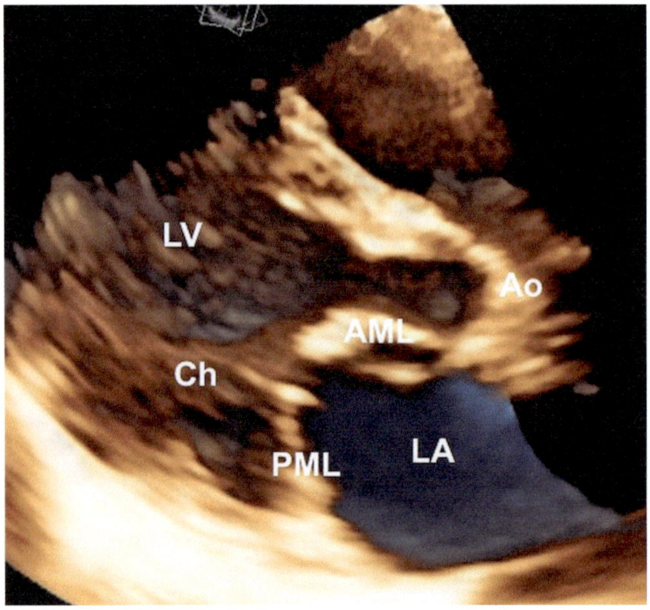

Fig. 8.15 Transthoracic 3DE obtained from the parasternal approach in a patient with severe mitral stenosis. Longitudinal cut plane showing thickened, fused and shortened chordae tendineae (Ch) (Video 8.13). *AML* anterior mitral leaflet, *PML* posterior mitral leaflet, *Ao* aortic valve, *LA* left atrium, *LV* left ventricle

the MV is included in the data set); (2) the position and the orientation of the cut plane can be controlled in order to have it in the narrowest portion of the funnel created by mitral leaflets and oriented perpendicular to the opening axis of the stenosis (Fig. 8.16); (3) The planimetry can be performed either on the volume rendered image or on a two-dimensional cut plane obtained at the level of the narrowest orifice. The latter is preferred to avoid to trace on images in which there are structures at different depths and because the two-dimensional images are less dependent on the gain settings than volume rendering (Fig. 8.17, Video 8.14).

The 3DE planimetered MV area has been shown to be well correlated both with the one calculated invasively with the Gorlin formula [38], and to be superior to MV area planimetered using two-dimensional echocardiography as well as calculated with the pressure half-time method [38, 39].

Mitral Valve Scoring

Echocardiographic assessment of MV apparatus in rheumatic mitral stenosis is pivotal to plan treatment and predict outcomes.

Rheumatic involvement of the MV apparatus includes progressive leaflet thickening and calcification, commissural fusions and/or calcification, cordal thickening, fusion and/or shortening. All of them contribute to the global narrowing of the MV orifice and the funnel shaped appearance of the MV apparatus [40].

Different scoring systems have been developed to assess the suitability of the rheumatic mitral stenosis for percutaneous mitral balloon valvuloplasty by evaluating and scoring the MV leaflet mobility and flexibility, extent of leaflet thickening and calcification, subvalvular thickening and fusion, and extent of commissural fusion and calcification. The latter being one of the strongest predictors of outcome after percutaneous mitral balloon valvuloplasty as it affects the degree of commissural splitting [41]. Among the different scoring systems, the most widely used is the Wilkins's scoring system computed using two-dimensional echocardiography [42].

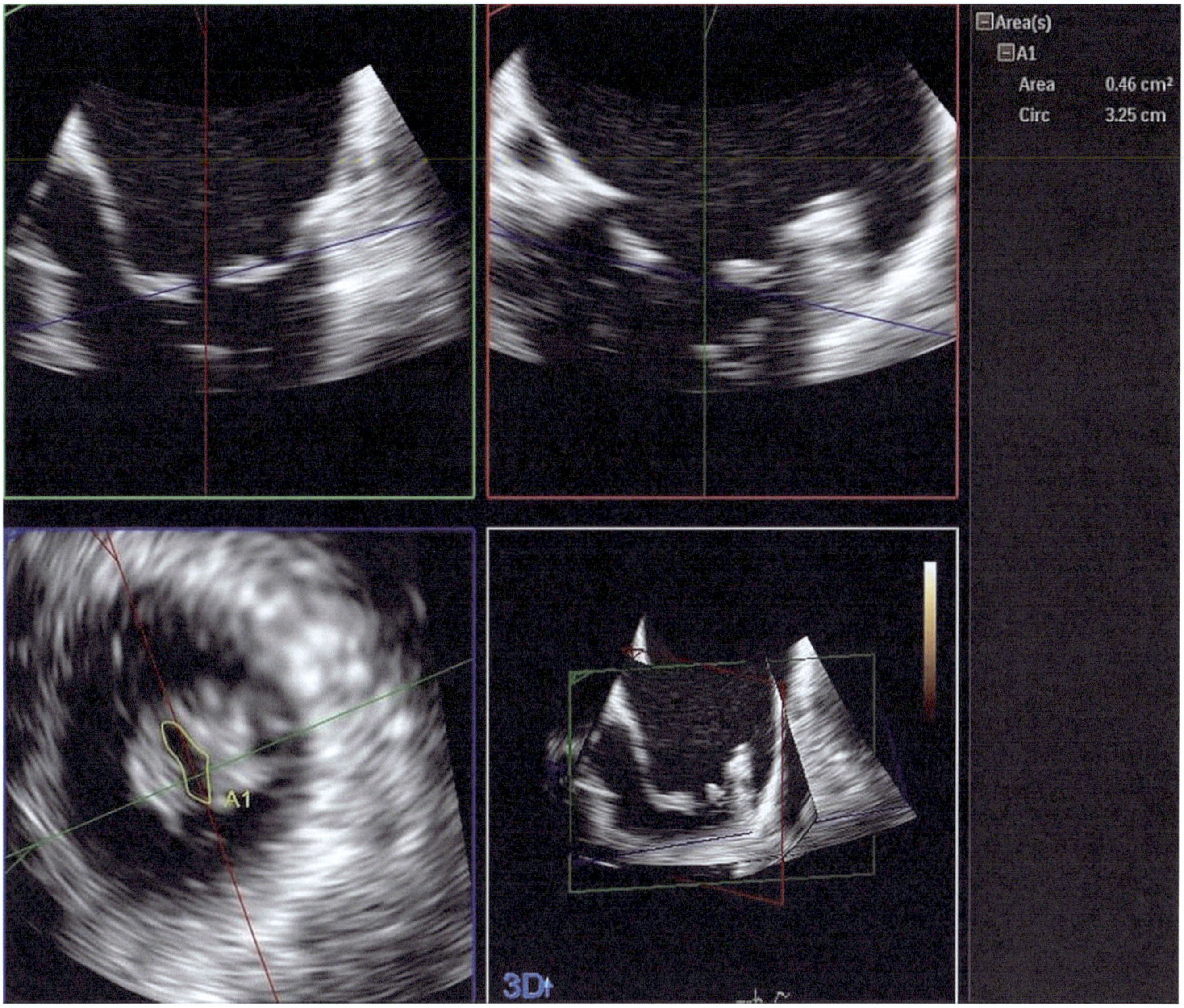

Fig. 8.16 Multi-planar reformatting (MPR) mode during offline analysis of a full-volume obtained from a patient with stenotic rheumatic mitral valve. The blue plane is positioned at the tip of the thickened mitral leaflet perpendicular to the opening direction of the stenotic orifice. Position and orientation of the blue plane is controlled in the two orthogonal longitudinal planes (red and green planes). The planimetry of the residual orifice area can be performed in the blue plane (left lower panel) where a transversal cut plane of the mitral valve orifice is shown

Anwar et al. [33] introduced a score obtained using 3DE to assess the patients with mitral stenosis before percutaneous mitral balloon valvuloplasty. This score includes the evaluation of both mitral leaflets as well as the subvalvular apparatus. The 3DE score was shown to be feasible and highly reproducible with good interobserver and intraobserver agreement in the assessment of MV in patients with mitral stenosis [33]. Leaflet mobility and the involvement of the subvalvular apparatus were found to be the best predictors of optimal percutaneous mitral balloon valvuloplasty results. High 3DE calcification score was associated with the incidence and severity of post-procedural mitral regurgitation (Table 8.1).

Following the general principles of the Wilkins's score, the 3DE score was developed to include both MV leaflets as well as the subvalvular apparatus (Table 8.1). Each scallop of both MV leaflets was separately assessed and scored in terms of thickness, mobility, and calcification as follows: normal thickness and mobility were scored as 0; whereas abnormal thickness or restricted mobility was scored 1. Absence of calcification was scored 0, whereas calcification in middle portion (A2 or P2) was scored 1. Calcification of the commissural scallops of both leaflets (A1, A3, P1, and P3) was scored 2, because commissural calcification carries higher risk than middle scallop calcification.

The subvalvular apparatus was divided into three levels, proximal (at the valve level), middle, and distal (at the papillary muscle level) and it assessed in terms of chordal thickness and separation. Normal chordal thickness was scored 0,

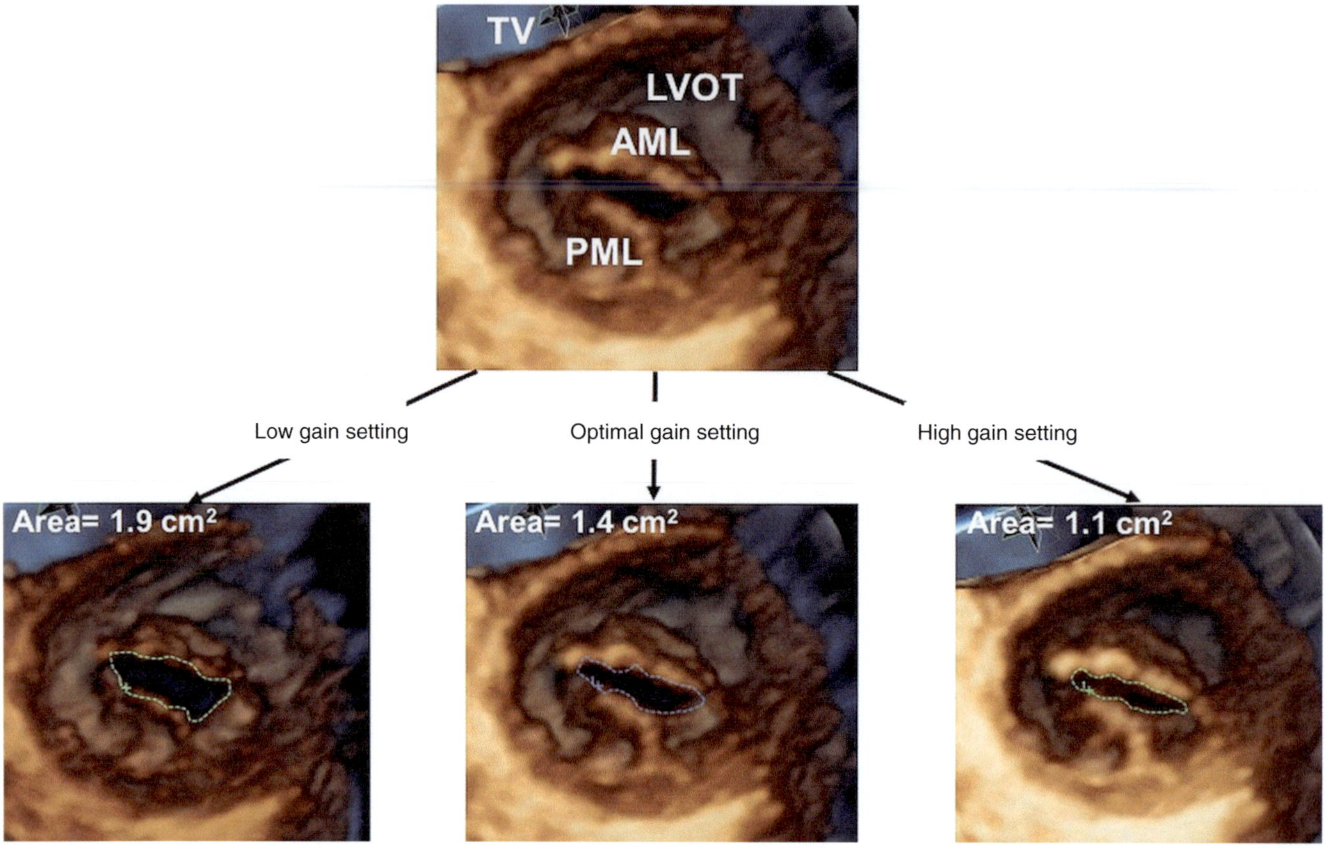

Fig. 8.17 Effects of gain settings on mitral valve area planimetered on 3DE volume rendered images. *Top panel*, the orifice is clearly delimited by leaflet margins that are at different depth in the data set whereas the planimetry occurs on a flat plane that cannot account for it (Video 8.14). *Lower left panel*, gain setting is too low (the left atrial wall almost disappear) and a 36% overestimation of actual residual mitral valve orifice area occurred. *Lower central panel*, optimal gain setting allows the correct measurement of residual mitral valve orifice area (1.4 cm^2); *Lower right panel*, gain setting is too high and a 21% underestimation of actual residual mitral valve orifice area occurred

Table 8.1 3DE score for the assessment of mitral stenosis

	Anterior mitral leaflet			Posterior mitral leaflet		
	A1	A2	A3	P1	P2	P3
Thickness (0–6) (0 = normal, 1 = thickened)[a]	0–1	0–1	0–1	0–1	0–1	0–1
Mobility (0–6) (0 = normal, 1 = limited)[a]	0–1	0–1	0–1	0–1	0–1	0–1
Calcification (0–10) (0 = no, 1–2 = calcified)[b]	0–2	0–1	0–2	0–2	0–1	0–2
Subvalvular apparatus						
	Proximal third		**Middle third**		**Distal third**	
Thickness (0–3) (0 = normal, 1 = thickened)	0–1		0–1		0–1	
Separation (0–6) (0 = normal, 1 = partial, 2 = no)	0, 1, 2		0, 1, 2		0, 1, 2	

Modified from Anwar et al. [33] with permission from Elsevier. Reprinted from Journal of the American Society of Echocardiography, Vol. 23/No. 1, Anwar AM, Attia WM, Nosir YF, Soliman OI, Mosad MA, Othman M, et al., Validation of a New Score for the Assessment of Mitral Stenosis Using Real-Time Three-Dimensional Echocardiography, pp. 13–22, © 2010, with permission from Elsevier

[a]Normal = 0, mild = 1–2, moderate = 3–4, severe ≥ 5

[b]Normal = 0, mild = 1–2, moderate = 3–5, severe ≥ 6

whereas chordal thickening was scored 1. Normal chordal separation (distance in between >5 mm) was scored 0, partial chordal separation (distance in between <5 mm) was scored 1, and a score of 2 was given to absence of chordal separation.

Final 3DE score will be obtained by summing up the individual scores of leaflets and subvalvular apparatus and it will range from 0 to 31 points. Mild MV involvement was defined as 3DE score <8, moderate MV involvement as 3DE score between 8 and 13, and severe MV involvement as 3DE score ≥14 points [33].

Non-rheumatic Mitral Stenosis

Other less common causes of mitral stenosis include congenital mitral stenosis which also shows diastolic doming of MV leaflets, and degenerative, calcific mitral stenosis. Unlike rheumatic mitral stenosis, degenerative, calcific mitral stenosis is characterized by marked mitral annular calcification that encroaches on the bases of the mitral leaflets with a lesser effect on the leaflet tips causing no diastolic doming (Fig. 8.18, Videos 8.15a, 8.15b, and 8.15c).

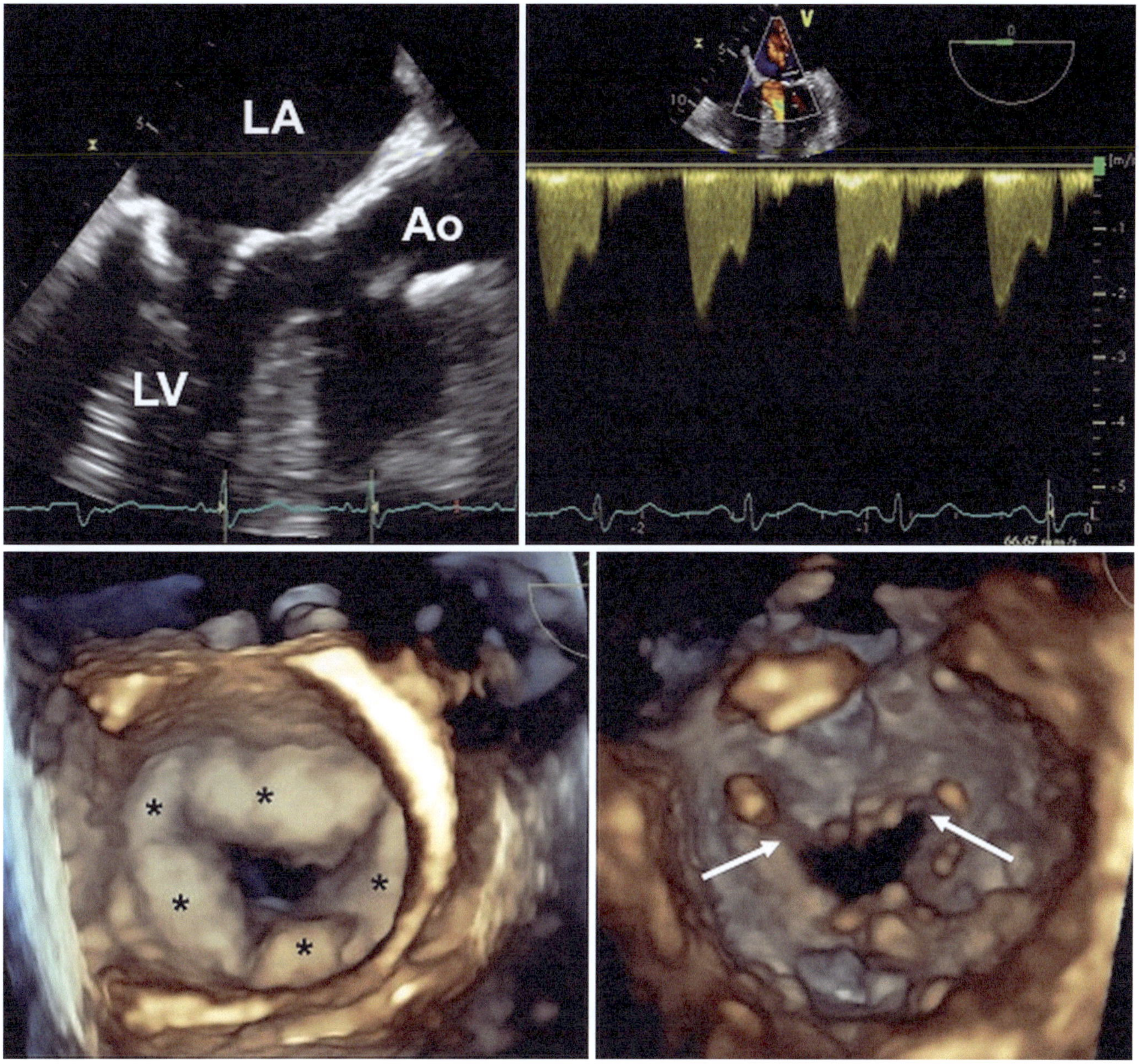

Fig. 8.18 Degenerative, calcific mitral stenosis. *Left upper panel*, transesophageal two-dimensional long axis view showing the extensive calcification of the annulus involving the basal two thirds of the mitral leaflets (Video 8.15a Upper). *Left lower panel*, Transesophageal 3DE *en face* view of the mitral valve from the atrial perspective showing the massive calcifications of the annulus (black asterisks) narrowing the mitral valve orifice (Video 8.15b Left). *Right lower panel*, Transesophageal 3DE *en face* view of the mitral valve from the ventricular perspective showing the normal opening of both the commissures (white arrows) (Video 8.15c Right)

Usually, the degenerative calcification involves the posterior annulus, with minimal extension to leaflets and chordae. Reduction of normal mitral annular dilatation during diastole and the addition of impaired anterior mitral leaflet mobility appeared to be possible mechanisms for the significant functional stenosis. Transvalvular mean gradient is not the best marker of the severity of mitral stenosis because it is also influenced by other factors (heart rate, presence of regurgitation etc.). The values of mean gradient and systolic pulmonary artery pressure should be only supportive signs. Continuity equation method is an independent standard for measuring the effective MVA in degenerative MS, correlating well with invasive methods. Both two- and 3DE planimetry of residual orifice area have limitations, in regard to the irregularity and non planarity of the orifice due to calcifications (Fig. 8.18) [43].

To differentiate degenerative from rheumatic mitral stenosis we have proposed four criteria: (1) presence of significant transvalvular gradient; (2) circular mitral annular calcification with calcific involvement of the leaflets which are not thickened, (3) absence of commissural fusion; (4) absence of involvement of the subvalvular apparatus. 3DE is pivotal to assess the extent of calcifications, commissural and subvalvular apparatus involvement (Fig. 8.18).

Percutaneous Mitral Balloon Valvuloplasty

In 1984, Inoue introduced his new balloon for percutaneous mitral commissurotomy [44]. His procedure showed a huge success rate (>95%) with very low hospital mortality rates [31], and became the first-line treatment for anatomically suitable symptomatic patients with severe rheumatic MV stenosis.

The detailed description of the procedural steps is beyond the scope of this book. In short, it starts with transseptal puncture through which the balloon catheter will be introduced into the left atrium. Then the balloon will be positioned across the stenotic mitral valve and the distal part of the balloon will be inflated and pulled back till it touches the ventricular side of the MV orifice. Finally, the proximal portion of the balloon will be inflated to split MV commissures. Then, echocardiography will be used to assess the results of the procedure by measuring the residual MV area and transvalvular gradients, and to identify complications if any.

Although many centers use fluoroscopy as the sole guiding modality during percutaneous mitral balloon valvuloplasty, yet transesophageal two- 3DE has been shown to have an incremental value in different procedural steps.

Transeptal puncture can really be challenging in patients with previous transeptal puncture, cardiac surgery, markedly dilated left atrium or in patients suffering from scoliosis. In those patients, transesophageal two- 3DE can give more confidence in determining the suitable puncture site and to avoid complications. However, two-dimensional transesophageal echocardiography has the inherent disadvantage of being a tomographic imaging technique and it is not uncommon for the echocardiographer to lose the view of the catheter if it moves few millimeters out of the very thin imaging plane.

Transesophageal 3DE was shown to have an incremental value over its two-dimensional counterpart during the transeptal puncture as it has the potential to shorten both the fluoroscopy time and radiation exposure. These results are due to the ability of 3DE to provide anatomically oriented *en face* view for the inter-atrial septum from the right atrial perspective to allow the interventionist to visualize the position of the puncture catheter and needle in relationship to the fossa ovalis, giving an easier and more confident reference compared to fluoroscopy where the interventionist can only see the catheters [45].

RATLe-90 maneuver "**R**otate **A**nti-clockwise **T**ilt **Le**ft for **90** degrees", was described as a 3DE step-by-step approach to get the anatomically oriented view for the inter-atrial septum from the right atrial perspective in order to use it for monitoring the transeptal puncture (Figs. 8.19, 8.20, and 8.21, Videos 8.16 and 8.17).

One of the challenges encountered with transesophageal 3DE is the appreciation of the septal tenting, and that can be overcome with mild tilting of the 3D volume in order to be able to see the tenting point from a side [46] (Fig. 8.22, Video 8.18). For most of the cases, the preferred transeptal puncture site is the infero-posterior part of the fossa (Fig. 8.22).

The 3DE anatomically oriented view for the MV from the left atrial perspective, acquired in zoom mode, is usually optimum for monitoring and guiding the balloon positioning across the stenotic MV (Fig. 8.23, Video 8.19).

Although 3DE is not yet proven to shorten the time of this step, the anatomically oriented wide sector live images it provides are easily understood and create a common language between the echocardiographer and the interventionist. At the same time, 3DE has the potential to decrease the number of transesophageal probe manipulations needed to obtain the different views with two-dimensional echocardiography. Differently from two-dimensional echocardiography, the 3DE wide sector live image will keep both the balloon and the catheter within the view field even if they swing from side to side within the left atrium.

Transesophageal 3DE can also help to monitor the behaviour of the inflating balloon within the MV orifice. However, this can often be done using two-dimensional or X-plane imaging in order to be able to visualize both the distal and the proximal parts of the balloon (Fig. 8.24, Video 8.20).

After balloon withdrawal, the echocardiographer will check the expected increase in the MV area, the increase in commissural splitting which is the main target of the procedure, assess the presence and severity of mitral regurgitation if any, evaluate the mechanism of mitral regurgitation and exclude MV leaflet tear.

Transesophageal 3DE provides more accurate planimetry of residual MV orifice area using the multiplanar reformatting compared with two-dimensional transesophageal in the immediate post-procedural setting [47].

Transesophageal 3DE was also shown to be more accurate than either two-dimensional transesophageal echocardiography or intracardiac echocardiography to detect the presence and extent of MV leaflet tears [48] and to assess the extent of commissural splitting.

Assessment of commissural splitting using transesophageal 3DE is also more superior than with two-dimensional transesophageal and it has an important prognostic value of the clinical success of the procedure [49] (Fig. 8.25).

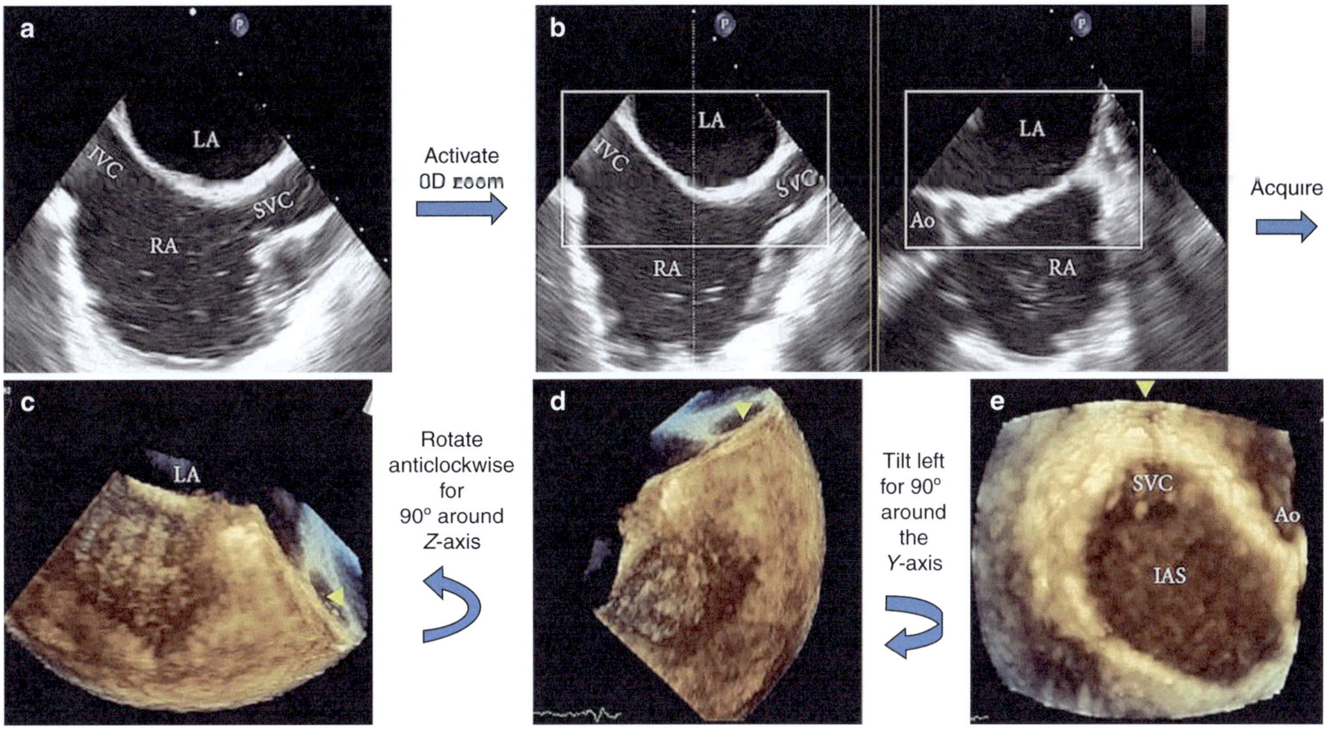

Fig. 8.19 RATLe-90 Maneuver; starting by 2D-mid-esophageal 90° bicaval view (**a**), activate the 3D-zoom mode. The zoom box should be optimized to include the openings of the superior vena cava (SVC), inferior vena cava (IVC), and aortic root (Ao), with enough depth to include the whole interatrial septum (IAS) from both atrial perspectives excluding extra atrial tissues (**b**). Then, acquiring this volume will give us a truncated volume with the SVC (arrow head) pointing to the right of the screen, IVC pointing to the left, left atrial perspective of the IAS is up, and right atrial perspective is down (**c**). Then we will rotate anticlockwise this volume for 90° around the *z*-axis to have the SVC pointing superiorly (arrow head) and the IVC pointing inferiorly (**d**). Then we will Tilt-Left this volume for 90° around the *y*-axis to have the anatomically oriented en face view of the IAS from the right atrial (RA) perspective (**e**) (Video 8.16) [46]. Figure and video reproduced from Mahmoud HM, Al-Ghamdi MA, Ghabashi AE Anwar AM. A Proposed Maneuver to Guide Transseptal Puncture Using Real-Time Three-Dimensional Transesophageal Echocardiography: Pilot Study. Cardiol Res Practice. 2015;2015, Article ID 174051, 4 pages

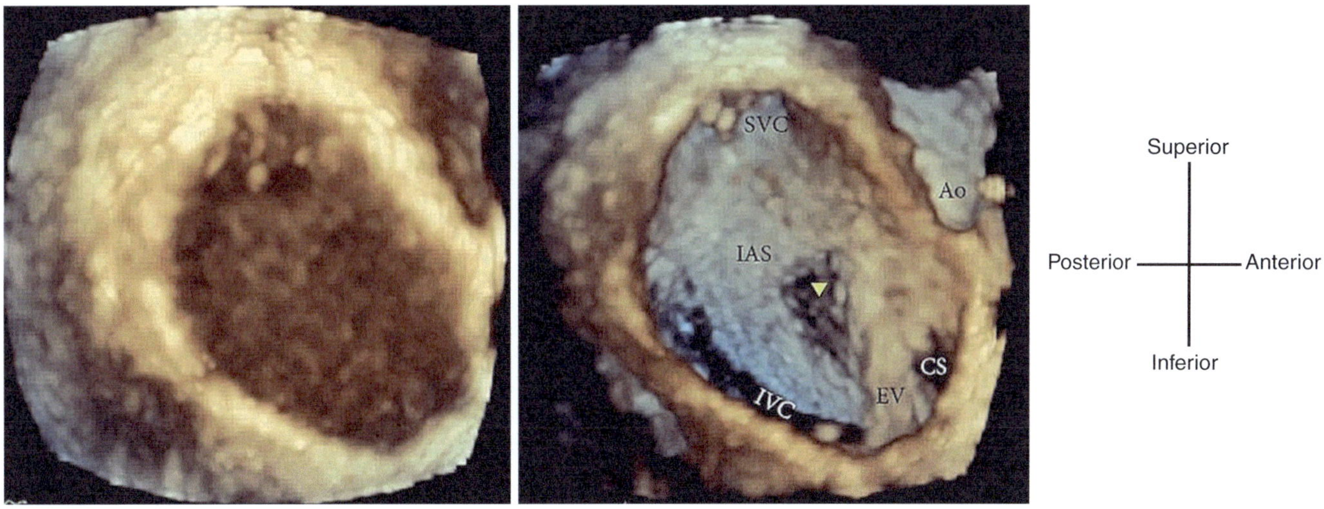

Fig. 8.20 Reducing the gain will remove the noise and will allow clear identification of the right atrial structures, for example, superior (SVC) and inferior (IVC) vena cava opening, Eustachian valve (EV), coronary sinus (CS) opening, and aortic root (Ao). Further gain reduction will cause dropout artifact in the thin area of the fossa ovalis (arrow head) that will help determining its location to guide septal puncture (Video 8.17) [46]. Figure and video reproduced from Mahmoud HM, Al-Ghamdi MA, Ghabashi AE Anwar AM. A Proposed Maneuver to Guide Transseptal Puncture Using Real-Time Three-Dimensional Transesophageal Echocardiography: Pilot Study. Cardiol Res Practice. 2015;2015, Article ID 174051, 4 pages

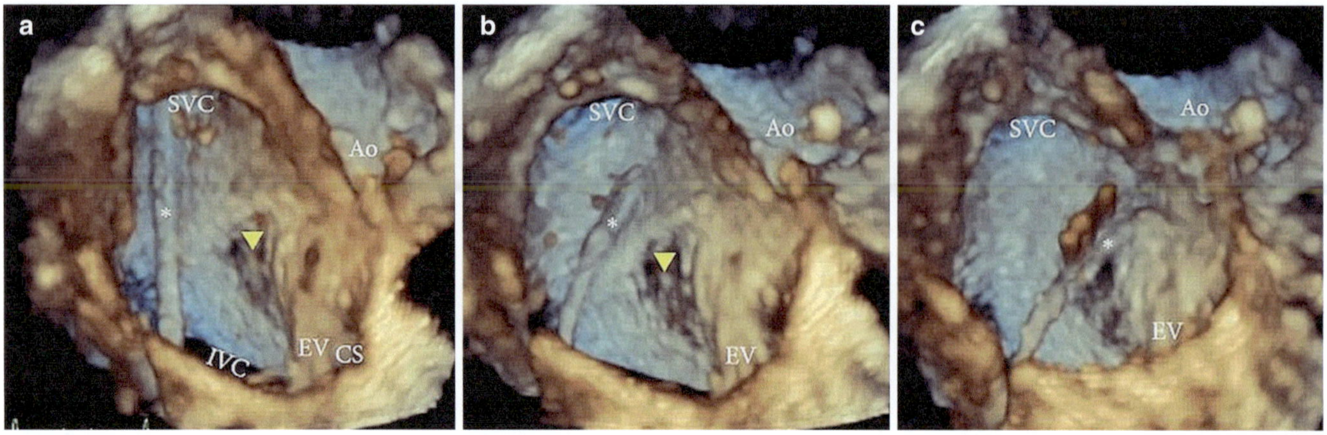

Fig. 8.21 Transesophageal 3DE anatomically oriented view of the interatrial septum from the right atrial perspective during guidance of transseptal puncture. The puncture catheter (asterisk) was introduced through the inferior vena cava (IVC) into the superior vena cava (SVC) (**a**). Then the catheter (asterisk) was pulled inferiorly and anteriorly towards the thin part of the interatrial septum (the arrow head points to the "fossa ovalis") (**b**, **c**) [46]. Figure reproduced from Mahmoud HM, Al-Ghamdi MA, Ghabashi AE Anwar AM. A Proposed Maneuver to Guide Transseptal Puncture Using Real-Time Three-Dimensional Transesophageal Echocardiography: Pilot Study. Cardiol Res Practice. 2015;2015, Article ID 174051, 4 pages

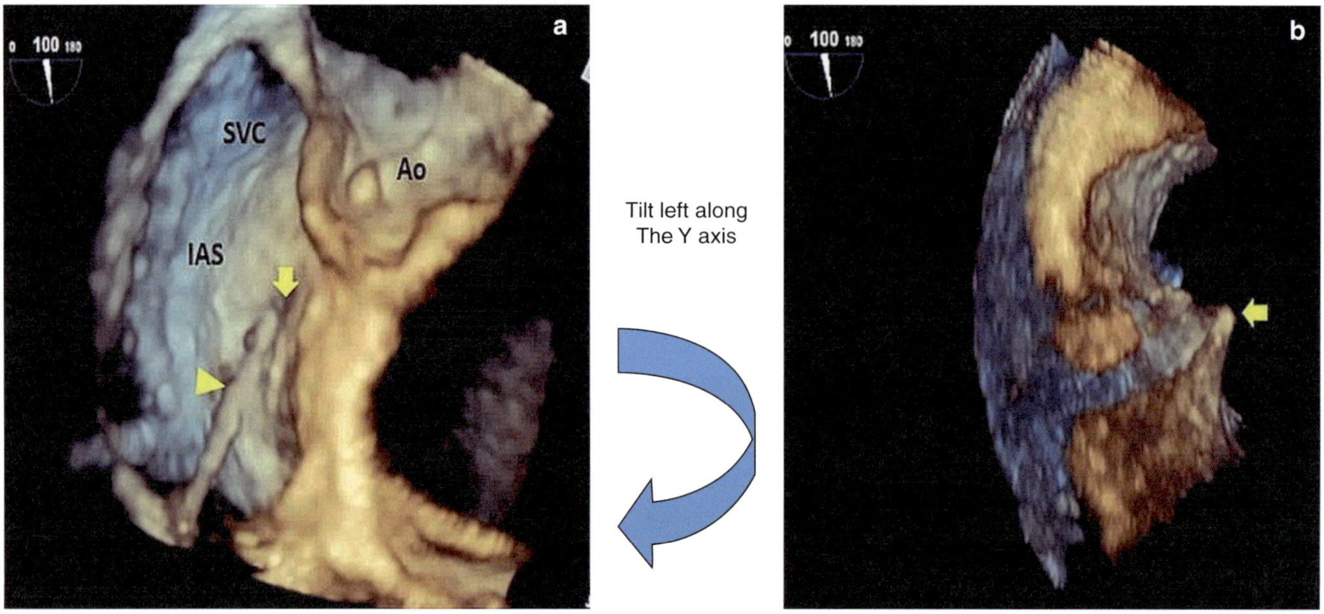

Fig. 8.22 Transesophageal 3DE anatomically oriented view of the interatrial septum (IAS) from the right atrial perspective during guidance of transseptal puncture. The puncture catheter (arrow head) is tenting (arrow) the IAS (**a**). With tilting the volume to the left along the Y axis, the tenting (arrow) could be clearly appreciated from the left atrial side (**b**) (Video 8.18). *SVC* Superior vena cava, *Ao* Aorta

Future Perspectives

Measuring the Residual Orifice Area by 3DE

Neither two- nor 3DE planimetry methods takes the mitral commissures into account. Thus, if the commissures are not completely fused, the diastolic MV orifice will not be planar and underestimation of the MV area may occur by planimetering on a tomographic frame.

The Mitral Valve Navigation (MVN) software package (Q-Lab-10, Philips Medical Systems, Andover, USA) was originally dedicated to assess MV prolapse and/or flail in a systolic frame.

It has been reported that using MVN in a diastolic frame, that shows the maximum diastolic opening of the MV, with manual editing and tracing of the commissures and leaflet tips may provide a more accurate measure of the residual MV orifice area. Residual MV orifice area is reported by the software as the "MV MR orifice area"

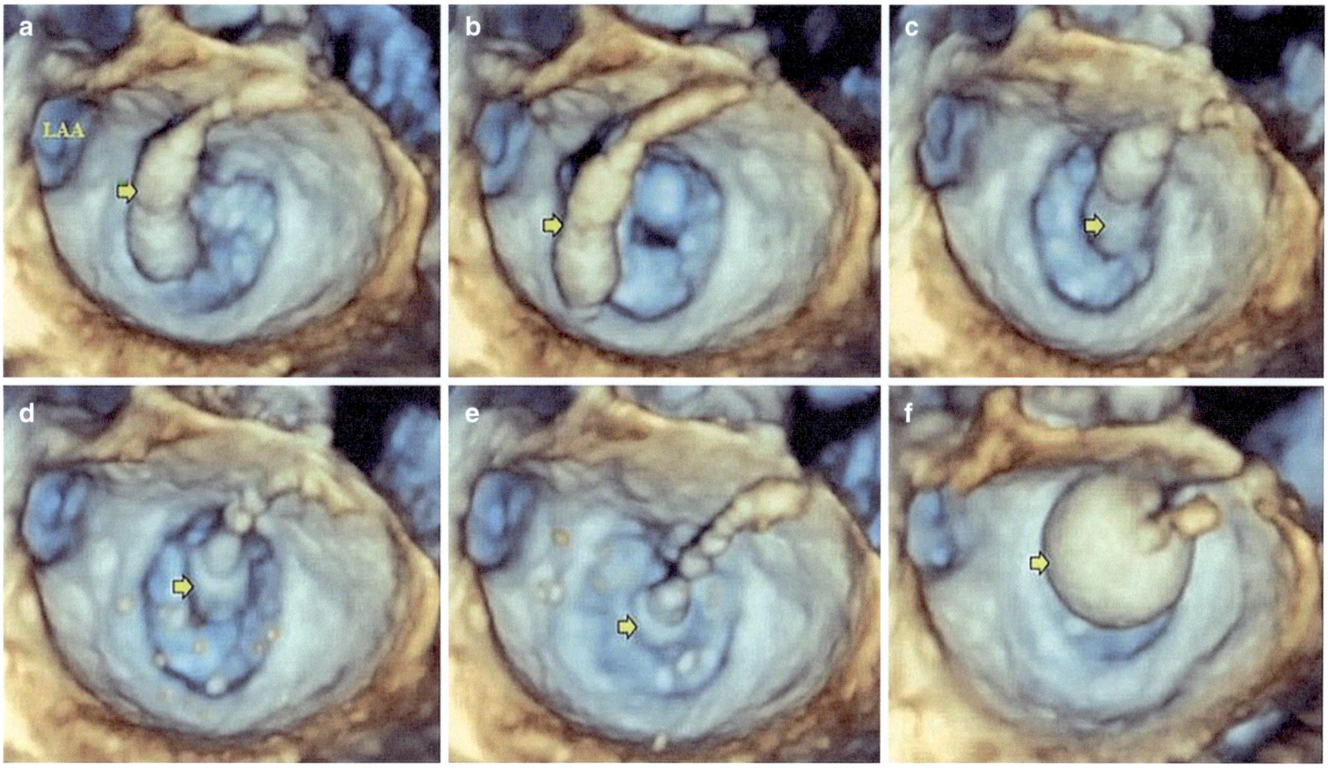

Fig. 8.23 Transesophageal 3DE (zoom mode) anatomically oriented view of MV from the left atrial perspective showing serial images of the positioning of the balloon (arrow) inside the left atrium while crossing the stenosed MV (**a**–**e**), then during balloon inflation (**f**) (Video 8.19). *LAA* left atrial appendage

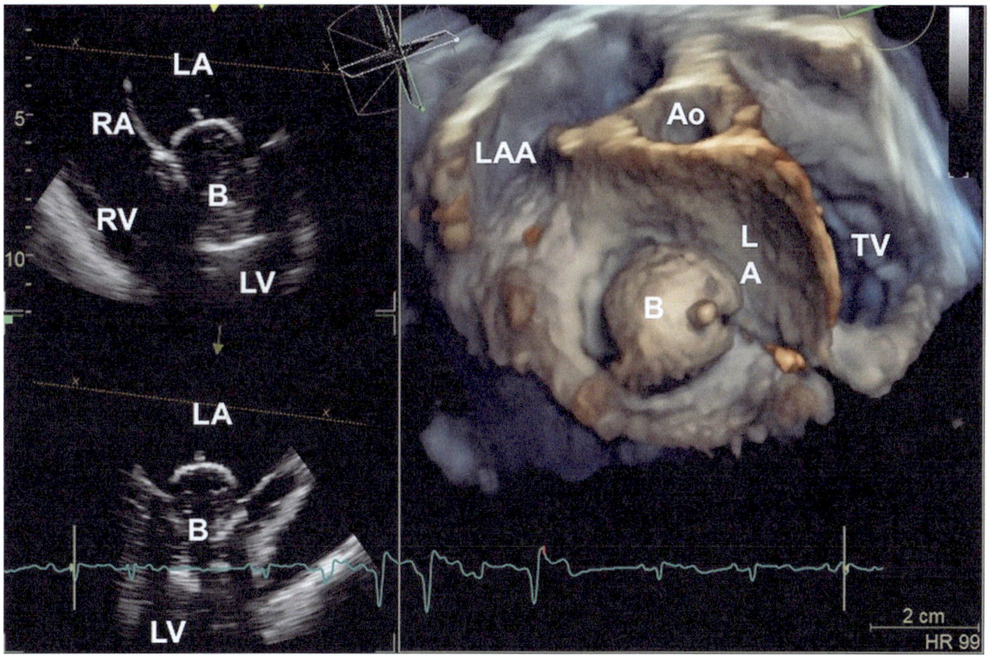

Fig. 8.24 Live/real-time transesophageal 3DE during balloon inflation. The simultaneous visualization of two orthogonal two-dimensional views (four-chamber, *upper left panel,* and bicommissural, *lower left panel*) together with the volume rendered *en face* view from the left atrium allows the full control of balloon positioning during inflation (Video 8.20). *Ao* aorta, *B* balloon, *LA* left atrium, *LAA* left atrial appendage, *LV* left ventricle, *RA* right atrium, *RV* right ventricle, *TV* tricuspid valve

because MVN was originally developed to measure the mitral regurgitation gap in a systolic frame (Fig. 8.26).

Measurement of the residual MV orifice area by the MVN method was shown to be feasible and more correlated to the invasive Gorlin's area than the 3DE-planimetry method. This is the first method of calculating the MVA that takes MV commissures into account [50].

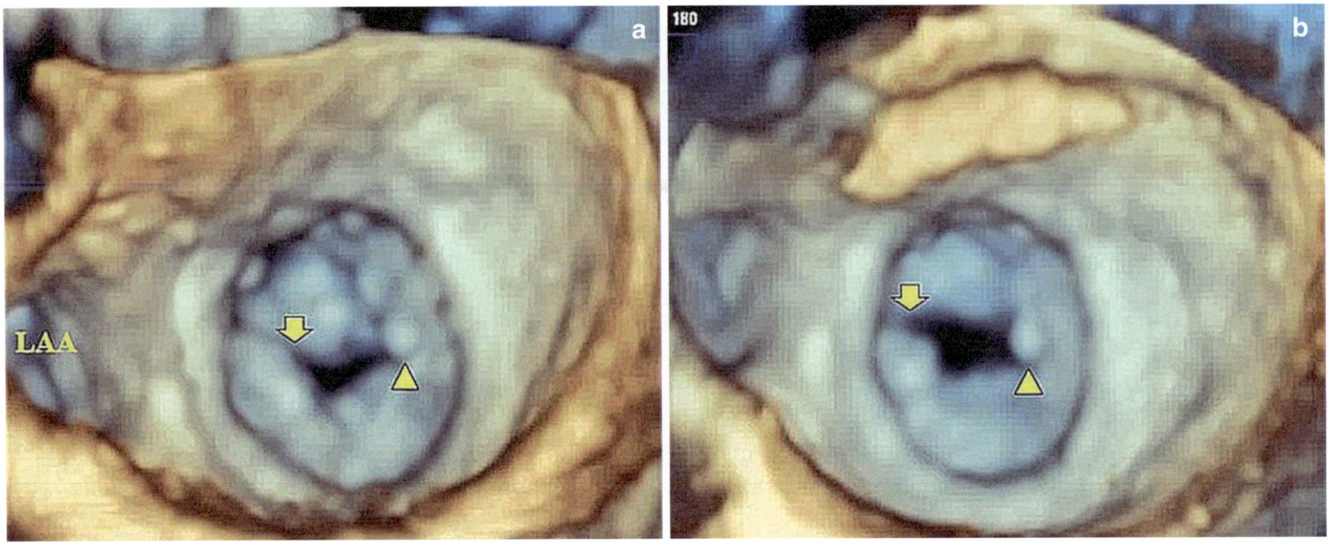

Fig. 8.25 Transesophageal 3DE (3D-zoomed) anatomically oriented view of MV from the left atrium perspective showing (**a**) the MV diastolic opening before balloon inflation, and (**b**) after balloon inflation where there is clear increase the diastolic opening with splitting of the lateral commissure (arrow), while the medial calcified commissure (arrow head) did not show significant splitting. *LAA* left atrial appendage

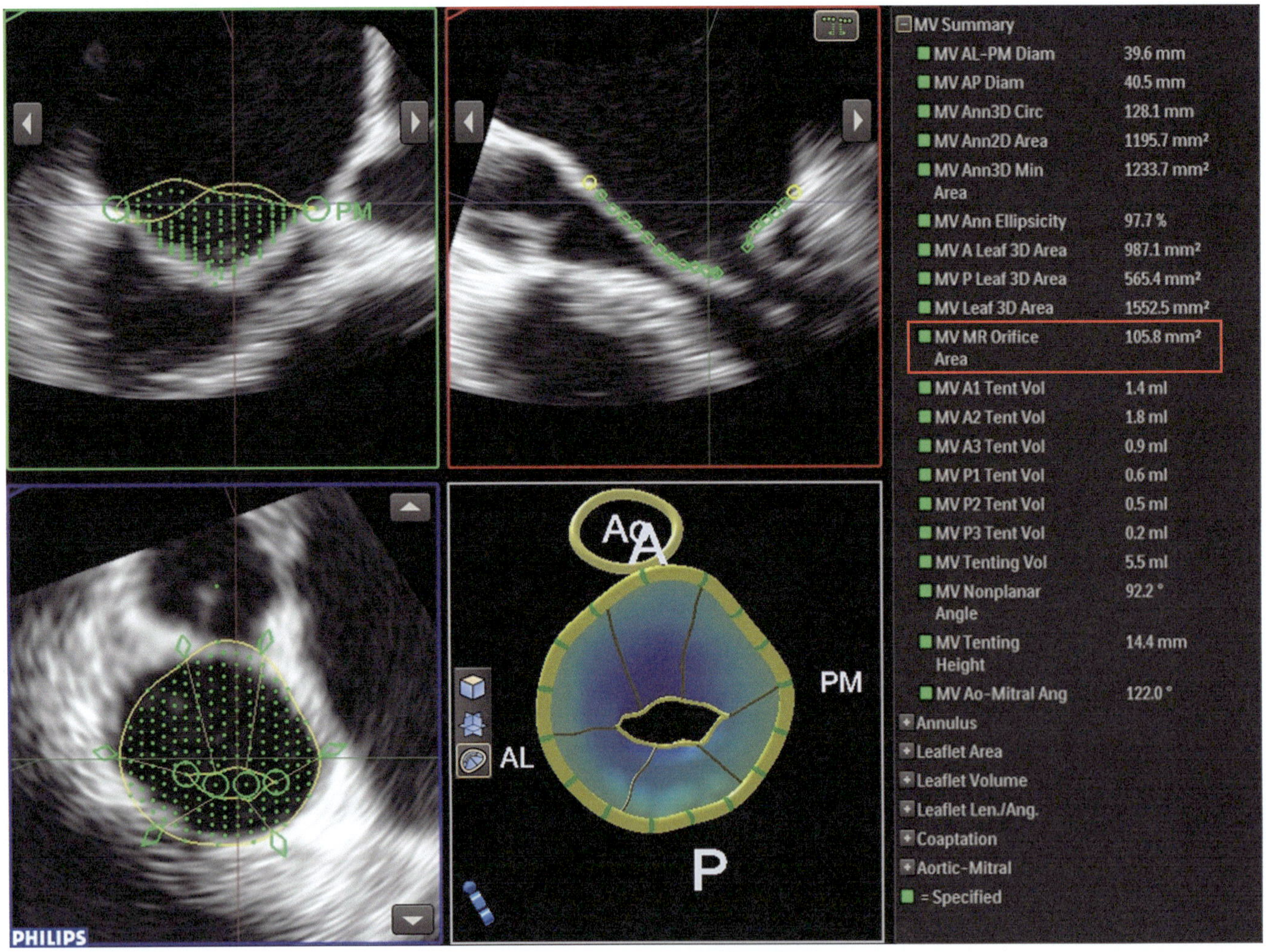

Fig. 8.26 Offline analysis of the 3D-TEE dataset using the Mitral Valve Navigation (MVN) software in a diastolic frame that shows the maximum diastolic opening of the MV with manual editing and tracing of the commissures and leaflet

References

1. Seguela PE, Houyel L, Acar P. Congenital malformations of the mitral valve. Arch Cardiovasc Dis. 2011;104:465–79.
2. Banerjee A, Kohl T, Silverman NH. Echocardiographic evaluation of congenital mitral valve anomalies in children. Am J Cardiol. 1995;76:1284–91.
3. Oppido G, Davies B, McMullan DM, et al. Surgical treatment of congenital mitral valve disease: midterm results of a repair oriented policy. J Thorac Cardiovasc Surg. 2008;135:1313–20.
4. Mantovani F, Clavel MA, Vatury O, et al. Cleft-like indentations in myxomatous mitral valves by three-dimensional echocardiographic imaging. Heart. 2015;101:1111–7.
5. McCarthy KP, Ring L, Rana BS. Anatomy of the mitral valve: understanding the mitral valve complex in mitral regurgitation. Eur J Echocardiogr. 2010;11:i3–9.
6. Agricola E, Oppizzi M, Maisano F, et al. Detection of mechanisms of immediate failure by transesophageal echocardiography in quadrangular resection mitral valve repair technique for severe mitral regurgitation. Am J Cardiol. 2003;91:175–9.
7. Manganaro R, Zito C, Khandheria BK, et al. Accessory mitral valve tissue: an updated review of the literature. Eur Heart J Cardiovasc Imaging. 2014;15:489–97.
8. Prifti E, Bonacchi M, Bartolozzi F, Frati G, Leacche M, Vanini V. Postoperative outcome in patients with accessory mitral valve tissue. Med Sci Monit. 2003;9:RA146–53.
9. Anderson RH, Zuberhuler JR, Penkoske PA, Neches WH. Of clefts, commissures, and things. J Thorac Cardiovasc Surg. 1985;90:605–10.
10. Miglioranza MH, Muraru D, Mihaila S, Haertel JC, Iliceto S, Badano LP. Isolated anterior mitral valve leaflet cleft: 3D transthoracic echocardiography-guided surgical strategy. Arq Bras Cardiol. 2015;104:e49–52.
11. Seguela P-E, Brosset P, Acar P. Isolated cleft of the posterior mitral valve leaflet assessed by real-time 3D echocardiography. Arch Cardiovasc Dis. 2011;104:365–6.
12. Wyss CA, Enseleit F, van der Loo B, et al. Isolated cleft of the posterior mitral valve leaflet: a congenital form of mitral regurgitation. Clin Cardiol. 2009;32:553–60.
13. Kent SM, Markwood TT, Vernalis MN, et al. Cleft posterior mitral valve leaflet associated with counterclockwise papillary muscle rotation. J Am Soc Echocardiogr. 2001;14:303–4.
14. Ziani AB, Latcu DG, Abadir S, et al. Assessment of proximal isovelocity surface area (PISA) shape using three-dimensional echocardiography in a paediatric population with mitral regurgitation or ventricular shunt. Arch Cardiovasc Dis. 2009;102:185–91.
15. Zalstein E, Hamilton R, Zucker N, Levitas A, Gross GJ. Presentation, natural history, and outcome in children and adolescents with double orifice mitral valve. Am J Cardiol. 2004;93:1067–9.
16. Ermacora D, Muraru D, Cecchetto A, Cucchini U, Badano LP. Transthoracic three-dimensional echocardiography visualization of functional anatomy of double orifice mitral regurgitation. Eur Heart J Cardiovasc Imaging. 2015;16:862.
17. Trowitzsch E, Bano-Rodrigo A, Burger BM, Colan SD, Sanders SP. Twodimensional echocardiographic findings in double orifice mitral valve. J Am Coll Cardiol. 1985;6:383–7.
18. Séguéla P-E, Dulac Y, Acar P. Double-orifice mitral valve assessed by two- and three-dimensional echocardiography in a newborn. Arch Cardiovasc Dis. 2011;104:361–2.
19. Shone JD, Sellers RC, Anderson RC, et al. The developmental complex of "parachute mitral valve" supravalvular ring of left atrium, subaortic stenosis and coartaction of aorta. Am J Cardiol. 1963;11:714–25.
20. Marino BS, Kruge LE, Cho CJ, Tomlinson RS, Shera D, Weinberg PM, et al. Parachute mitral valve: morphologic descriptors, associated lesions, and outcomes after biventricular repair. J Thorac Cardiovasc Surg. 2009;137:385–93.e4.
21. Purvis JA, Smyth S, Barr SH. Multi-modality imaging of an adult parachute mitral valve. J Am Soc Echocardiogr. 2011;24:351.e1–3.
22. Wood P. An appreciation of mitral stenosis. I: clinical features. Br Med J. 1954;4870:1051.
23. Marijon E, Ou P, Celermajer DS, et al. Prevalence of rheumatic heart disease detected by echocardiographic screening. N Engl J Med. 2007;357:470–6.
24. Rusted IE, Scheifley CH, Edwards JE. Studies of the mitral valve: II. Certain anatomic features of the mitral valve and associated structures in mitral stenosis. Circulation. 1956;14:398–406.
25. Faletra FF, Perk G, Pandian NG, Nesser H-J, Kronzon I. Real-time 3D interventional echocardiography. London, Heidelberg, New York, Dordrecht: Springer; 2014. https://doi.org/10.1007/978-1-4471-4745-9.
26. Lang RM, Badano LP, Tsang W, et al. EAE/ASE recommendations for image acquisition and display using three-dimensional echocardiography. J Am Soc Echocardiogr. 2012;25:3–46.
27. Pérez de Isla L, Casanova C, Almería C, Rodrigo JL, Cordeiro P, Mataix L, Aubele AL, Lang R, Zamorano JL. Which method should be the reference method to evaluate the severity of rheumatic mitral stenosis? Gorlin's method versus 3D-echo. Eur J Echocardiogr. 2007;8:470–3.
28. Baumgartner H, Falk V, Bax JJ, et al. 2017 ESC/EACTS guidelines for the management of valvular heart disease. Eur Heart J. 2017;38:2739–91.
29. Nishimura RA, Otto CM, Bonow RO, et al. 2017 AHA/ACC focused update of the 2014 AHA/ACC guideline for the management of patients with valvular heart disease: a report of the American College of Cardiology/American Heart Association Task Force on Practice Guidelines. J Am Coll Cardiol. 2017;70:252–89.
30. Mannaerts HF, Kamp O, Visser CA. Should mitral valve area assessment in patients with mitral stenosis be based on anatomical or on functional evaluation? A plea for 3D echocardiography as the new clinical standard. Eur Heart J. 2004;25:2073–4.
31. Langerveld J, Valocik G, Plokker HW, et al. Additional value of three-dimensional transesophageal echocardiography for patients with mitral valve stenosis undergoing balloon valvuloplasty. J Am Soc Echocardiogr. 2003;16:841–9.
32. Zamorano J, de Augustn JA. Three-dimensional echocardiography for assessment of mitral valve stenosis. Curr Opin Cardiol. 2009;24:415–9.
33. Anwar AM, Attia WM, Nosir YF, et al. Validation of a new score for the assessment of mitral stenosis using real-time three-dimensional echocardiography. J Am Soc Echocardiogr. 2010;23:13–22.
34. Hildick-Smith DJ, Taylor GJ, Shapiro LM. Inoue balloon mitral valvuloplasty: long-term clinical and echocardiographic follow-up of a predominantly unfavourable population. Eur Heart J. 2000;21:1690–7.
35. Chu JW, Levine RA, Chua S, et al. Assessing mitral valve area and orifice geometry in calcific mitral stenosis: a new solution by real-time three-dimensional echocardiography. J Am Soc Echocardiogr. 2008;21:1006–9.
36. Gorlin R, Gorlin SG. Hydraulic formula for calculation of the area of the stenotic mitral valve, other cardiac valves, and central circulatory shunts. Am Heart J. 1951;41:1–29.
37. Cannan CR, Nishimura RA, Reeder GS, Ilstrup DR, Larson DR, Holmes DR, et al. Echocardiographic assessment of commissural calcium: a simple predictor of outcome after percutaneous mitral balloon valvotomy. J Am Coll Cardiol. 1997;29:175–80.
38. Zamorano J, Perez de Isla L, Sugeng L, et al. Real-time three-dimensional echocardiography for rheumatic mitral valve stenosis evaluation: an accurate and novel approach. J Am Coll Cardiol. 2004;43:2091–6.

39. Xie MX, Wang XF, Cheng TO, Wang J, Lu Q. Comparison of accuracy of mitral valve area in mitral stenosis by real-time, three-dimensional echocardiography versus two-dimensional echocardiography versus Doppler pressure half-time. Am J Cardiol. 2005;95:1496–9.
40. Roberts WC, Perloff JK. Mitral valvular disease: a clinicopathologic survey of the conditions causing the mitral valve to function abnormally. Ann Intern Med. 1972;77:939–75.
41. Turgeman Y, Atar S, Rosenfeld T. The subvalvular apparatus in rheumatic mitral stenosis: methods of assessment and therapeutic implications. Chest. 2003;124:1929–36.
42. Wilkins GT, Weyman AE, Abascal VM, et al. Percutaneous balloon dilatation of the mitral valve: an analysis of echocardiographic variables related to outcome and the mechanism of dilatation. Br Heart J. 1988;60:299–308.
43. Carpentier A, Pellerin M, Fuzellier J, Relland J. Extensive calcification of the mitral valve annulus: pathology and surgical management. J Thorac Cardiovasc Surg. 1996;11:718–30.
44. Inoue K, Owaki T, Nakamura T, Kitamura F, Miyamoto N. Clinical application of transvenous mitral commissurotomy by a new balloon catheter. J Thorac Cardiovasc Surg. 1984;87:394–402.
45. Iung BL, Garbarz E, Michaud P, et al. Late results of percutaneous mitral commissurotomy in a series of 1024 patients: analysis of late clinical deterioration: frequency, anatomic findings and predictive factors. Circulation. 1999;99:3272–8.
46. Mahmoud HM, Al-Ghamdi MA, Ghabashi AE, Anwar AM. A proposed maneuver to guide transseptal puncture using real-time three-dimensional transesophageal echocardiography: pilot study. Cardiol Res Pract. 2015;174051.
47. Zamorano J, Perez de Isla L, Sugeng L, et al. Non-invasive assessment of mitral valve area during percutaneous balloon mitral valvuloplasty: role of real-time 3D echocardiography. Eur Heart J. 2004;25:2086–91.
48. Applebaum RM, Kasliwal RR, Kanojia A, Seth A, Bhandari S, Trehan N, et al. Utility of three-dimensional echocardiography during balloon mitral valvuloplasty. J Am Coll Cardiol. 1998;32:1405–9.
49. Messika-Zeitoun D, Blanc J, Iung B, et al. Impact of degree of commissural opening after percutaneous mitral commissurotomy on long-term outcome. J Am Coll Cardiol Img. 2009;2:1–7.
50. Mahmoud Elsayed HM, Hassan M, Nagy M, et al. A novel method to measure mitral valve area in patients with rheumatic mitral stenosis using three dimensional transesophageal echocardiography: feasibility and validation. Echocardiography. 2018;35(3):368–74.

Degenerative Mitral Regurgitation

9

Wendy Tsang and Roberto M. Lang

Abstract

Degenerative mitral valve disease consists of a spectrum, with the mildest form recognized as fibroelastic deficiency and the most severe form as Barlow's disease. Both forms, through different mechanisms, result in thickened leaflet segments that prolapse and billow resulting in mitral regurgitation. These disease processes also lead to changes in mitral annular shape and function. Management of these diseases will differ depending on the extent of valve involvement. Most surgeons can surgically correct mild disease affecting a single P2 segment whereas complex disease affecting both the anterior and posterior leaflets or multiple segments requires an expert mitral valve surgeon. Three-dimensional echocardiography helps determine the location and extent of the lesion. Parametric models are color-encoded topographic displays of mitral valve anatomy from three-dimensional echocardiographic images. These models improve assessment of valve anatomy and provide quantitative measurements that can be used to determine the etiology of the valve abnormality and can therefore be used to direct treatment. Three-dimensional echocardiography also improves quantification of mitral regurgitation severity. This is especially true for degenerative mitral valve disease where the regurgitant orifice is frequently eccentric resulting in an eccentric regurgitant jet. This is achieved by improving the calculation of the effective regurgitant orifice area with vena contracta area or proximal isovelocity surface area, and/or by measuring the true 3D anatomical regurgitant orifice area. Overall, three-dimensional echocardiography improves diagnosis and management of patients with degenerative mitral valve disease.

Keywords

Mitral valve · Regurgitation severity quantification
Barlow's disease · Fibroelastic deficiency
Mitral annulus anatomy · Mitral leaflet anatomy
Degenerative mitral regurgitation

Introduction

Degenerative or myxomatous mitral valve (MV) disease is the most common cause of mitral regurgitation in developed countries [1]. It is comprised of a spectrum of valvular involvement with its mildest form known as fibroelastic deficiency and its' most severe as Barlow's disease (Table 9.1). In this chapter we will discuss the changes to valve and annular morphology with degenerative MV disease, quantification of mitral regurgitation and present some cases.

Mitral Valve Morphology

Valve morphology is greatly affected by the form of degenerative MV disease that is present. With fibroelastic deficiency, there is an impairment in the production of connective tissue that affects the mechanical integrity of the MV leaflets and chords [3]. Typically a single leaflet segment is affected and due to the abnormalities in connective tissue structure and function, this leaflet segment is usually thickened and prolapsing. The chordal structures attached to this segment are also

Electronic Supplementary Material The online version of this chapter (https://doi.org/10.1007/978-3-030-14032-8_9) contains supplementary material, which is available to authorized users.

W. Tsang (✉)
Cardiology, Toronto General Hospital, University Health Network, University of Toronto, Toronto, ON, Canada
e-mail: wendy.tsang@uhn.ca

R. M. Lang
Noninvasive Cardiac Imaging Laboratories, Department of Medicine/Section of Cardiology, University of Chicago Medical Center, Chicago, IL, USA
e-mail: rlang@bsd.uchicago.edu, rlang@medicine.bsd.uchicago.edu

L. P. Badano et al. (eds.), *Textbook of Three-Dimensional Echocardiography*, https://doi.org/10.1007/978-3-030-14032-8_9

elongated and due to their tissue abnormality can suffer an acute loss of mechanical integrity resulting in chordal rupture with a flail leaflet (Fig. 9.1a). Thus, patients most commonly present in the sixth decade of life with a relatively short history of acute onset of symptoms from the rupture of a single mitral chordae tendineae with resulting mitral regurgitation.

In comparison, Barlow's disease results from an abnormal accumulation of mucopolysaccharides [3]. This myxoid infiltration leads to thick, bulky, redundant billowing leaflets and thick, elongated chordae. Thus, involvement of multiple segments of one or both leaflets is often seen on examination of the valve (Fig. 9.1b). As this is a chronic process, Barlow's disease is usually diagnosed in young adulthood and patients are typically followed for many decades with well-preserved left ventricular size until indications for surgery are met in the fourth or fifth decade of life. Females are predominantly affected with Barlow's disease.

The specific diagnosis of fibroelastic deficiency versus Barlow's disease is often difficult to definitively determine by either the gross or histologic appearance of the MV. This is because degenerative MV disease is a spectrum and there may be an overlap of these forms. For instance, there is a *forme-fruste* of Barlow's disease that may morphologically appear as fibroelastic deficiency [4]. Only histological examination may differentiate these valves. However, differentiation is crucial in management of these patients for

Table 9.1 Differences between Barlow's disease and fibroelastic deficiency [2]

Differentiating characteristics	Fibroelastic deficiency	Barlow's disease
Pathology	Impaired production of connective tissue resulting in loss of mechanical integrity	Mucopolysaccharide accumulation resulting in excess leaflet tissue
Typical age of diagnosis	>60 years old	<40 years
Duration of disease	Days to months	Years to decades
Physical exam	Holosystolic murmur	Late systolic murmur Midsystolic click
Leaflet	Single segment involved Involved segment is thick Remaining leaflets are normal	Multiple segments involved Thick, billowing leaflets
Chordae lesions	Chordal elongation and chordal rupture	Chordal thickening and elongation
Carpentier classification	Type II	Type II
Type of dysfunction	Prolapse and/or flail	Bileaflet prolapse
Complexity of valve repair	Typically not complex	Typically complex

Reprinted from Three-Dimensional Anatomy of the Aortic and Mitral Valves, Tsang W, Freed BH, Lang RM, in Valvular Heart Disease: A Companion to Braunwald's Heart Disease, 4th Edition, Editors Otto CM, Bonow R, Philadelphia: Saunders Elsevier, 2014, 488 pages, with permission from Elsevier

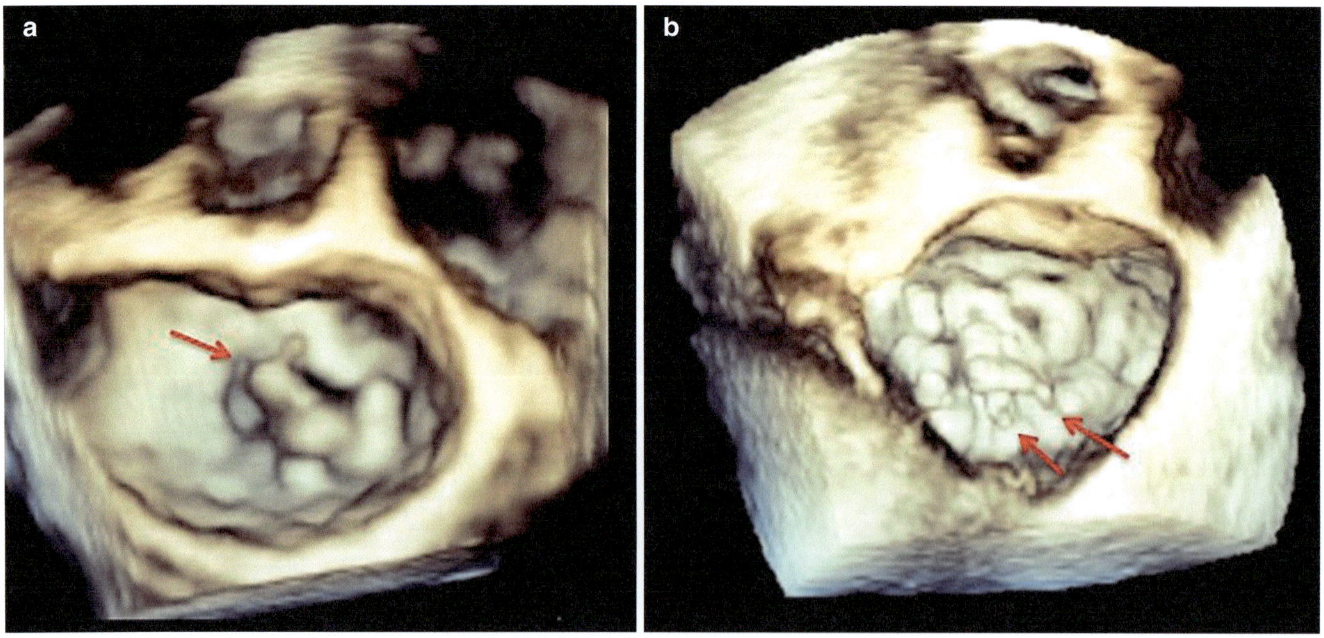

Fig. 9.1 Three-dimensional transesophageal echocardiographic images of the mitral valve demonstrating fibroelastic deficiency (**a**) with P3 prolapse and chordal rupture (red arrow) and Barlow's disease (**b**) with bileaflet, multi-segmental prolapse and A2 segment flail (red arrows)

surgeon-specific referral and determining the optimal surgical strategy, which affects post-operative outcome. As described previously, patients with fibroelastic deficiency typically have a single MV segment lesion. These can be repaired using simple techniques that can be performed by most cardiothoracic surgeons. Patients with Barlow's Disease often have multi-segmental leaflet involvement, which requires an expert mitral valve surgeon to attain a successful repair. Poor pre-surgical planning may lead to either unsuccessful repair or conversion to valve replacement with less favorable outcomes in patients with complex valvular disease [5, 6].

Three-dimensional echocardiography (3DE) can improve the ability to differentiate between forms of degenerative MV disease and has been demonstrated to be superior to two-dimensional echocardiographic (2DE) examinations [4, 7–10]. 3DE not only improves accuracy of lesion localization but is less operator-dependent, and more reproducible than 2DE at any expertise level. For instance, the use of transesophageal 3DE results in correct identification of the prolapsed segment in 92% of patients versus 78% of patients using transesophageal 2DE.

Parametric models transform the 3DE images of the MV into color-encoded topographic displays of mitral valve anatomy (Fig. 9.2). The color gradations on the parametric maps indicate the distance of the leaflet from the mitral annular plane toward the left atrium, which helps improve lesion localization diagnostic accuracy [9]. These maps also allow quantitation of MV parameters such as leaflet height and annular area, which have been used to differentiate Barlow's disease from fibroelastic deficiency. 3DE quantification of billowing height with a cutoff value of 1.0 mm can differentiated between normal and MV prolapse without overlap, while 3DE billowing volume with a cutoff value of 1.15 mL can differentiated between Barlow's disease and fibroelastic deficiency without overlap [8].

Regardless of the etiology of the MV disease, each disease process frequently results in one or more lesions. For example, degenerative diseases such as Barlow's disease and fibroelastic deficiency result in multiple types of lesions including excess myomatous leaflet tissue, chordal elongation, thinning, and rupture that leads to mitral regurgitation. Instead of classifying this dysfunction as simply MV stenosis or regurgitation, the Carpentier classification scheme has been developed to aid in the surgical strategy based on the type of leaflet motion (Table 9.2) [11]. Patients with mitral annular dilatation or leaflet perforation usually have normal leaflet motion and are categorized as Type I dysfunction. Type II dysfunction includes patients with prolapse (free edge of one or both leaflets overriding the plane of the annulus during valve closure) and flail (excessive motion of the leaflet margin above the plane of the annulus) due to excessive and redundant leaflet tissue or chordal rupture, respectively (Fig. 9.2). Leaflet restriction during valve closure due to fusion of various components of the MV apparatus is defined as Type IIIa dysfunction while leaflet restriction during valve opening resulting from leaflet tethering, is defined as Type IIIb dysfunction. In addition to the Carpentier classification, a modified version has been developed that accounts for systolic anterior motion of the leaflets (Type IVa) and hybrid conditions (Type V) [12].

It has been recognized that the Carpentier classification has many weaknesses. For instance, it neglects to include papillary muscle motion abnormalities in the list of lesions involved in MV disease [12]. As described above, 3DE improves assessment of the MV. This allows a tailored approach rather than a standard approach in which a pre-established operation is performed according to the Carpentier classification system.

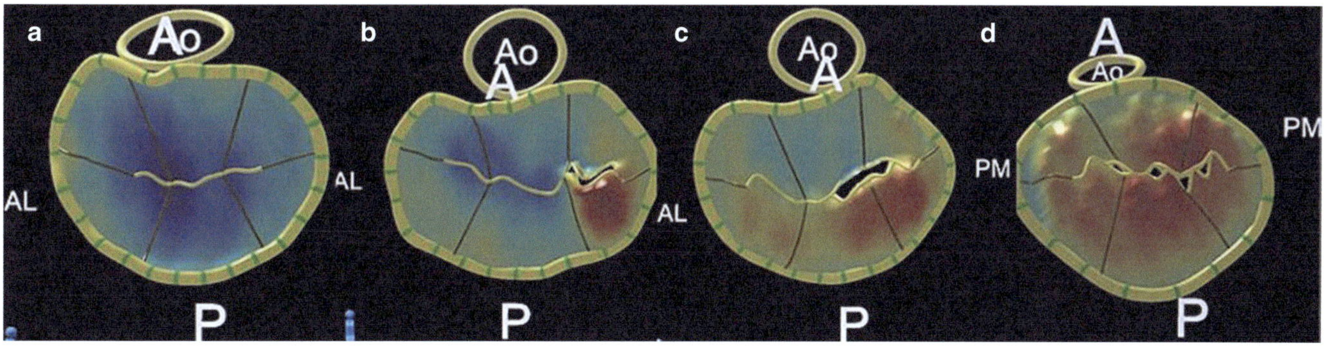

Fig. 9.2 Three-dimensional parametric maps of the mitral valve demonstrating (**a**) normal anatomy, (**b**) P3 flail scallop, (**c**) P2 and P3 prolapse, and (**d**) Barlow's disease [9]. Reprinted from Journal of the American Society of Echocardiography, Vol. 24/Issue 8, Tsang W, Weinert L, Sugeng L, Chandra S, Ahmad H, Spencer K, et al., The Value of Three-Dimensional Echocardiography Derived Mitral Valve Parametric Maps and the Role of Experience in the Diagnosis of Pathology, pp. 860–7, ©2011, with permission from Elsevier

Table 9.2 Carpentier classification of mitral valve dysfunction with modification [12]

	Type 1	Type 2	Type IIIA	Type IIIB	Type IVA	Type V
Motion of leaflet margin	Normal	Prolapse or flail	Restricted leaflet opening	Restricted leaflet closure	Systolic anterior leaflet motion	Hybrid conditions
Associated disease processes	• Chronic atrial fibrillation • Bacterial endocarditis	• Degenerative disease (Barlow's disease or fibroelastic deficiency)	• Rheumatic disease	• Myocardial infarction • Dilated cardiomyopathy	• Hypertrophic cardiomyopathy • Post-mitral valve repair • Hemodynamic-induced (e.g. hypovolemia, tachycardia)	• Combined rheumatic valve disease and infective endocarditis
Associated lesions	• Annular dilatation • Leaflet perforation	• Leaflet thickening • Leaflet billowing • Leaflet elongation • Chordal thickening • Chordal rupture	• Commissure fusion • Leaflet thickening • Chordae thickening	• Papillary displacement • Chordae tethering • Annular dilatation	• Asymmetric septal hypertrophy • Anterior leaflet enlargement • Undersized mitral annuloplasty ring	• Tethered, restricted small posterior leaflet with flail anterior leaflet • Anterior leaflet systolic anterior motion with flail or prolapsing posterior leaflet

3DE Study of Mitral Valve Anatomy and Pathology of Degenerative Mitral Valve Disease

Unlike 2DE, which requires several views to examine the different scallops of the MV leaflets, 3DE provides a comprehensive assessment of the MV in one data set acquisition. The 3DE data set can be acquired from either a transthoracic or a transesophageal approach and, depending on the size of the data set, the patient's characteristics (ability to cooperate, heart rhythm etc.) and the clinical scenario, either the zoom (single or multibeat) or the full volume (usually multibeat) modes could be used. Typically, a temporal resolution of around 10 vps is sufficient for qualitative assessment of pathological anatomy. For quantitative assessment of leaflet or annular function, 3DE data sets with temporal resolution that is greater than 20 vps are needed. The best spatial resolution (image quality) is usually obtained using the transesophageal approach because of the higher frequency of the transesophageal transducer and the close position of the MV to the probe. However, diagnostic images can be obtained from transthoracic images in patients with good acoustic window (Fig. 9.3, Videos 9.1a and 9.1b) and these transthoracic data sets are of sufficient quality to be used to plan the reparative strategy [13–15]. Indeed, transthoracic 3DE has been reported to be more accurate than transesophageal 2DE, when compared to surgical inspection of the MV. While the information provided by transesophageal 3DE is significant, it provides only a little additional informative content to transthoracic 3DE [16].

Using both the transthoracic and the transesophageal approach, it is important to select the smallest region of interest that encompasses all the components of the MV apparatus in order to maximize both temporal and spatial resolution. The acquired data set is then cropped to visualize the mitral valve from the atrial perspective and rotated in order to show the aortic valve on top of the anterior leaflet, at about 12 o'clock. Using the *en face* view from the atrial perspective (also called "surgical view" because it is quite similar to the way the cardiac surgeon visualizes the mitral valve after opening the left atrium), cleft-like indentations of the posterior leaflet, defined as visible tissue defect seen during systole, divide it into three scallops (P1, the lateral one, closest to the left atrial appendage; P2, the central one; and P3, the medial one, closest to interatrial septum) (Fig. 9.4). Usually, the anterior leaflet does not have any indentations and the segments are identified as the portions of the anterior leaflet facing the corresponding scallop of the posterior leaflet. Both transverse (*en face* views) and longitudinal cut planes are used to localize and assess the extent of displacement of the various scallops (Fig. 9.5, Videos 9.2a and 9.2b). At the beginning of the 3DE experience, it is useful to play the data sets of the MV at a slow speed or frame by frame to better identify the prolapsing scallops and chordal anatomy. Alternatively, the volume rendered data set can be sliced to obtain two-dimensional views at the level of the lesion in order to display it in a more comfortable two-dimensional display (Fig. 9.6). Once the lesion has been identified, the data set can be played at normal speed to gain confidence in 3DE anatomy (Figs. 9.7, 9.8, 9.9, 9.10, 9.11 and 9.12, Videos 9.3, 9.4a, 9.4b, 9.5, 9.6, 9.7, and 9.8).

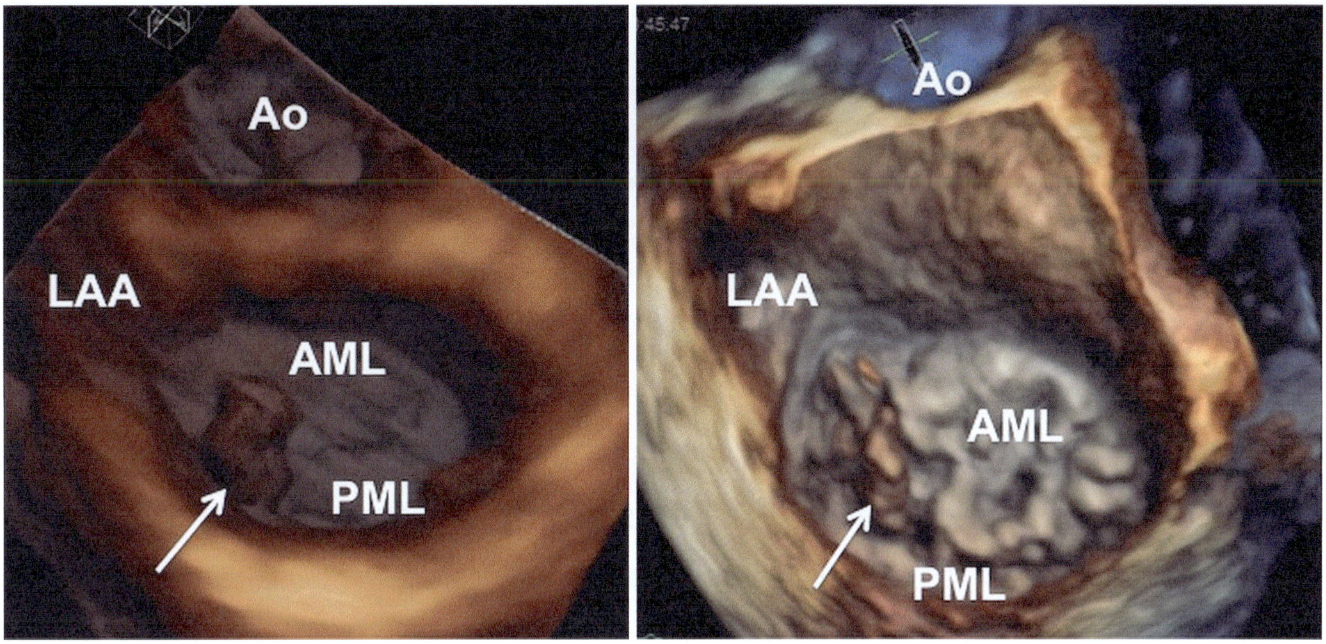

Fig. 9.3 Comparison of transthoracic and transesophageal 3DE visualization of a flail P1 (white arrow) scallop with ruptured chordae using a volume rendered *en face* view of the mitral valve from the atrial perspective. *Left panel*, transthoracic 3DE acquisition from the apical approach (Video 9.1a Left). *Right panel*, transesophageal 3DE acquisition using zoom mode (Video 9.1b Right). Despite the fact that the transesophageal images have better spatial resolution (the thin ruptured chorda is clearly visualized) the pathological lesion was equally identified on the data set acquired from the transthoracic approach. *Ao* aorta, *AML* anterior mitral leaflet, *LAA* left atrial appendage, *PML* posterior mitral leaflet

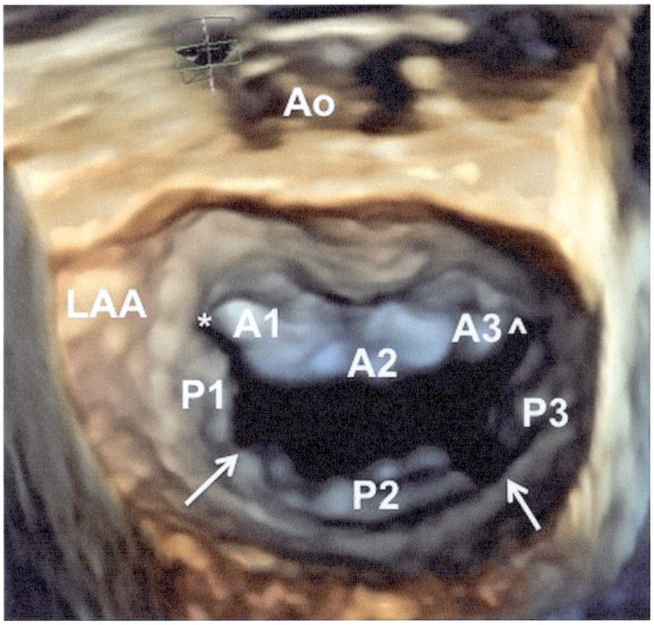

Fig. 9.4 Segmentation of a normal mitral valve. The two indentations (white arrows) divide the posterior leaflet in three scallops. The one next to the anterior-lateral commissure (*, close to left atrial appendage) is P1. The central one is P2. The one next to the posterior-medial commissure (^, close to interatrial septum) is P3. By analogy to posterior leaflet and despite the absence of indentations, the portions of the anterior leaflet facing the corresponding ones on the posterior leaflet are named A1, A2, A3. *Ao* aorta, *AML* anterior mitral leaflet, *LAA* left atrial appendage, *PML* posterior mitral leaflet

Mitral Annulus

The mitral annulus is a fibro-muscular ring to which the anterior and posterior mitral valve leaflets attach. It normally has a 3D saddle shape with its "lowest points" at the level of the valve commissures, which allows leaflet apposition during systole and minimizes leaflet stress [17]. The annulus is a dynamic structure that needs to undergo 3D deformation in its circumference, excursion, curvature, shape, and size to maintain proper function [4, 18–21]. The posterior portion of the annulus is less developed due to the discontinuity of the fibrous skeleton in this region and is therefore susceptible to pathologic dilatation [22].

Volumetric 3DE quantification in patients with degenerative MV disease has determined that as the annulus enlarges it loses its 3D saddle shape [23, 24]. Specifically, patients have larger annular dimensions during diastole and annular dimensions fail to change during systole. This combination of annular enlargement and distortion is thought to be one of the driving forces for valve incompetence in patients with degenerative MV disease [24]. This has led to the development of multiple types of annuloplasty rings for use in MV repair. 3DE has been used to demonstrate that the rigidity of these rings may affect the restoration of normal annular function after MV repair surgery [25]. For instance post-repair surgery, the annulus is smaller but continues to lack systolic saddle-shape accentuation [26].

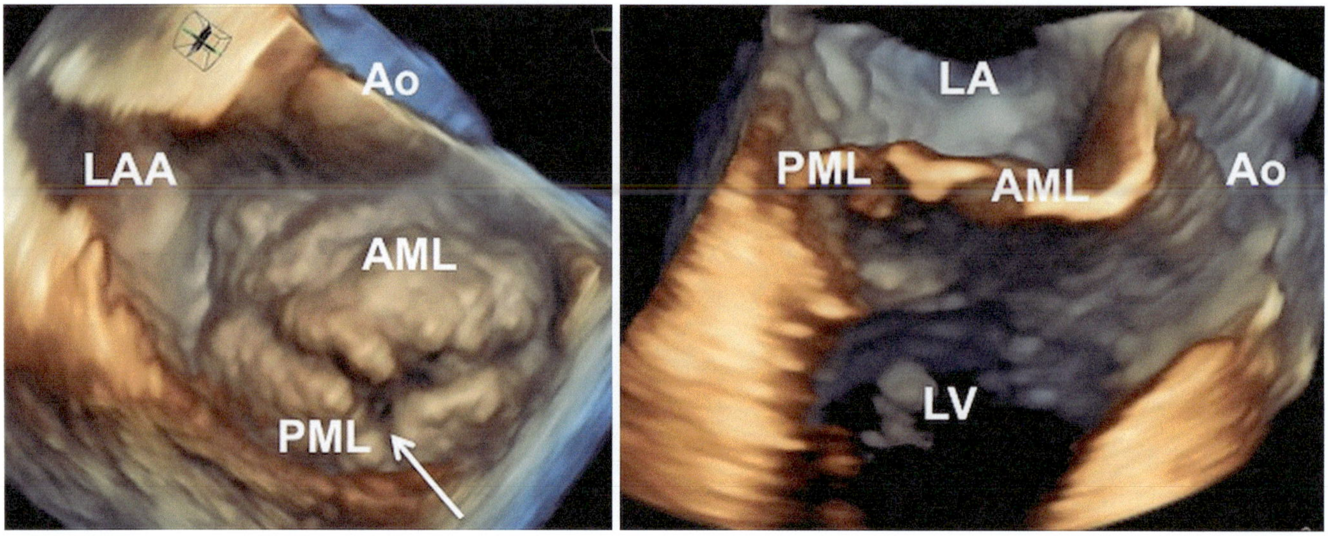

Fig. 9.5 Use of different cut planes to assess the functional anatomy of mitral valve in a patient with Barlow's disease. *Left panel*, volume rendered *en face* view from the atrial perspective of a transesophageal 3DE data set of the mitral valve (Video 9.2a Left). A cleft-like indentation of the posterior leaflet is present in P2 (arrow). *Right panel*, volume rendered longitudinal cut plane at A2-P2 level (Video 9.2b Right). *LA* left atrium, *LV* left ventricle, *Ao* aorta, *AML* anterior mitral leaflet, *LAA* left atrial appendage, *PML* posterior mitral leaflet

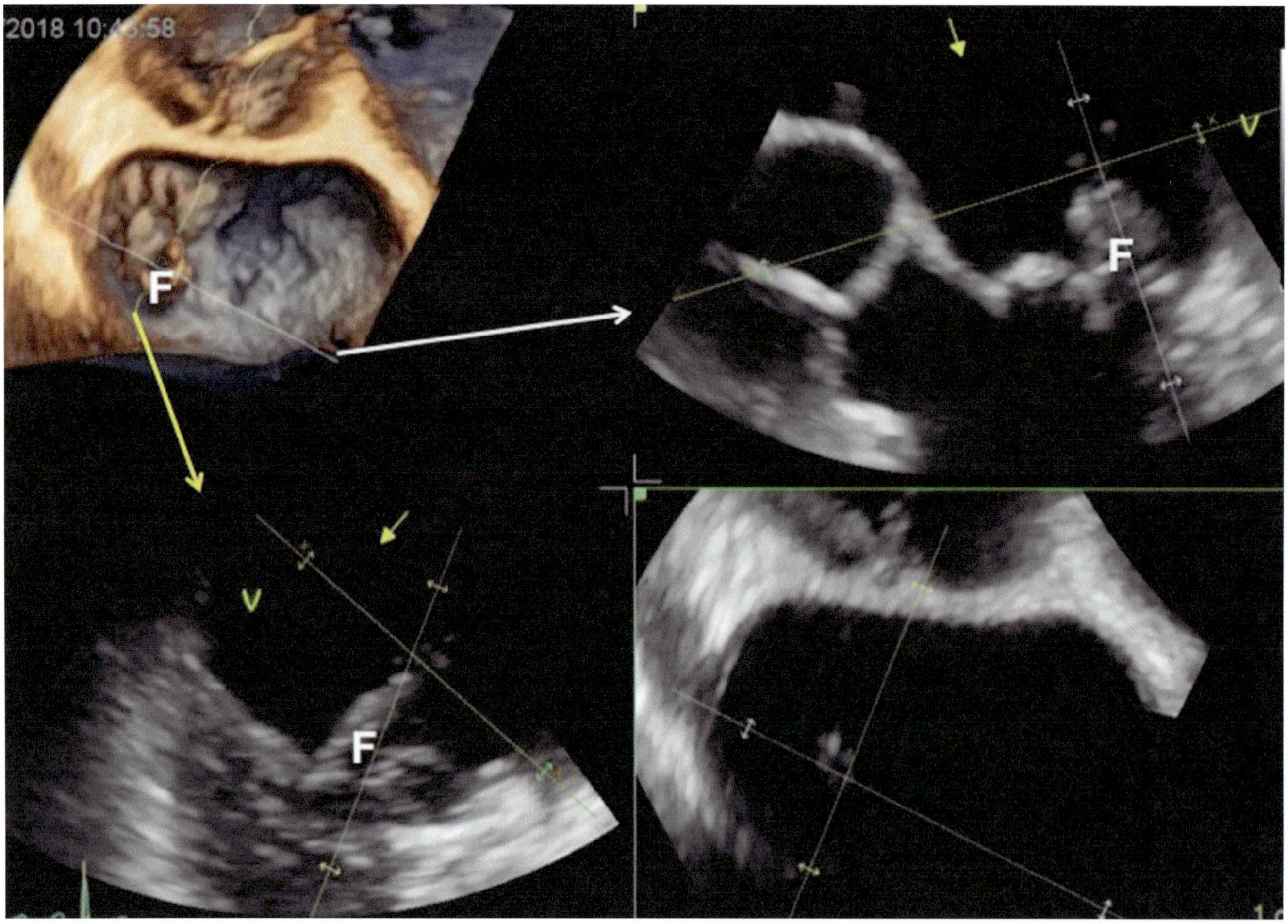

Fig. 9.6 Slicing of a 3DE data set to obtain two-dimensional views of a lesion. The flailing P1 (F), visualized on the volume rendered image (left upper panel, Video 9.1b, Right) has been sliced into two longitudinal tomographic views to appreciate the flail in a more conventional manner for novice 3DE interpreters/operators. The orientation of the tomographic views is shown on the volume rendered images with two lines: the white line corresponding to the view in the white (right upper) panel, and the yellow one, corresponding to the yellow (left lower) panel (FlexiSlice®, GE Vingmed, Horten, NO)

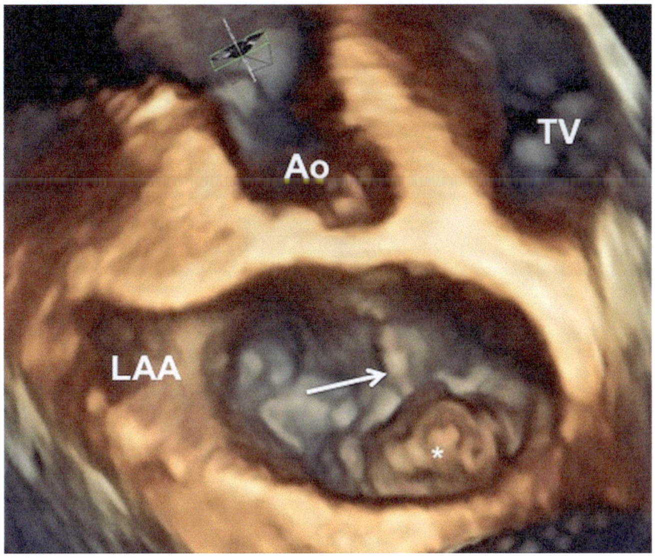

Fig. 9.7 Volume rendered *en face* view from the atrial perspective of a transesophageal 3DE data set of the mitral valve in a patient with P2 P3 prolapse (*) and ruptured chords (arrow) (Video 9.3). *Ao* aorta, *AML* anterior mitral leaflet, *LAA* left atrial appendage, *PML* posterior mitral leaflet, *TV* tricuspid valve

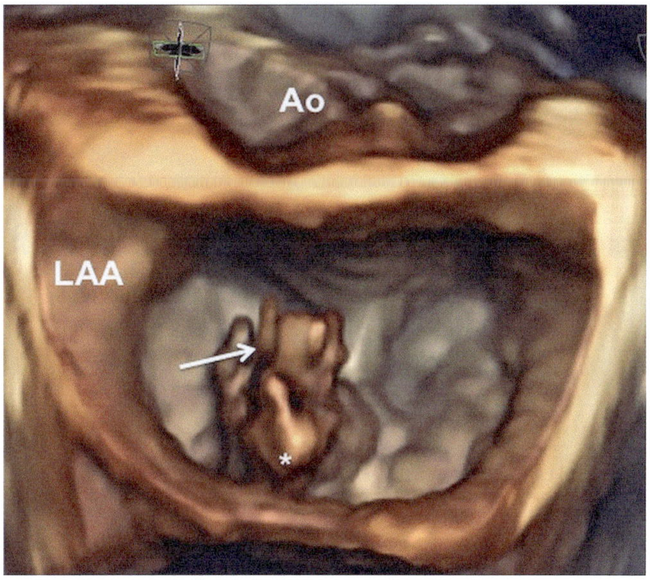

Fig. 9.9 Volume rendered transesophageal 3DE data set of the mitral valve in a patient with P2 flail (*) and multiple ruptured chords (arrow) (Video 9.5). *Ao* aorta, *LAA* left atrial appendage

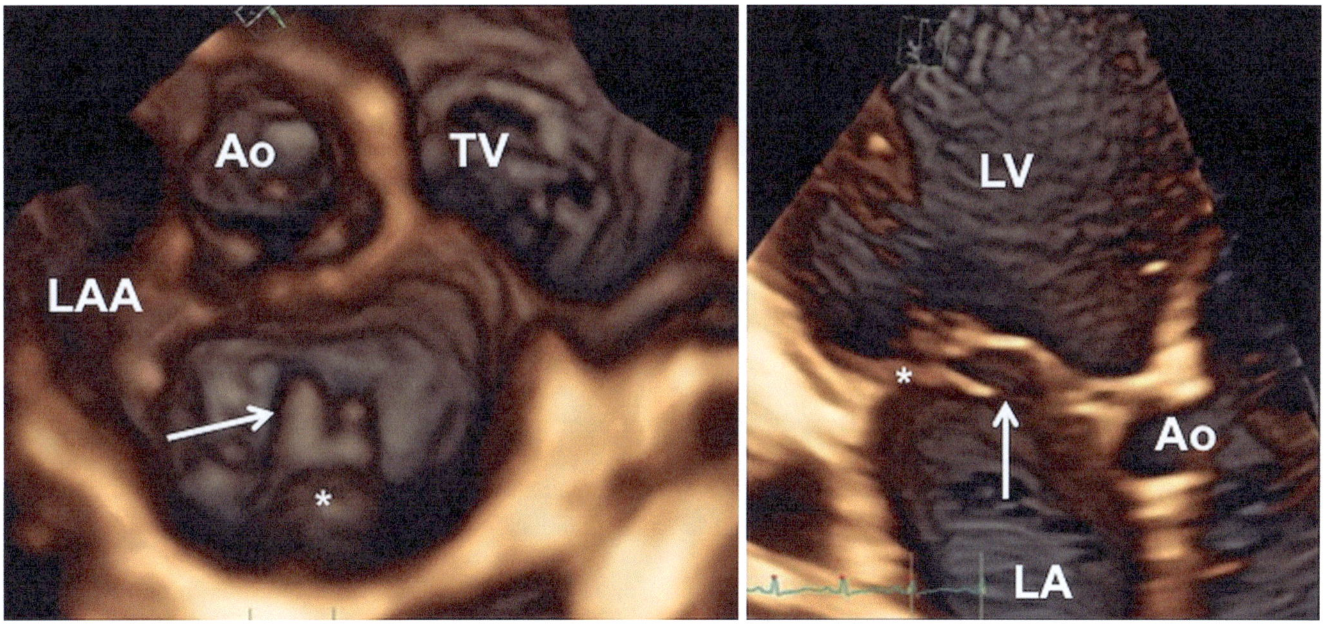

Fig. 9.8 Volume rendered transthoracic 3DE data set of the mitral valve in a patient with P2 flail (*) and ruptured chords (arrow). *Left panel*, *en face* view from the atrial perspective (Video 9.4a Left). *Right panel*, Longitudinal cut plane at the level of A2-P2 (Video 9.4b Right). *TV* tricuspid valve, *Ao* aorta, *LA* left atrium, *LAA* left atrial appendage, *LV* left ventricle

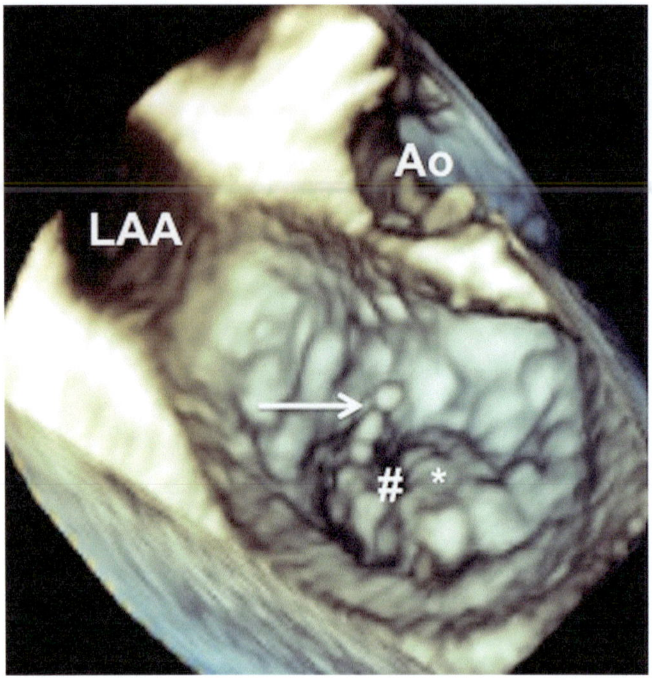

Fig. 9.10 Volume rendered transesophageal 3DE data set of the mitral valve in a patient with ruptured chords (arrow) and a cleft-like indentation (#) splitting a large P2 prolapse (*) (Video 9.6). *Ao* aorta, *LAA* left atrial appendage

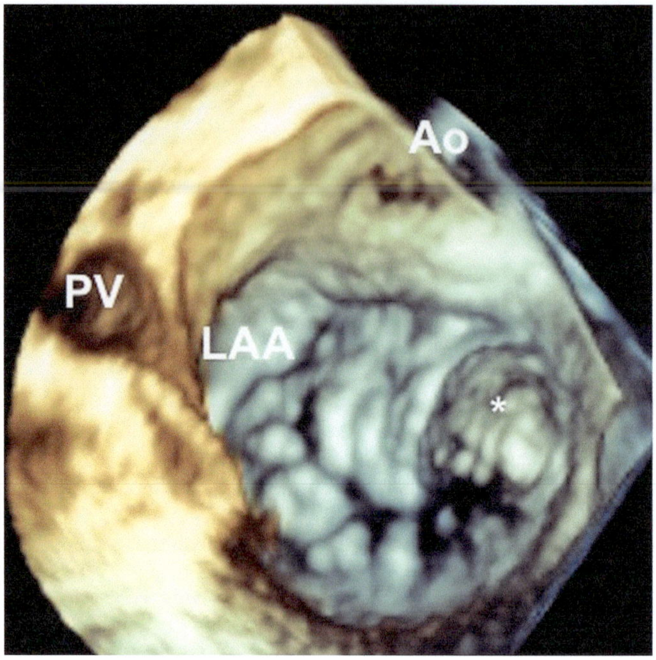

Fig. 9.12 Volume rendered transesophageal 3DE data set of the mitral valve in a patient with Barlow disease, medial commissural flail (*) and multiple ruptured chords (Video 9.8). *PV* pulmonary vein, *Ao* aorta, *LAA* left atrial appendage

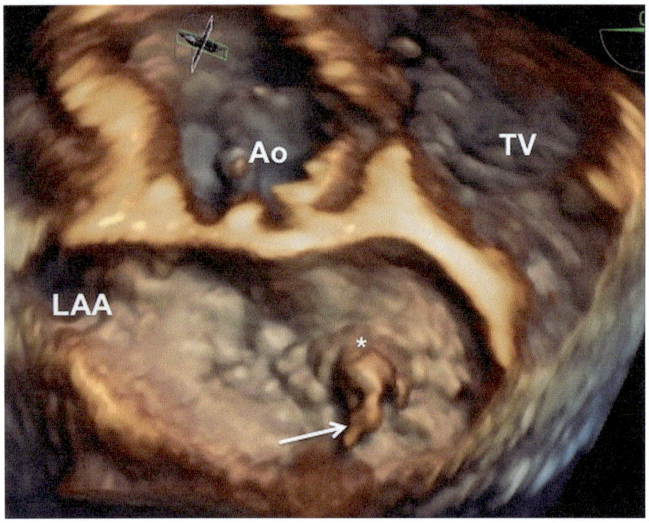

Fig. 9.11 Volume rendered transesophageal 3DE data set of the mitral valve in a patient with A2 flail (*) and multiple ruptured chords (arrow) (Video 9.7). *TV* tricuspid valve, *Ao* aorta, *LAA* left atrial appendage

Assessment of Regurgitation Severity

Assessment of mitral regurgitation severity is critical in the management of patients with degenerative MV disease. Current guidelines recommend the use of quantitative methods such as effective regurgitant orifice area, regurgitant volume and regurgitant fraction. These guidelines have provided cut-off values for the determination of the presence of severe regurgitation (Table 9.3) [27]. It must be noted that in previous guidelines, there was a difference in cut-off values between secondary mitral regurgitation, where degenerative mitral valve disease would be classified, and primary mitral regurgitation.

The leaflet and chordal changes in degenerative MV disease result in effective regurgitant orifice areas, vena contracta area, proximal isovelocity surface areas, and anatomical regurgitant surface areas with complex 3D geometry. While 2DE methods are recommended for quantitation of mitral regurgitation, these 2DE methods fail to account for the complex 3D geometry of the mitral orifice or of the regurgitant jet due to its planar nature. 3DE improves the assessment of mitral regurgitation by improving the calculation of the effective regurgitant orifice area with vena contracta area or proximal isovelocity surface area and by measuring the true 3D anatomical regurgitant orifice area (Table 9.4) [28].

3D Vena Contracta Area

Degenerative MV disease often results in eccentric regurgitant jets with asymmetric vena contracta areas, which are better assessed by 3DE. 3DE has demonstrated that less than 10% of patients have truly circular vena contracta areas. This

Table 9.3 Quantitative assessment of severe mitral regurgitation

Parameter	Primary mitral regurgitation	Secondary mitral regurgitation
Vena contracta	≥0.7 cm	Not recommended
Effective regurgitant orifice area	≥0.4 cm^2	≥0.2 cm^2
Regurgitant volume	≥60 mL	≥30 mL
Regurgitant fraction	0%	≥50%

Table 9.4 Strengths and weaknesses of 3DE quantitative assessment of mitral regurgitation

	2DE weakness	3DE strengths	3DE weakness
Vena Contracta	• Degenerative mitral leaflets form an asymmetric jet resulting in a non-circular vena contracta	• True cross-sectional vena contracta measurement • Multi-planar, cross-sectional width assessment • Direct measure of effective regurgitant orifice area avoiding geometric assumptions • More accurate and reproducible	• Requires proper selection of the systolic frame • Displayed area is affected by user settings • Poor correlation with mild regurgitant flows • 3DE color Doppler limitations (limited spatial and temporal resolution, risk of stitch artifact)
Proximal isovelocity surface area	• Asymmetric orifice formed by the degenerative mitral valve leaflets results in non-hemispheric proximal isovelocity surface area	• Convergence is non-hemispherical • More accurate assessment of radius without geometric assumptions	• Greater Doppler angle dependence defines the lateral margins of the isovelocity surface area • Not validated for multiple jets • Requires significant off-line processing • 3DE color Doppler limitations (see above)
Regurgitant orifice area	• Degenerative mitral valve leaflets result in asymmetric, non-planar anatomic orifice	• Direct *en face* visualization of the mitral valve regurgitant orifice • Can be measured in real-time	• Requires proper selection of the systolic frame
Stroke volume		• Integration of flow velocities throughout the entire cardiac cycle • More accurate and reproducible	• Not valid with concomitant valvular disease or intra-cardiac shunting

explains why 2DE single-plane vena contracta width measurements underestimate effective regurgitant orifice area [29]. Where the 2DE cut-plane passes through the vena contracta determines the vena contracta width. If the vena contracta area is asymmetrical, then it will be wider in some views than in others (Fig. 9.13). 3DE allows direct visualization and measurement of the vena contracta area, which has been demonstrated to be not only reliable but also accurate [30]. Comparisons of vena contracta area measured by 3DE to various 2D quantitative parameters have consistently reported that accuracy and reproducibility for MR severity is superior with 3DE vena contracta area measurements [31–33]. Measurement of 3DE vena contracta area is performed from an *en face* cut plane (Fig. 9.13), which has been shown to classify mitral regurgitation severity comparable to recommended 2DE integrative method [30]. A 3DE vena contracta area cutoff of 0.41 cm^2 is 82% sensitive and 97% specific in differentiating moderate from severe mitral regurgitation, regardless of whether the mitral regurgitation etiology is ischemic or degenerative [31].

3D Proximal Isovelocity Surface Area

The 2DE based formula used to calculate effective regurgitant orifice area assumes that the proximal flow convergence region is hemispherical and that the regurgitant orifice is circular and flat. However, an asymmetric regurgitant orifice area is commonly present in degenerative mitral valve disease patients, which results in a non-hemipherical proximal flow convergence region [34]. Three-dimensional computational fluid dynamics models have demonstrated that the convergence region becomes spheroidal (flattened) near the orifice and ellipsoidal (elongated) farther from the orifice in asymmetric orifices [34]. Thus, the use of a formula, which assumes an underlying hemispheric shape to calculate effective regurgitant orifice area, is inherently inaccurate. By substituting hemi-ellipsoidal formulas into 2DE formulas for calculating effective regurgitant orifice area, more accurate estimations of effective regurgitant orifice area have been demonstrated [35, 36].

The use of multi-planar reconstruction techniques to obtain the largest radius of the proximal isovelocity surface from a 3DE color Doppler dataset can also improve the accuracy in calculating effective regurgitant orifice area. While this method improves effective regurgitant orifice area assessment, it still relies on geometric assumptions regarding the proximal flow convergence region. These assumptions can be avoided by directly measuring the area of the proximal isovelocity surface from the 3DE dataset [35, 37].

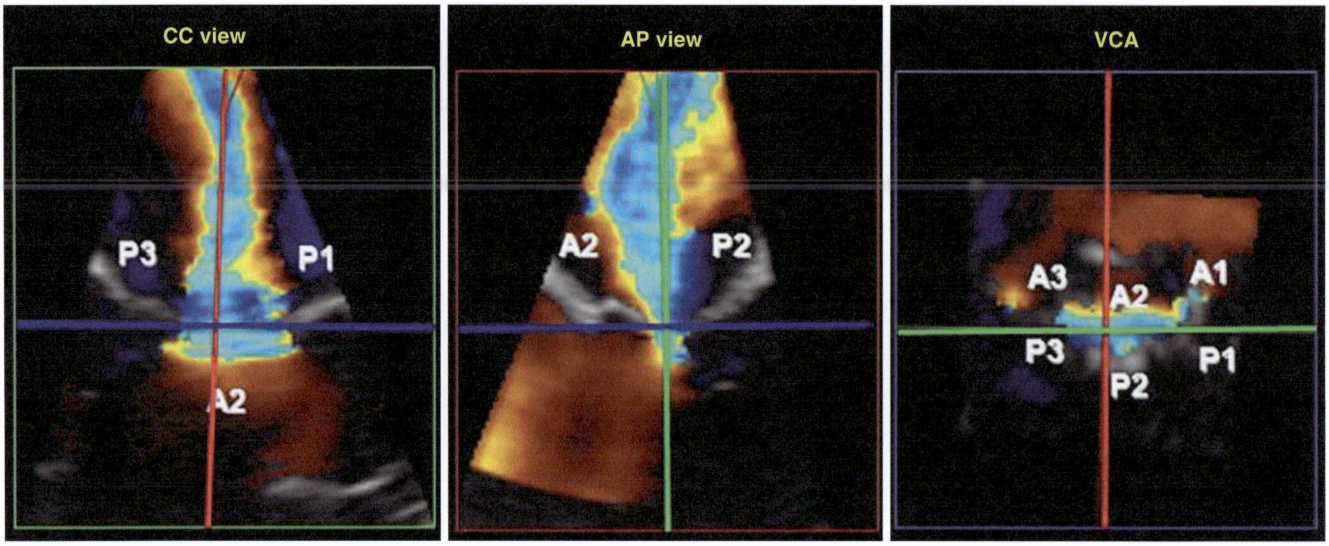

Fig. 9.13 Multi-planar analysis of mitral regurgitation from a three-dimensional color Doppler dataset. The true cross-sectional vena contracta area can be measured from the *en face* plane (blue plane) identified using orthogonal cut planes (green, red and blue planes). Note the difference in vena contracta width between the green plane (CC view) and the red plane (AP view). *CC* commissure-to-commissure, *AP* anterior-posterior

3D Anatomic Regurgitant Orifice Area

In patients with degenerative MV disease, 3D anatomic regurgitant orifice area measurement may provide a reasonable alternative to determine the severity of mitral regurgitation over 2DE planimetry of the effective regurgitant orifice area [38]. There are several methods for determining the anatomic regurgitant orifice area (Fig. 9.14). One method requires manual tracing of the leaflet edges within a 3DE data set. This method demonstrates good correlation with 2DE proximal isovelocity surface area-derived effective regurgitant orifice area but with better reproducibility [38]. Another method that does not fully account for the 3D shape of the anatomic regurgitant orifice area is to use multi-planar analysis of the 3DE dataset of the MV to identify the anatomic regurgitant orifice area and obtain a planar measurement [39].

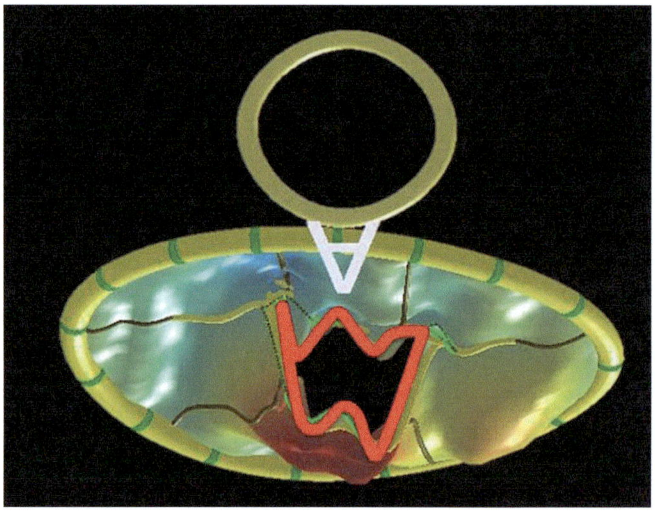

Fig. 9.14 Three-dimensional parametric map of the mitral valve demonstrating the non-planar, asymmetric anatomic regurgitant orifice (red outline) in a patient with P2 leaflet prolapse. Upside down *A* anterior

3D Mitral Inflow and Left Ventricular Outflow Tract Stroke Volume

An alternative to estimating the effective regurgitant orifice area or measuring the anatomic regurgitant orifice area in patients with degenerative MV disease is to determine mitral regurgitation severity by quantitating the regurgitant volume. This eliminates the need to assess the complex geometry of the degenerative MV orifice area and resultant jet. 3DE is superior to 2DE in obtaining regurgitant volume because it allows stroke volume quantification without geometric or flow profile assumptions, or reliance on single plane measurements. This technique uses 3DE color Doppler data within a region of interest to calculate the stroke volume (Fig. 9.15). Studies have demonstrated the accuracy of 3D-derived left ventricular outflow and mitral inflow stroke volume measurements [40, 41]. A different method for quantifying MV regurgitant volume uses a single transthoracic 3DE volume data set to obtain both 3D-derived left ventricular outflow and mitral valve inflow stroke volumes [42]. Publications on this method reported that left ventricular outflow and mitral valve inflow stroke volume measurements, using real-time 3DE, were significantly more accurate and reproducible than those obtained with 2DE. Additionally,

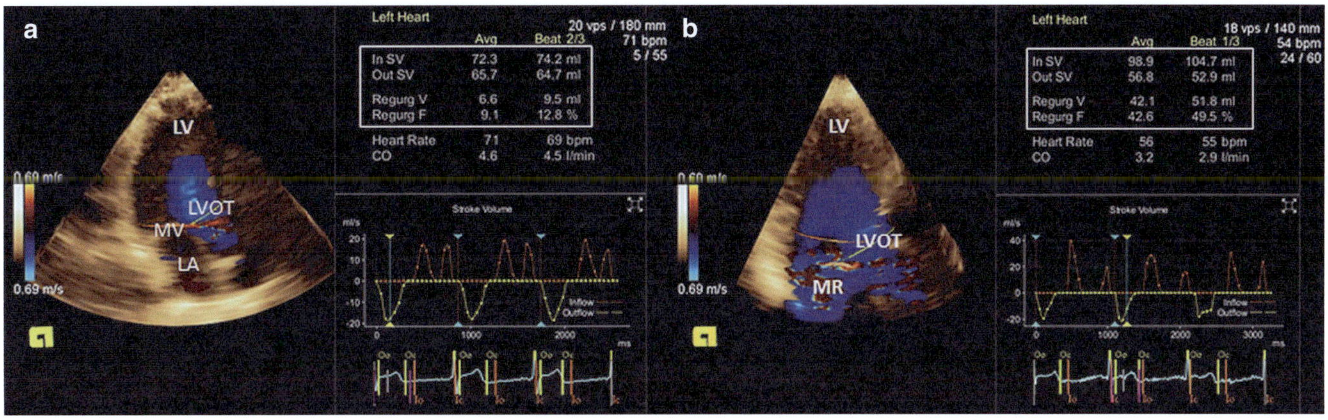

Fig. 9.15 3DE measurement of the regurgitant volume. (**a**) Visualization of volume color Doppler across the LVOT during Systole. The summarized report displays inflow and outflow stroke volume with the derived regurgitant volume and fraction. Cardiac Output is also displayed. The orange, curve on the graph above the baseline, represents the integrated velocities of the orange disc (mitral inflow) tracked over three cardiac cycles. The yellow curve, on the graph below the baseline, represents the integrated velocities of the yellow (outflow) disc tracked over three cardiac cycles. The Inflow–Outflow difference is less than 10 mL and is representative of normal flow without mitral regurgitation. (**b**) Visualization of volume color Doppler across the LVOT during systole with reverse flow into the left atrium. The summarized report displays inflow and outflow stroke volume with the derived regurgitant volume and fraction. Cardiac Output is also displayed. The orange, curve on the graph above the baseline, represents the integrated velocities of the orange disc (mitral inflow) tracked over three cardiac cycles. The yellow curve, on the graph below the baseline, represents the integrated velocities of the yellow (outflow) disc tracked over three cardiac cycles. The Inflow–Outflow difference is above 40 mL considered severe mitral regurgitations

this technique was highly feasible and post-processing data required less than one minute.

Limitations of 3D-Derived Quantitative Measurements for MR

While there are advantages to using 3DE to assess degenerative MV disease regurgitation severity, there are still limitations for each technique. 3DE-derived vena contracta area is subject to color Doppler gain settings and is also dependent on the proper selection of the systolic frame, which affects measurement accuracy and reproducibility [43]. Proximal isovelocity surface area still requires significant off-line processing and is not practical in a busy clinical setting. While 3D proximal velocity flow convergence is angle-independent, the lower temporal resolution of 3DE color Doppler might affect proper selection of the largest flow convergence region. Anatomic regurgitant orifice area also requires proper selection of the systolic frame and is limited by the relatively poor temporal resolution of 3DE. 3D mitral inflow and left ventricular outflow tract stroke volume holds great promise, but this method still requires further validation in patients with mitral regurgitation.

Anatomy

All assessments of degenerative mitral regurgitation should include assessment of mitral valvular and sub-valvular anatomy, left ventricular function and left atrial size. Severe mitral regurgitation rarely occurs in the presence of a normal mitral apparatus and left ventricular structure. Changes to left ventricular function and left atrial size also allow determination of mitral regurgitation chronicity and the severity of changes to the left ventricle and atrium have been associated with poorer outcomes [44–47]. Thus, it has been recommended that patients with left ventricular ejection fraction ≤60% be considered for surgery [27]. 3DE has been demonstrated to have superior accuracy and reproducibility in the assessment of left ventricular and left atrial volumes and should be used to follow patients if possible [48–50].

Cases

Case 9.1

A 63-year-old male presented with acute shortness of breath. He has previously been well. His past medical history was significant for hypertension, atrial fibrillation and smoking. On examination he was found to be tachypneic. His heart rate was irregular ranging between 110 and 131 bpm. Oxygen saturation was 80% on RA and improved to 95% with oxygen supplementation. Blood pressure was 150/85 mmHg. Jugular venous distension was present and auscultation revealed a 4/6 apical holosystolic murmur that radiated to the axilla.

Transthoracic echocardiography was performed and demonstrated the presence of a flail leaflet with an eccentric jet of

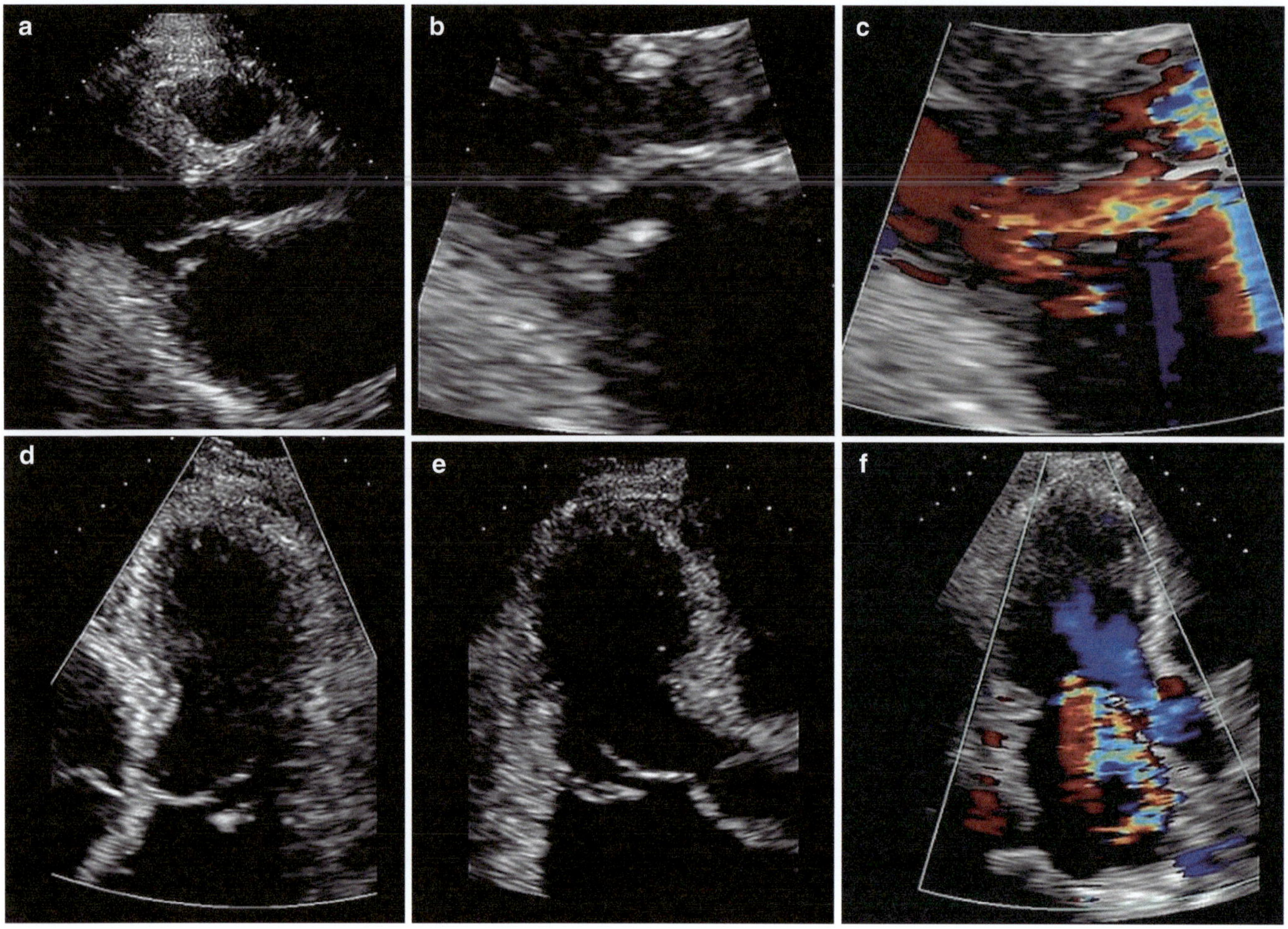

Fig. 9.16 Transthoracic two-dimensional echocardiographic images demonstrating a posterior mitral leaflet flail in the parasternal long axis views (**a**, **b**). An eccentric, wall-hugging jet of severe regurgitation accompanied the valve abnormality (**c**). In the apical 4- and 3-chamber views, the flail leaflet can also be seen (**d**, **e**) as can the regurgitant jet (**f**)

severe mitral regurgitation (Fig. 9.16). The left atrium was dilated and left ventricular function was normal. Transesophageal echocardiography was subsequently performed in preparation for surgery. This demonstrated P2 segment flail and prolapse of P2 and P3 on two-dimensional (Fig. 9.17) and three-dimensional (Fig. 9.18) interrogation of the mitral valve. From the two-dimensional echocardiographic images, a complex, multidirectional eccentric wall hugging jet is appreciated. The three-dimensional parametric models demonstrate the asymmetric shape of the regurgitant orifice that resulted in this jet. At the time of surgery, the echocardiographic findings were confirmed.

This patient has Barlow's disease with chronic mitral regurgitation and an acute rupture of the chord of the P2 segment of his posterior leaflet resulting in mitral regurgitation. The increased left atrial size suggests some chronicity under his acute presentation. The transthoracic and transesophageal two-dimensional echocardiogram allow identification of the mitral leaflet pathology. However, the three-dimensional transesophageal echocardiogram simplifies identification of the lesion and increases the appreciation for the mechanism for the complexity of the jet. From the two- and three-dimensional echocardiographic images, the prolapse is mainly located to the P2 segment with some P3 segment involvement. The parametric model also reveals that the saddle shape of the mitral annulus is relatively preserved.

Three-dimensional modeling of the mitral valve reported a prolapse height of 12.2 mm and a prolapse volume of 5.7 mL. The prolapse height is greater than 1 mm, which confirms that this is degenerative mitral valve disease and the prolapse volume is greater than 1.2 mL suggests that this is Barlow's disease. While the age and acuteness of symptoms at presentation would have suggested fibroelastic deficiency, the combination of chronicity suggested by left atrial enlargement with atrial fibrillation and the multi-segmental involvement resulting in a significant prolapsing volume are more consistent with Barlow's disease.

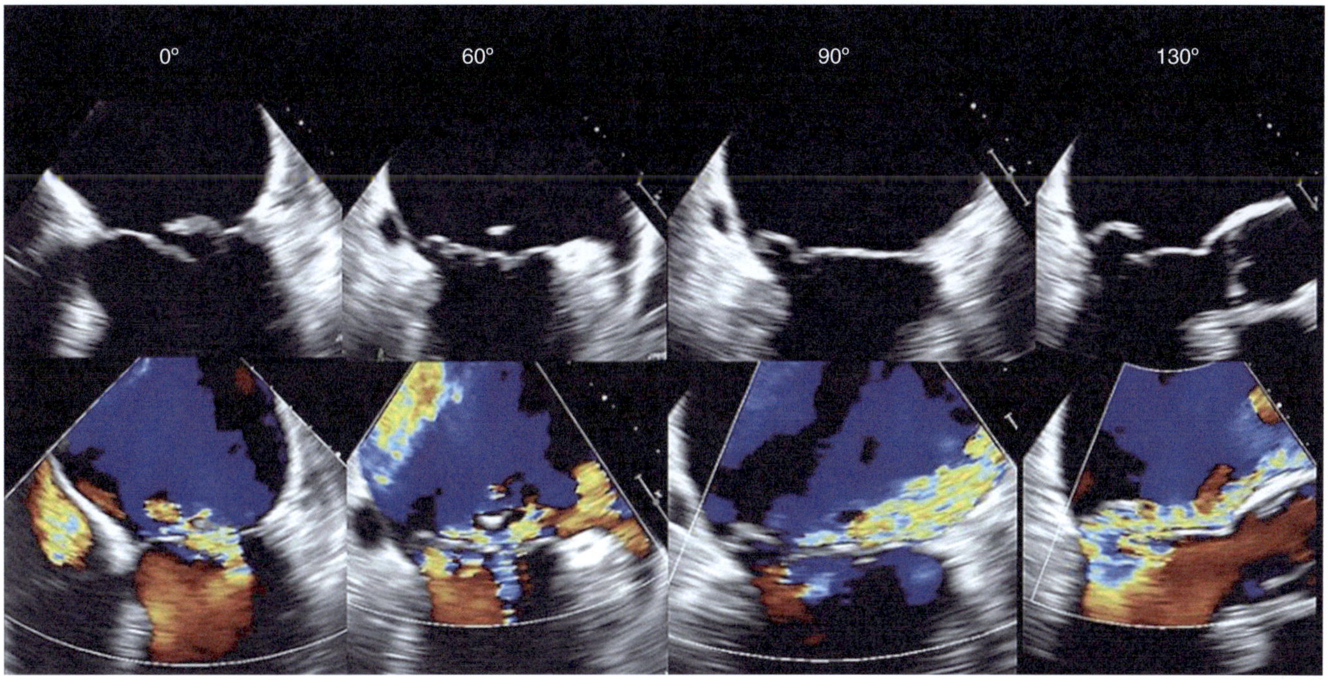

Fig. 9.17 Transesophageal two-dimensional echocardiographic images of the mitral valve at 0°, 60°, 90° and 130°, demonstrating that the posterior flail involves segment P2. There is prolapse of segments P2 and P3

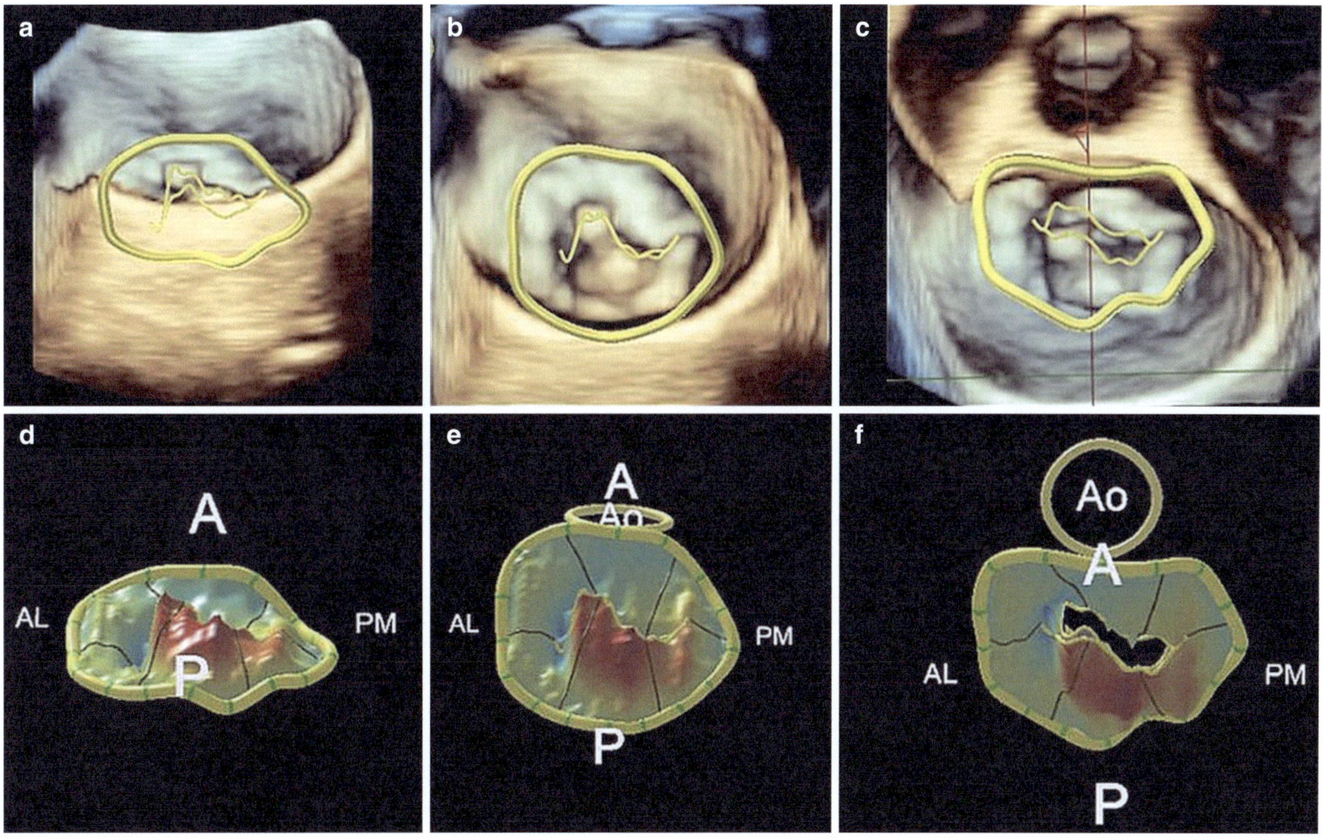

Fig. 9.18 These images display peak systolic transesophageal three-dimensional echocardiographic volumes with an embedded mitral valve models (**a**–**c**) and parametric mitral valve models (**d**–**f**) rotated from a left atrial posterior tilt perspective (**a**, **d**), to a left atrial *en-face* perspective (**b**, **e**) and a left atrial anterior tilt perspective (**c**, **f**). They demonstrate both the location and severity of the prolapse/flail segment. As well, the left atrial anterior tilt perspective of the parametric model allows us to appreciate the asymmetric nature of the regurgitant orifice

Case 9.2

A 55-year-old male presents with shortness of breath. His shortness of breath has been worsening over a period of 4 months. His past medical history was significant for a murmur that had been present for many years. On examination his heart rate was regular at 86 bpm. Oxygen saturation was 96% on RA and blood pressure was 135/80 mmHg. Jugular venous distension was present and auscultation revealed a 4/6 apical holosystolic murmur that radiated to the axilla.

Transthoracic echocardiography was performed and demonstrated the presence of a bileaflet mital valve prolapse resulting in an eccentric jet of severe regurgitation (Fig. 9.19). The left atrium was dilated and left ventricular function was normal. Transesophageal echocardiography demonstrated multisegmental mitral leaflet thickening and prolapse (Fig. 9.20) with a gap along the P1-P2-A1-A2 leaflets resulting in an eccentric jet of severe mitral regurgitation. These finding were more easily demonstrated with three-dimensional echocardiography (Fig. 9.21). The three-dimensional parametric models allow easy appreciation of the regurgitant orifice.

This patient has Barlow's disease resulting in chronic mitral regurgitation. The chronic mitral regurgitation results in increased left atrial size. The transthoracic and transesophageal two-dimensional echocardiogram demonstrate multi-segmental thickening and prolapse of the mitral valve. The three-dimensional transesophageal echocardiogram allows identification of the flail segment with resulting regurgitant orifice.

The three-dimensional model reveals that the mitral annulus is enlarged and that the normal saddle shape has been lost. Three-dimensional modeling of the mitral valve reported a prolapse height of 16 mm and a prolapse volume of 20 mL. While the valve clearly appears myxomatous, the measurements from the model confirm these findings.

Summary

Overall, 3DE has improved our quantification of mitral valve anatomy and regurgitation severity in patients with degenerative mitral valve disease. While there are limitations, it is a methodology that will continue to improve with future hardware and software developments. As well, automation of analysis and integration into echocardiographic carts will allow it to be integrated into clinical practice.

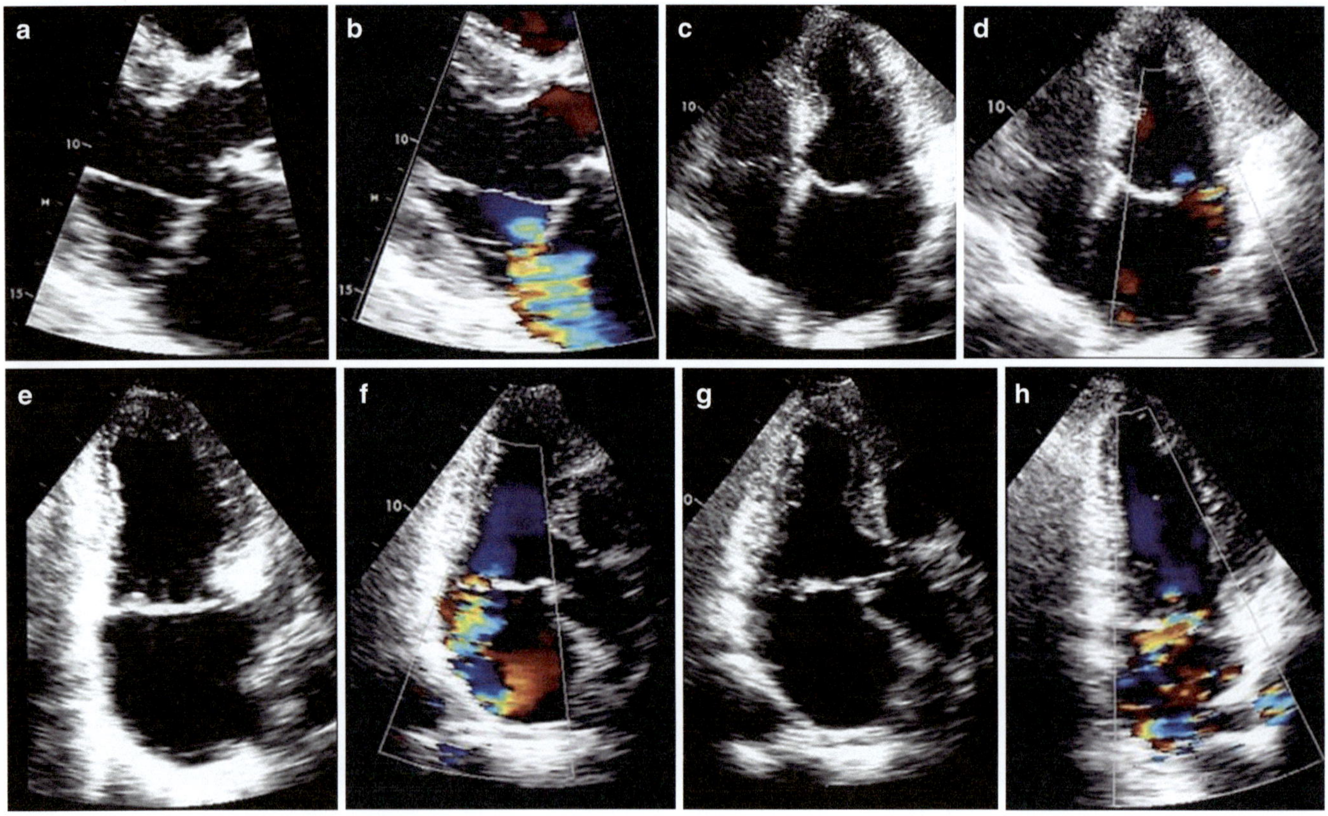

Fig. 9.19 Transthoracic two-dimensional echocardiographic images demonstrating a bileaflet mitral valve prolapse with a flail segment in the parasternal long axis views (**a**). An eccentric jet of severe regurgitation accompanied the abnormality (**b**). While the degree of prolapse and leaflet involvement is not well appreciated on the apical 4-, 2- and 3-chamber views (**c–h**), the eccentricity of regurgitant jet is clearly demonstrated

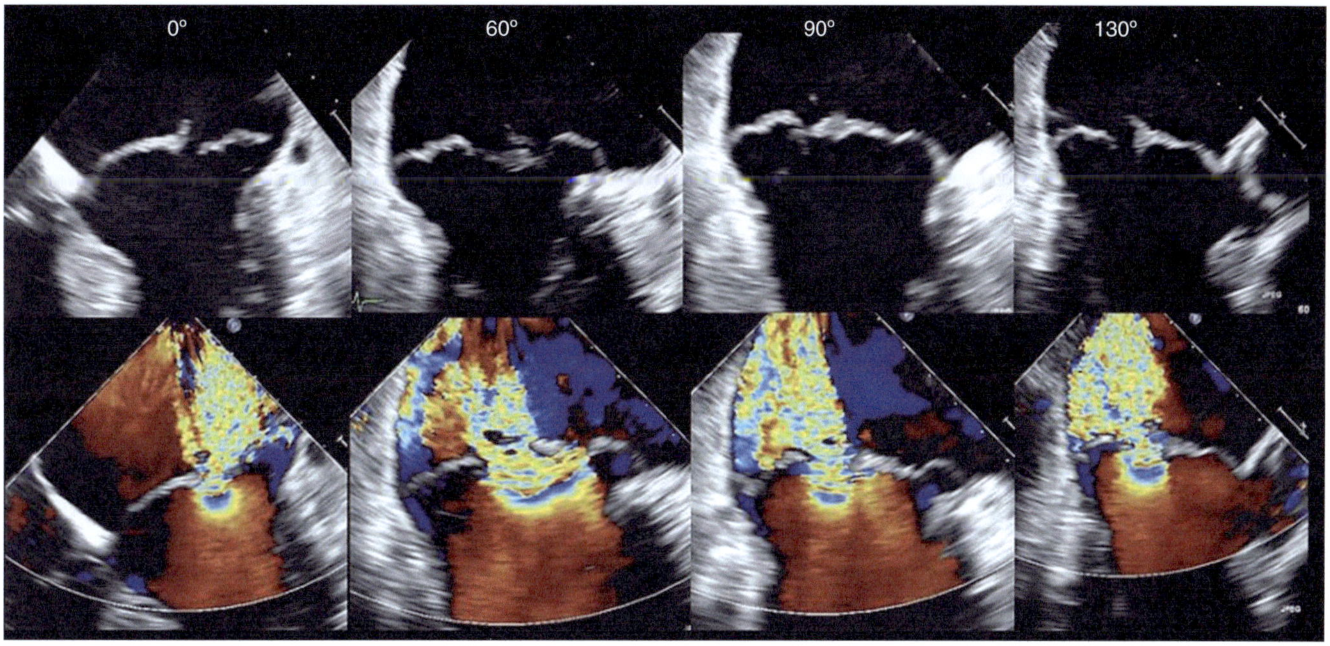

Fig. 9.20 Transesophageal two-dimensional echocardiographic images of the mitral valve at 0°, 60°, 90° and 130°, demonstrating bileaflet myomatous disease with a flail segment involving the A2 segment

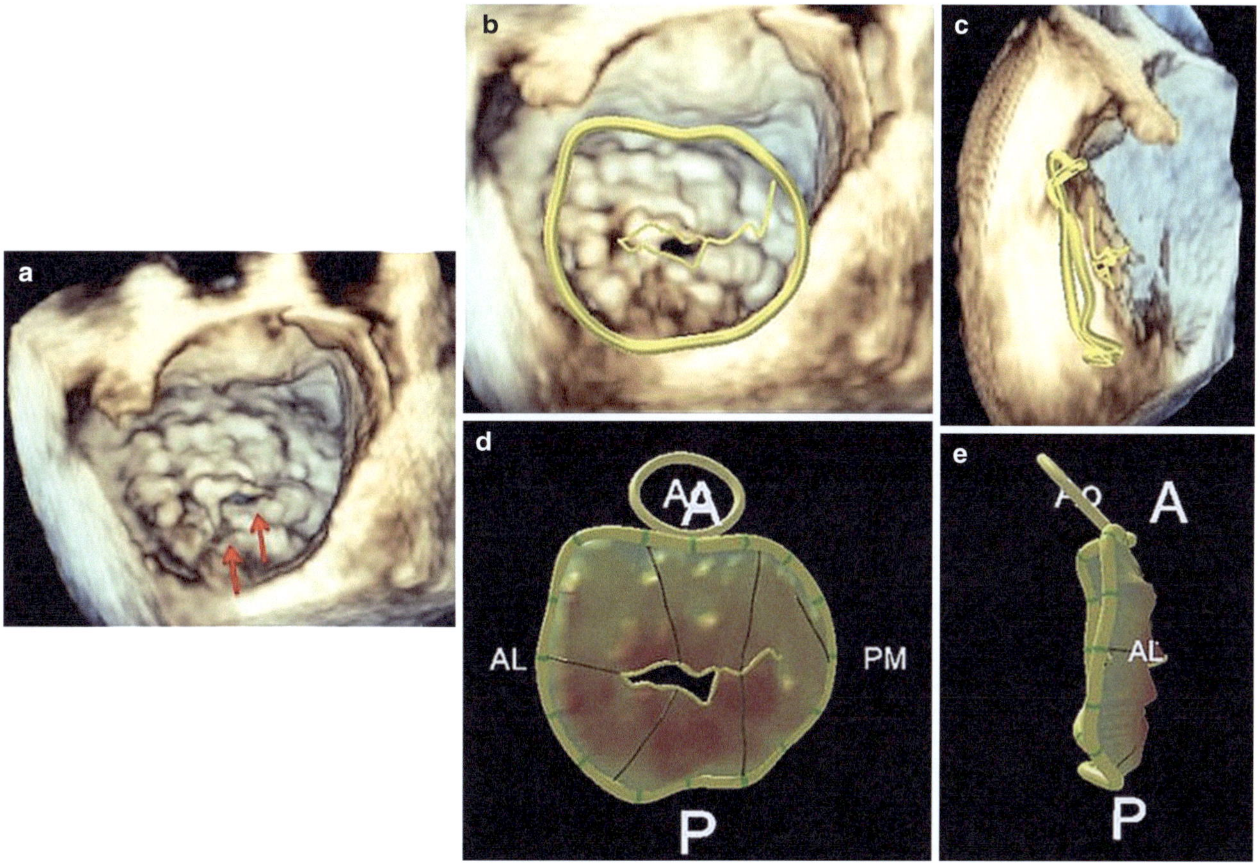

Fig. 9.21 A peak systolic transesophageal three-dimensional volume rendered image of the mitral valve demonstrating the bileaflet prolapse with ruptured chords (**a**, arrows). Images (**b**, **c**) are of three-dimensional volume rendered images of the mitral valve with embedded mitral valve models. Image (**b**) is viewed *en face* from the left atrial perspective and image (**c**) is rotated leftward for a profile view. The corresponding parametric mitral valve models are displaced in images (**d**, **e**). These images demonstrate the severity and extent of the bi-leaflet prolapse. The mitral annulus is enlarged and in the profile shot, the loss of the normal saddle shape is revealed. The parametric maps help localize the origin of the regurgitant jet given the extent of disease. It also allows us to appreciate the asymmetric nature of the regurgitant orifice

References

1. Griffin BP. Myxomatous mitral valve disease. In: Otto CM, Bonow RO, editors. Valvular heart disease. Philadelphia: Saunders Elsevier; 2009. p. 243–59.
2. Tsang W, Freed BH, Lang RM. Three-dimensional anatomy of the aortic and mitral valves. In: Otto CM, Bonow R, editors. Valvular heart disease: a companion to Bruanwald's heart disease. 4th ed. Philadelphia: Saunders Elsevier; 2014. p. 488.
3. Anyanwu AC, Adams DH. Etiologic classification of degenerative mitral valve disease: Barlow's disease and fibroelastic deficiency. Semin Thorac Cardiovasc Surg. 2007;19:90–6.
4. Adams DH, Anyanwu AC, Sugeng L, Lang RM. Degenerative mitral valve regurgitation: surgical echocardiography. Curr Cardiol Rep. 2008;10:226–32.
5. Gillinov AM, Cosgrove DM, Blackstone EH, et al. Durability of mitral valve repair for degenerative disease. J Thorac Cardiovasc Surg. 1998;116:734–43.
6. Lee EM, Shapiro LM, Wells FC. Superiority of mitral valve repair in surgery for degenerative mitral regurgitation. Eur Heart J. 1997;18:655–63.
7. Sugeng L, Shernan SK, Salgo IS, et al. Live 3-dimensional transesophageal echocardiography initial experience using the fully-sampled matrix array probe. J Am Coll Cardiol. 2008;52:446–9.
8. Chandra S, Salgo IS, Sugeng L, et al. Characterization of degenerative mitral valve disease using morphologic analysis of real-time three-dimensional echocardiographic images: objective insight into complexity and planning of mitral valve repair. Circ Cardiovasc Imaging. 2011;4:24–32.
9. Tsang W, Weinert L, Sugeng L, et al. The value of three-dimensional echocardiography derived mitral valve parametric maps and the role of experience in the diagnosis of pathology. J Am Soc Echocardiogr. 2011;24(8):860–7.
10. La Canna G, Arendar I, Maisano F, et al. Real-time three-dimensional transesophageal echocardiography for assessment of mitral valve functional anatomy in patients with prolapse-related regurgitation. Am J Cardiol. 2011;107:1365–74.
11. Carpentier A. Cardiac valve surgery—the "French correction". J Thorac Cardiovasc Surg. 1983;86:323–37.
12. Shah PM, Raney AA. Echocardiography in mitral regurgitation with relevance to valve surgery. J Am Soc Echocardiogr. 2011;24:1086–91.
13. Tamborini G, Muratori M, Maltagliati A, Galli CA, Naliato M, Zanobini M, Alamanni F, Salvi L, Sisillo E, Fiorentini C, Pepi M. Preoperative transthoracic real-time three-dimensional echocardiography in patients undergoing mitral valve repair: accuracy in cases with simple vs complex prolapse lesion. Eur J Echocardiogr. 2010;11:778–85.
14. Gutierrez-Chico JL, Zamorano Gomez JL, Rodrigo-Lopez JL, et al. Accuracy of real time 3-dimensional echocardiography in the assessment of mitral prolapse: is transesophageal echocardiography still mandatory? Am Heart J. 2008;155:694–8.
15. Gripari P, Mapelli M, Bellacosa I, et al. Transthoracic echocardiography in patients undergoing mitral valve repair: comparison of new transthoracic techniques to 2D transesophageal echocardiography in the localization of mitral valve prolapse. Int J Cardiovasc Imaging. 2018;34(7):1099–107. https://doi.org/10.1007/s10554-018-1324-2.
16. Pepi M, Tamborini G, Maltagliati A, et al. Head-to head comparison of two- and three-dimensional transthoracic and transesophageal echocardiography in the localization of mitral valve prolapse. J Am Coll Cardiol. 2006;48:2424–30.
17. Salgo IS, Gorman JH 3rd, Gorman RC, et al. Effect of annular shape on leaflet curvature in reducing mitral leaflet stress. Circulation. 2002;106:711–7.
18. Levine RA, Handschumacher MD, Sanfilippo AJ, et al. Three-dimensional echocardiographic reconstruction of the mitral valve, with implications for the diagnosis of mitral valve prolapse. Circulation. 1989;80:589–98.
19. Watanabe N, Ogasawara Y, Yamaura Y, et al. Mitral annulus flattens in ischemic mitral regurgitation: geometric differences between inferior and anterior myocardial infarction: a real-time 3-dimensional echocardiographic study. Circulation. 2005;112:1458–62.
20. Lang RM, Mor-Avi V, Dent JM, Kramer CM. Three-dimensional echocardiography: is it ready for everyday clinical use? JACC Cardiovasc Imaging. 2009;2:114–7.
21. Gorman JH 3rd, Gupta KB, Streicher JT, et al. Dynamic three-dimensional imaging of the mitral valve and left ventricle by rapid sonomicrometry array localization. J Thorac Cardiovasc Surg. 1996;112:712–26.
22. Lang RM, Adams DH. 3D echocardiographic quantification in functional mitral regurgitation. JACC Cardiovasc Imaging. 2012;5:346–7.
23. Little SH, Ben Zekry S, Lawrie GM, Zoghbi WA. Dynamic annular geometry and function in patients with mitral regurgitation: insight from three-dimensional annular tracking. J Am Soc Echocardiogr. 2010;23:872–9.
24. Jassar AS, Vergnat M, Jackson BM, et al. Regional annular geometry in patients with mitral regurgitation: implications for annuloplasty ring selection. Ann Thorac Surg. 2014;97:64–70.
25. Ben Zekry S, Lang RM, Sugeng L, et al. Mitral annulus dynamics early after valve repair: preliminary observations of the effect of resectional versus non-resectional approaches. J Am Soc Echocardiogr. 2011;24:1233–42.
26. Grewal J, Suri R, Mankad S, et al. Mitral annular dynamics in myxomatous valve disease: new insights with real-time 3-dimensional echocardiography. Circulation. 2010;121:1423–31.
27. Nishimura RA, Otto C. 2014 ACC/AHA valve guidelines: earlier intervention for chronic mitral regurgitation. Heart. 2014;100(12):905–7.
28. Bhave NM, Lang RM. Quantitative echocardiographic assessment of native mitral regurgitation: two- and three-dimensional techniques. J Heart Valve Dis. 2011;20:483–92.
29. Kahlert P, Plicht B, Schenk IM, Janosi RA, Erbel R, Buck T. Direct assessment of size and shape of noncircular vena contracta area in functional versus organic mitral regurgitation using real-time three-dimensional echocardiography. J Am Soc Echocardiogr. 2008;21:912–21.
30. Little SH, Pirat B, Kumar R, et al. Three-dimensional color Doppler echocardiography for direct measurement of vena contracta area in mitral regurgitation: in vitro validation and clinical experience. JACC Cardiovasc Imaging. 2008;1:695–704.
31. Zeng X, Levine RA, Hua L, et al. Diagnostic value of vena contracta area in the quantification of mitral regurgitation severity by color Doppler 3D echocardiography. Circ Cardiovasc Imaging. 2011;4:506–13.
32. Marsan NA, Westenberg JJ, Ypenburg C, et al. Quantification of functional mitral regurgitation by real-time 3D echocardiography: comparison with 3D velocity-encoded cardiac magnetic resonance. JACC Cardiovasc Imaging. 2009;2:1245–52.
33. Yosefy C, Hung J, Chua S, et al. Direct measurement of vena contracta area by real-time 3-dimensional echocardiography for assessing severity of mitral regurgitation. Am J Cardiol. 2009;104:978–83.
34. Shiota T, Jones M, Delabays A, et al. Direct measurement of three-dimensionally reconstructed flow convergence surface area and regurgitant flow in aortic regurgitation: in vitro and chronic animal model studies. Circulation. 1997;96:3687–95.
35. Matsumura Y, Saracino G, Sugioka K, et al. Determination of regurgitant orifice area with the use of a new three-dimensional flow convergence geometric assumption in functional mitral regurgitation. J Am Soc Echocardiogr. 2008;21:1251–6.

36. Shiota T, Sinclair B, Ishii M, et al. Three-dimensional reconstruction of color Doppler flow convergence regions and regurgitant jets: an in vitro quantitative study. J Am Coll Cardiol. 1996;27:1511–8.
37. Little SH, Igo SR, Pirat B, et al. In vitro validation of real-time three-dimensional color Doppler echocardiography for direct measurement of proximal isovelocity surface area in mitral regurgitation. Am J Cardiol. 2007;99:1440–7.
38. Chandra S, Salgo IS, Sugeng L, et al. A three-dimensional insight into the complexity of flow convergence in mitral regurgitation: adjunctive benefit of anatomic regurgitant orifice area. Am J Physiol Heart Circ Physiol. 2011;301(3):H1015–24.
39. Altiok E, Hamada S, van Hall S, et al. Comparison of direct planimetry of mitral valve regurgitation orifice area by three-dimensional transesophageal echocardiography to effective regurgitant orifice area obtained by proximal flow convergence method and vena contracta area determined by color Doppler echocardiography. Am J Cardiol. 2011;107:452–8.
40. Lodato JA, Weinert L, Baumann R, et al. Use of 3-dimensional color Doppler echocardiography to measure stroke volume in human beings: comparison with thermodilution. J Am Soc Echocardiogr. 2007;20:103–12.
41. Pemberton J, Jerosch-Herold M, Li X, et al. Accuracy of real-time, three-dimensional Doppler echocardiography for stroke volume estimation compared with phase-encoded MRI: an in vivo study. Heart. 2008;94:1212–3.
42. Thavendiranathan P, Liu S, Datta S, et al. Automated quantification of mitral inflow and aortic outflow stroke volumes by three-dimensional real-time volume color-flow Doppler transthoracic echocardiography: comparison with pulsed-wave Doppler and cardiac magnetic resonance imaging. J Am Soc Echocardiogr. 2012;25:56–65.
43. Buck T, Plicht B, Kahlert P, Schenk IM, Hunold P, Erbel R. Effect of dynamic flow rate and orifice area on mitral regurgitant stroke volume quantification using the proximal isovelocity surface area method. J Am Coll Cardiol. 2008;52:767–78.
44. Le Tourneau T, Messika-Zeitoun D, Russo A, et al. Impact of left atrial volume on clinical outcome in organic mitral regurgitation. J Am Coll Cardiol. 2010;56:570–8.
45. Rusinaru D, Tribouilloy C, Grigioni F, et al. Left atrial size is a potent predictor of mortality in mitral regurgitation due to flail leaflets: results from a large international multicenter study. Circ Cardiovasc Imaging. 2011;4:473–81.
46. Tribouilloy C, Grigioni F, Avierinos JF, et al. Survival implication of left ventricular end-systolic diameter in mitral regurgitation due to flail leaflets a long-term follow-up multicenter study. J Am Coll Cardiol. 2009;54:1961–8.
47. Tribouilloy C, Rusinaru D, Grigioni F, et al. Long-term mortality associated with left ventricular dysfunction in mitral regurgitation due to flail leaflets: a multicenter analysis. Circ Cardiovasc Imaging. 2014;7:363–70.
48. Wu VC, Takeuchi M, Kuwaki H, et al. Prognostic value of LA volumes assessed by transthoracic 3D echocardiography: comparison with 2D echocardiography. JACC Cardiovasc Imaging. 2013;6:1025–35.
49. Mor-Avi V, Jenkins C, Kuhl HP, et al. Real-time 3-dimensional echocardiographic quantification of left ventricular volumes: multicenter study for validation with magnetic resonance imaging and investigation of sources of error. JACC Cardiovasc Imaging. 2008;1:413–23.
50. Thavendiranathan P, Grant AD, Negishi T, Plana JC, Popovic ZB, Marwick TH. Reproducibility of echocardiographic techniques for sequential assessment of left ventricular ejection fraction and volumes: application to patients undergoing cancer chemotherapy. J Am Coll Cardiol. 2013;61:77–84.

Functional Mitral Regurgitation

10

Timothy C. Tan, Xin Zeng, and Judy Hung

Abstract

Mitral valve regurgitation is one of the most common valve lesions. Clinical decision making for mitral regurgitation depends on accurate assessment of the mechanism and quantitation of mitral regurgitation. The mechanism of mitral regurgitation in a significant proportion of patients especially in the developed countries is functional. The mechanism underlying functional mitral regurgitation is due to left ventricular dilation. Furthermore, as functional mitral regurgitation is by nature a dynamic problem, accurate assessment of severity can be challenging. Echocardiography which enables real time imaging of the heart is the primary imaging modality in the diagnosis and assessment of functional mitral regurgitation. Important information can be obtained from a systematic echocardiographic assessment of the whole mitral apparatus and the underlying ventricular myocardium. Due to the complex spatial and dynamic pattern of flow across the mitral valve in patients with functional mitral regurgitation, obtaining accurate flow quantification using standard two-dimensional measures can be challenging. Three-dimensional echocardiographic techniques have been successful in overcoming some of the inherent geometric limitations of two-dimensional imaging. This chapter outlines the key aspects of functional mitral regurgitation and includes an overview of the anatomy of the mitral valve in the context of functional mitral regurgitation and standard flow measures as assessed using two- and three dimensional echocardiography.

Keywords

Mitral regurgitation · Functional · Ischemic Echocardiography · Severity · Three-dimensional echocardiography

Introduction

Mitral valve regurgitation is one of the most common valve lesions, representing nearly one-third of acquired left-sided valve pathology [1, 2]. This constitutes a significant disease burden considering that the prevalence of significant regurgitation (moderate to severe and severe) in the general population has been estimated at 2–3% and predicted to become increasingly more prevalent as the population ages [2]. Mitral regurgitation can arise from abnormalities in the function of the mitral valve which can be broadly classified into mitral regurgitation due to pathology or damage to the mitral valve leaflets or the associated valvular structures (primary mitral regurgitation); or mitral regurgitation due to left ventricular (LV) dilation resulting in failure of coaptation of the mitral valve leaflets without coexisting structural abnormalities of the valve or its associated valvular apparatus (functional mitral regurgitation, FMR). FMR, or secondary mitral regurgitation, makes up a large proportion of the cases of mitral regurgitation and has been independently associated with poor long-term survival, excessive morbidity and mortality. Hence, timely diagnosis and accurate grading of the severity of FMR are critical for appropriate patient management, particularly timing of surgical intervention [3–8]. Population studies also indicate that the incidence of FMR is expected to increase due to predicted demographic changes,

Electronic Supplementary Material The online version of this chapter (https://doi.org/10.1007/978-3-030-14032-8_10) contains supplementary material, which is available to authorized users.

T. C. Tan
Department of Cardiology, Westmead Hospital, Westmead, NSW, Australia
e-mail: tim.tan@sydney.edu.au

X. Zeng · J. Hung (✉)
Department of Medicine/Cardiology, Massachusetts General Hospital, Boston, MA, USA
e-mail: xzeng@mgh.harvard.edu; jhung@mgh.harvard.edu

L. P. Badano et al. (eds.), *Textbook of Three-Dimensional Echocardiography*, https://doi.org/10.1007/978-3-030-14032-8_10

progressively higher and longer survival to acute and chronic cardiac diseases affecting LV geometry and function. Factors such as an aging population and greater life expectancy, are expected to contribute to an increase in the incidence of ischaemic heart disease and dilated cardiomyopathy (the two most common causes of FMR) [2, 3].

FMR essentially results from failure of systolic coaptation of the mitral valve leaflets due to pathology affecting the LV. Most typically, the initiating insult relates to ventricular remodeling following myocardial infarction or ischemia, or dilated non-ischemic cardiomyopathy. Up to 40% of patients with heart failure caused by dilated cardiomyopathy are estimated to go on to develop FMR [9, 10]. Symptoms arising from FMR typically progresses slow and also often ends in contributing towards irreversible LV dysfunction.

Pathophysiology of Functional Mitral Regurgitation

FMR results from an altered force balance between tethering forces on the mitral leaflets from ventricular dilation and decreased closing forces (Fig. 10.1). With adverse LV remodeling that occurs with myocardial infarction or cardiomyopathy, the myocardium underlying the papillary muscles dilates and the mitral leaflets are pulled apically into the LV as a consequence of the outward displacement of the papillary muscles resulting from LV dilation. This results in increased tethering forces on the mitral leaflets resulting in incomplete mitral leaflet closure. Closing forces generated from LV contraction which act to close the leaflets are typically diminished in setting of LV cardiomyopathy and contribute to development of FMR [11]. FMR has also been proposed to occur in LV dyssynchrony. In this instance, the mechanism is believed to be due to a combination of reduced closing force and discoordination of contraction of the papillary muscles, which results in dynamic tethering of the leaflets [12].

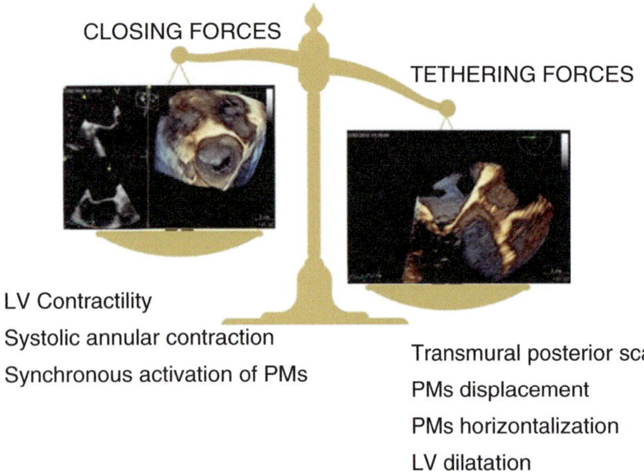

Fig. 10.1 Mechanism of functional mitral regurgitation. In patients with functional mitral regurgitation, the tethering forces on the mitral leaflets from ventricular dilation and or regional dysfunction prevail on the closing forces which are decreased. *LV* left ventricular, *PM* papillary muscles

Mitral Valve Anatomy and the Underlying Mechanism of Functional Mitral Regurgitation

To understand the underlying pathophysiology associated with FMR and to diagnose FMR require an understanding of the normal mitral valve anatomy. This is important as treatment approaches are different in patients with primary versus FMR. In the case of primary mitral regurgitation, treatment strategies will target the mitral valve as opposed to FMR where the target strategies will predominantly be focused on the left ventricle. The anatomic structure of the mitral valve apparatus is complex and is composed of several components working in synchrony to open during diastole and close in systole effectively within the high-pressure systemic environment (see also Chap. 7). Essentially, the mitral valve is comprised of: (1) annulus, (2) leaflets, (3) chordae tendinae, and (4) papillary muscles. These will now be individually examined in the context of FMR.

Mitral Annulus

The mitral annulus is the anatomical poorly defined junctional zone, which separates the left atrium and left ventricle, to which the mitral leaflets are attached. It is oval in shape with the intercommissural diameter being larger than the anteroposterior diameter (Fig. 10.2). There is evidence that the mitral annulus is not simply a rigid fibrous ring but is pliable, and has been shown to undergo dynamic changes in shape and area throughout the cardiac cycle. Three-dimensional echocardiography (3DE) has revealed that the mitral annulus adopts a non-planar saddle-shape (Fig. 10.3). The anterior portion of the mitral annulus, which continuous with the aortic annulus, serves as the highest point (most atrial) of the mitral annulus and is more fibrous compared to the rest of the annulus, thus less prone to dilatation. On the other hand, the posterior annulus, which comprises of the remaining two-thirds of the annulus is more muscular, includes the low points of the saddle close to the lateral and medial commissures which are more loosely anchored to the surrounding tissue, hence able to move more freely with myocardial contraction and relaxation [13]. The posterior annulus is often the part of the mitral annulus, which dilates with significant mitral regurgitation, and is more prone to calcification [14]. The dynamic pliable nature of the mitral annu-

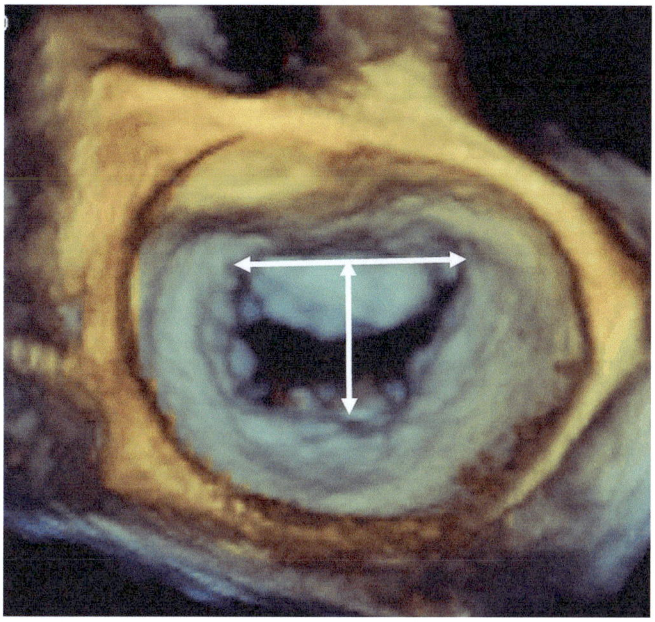

Fig. 10.2 3DE image of the mitral valve as viewed from the left atrium showing the D shape of the mitral annulus. The intercommissural diameter (horizontal arrow) is larger than the anteroposterior diameter (vertical arrow)

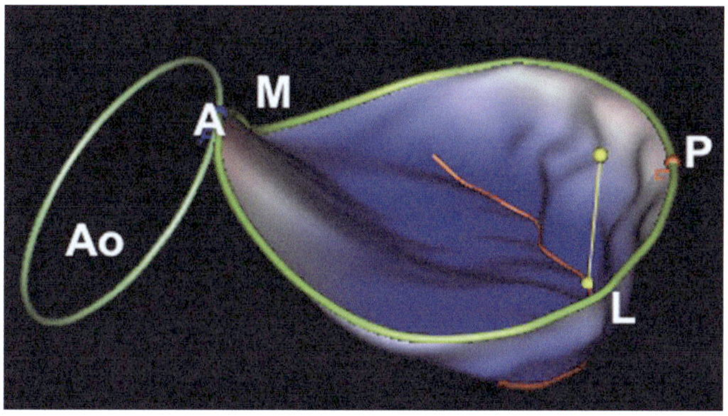

Fig. 10.3 3DE reconstruction of normal mitral valve annulus showing bimodal shape with high points (superiorly directed toward left atrium) located anterior-posterior orientation and low points located in medial-lateral orientation. *A* anterior, *Ao* aortic annulus, *L* lateral, *M* medial, *P* posterior

lus allows for systolic apical bending along a mediolateral commissure axis, and reciprocal systolic and diastolic changes in mitral annulus area [15–17]. Dynamic changes in the shape and area throughout the cardiac cycle have been shown to play an important role in maintaining the geometry of the mitral leaflets, aiding leaflet coaptation, reduce leaflet tissue stress and preventing unfavorable mitral leaflet remodeling [18–25]. Hence, morphological changes of the valve may potentially affect mechanical integrity of the total valve structure, resulting in abnormal leaflet closure and regurgitation of blood back into the left atrium. Interestingly, various

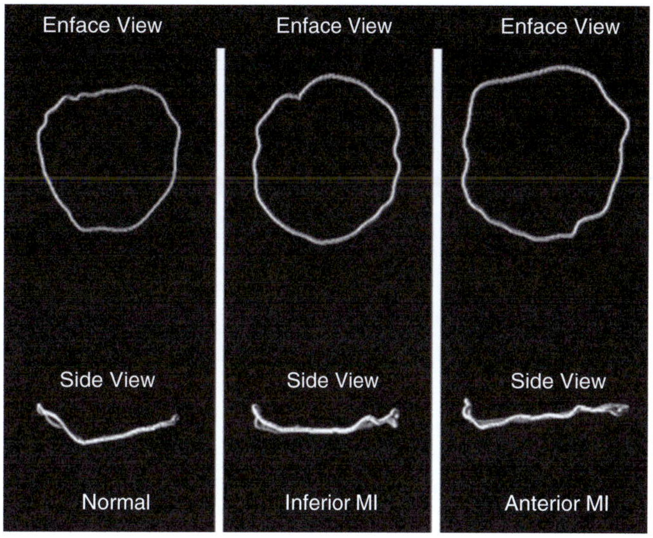

Fig. 10.4 Loss of saddle shape with infarction [33]. Adapted from Watanabe et al. Circulation 2005;112 9 Suppl:I458–I462

imaging modalities have quantified the average mitral annular area in healthy subjects to be approximately 10 cm^2 [26–31]. In pathological states such as in the case of dilatation of the LV, a significant increase in mitral annular area [26–28], decrease and delay of mitral annular area reduction during systole [28, 32] and flattening [28, 33] of its shape has been demonstrated [28, 32]. While mitral annular flattening has also been described in myxomatous valve disease, associated with more severe mitral regurgitation and chordal rupture, these are potentially though to be more likely related to increased out-of-plane stresses [18, 34]. Studies have demonstrated that the mitral annulus dilates and becomes flatter in response to development of FMR (Fig. 10.4) [35, 36].

Mitral Leaflets

The mitral valve comprises of two leaflets with variable commissural scallops to occlude medial and lateral gap, which lie within the ventricular inlet portion and have inherent differences in structure. The leaflets attach to the mitral annulus circumferentially with a minimum tissue length of 0.5–1 cm [37]. The anterior leaflet is trapezoid- or dome-shaped and much broader, longer and thicker but is attached to only one third of the annular circumference as compared to the narrower crescentic posterior leaflet with a long circumferential base [13] and relatively short radial length, which extends the remaining two-thirds of the annular diameter. Even though the posterior mitral leaflet appears smaller compared to the anterior leaflet, it has a larger area i.e. approximately 5 vs. 3 cm^2 respectively. The predominant feature of the anterior leaflet is the fibrous continuity with the left and non-coronary cusps of the aortic valve and with the interleaflet triangle between the aortic cusps that abuts onto the membranous septum [14]. It is also thicker and thus allows the leaflet to withstand a significantly higher tensile load without tissue disruption compared to the posterior leaflet which is thinner and more flexible [38, 39]. The anterior leaflet is divided into three arbitrary segments (scallops), A1, A2 and A3, which correspond to adjacent regions on the posterior leaflet, P1, P2 and P3 delineated by 2 clefts (partial indentations in the leaflet which do not typically extend all the way through the leaflet). A1 and P1 being the most lateral segments, lie adjacent to the anterolateral commissure while A3 and P3 being the most medial, is adjacent to the posteromedial commissure. One other key point to note is that the nomenclature of the leaflets can be different based on whether the Carpentier numbering system (A1, A2, A3, P1, P2, P3; defined by where P1, P2, and P3, co-apt with the anterior leaflet) or the ASE/SCA anatomic nomenclature system (where there is a random division of the anterior leaflet into thirds; A1, the lateral third of the anterior leaflet; A2, the middle third of the anterior leaflet; A3, the medial third of anterior leaflet; P1, lateral scallop of posterior leaflet; P2, middle scallop of posterior leaflet; P3 medial scallop of posterior leaflet) is used [40, 41]. The commissural portions remain as the anterolateral commissure and posteromedial commissure in both nomenclature systems. Each of the leaflets can be characterized into three zones (basal, clear and rough zones), from their attachment point at the annulus to the free edge of the leaflet. The basal zone arises where the leaflet connects to the atrioventricular junction, followed by the thin, translucent central portion (body of the leaflet) known as the clear zone which then transitions into the rough zone, a hydrophilic protein rich zone measuring approximately 1 cm which incorporates the thicker free edge of the leaflets, and where chordal attachment, coaptation (i.e. where the leaflets meet) and apposition (overlap of the leaflet free edge) of the leaflets occur. Some redundant leaflet tissue is critically important for adequate leaflet apposition and tight leaflet coaptation while the irregular surface of the rough zone helps to maintain and ensure a seal during leaflet coaptation. A minimum leaflet to mitral annular area ratio of 1.5–2 has been shown to be necessary to prevent significant mitral regurgitation [27, 37]. In the case of FMR, dilatation of the left ventricle and thus the annulus significantly reduces the minimum leaflet to mitral annular ratio. Interestingly, physiologic or pathologic-induced leaflet stress can induce mitral leaflet adaptation as evidenced by the wide range of total leaflet area seen in various cardiac pathologies. Recently, 3DE have been used to provide valuable insight into the potential of the mitral leaflets to adapt i.e. mitral valve leaflets may be elongated in response to the stress imposed by increased tethering caused by dilated cardiomyopathy or inferior myocardial infarction [27, 42, 43]. However, the underlying cellular mechanisms underpinning the adaptive changes seen in the mitral leaflets are still not well understood. One study demonstrated that in patients with FMR and symmetrical tethering, mitral leaflet coaptation decreases proportionally to the bilateral papillary muscle displacement, despite the presence of increased total leaflet area. This study also found that the coaptation area was a strong determinant of mitral regurgitation severity [27].

Chordae Tendineae

The chordae tendinae are fan-shaped fibrous chords running from the papillary muscles and attaching into the anterior and posterior leaflets in an organized manner which serve to dampen the papillary muscle-leaflet force transmission [44]. Chordae arising from the anterolateral papillary muscle attach to A1, anterolateral commissure, P1, and the lateral half of P2 and A2. Chordae arising from the posteromedial papillary muscle attach to, A3, posteromedial commissure, P3, and medial half of P2, and A2. The chordae can also be categorized into three types based on their area of attachments on the leaflets: primary chordae attach to the free edge of both leaflets within the rough zone; secondary chordae attach to the ventricular surface in the region of the rough zone in the case of the anterior leaflet and throughout the posterior leaflet body [45], and tertiary chordae found associated with in the basal zone posterior leaflet only. Primary chordae are thinner and shorter (average length approximately 1–2 mm) compared to secondary chordae (average length approximately 20 mm), have limited extensibility [46] and serve predominantly to prevent leaflet edge eversion [45, 47–49]. Secondary chordae being thicker than primary chordae, are also more extensible than the primary chordae [46]. Of particular note are a pair of prominent thick secondary chordae thought to be the strongest chordae, termed strut chordae, arising from the tip of each papillary muscle and inserting into the ventricular aspect of the anterior leaflet [14]. Typically one arises from the anterior papillary muscle and attaches to A1/A2 area of the anterior leaflet; one arises from the posterior papillary muscle and attaches to the A2/A3 portion of the anterior leaflet although additional strut chords, including to the posterior leaflet have been described. Similar to mitral leaflets, the chordae tendinae also have the ability to adapt to altered loading conditions [47]. Interestingly, pathologic apical leaflet tethering can be relieved and mitral leaflet coaptation restored in patients with functional/ischemic mitral regurgitation, by cutting selected secondary chordae without deleterious effects on LV function [50–52].

Papillary Muscles

In a normal mitral valve, there are usually two associated papillary muscles named, based on their position, i.e. anterolateral and posteromedial papillary muscles. These are essentially large trabeculae originating along the mid to apical segments of the left ventricular wall in a plane posterior to the inter-commissural plane in diastole and usually only have one head (although double, triple or multiple heads are also possible variants) [53]. More specifically, the anterolateral papillary muscle is usually seen to attach at the border of the anterolateral (lateral) free wall of the LV and the posteromedial over the inferior wall of the LV at the junction of the inferior left ventricular free wall and the muscular ventricular septum with both papillary muscles extending into the upper third of the ventricular cavity below the commissural tissue. In terms of blood supply, there is common dual supply to the anterolateral papillary muscle, i.e. the first obtuse marginal arising from the left circumflex and the first diagonal arising from the anterior descending artery as opposed to the posteromedial which is only supplied by a single artery (usually from the right coronary artery or the third obtuse marginal of the left circumflex). The papillary muscle contraction maintains the systolic spatial relationship between the mitral annulus and the papillary muscle heads as the myocardium contracts, thereby preventing leaflet prolapse [54–56]. The papillary muscle head positions and relative distance to each other keep both leaflets under outwardly-directed tension and therefore posteriorly restrained to prevent anterior motion. Any damage sustained by the papillary muscles such as a localized area of infarction may result in remodeling and subsequent tethering of the leaflets by outward displacement of the myocardium underlying the papillary muscle (Fig. 10.5). On the other hand, global left ventricular dilatation and increased LV sphericity potentially restricts leaflet closure by displacing the papillary muscles potentially increasing the distance from the papillary muscle to the leaflet and thus causing tethering [57]. However, ischemic and/or systolic papillary muscle dysfunction itself does not seem to contribute to FMR on top of the contribution of papillary muscle displacement. This is evidenced by results from a sheep model of chronic ischemic mitral regurgitation which demonstrated that papillary ischemia as measured by decreased strain rate correlated with diminished tethering distances and reduced mitral regurgitation [58]. Similarly, in humans, there is also some evidence that papillary muscle dysfunction, as measured by longitudinal systolic strain, actually reduces mitral regurgitation observed after inferior myocardial infarction highlighting that impairment of papillary muscle contraction presumably reduces tension on the chordae and paradoxically compensates for the tethering forces exerted by papillary muscle misalignment and/or left ventricular dilatation. These observations support the hypothesis that geometric papillary muscle displacement, and not necessarily systolic function, is the key factor in determining functional mitral regurgitation.

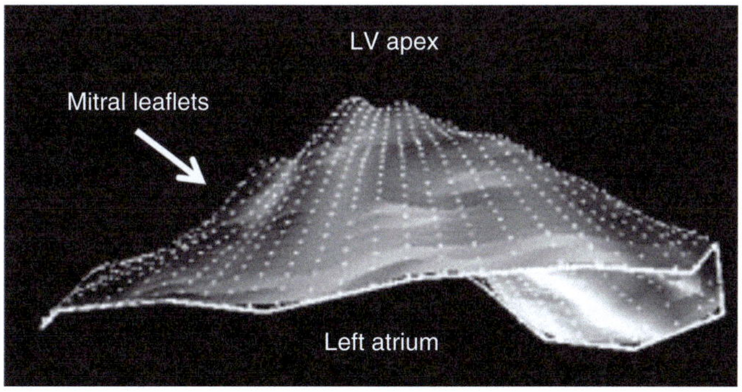

Fig. 10.5 Tethered leaflets (white arrow) with apically displaced coaptation line and increased tenting volume in a patient with functional mitral regurgitation

3DE has been applied to measure quantitative mitral valve geometric parameters such as mitral annular area and shape, leaflet area, tenting volume (volume underneath leaflets to mitral annular plane in systole) (Fig. 10.6, left panel), and tethering distances (distance from papillary muscle tips to mitral valve trigone) (Fig. 10.6, right panel). These quantitative measures of mitral valve geometry can be valuable tools to demonstrate mechanism and clinical outcome associations [59].

Assessment of Severity of Functional Mitral Regurgitation

There have been a number of methods used to assess the severity of FMR. Direct surgical measurements have been proposed as the gold standard for the assessment of the severity of FMR. However, direct surgical measurements are impractical in the clinical setting as they can only be performed on the arrested heart and do not accurate reflect physiological conditions. There are also a number of non-invasive methods such as echocardiography, cardiac computed tomography [60, 61] and cardiac magnetic resonance [62, 63] that have been used successfully to assess and characterize FMR but none have been identified as the gold standard. Hence a true gold standard technique for assessment of FMR is presently still lacking [64, 65]. Of all these imaging modalities, echocardiography is recommended as the first line investigation. Echocardiography is more readily available and relatively cheaper compared to the other imaging modalities. It has the ability to provide live images of the beating heart, allowing for dynamic quantification from moving images, quantitative analysis on frozen frames throughout the cardiac cycle and,

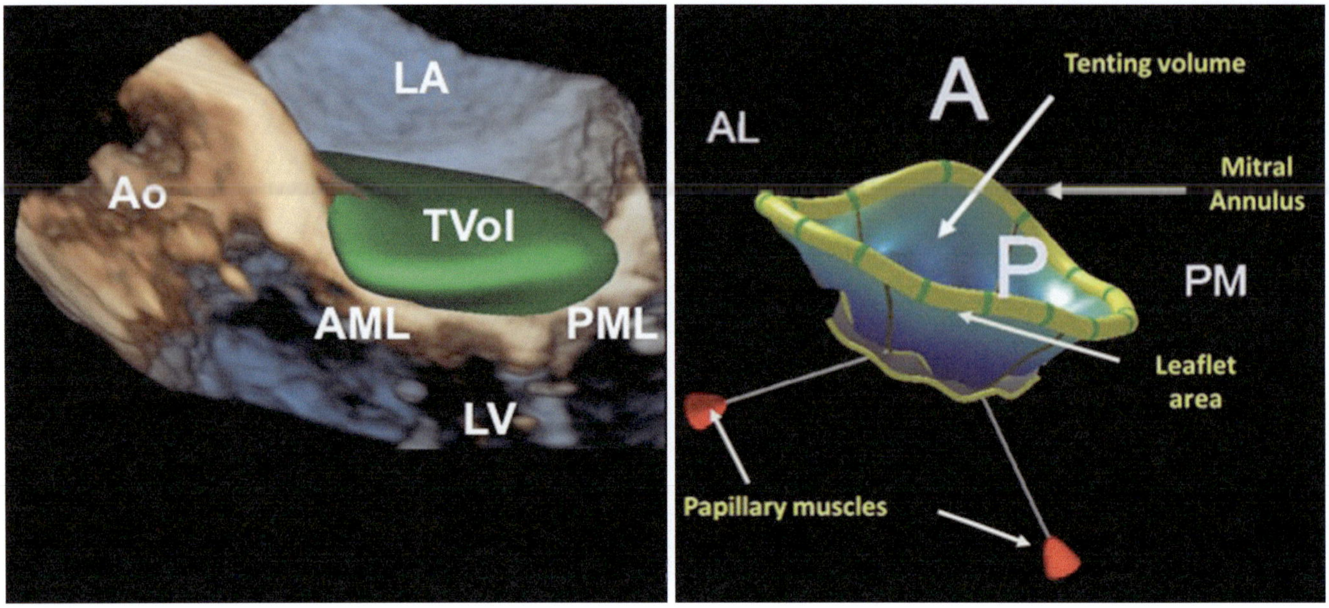

Fig. 10.6 Mitral valve geometry in functional mitral regurgitation. *Left panel*, the tenting volume is the space between the atrial surface of mitral valve leaflets and the mitral annulus. *Right panel*, quantitative measures including tenting volume, mitral annulus and leaflet area can be obtained from 3DE dataset of mitral valve using commercially available software package (Mitral Valve Navigator in QLab 10, Philips Medical Systems, Andover, USA). *A* anterior, *AML* anterior mitral leaflet, *AL* anterolateral, *Ao* aortic root, *LA* left atrium, *LV* left ventricle, *P* posterior, *PM* posteromedial, *TVol* tenting volume

measurements which are performed under more physiologic loading condition. Furthermore echocardiography, which does not utilise ionising radiation and is more readily available, can also be used to perform serial assessments allowing for characterization of progressive morphological changes induced by disease particularly those to the ventricle and allows for better understanding of the temporal trends of the underlying disease process [13, 66, 67]. Current guidelines recommend that asymptomatic patients with significant mitral regurgitation undergo serial echocardiography every 6–12 months to assess LV size and systolic function as this information is important for informing optimal timing for surgery intervention (Class I) [68]. One key point to note is that FMR occurs due to a complex interplay of geometric and contractile abnormalities, its severity can vary during the cardiac cycle and with ventricular loading conditions hence assessment of FMR can be very challenging [69]. FMR must always be interpreted in the context of loading conditions. Ambient preload and afterload conditions such as patient's volume status, systemic blood pressure, and medications may affect the observed degree of mitral regurgitation. Hence the blood pressure and medications at the time of assessment should always be considered and factored in the assessment of the severity of regurgitation.

Echocardiographic Assessment of Severity Functional Mitral Regurgitation

The echocardiographic assessment of FMR can be categorised into the assessment of the morphology of the mitral valve leaflets and the associated structures (in order to help delineate the aetiology of the mitral regurgitation) and severity of valve disease, which is essential for management planning [66, 67, 70, 71]. Assessment of mitral valve morphology is important as it also allows for determination of clinical or haemodynamic consequences. The presence of the "seagull" sign due to chordal tethering and kinking of the anterior leaflet in its mid-belly can be helpful in identifying FMR. The tethering of the leaflets can potentially also be quantified by the measures of tenting height (also named coaptation height or coaptation depth). The tenting height represents the distance from the annulus plane of the mitral valve to the leaflet coaptation point whereas the tenting area and volume represent more global measures of tethering of the leaflets [72–75] (Fig. 10.7, Video 10.1). The tethering angles can also be used to quantify individual leaflet tethering [74]. In terms of the tethering angles, the anterior leaflet can be characterised by two angles, a proximal tethering angle and a distal tethering angle, as being more prone to tethering forces can bend a wider range of compared to the posterior leaflet.

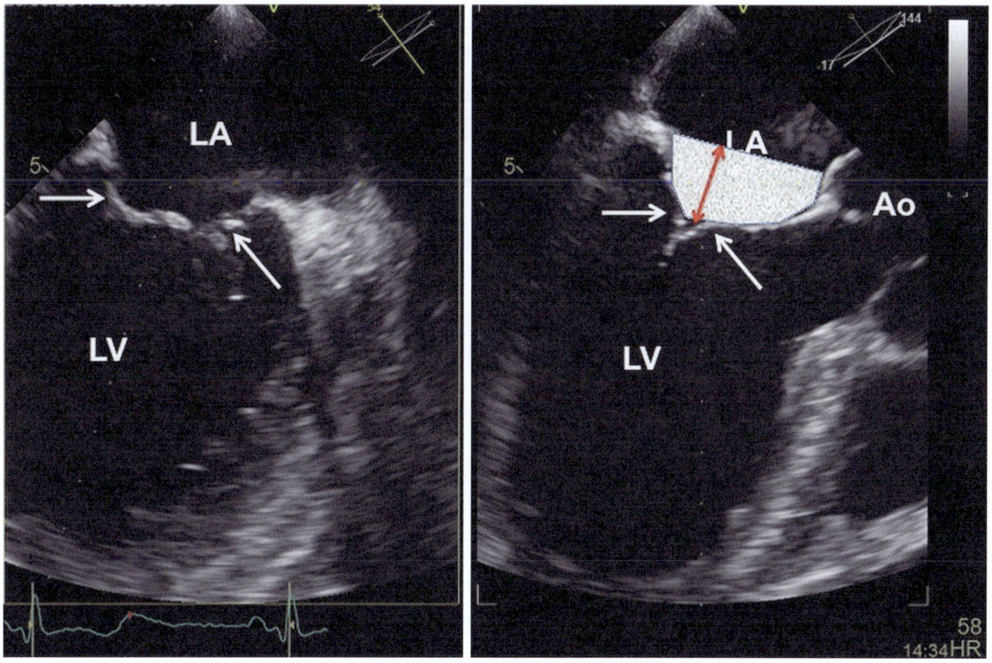

Fig. 10.7 Biplane image of dilated left ventricle showing tethering (white arrows) of the mitral leaflets resulting in incomplete coaptation. Tethering is the fundamental mechanism of functional mitral regurgitation (Video 10.1). The gray area is the tenting area and the coaptation depth is shown by the double head red arrow. *Ao* aortic root, *LA* left atrium, *LV* left ventricle

Current American College of Cardiology/American Heart Association guidelines recommend that two-dimensional and Doppler echocardiography be used to assess all patients with suspected mitral regurgitation to confirm its presence and determine its severity (according to the Functional Class), i.e. assessment of severity should based on a combination of echocardiographic and symptomatic parameters, with stages of "at risk" to "progressive" to "asymptomatic severe" to "symptomatic severe" [68]. Quantitative analysis is also an integral part of the assessment and provides objective evidence for the classification of the degree of severity of the mitral regurgitation. Current guidelines also recommend the integration of a number of specific, supportive, and quantitative features including cardiac chamber size and volume, regurgitant jet size by color Doppler, regurgitant jet density by continuous-wave Doppler, and pulmonary vein and mitral valve inflow by pulse-wave Doppler in classifying the severity of the mitral regurgitation [1, 65]. Additionally, Doppler echocardiography allow for quantitative measurement of mitral regurgitation, including the regurgitant volume and the regurgitant orifice area. In addition to semi-quantitative and quantitative Doppler techniques, it is important to integrate supportive and complementary data into the overall severity grading. Pulmonary venous flow reversal is specific for severe mitral regurgitation although of lower sensitivity. Chamber enlargement (left atrium and LV), dense continuous wave mitral regurgitation Doppler profile, and elevated E wave peak velocity >1.2 m/s are all suggestive of severe mitral regurgitation [76].

However, defining FMR and quantification of the severity of FMR can be very challenging using standard two-dimensional echocardiographic techniques due to the considerable clinical heterogeneity seen. Furthermore, the geometric distortions underlying FMR result in failure of the coaptation along the closure line of the valve in a variable manner such that the regurgitant orifice is non-circular but elliptical or slit-like. Additionally, mitral regurgitation may be complex with several separate regurgitant orifices along the closure line. This potentially impacts on the accuracy of standard recommended two-dimensional measures used in the quantification of the severity of mitral regurgitation, particularly measures dependent on flow or flow quantification, due to the complex spatial and dynamic patterns of flow across the mitral valve. While these quantitative techniques can be accurate and reproducible in single centers [77, 78], there can be significant interobserver variability among centers [79]. The application of 3DE has allowed some of the geometric limitations seen with two-dimensional echocardiography to potentially be overcome.

Assessment of Effective Regurgitant Orifice Area and Regurgitant Volume

The effective regurgitant orifice area and regurgitant volume can be assessed using a number of approaches. Evaluation of both the effective regurgitant orifice area and regurgitant volume are currently also recommended in current guidelines in the assessment of mitral regurgitation [1, 65]. However, all methods outlined below, if performed with two-dimensional echocardiography imaging have limitations and are often inaccurate due to the multiple indirect measurements required, imprecise hemodynamic assumptions frequently lead to inaccurate assessments [64, 78, 80, 81].

Vena Contracta

Given that the vena contracta area is also the effective orifice area, vena contracta width is an accepted direct assessment of the effective regurgitant orifice area. It is defined as the narrowest cross section of the regurgitant jet [65, 77, 82] and assumes that the regurgitant orifice is virtually circular. Measurements made from transesophageal echo images are more accurate than those made from transthoracic echo images [65]. Vena contracta width measurements appear to be less influenced by instrument settings compared to other quantitative techniques [65] and appear to be reasonably accurate indicators severity of mitral regurgition, regardless of the mitral regurgitation etiology and jet direction [76]. However, limitations of this method include the fact that small measurement errors can also result in the misclassification of MR severity. Furthermore, the exact shape and size of the regurgitant orifice is not accurately assessed nor factored into this measurement due to the limited scan plane orientation of two-dimensional echocardiography. Traditionally, the vena contracta is assessed in the parasternal long-axis view or apical three-chamber view and is measured as the diameter of the narrowest part of the regurgitant jet as it passes through the regurgitant orifice and is a reasonable estimate of severity [1]. However in the instance of an elliptical orifice, the extent of regurgitation may be underestimated or overestimated dependent on the view where the measurement is made [83].

3DE allows for direct visualization of the effective regurgitant orifice thus allowing direct planimetry of the vena contracta area. (Fig. 10.8, Video 10.2a Left and 10.2b Right) This is particularly relevant for patients with FMR, where the effective regurgitant orifice geometry is usually complex and asymmetric [84, 85] therefore measurements done using 3DE greatly improves the accuracy of the assessment of the effective regurgitant orifice area in this patient group. Using color Doppler 3DE image plane orientation can be adjusted to the true plane of the regurgitant orifice for direct quantification of the regurgitant area [83, 84, 86] (Fig. 10.9). Correlative studies with cardiac magnetic resonance have demonstrated a good correlation between regurgitant volume derived from effective regurgitant orifice measured by 3DE planimetry and that measured using velocity-encoded cardiac magnetic resonance imaging compared to two-dimensional echocardiography measures which consistently underestimated both effective regurgitant orifice area and regurgitant volume [69]. Additionally, the vena contracta area has also been shown to frequently not to be circular as assumed but asymmetric in the majority of patients and etiologies. (Fig. 10.10, Video 10.3) Nonetheless, a true

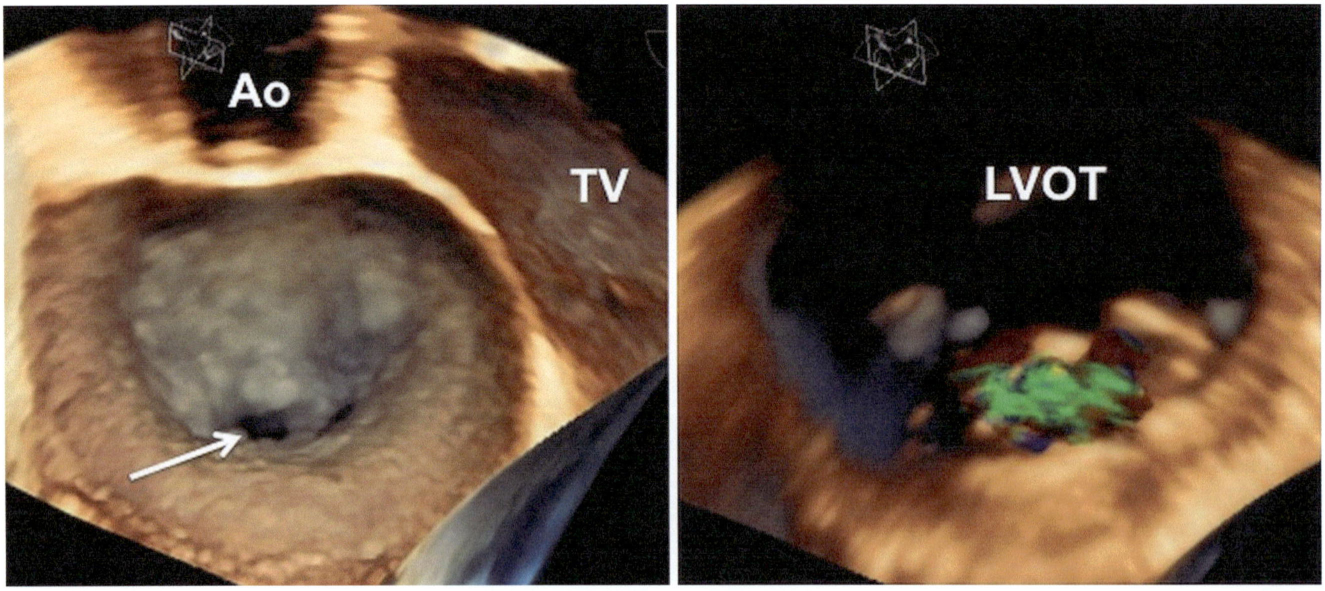

Fig. 10.8 Incomplete closure due to leaflet tethering. *Left panel*: transesophageal 3DE image of the mitral valve viewed from left atrium in a patient with functional mitral regurgitation. There is a visible gap along the coaptation line due to tethered mitral leaflets (white arrow, Video 10.2a Left). *Right panel*: Corresponding 3DE color Doppler image of the mitral valve seen from the left ventricular perspective showing origin of functional mitral regurgitation jet is through this gap (Video 10.2b Right). *Ao* aortic valve, *LVOT* left ventricular outflow tract, *TV* tricuspid valve

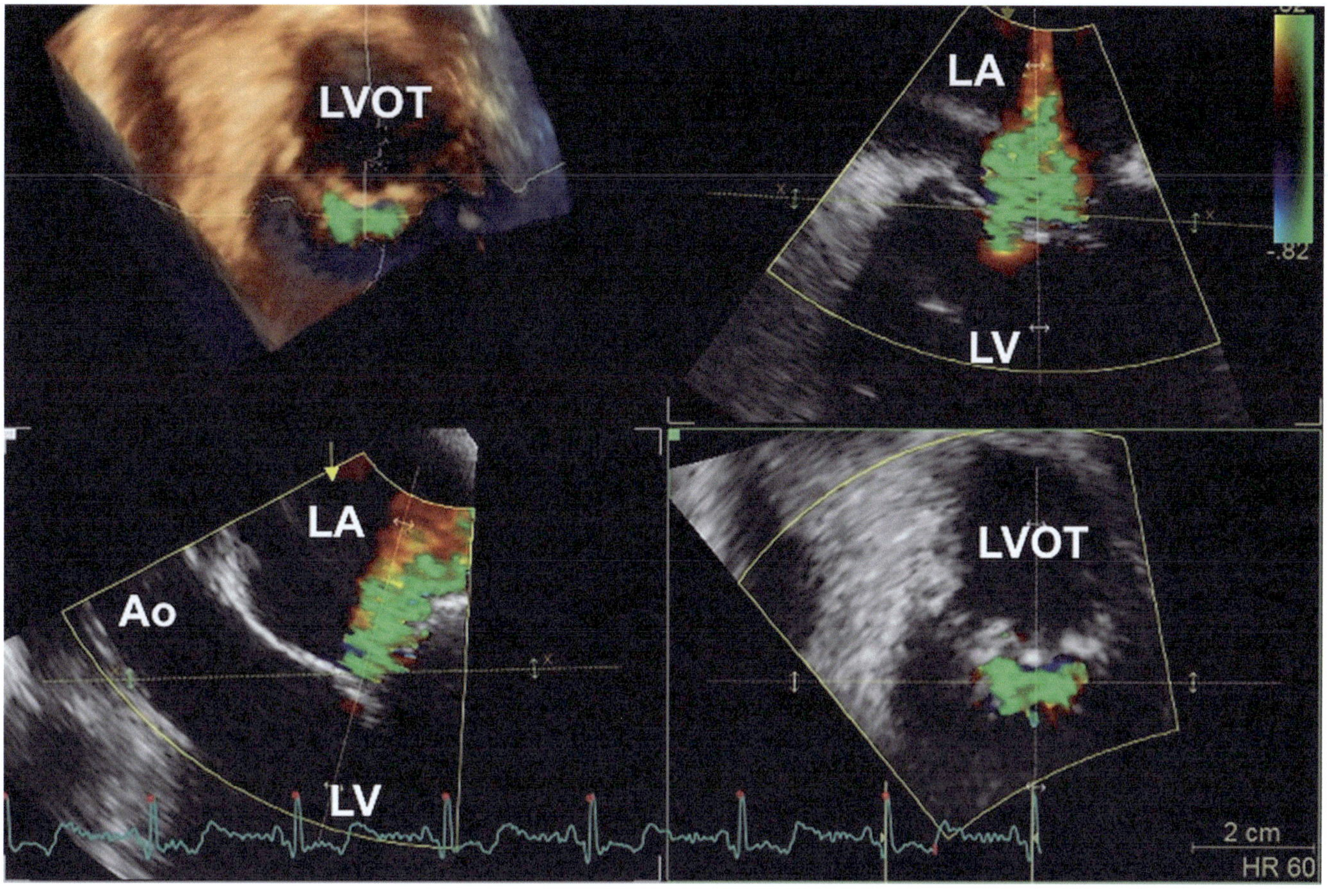

Fig. 10.9 Complexity of the geometry of the regurgitant orifice in functional mitral regurgitation. In most of the patients with functional mitral regurgitation, the valve leaks along part or the entire coaptation line as shown in the transesophageal 3DE color Doppler data set of the mitral valve seen *en face* from the ventricular perspective (*upper left panel*). This means that the shape of the regurgitant orifice is more oval or slit like than rounded, and measurement of a single diameter of the vena contracta may be misleading. Erroneously small if measured perpendicular to the coaptation line (*lower left panel*), or very large if measured along the coaptation line (*upper right panel*). A cut plane (green dotted line) positioned at the level of the narrowest part of the regurgitant orifice, and perpendicular to the direction of the jet, allows to visualize the actual vena contracta shape and size (*lower right panel*). *Ao* aortic valve, *LA* left atrium, *LV* left ventricle, *LVOT* left ventricular outflow area

validation study of 3DE measurements of effective regurgitant orifice area is lacking [83, 84, 87].

Proximal Isovelocity Surface Area

Calculation of effective regurgitant orifice area and regurgitant volumes can also be obtained by using Doppler techniques such as the proximal flow convergence method using color Doppler. The proximal isovelocity surface area (PISA) method provides a quantitative method for grading of mitral regurgitation. In this approach the following formula are used to calculate the effective regurgitant orifice area and regurgitant volume respectively.

$$\text{EROA} = 2\text{pR}^2 \times \text{Aliasing Velocity} \div \text{Peak Velocity of mitral regurgitation}$$

where R is the radius of the hemispheric PISA zone

$$\text{Regurgitant Volume} = \text{EROA} \times \text{TVI of the continuous wave Doppler profile of the mitral regurgitation}$$

The dynamic nature of FMR is also a major challenge to quantification using standard flow convergence methods utilizing the proximal isovelocity area (Video 10.4). Traditionally, the mid-systolic PISA coincident with the peak regurgitant velocity is used to estimate peak regurgitant flow rate and from that the maximal effective regurgitant orifice area and the regurgitant stroke volume. However, this approach is based on the assumption that the mid-systolic PISA is truly maximal (i.e. that the effective regurgitant orifice area is largest and mitral regurgitation the worst) [1]. In functional mitral regurgitation, the mid-systolic PISA is generally the smallest as there is improved coaptation due

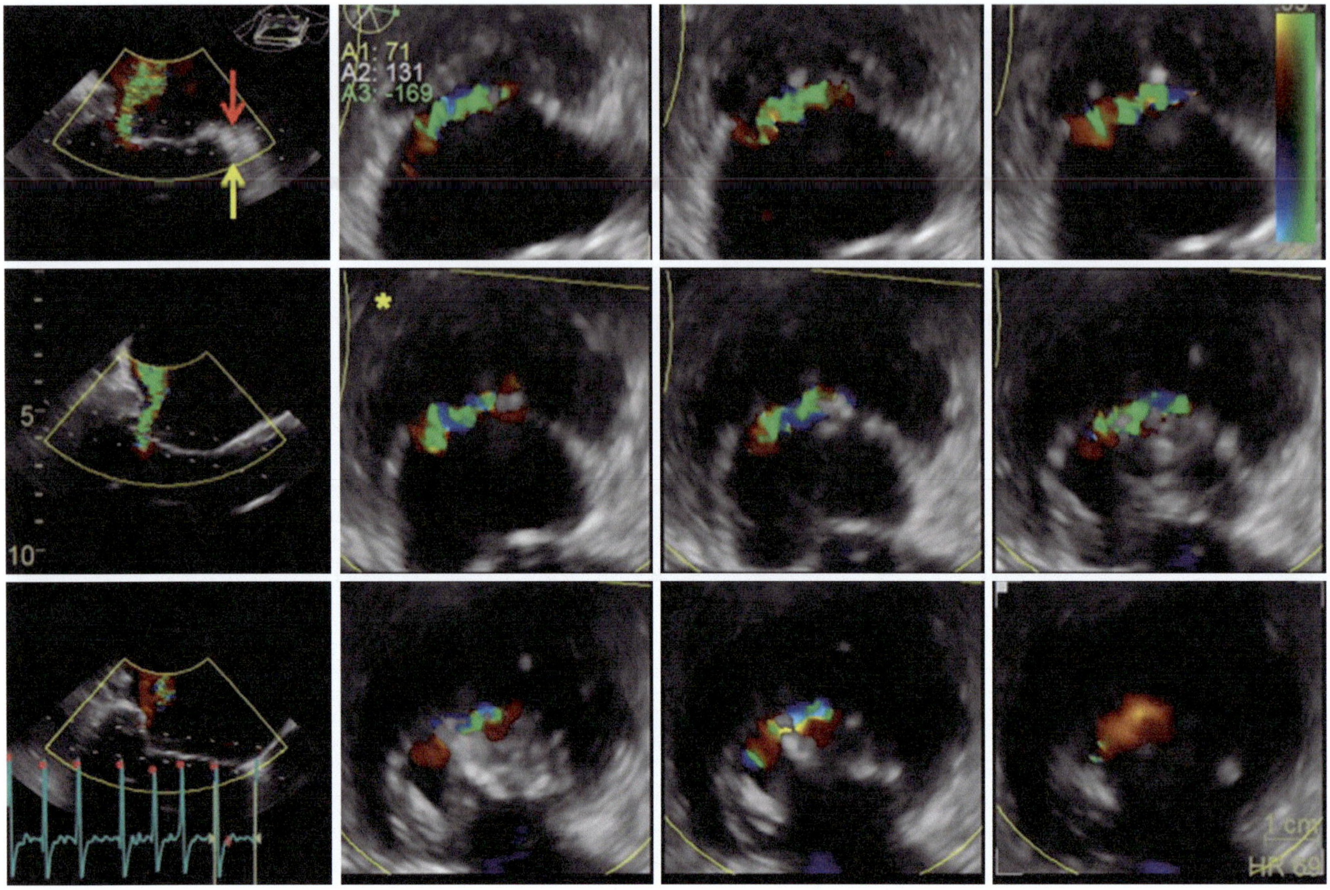

Fig. 10.10 Methodology to identify the vena contracta of the regurgitant mitral jet using transesophageal 3DE color Doppler. The 3DE color Doppler is displayed in multislice mode. The upper (yellow dotted line showed by the red arrow) and the lower (yellow dotted line showed by the yellow arrow) cut plane are positioned in order to include the proximal isovelocity area and the proximal part of the jet, perpendicular to the direction of the jet, in order to have multiple slice in the proximal part of the jet (Video 10.3). The smallest among the color Doppler area displayed in the multislice will be the true vena contracta and its area can be planimetered (yellow asterisk)

to maximal closing forces hence the effective regurgitant orifice is smaller. Hence the haemodynamic workload is underestimated if only a single mid-systolic point is used. Similarly, the effective regurgitant orifice area is likely to be overestimated if a maximal PISA in early or late systole is selected which does not coincide with the mid-systolic peak regurgitant velocity [69, 84]. Characterization of the PISAs in a population of patients with mitral regurgitation also revealed a heterogeneous spread of PISAs with the location and nature of the PISA dependent on the underlying geometry of the valve (Fig. 10.11). This study revealed that approximately 50% have a PISA away from the mid-point of the closure line, 35% have PISAs that are dominant in both the medial and lateral aspects of the closure line and relatively small in the centre, and approximately 25% have multiple separate PISAs suggesting that the standard two-dimensional echocardiography techniques do not provide an accurate estimate of the severity of regurgitation [88]. Another study which compared four different PISA methods against volumetric cardiac magnetic resonance as the gold standard highlighted that mid-systolic single time point estimates of PISA substantially underestimate the severity of FMR compared with cardiac magnetic resonance [88]. 3DE assessment of PISA shape has demonstrated that the hemispherical assumption is often not present-especially in functional mitral regurgitation where it is often hemielliptical (Fig. 10.12). Adoption of a hemisphere likely accounts for the underestimation of effective regurgitant orifice area in two-dimensional PISA methods of measuring effective regurgitant orifice area [76].

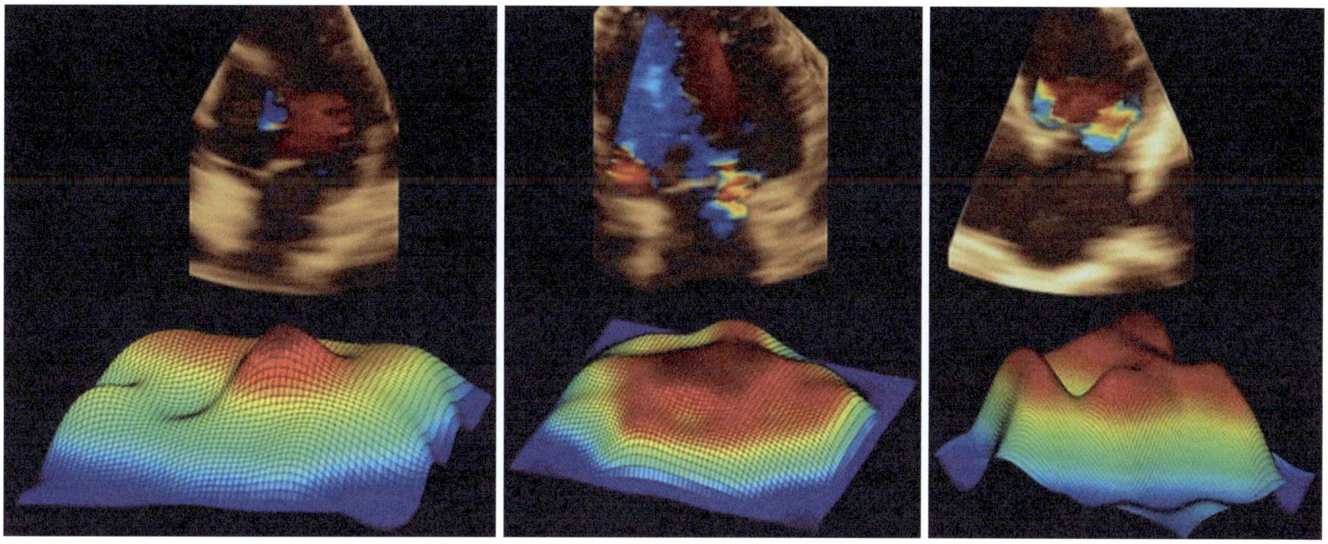

Fig. 10.11 3DE computerized reconstruction of the actual geometry of the proximal isovelocity surface are in three patients with various degrees and causes of functional mitral regurgitation. Actually, proximal isovelocity surface is almost never a hemisphere and calculations of its area based on a single diameter may be misleading

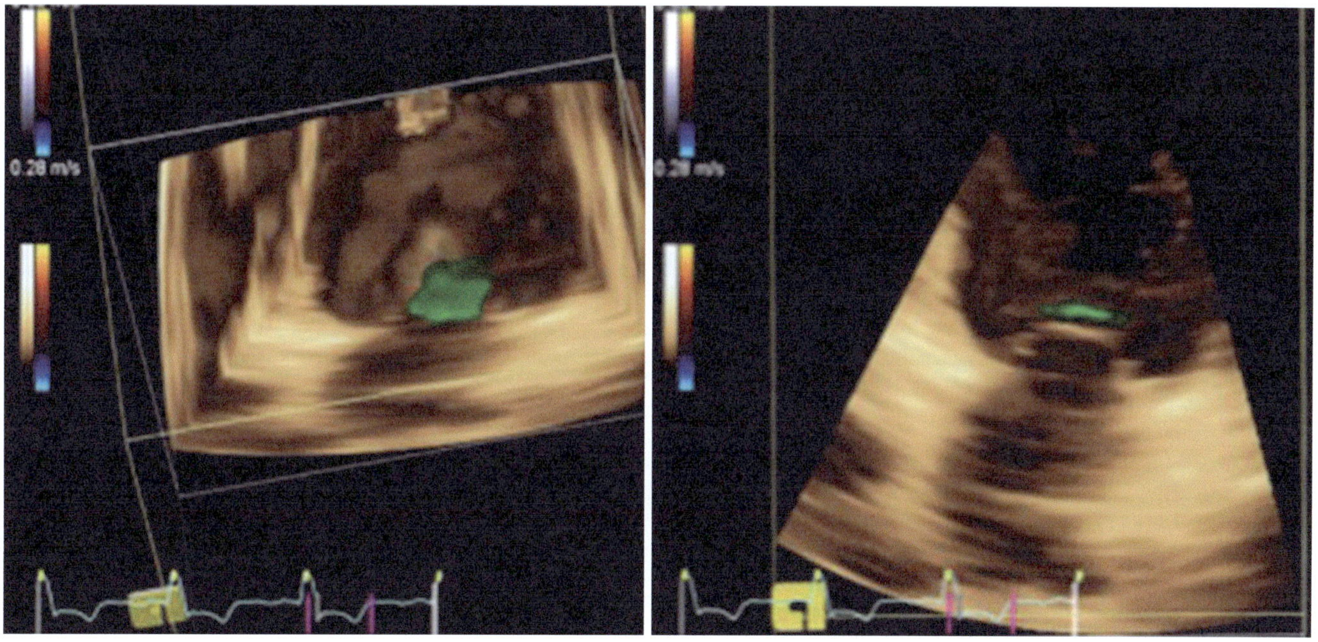

Fig. 10.12 3DE geometry of the actual proximal isovelocity surface area/volume in a patient with functional mitral regurgitation seen an face (*left panel*) and from a side (*right panel*)

Alternative Methods for Quantification of Mitral Regurgitant Volume

Another method to calculate the mitral regurgitant volume is the pulsed Doppler volumetric method, which determines the mitral regurgitant volume by subtracting the aortic forward stroke volume from the total stroke volume through the mitral annulus [1, 65]. This method requires two non-stenotic valves without significant aortic regurgitation.

Stress Echocardiography

Exercise stress echocardiography may also be useful in the assessment of FMR particularly in the context of determining clinical significance i.e. objective measure of exercise tolerance in a patient, worsening in the severity of mitral regurgitation, pulmonary pressure, and contractile reserve to exercise (Class IIa) [68]. Exercise may provoke hemodynamically significant mitral regurgitation in patients who have a degree of exertional dyspnea is out of keeping with the extent of LV dysfunction or degree of regurgitation at rest and pulmonary edema without an obvious cause [89]. Furthermore, an exercise-induced increase in effective regurgitant orifice area of ≥13 mm^2 is associated with increased morbidity and mortality [90]. Dobutamine stress echo may also be useful to determine the extent of viable myocardium that might recover with revascularization, effectiveness of medical treatment, or possibly resynchronization but is not so useful in assessing the severity of FMR as it has direct effects on loading conditions [91].

References

1. Lancellotti P, Moura L, Pierard LA, Agricola E, Popescu BA, Tribouilloy C, et al. European Association of Echocardiography recommendations for the assessment of valvular regurgitation. Part 2: mitral and tricuspid regurgitation (native valve disease). Eur J Echocardiogr. 2010;11:307–32.
2. Nkomo VT, Gardin JM, Skelton TN, Gottdiener JS, Scott CG, Enriquez-Sarano M. Burden of valvular heart diseases: a population-based study. Lancet. 2006;368:1005–11.
3. Bursi F, Enriquez-Sarano M, Nkomo VT, Jacobsen SJ, Weston SA, Meverden RA, et al. Heart failure and death after myocardial infarction in the community: the emerging role of mitral regurgitation. Circulation. 2005;111:295–301.
4. Grigioni F, Detaint D, Avierinos JF, Scott C, Tajik J, Enriquez-Sarano M. Contribution of ischemic mitral regurgitation to congestive heart failure after myocardial infarction. J Am Coll Cardiol. 2005;45:260–7.
5. Grigioni F, Enriquez-Sarano M, Zehr KJ, Bailey KR, Tajik AJ. Ischemic mitral regurgitation: long-term outcome and prognostic implications with quantitative Doppler assessment. Circulation. 2001;103:1759–64.
6. Iung B, Baron G, Butchart EG, Delahaye F, Gohlke-Barwolf C, Levang OW, et al. A prospective survey of patients with valvular heart disease in Europe: The Euro Heart Survey on Valvular Heart Disease. Eur Heart J. 2003;24:1231–43.
7. Enriquez-Sarano M, Avierinos JF, Messika-Zeitoun D, Detaint D, Capps M, Nkomo V, et al. Quantitative determinants of the outcome of asymptomatic mitral regurgitation. N Engl J Med. 2005;352:875–83.
8. Rosenhek R, Rader F, Klaar U, Gabriel H, Krejc M, Kalbeck D, et al. Outcome of watchful waiting in asymptomatic severe mitral regurgitation. Circulation. 2006;113:2238–44.
9. Patel JB, Borgeson DD, Barnes ME, Rihal CS, Daly RC, Redfield MM. Mitral regurgitation in patients with advanced systolic heart failure. J Card Fail. 2004;10:285–91.
10. Blondheim DS, Jacobs LE, Kotler MN, Costacurta GA, Parry WR. Dilated cardiomyopathy with mitral regurgitation: decreased survival despite a low frequency of left ventricular thrombus. Am Heart J. 1991;122:763–71.
11. Levine RA, Hagege AA, Judge DP, Padala M, Dal-Bianco JP, Aikawa E, et al. Mitral valve disease--morphology and mechanisms. Nat Rev Cardiol. 2015;12:689–710.
12. Kanzaki H, Bazaz R, Schwartzman D, Dohi K, Sade LE, Gorcsan J 3rd. A mechanism for immediate reduction in mitral regurgitation after cardiac resynchronization therapy: insights from mechanical activation strain mapping. J Am Coll Cardiol. 2004;44:1619–25.
13. Dal-Bianco JP, Levine RA. Anatomy of the mitral valve apparatus: role of 2D and 3D echocardiography. Cardiol Clin. 2013;31:151–64.
14. McCarthy KP, Ring L, Rana BS. Anatomy of the mitral valve: understanding the mitral valve complex in mitral regurgitation. Eur J Echocardiogr. 2010;11:i3–9.
15. Hamdan A, Guetta V, Konen E, Goitein O, Segev A, Raanani E, et al. Deformation dynamics and mechanical properties of the aortic annulus by 4-dimensional computed tomography: insights into the functional anatomy of the aortic valve complex and implications for transcatheter aortic valve therapy. J Am Coll Cardiol. 2012;59:119–27.
16. Lansac E, Lim KH, Shomura Y, Goetz WA, Lim HS, Rice NT, et al. Dynamic balance of the aortomitral junction. J Thorac Cardiovasc Surg. 2002;123:911–8.
17. Veronesi F, Corsi C, Sugeng L, Caiani EG, Weinert L, Mor-Avi V, et al. Quantification of mitral apparatus dynamics in functional and ischemic mitral regurgitation using real-time 3-dimensional echocardiography. J Am Soc Echocardiogr. 2008;21:347–54.
18. Jensen MO, Hagege AA, Otsuji Y, Levine RA, Leducq Transatlantic MN. The unsaddled annulus: biomechanical culprit in mitral valve prolapse? Circulation. 2013;127:766–8.
19. Jensen MO, Jensen H, Levine RA, Yoganathan AP, Andersen NT, Nygaard H, et al. Saddle-shaped mitral valve annuloplasty rings improve leaflet coaptation geometry. J Thorac Cardiovasc Surg. 2011;142:697–703.
20. Jensen MO, Jensen H, Smerup M, Levine RA, Yoganathan AP, Nygaard H, et al. Saddle-shaped mitral valve annuloplasty rings experience lower forces compared with flat rings. Circulation. 2008;118:S250–5.
21. Jimenez JH, Liou SW, Padala M, He Z, Sacks M, Gorman RC, et al. A saddle-shaped annulus reduces systolic strain on the central region of the mitral valve anterior leaflet. J Thorac Cardiovasc Surg. 2007;134:1562–8.
22. Kunzelman KS, Reimink MS, Cochran RP. Annular dilatation increases stress in the mitral valve and delays coaptation: a finite element computer model. Cardiovasc Surg. 1997;5:427–34.
23. Padala M, Hutchison RA, Croft LR, Jimenez JH, Gorman RC, Gorman JH 3rd, et al. Saddle shape of the mitral annulus reduces systolic strains on the P2 segment of the posterior mitral leaflet. Ann Thorac Surg. 2009;88:1499–504.
24. Reimink MS, Kunzelman KS, Verrier ED, Cochran RP. The effect of anterior chordal replacement on mitral valve function and stresses. A finite element study. ASAIO J. 1995; 41:M754–62.
25. Salgo IS, Gorman JH 3rd, Gorman RC, Jackson BM, Bowen FW, Plappert T, et al. Effect of annular shape on leaflet curvature in reducing mitral leaflet stress. Circulation. 2002;106:711–7.
26. Alkadhi H, Desbiolles L, Stolzmann P, Leschka S, Scheffel H, Plass A, et al. Mitral annular shape, size, and motion in normals and in patients with cardiomyopathy: evaluation with computed tomography. Invest Radiol. 2009;44:218–25.
27. Chaput M, Handschumacher MD, Tournoux F, Hua L, Guerrero JL, Vlahakes GJ, et al. Mitral leaflet adaptation to ventricular remodeling: occurrence and adequacy in patients with functional mitral regurgitation. Circulation. 2008;118:845–52.
28. Flachskampf FA, Chandra S, Gaddipatti A, Levine RA, Weyman AE, Ameling W, et al. Analysis of shape and motion of the mitral annulus in subjects with and without cardiomyopathy by echocardiographic 3-dimensional reconstruction. J Am Soc Echocardiogr. 2000;13:277–87.
29. Maffessanti F, Gripari P, Pontone G, Andreini D, Bertella E, Mushtaq S, et al. Three-dimensional dynamic assessment of tricuspid and mitral annuli using cardiovascular magnetic resonance. Eur Heart J Cardiovasc Imaging. 2013;14:986–95.
30. Ormiston JA, Shah PM, Tei C, Wong M. Size and motion of the mitral valve annulus in man. I. A two-dimensional echocardiographic method and findings in normal subjects. Circulation. 1981;64:113–20.

31. Veronesi F, Corsi C, Sugeng L, Mor-Avi V, Caiani EG, Weinert L, et al. A study of functional anatomy of aortic-mitral valve coupling using 3D matrix transesophageal echocardiography. Circ Cardiovasc Imaging. 2009;2:24–31.
32. Daimon M, Saracino G, Fukuda S, Koyama Y, Kwan J, Song JM, et al. Dynamic change of mitral annular geometry and motion in ischemic mitral regurgitation assessed by a computerized 3D echo method. Echocardiography. 2010;27:1069–77.
33. Watanabe N, Ogasawara Y, Yamaura Y, Wada N, Kawamoto T, Toyota E, et al. Mitral annulus flattens in ischemic mitral regurgitation: geometric differences between inferior and anterior myocardial infarction: a real-time 3-dimensional echocardiographic study. Circulation. 2005;112:I458–62.
34. Lee AP, Hsiung MC, Salgo IS, Fang F, Xie JM, Zhang YC, et al. Quantitative analysis of mitral valve morphology in mitral valve prolapse with real-time 3-dimensional echocardiography: importance of annular saddle shape in the pathogenesis of mitral regurgitation. Circulation. 2013;127:832–41.
35. Watanabe N, Ogasawara Y, Yamaura Y, Kawamoto T, Akasaka T, Yoshida K. Geometric deformity of the mitral annulus in patients with ischemic mitral regurgitation: a real-time three-dimensional echocardiographic study. J Heart Valve Dis. 2005;14:447–52.
36. Kwan J, Qin JX, Popovic ZB, Agler DA, Thomas JD, Shiota T. Geometric changes of mitral annulus assessed by real-time 3-dimensional echocardiography: becoming enlarged and less nonplanar in the anteroposterior direction during systole in proportion to global left ventricular systolic function. J Am Soc Echocardiogr. 2004;17:1179–84.
37. Chiechi MA, Lees WM, Thompson R. Functional anatomy of the normal mitral valve. J Thorac Surg. 1956;32:378–98.
38. Kunzelman KS, Cochran RP, Chuong C, Ring WS, Verrier ED, Eberhart RD. Finite element analysis of the mitral valve. J Heart Valve Dis. 1993;2:326–40.
39. Kunzelman KS, Cochran RP, Murphree SS, Ring WS, Verrier ED, Eberhart RC. Differential collagen distribution in the mitral valve and its influence on biomechanical behaviour. J Heart Valve Dis. 1993;2:236–44.
40. Carpentier AF, Lessana A, Relland JY, Belli E, Mihaileanu S, Berrebi AJ, et al. The "physio-ring": an advanced concept in mitral valve annuloplasty. Ann Thorac Surg. 1995;60:1177–85; discussion 85–6.
41. Shanewise JS, Cheung AT, Aronson S, Stewart WJ, Weiss RL, Mark JB, et al. ASE/SCA guidelines for performing a comprehensive intraoperative multiplane transesophageal echocardiography examination: recommendations of the American Society of Echocardiography Council for Intraoperative Echocardiography and the Society of Cardiovascular Anesthesiologists Task Force for Certification in Perioperative Transesophageal Echocardiography. J Am Soc Echocardiogr. 1999;12:884–900.
42. Chaput M, Handschumacher MD, Guerrero JL, Holmvang G, Dal-Bianco JP, Sullivan S, et al. Mitral leaflet adaptation to ventricular remodeling: prospective changes in a model of ischemic mitral regurgitation. Circulation. 2009;120:S99–103.
43. Dal-Bianco JP, Levine RA. The mitral valve is an actively adapting tissue: new imaging evidence. Eur Heart J Cardiovasc Imaging. 2015;16:286–7.
44. Millington-Sanders C, Meir A, Lawrence L, Stolinski C. Structure of chordae tendineae in the left ventricle of the human heart. J Anat. 1998;192(Pt 4):573–81.
45. Degandt AA, Weber PA, Saber HA, Duran CM. Mitral valve basal chordae: comparative anatomy and terminology. Ann Thorac Surg. 2007;84:1250–5.
46. Liao J, Vesely I. A structural basis for the size-related mechanical properties of mitral valve chordae tendineae. J Biomech. 2003;36:1125–33.
47. Dal-Bianco JP, Aikawa E, Bischoff J, Guerrero JL, Handschumacher MD, Sullivan S, et al. Active adaptation of the tethered mitral valve: insights into a compensatory mechanism for functional mitral regurgitation. Circulation. 2009;120:334–42.
48. Lam JH, Ranganathan N, Wigle ED, Silver MD. Morphology of the human mitral valve. I. Chordae tendineae: a new classification. Circulation. 1970;41:449–58.
49. Obadia JF, Casali C, Chassignolle JF, Janier M. Mitral subvalvular apparatus: different functions of primary and secondary chordae. Circulation. 1997;96:3124–8.
50. Messas E, Guerrero JL, Handschumacher MD, Conrad C, Chow CM, Sullivan S, et al. Chordal cutting: a new therapeutic approach for ischemic mitral regurgitation. Circulation. 2001;104:1958–63.
51. Messas E, Pouzet B, Touchot B, Guerrero JL, Vlahakes GJ, Desnos M, et al. Efficacy of chordal cutting to relieve chronic persistent ischemic mitral regurgitation. Circulation. 2003;108(Suppl 1):II111–5.
52. Messas E, Yosefy C, Chaput M, Guerrero JL, Sullivan S, Menasche P, et al. Chordal cutting does not adversely affect left ventricle contractile function. Circulation. 2006;114:I524–8.
53. Rusted IE, Scheifley CH, Edwards JE. Studies of the mitral valve. I. Anatomic features of the normal mitral valve and associated structures. Circulation. 1952;6:825–31.
54. Gorman JH 3rd, Gupta KB, Streicher JT, Gorman RC, Jackson BM, Ratcliffe MB, et al. Dynamic three-dimensional imaging of the mitral valve and left ventricle by rapid sonomicrometry array localization. J Thorac Cardiovasc Surg. 1996;112:712–26.
55. Joudinaud TM, Kegel CL, Flecher EM, Weber PA, Lansac E, Hvass U, et al. The papillary muscles as shock absorbers of the mitral valve complex. An experimental study. Eur J Cardiothorac Surg. 2007;32:96–101.
56. Komeda M, Glasson JR, Bolger AF, Daughters GT 2nd, Ingels NB Jr, Miller DC. Papillary muscle-left ventricular wall "complex". J Thorac Cardiovasc Surg. 1997;113:292–300; discussion 1.
57. Kono T, Sabbah HN, Rosman H, Alam M, Jafri S, Goldstein S. Left ventricular shape is the primary determinant of functional mitral regurgitation in heart failure. J Am Coll Cardiol. 1992;20:1594–8.
58. Messas E, Guerrero JL, Handschumacher MD, Chow CM, Sullivan S, Schwammenthal E, et al. Paradoxic decrease in ischemic mitral regurgitation with papillary muscle dysfunction: insights from three-dimensional and contrast echocardiography with strain rate measurement. Circulation. 2001;104:1952–7.
59. Lang RM, Mor-Avi V, Sugeng L, Nieman PS, Sahn DJ. Three-dimensional echocardiography: the benefits of the additional dimension. J Am Coll Cardiol. 2006;48:2053–69.
60. Delgado V, Tops LF, Schuijf JD, de Roos A, Brugada J, Schalij MJ, et al. Assessment of mitral valve anatomy and geometry with multislice computed tomography. JACC Cardiovasc Imaging. 2009;2:556–65.
61. Shanks M, Delgado V, Ng AC, van der Kley F, Schuijf JD, Boersma E, et al. Mitral valve morphology assessment: three-dimensional transesophageal echocardiography versus computed tomography. Ann Thorac Surg. 2010;90:1922–9.
62. Kaji S, Nasu M, Yamamuro A, Tanabe K, Nagai K, Tani T, et al. Annular geometry in patients with chronic ischemic mitral regurgitation: three-dimensional magnetic resonance imaging study. Circulation. 2005;112:I409–14.
63. Myerson SG. Heart valve disease: investigation by cardiovascular magnetic resonance. J Cardiovasc Magn Reson. 2012;14:7.
64. Enriquez-Sarano M, Miller FA Jr, Hayes SN, Bailey KR, Tajik AJ, Seward JB. Effective mitral regurgitant orifice area: clinical use and pitfalls of the proximal isovelocity surface area method. J Am Coll Cardiol. 1995;25:703–9.
65. Zoghbi WA, Enriquez-Sarano M, Foster E, Grayburn PA, Kraft CD, Levine RA, et al. Recommendations for evaluation of the severity of native valvular regurgitation with two-dimensional and Doppler echocardiography. J Am Soc Echocardiogr. 2003;16:777–802.

66. Adams DH, Rosenhek R, Falk V. Degenerative mitral valve regurgitation: best practice revolution. Eur Heart J. 2010;31:1958–66.
67. Garbi M, Monaghan MJ. Quantitative mitral valve anatomy and pathology. Echo Res Pract. 2015;2:R63–72.
68. Nishimura RA, Otto CM, Bonow RO, Carabello BA, Erwin JP 3rd, Guyton RA, et al. 2014 AHA/ACC guideline for the management of patients with valvular heart disease: executive summary: a report of the American College of Cardiology/American Heart Association Task Force on Practice Guidelines. J Am Coll Cardiol. 2014;63:2438–88.
69. Buck T, Plicht B, Kahlert P, Schenk IM, Hunold P, Erbel R. Effect of dynamic flow rate and orifice area on mitral regurgitant stroke volume quantification using the proximal isovelocity surface area method. J Am Coll Cardiol. 2008;52:767–78.
70. Adams DH, Anyanwu AC. The cardiologist's role in increasing the rate of mitral valve repair in degenerative disease. Curr Opin Cardiol. 2008;23:105–10.
71. Chikwe J, Adams DH, Su KN, Anyanwu AC, Lin HM, Goldstone AB, et al. Can three-dimensional echocardiography accurately predict complexity of mitral valve repair? Eur J Cardiothorac Surg. 2012;41:518–24.
72. Agricola E, Oppizzi M, Maisano F, De Bonis M, Schinkel AF, Torracca L, et al. Echocardiographic classification of chronic ischemic mitral regurgitation caused by restricted motion according to tethering pattern. Eur J Echocardiogr. 2004;5:326–34.
73. Calafiore AM, Di Mauro M, Gallina S, Di Giammarco G, Iaco AL, Teodori G, et al. Mitral valve surgery for chronic ischemic mitral regurgitation. Ann Thorac Surg. 2004;77:1989–97.
74. Silbiger JJ. Mechanistic insights into ischemic mitral regurgitation: echocardiographic and surgical implications. J Am Soc Echocardiogr. 2011;24:707–19.
75. Yiu SF, Enriquez-Sarano M, Tribouilloy C, Seward JB, Tajik AJ. Determinants of the degree of functional mitral regurgitation in patients with systolic left ventricular dysfunction: a quantitative clinical study. Circulation. 2000;102:1400–6.
76. Zoghbi WA, Adams D, Bonow RO, Enriquez-Sarano M, Foster E, Grayburn PA, et al. Recommendations for noninvasive evaluation of native valvular regurgitation: a report from the American Society of Echocardiography developed in collaboration with the Society for Cardiovascular Magnetic Resonance. J Am Soc Echocardiogr. 2017;30:303–71.
77. Hall SA, Brickner ME, Willett DL, Irani WN, Afridi I, Grayburn PA. Assessment of mitral regurgitation severity by Doppler color flow mapping of the vena contracta. Circulation. 1997;95:636–42.
78. Schwammenthal E, Chen C, Benning F, Block M, Breithardt G, Levine RA. Dynamics of mitral regurgitant flow and orifice area. Physiologic application of the proximal flow convergence method: clinical data and experimental testing. Circulation. 1994;90:307–22.
79. Biner S, Rafique A, Rafii F, Tolstrup K, Noorani O, Shiota T, et al. Reproducibility of proximal isovelocity surface area, vena contracta, and regurgitant jet area for assessment of mitral regurgitation severity. J Am Coll Cardiol Imaging. 2010;3:235–43.
80. Utsunomiya T, Ogawa T, Doshi R, Patel D, Quan M, Henry WL, et al. Doppler color flow "proximal isovelocity surface area" method for estimating volume flow rate: effects of orifice shape and machine factors. J Am Coll Cardiol. 1991;17:1103–11.
81. Zoghbi WA, Quinones MA. Determination of cardiac output by Doppler echocardiography: a critical appraisal. Herz. 1986;11:258–68.
82. Mascherbauer J, Rosenhek R, Bittner B, Binder J, Simon P, Maurer G, et al. Doppler echocardiographic assessment of valvular regurgitation severity by measurement of the vena contracta: an in vitro validation study. J Am Soc Echocardiogr. 2005;18:999–1006.
83. Khanna D, Vengala S, Miller AP, Nanda NC, Lloyd SG, Ahmed S, et al. Quantification of mitral regurgitation by live three-dimensional transthoracic echocardiographic measurements of vena contracta area. Echocardiography. 2004;21:737–43.
84. Kahlert P, Plicht B, Schenk IM, Janosi RA, Erbel R, Buck T. Direct assessment of size and shape of noncircular vena contracta area in functional versus organic mitral regurgitation using real-time three-dimensional echocardiography. J Am Soc Echocardiogr. 2008;21:912–21.
85. Otsuji Y, Handschumacher MD, Schwammenthal E, Jiang L, Song JK, Guerrero JL, et al. Insights from three-dimensional echocardiography into the mechanism of functional mitral regurgitation: direct in vivo demonstration of altered leaflet tethering geometry. Circulation. 1997;96:1999–2008.
86. Irvine T, Li XN, Rusk R, Lennon D, Sahn DJ, Kenny A. Three dimensional colour Doppler echocardiography for the characterisation and quantification of cardiac flow events. Heart. 2000;84(Suppl 2):II2–6.
87. Iwakura K, Ito H, Kawano S, Okamura A, Kurotobi T, Date M, et al. Comparison of orifice area by transthoracic three-dimensional Doppler echocardiography versus proximal isovelocity surface area (PISA) method for assessment of mitral regurgitation. Am J Cardiol. 2006;97:1630–7.
88. Song JM, Kim MJ, Kim YJ, Kang SH, Kim JJ, Kang DH, et al. Three-dimensional characteristics of functional mitral regurgitation in patients with severe left ventricular dysfunction: a real-time three-dimensional colour Doppler echocardiography study. Heart. 2008;94:590–6.
89. Picano E, Pibarot P, Lancellotti P, Monin JL, Bonow RO. The emerging role of exercise testing and stress echocardiography in valvular heart disease. J Am Coll Cardiol. 2009;54:2251–60.
90. Lancellotti P, Gerard PL, Pierard LA. Long-term outcome of patients with heart failure and dynamic functional mitral regurgitation. Eur Heart J. 2005;26:1528–32.
91. Ray S. The echocardiographic assessment of functional mitral regurgitation. Eur J Echocardiogr. 2010;11:i11–7.

11 Assessment During and After Surgery or Interventional Procedures on the Mitral Valve

Muhamed Saric, Gila Perk, and Itzhak Kronzon

Abstract

This chapter provides an overview of the role of three-dimensional echocardiography (3DE) in surgical and percutaneous mitral valve procedures. Throughout the chapter, numerous still images and videos are provided to illustrate the incremental values of 3DE in these procedures. The chapter starts with the description of 3DE imaging of surgical mitral valve replacements and repairs. The 3DE appearance of major types of mechanical and bioprosthetic valves is given including Starr-Edwards, Medtronic Hall, St Jude, and Carpentier Edwards prosthetic valves. Thereafter, an overview of common surgical mitral valve repairs including the Alfieri stitch is discussed. Next, an overview of 3DE in percutaneous alternatives to surgical repairs of native and prosthetic mitral regurgitant lesions is provided including the mitral valve clipping and percutaneous closures of prosthetic paravalvular leaks. The chapter concludes with a description of the role of 3DE in percutaneous mitral balloon valvuloplasty of rheumatic mitral stenosis.

Keywords

3D echocardiography · Mitral valve · Percutaneous intervention · Valve surgery · Balloon valvuloplasty Valve repair · Valve replacement

Introduction

This chapter provides an overview of the role of three-dimensional echocardiography (3DE) in surgical and percutaneous mitral valve procedure. Surgical mitral valve replacement and repair procedures will be discussed first. Next, an overview of 3DE in percutaneous alternatives to surgical repairs of native and prosthetic mitral regurgitant lesions is provided. At the end of the chapter, the role of 3D echocardiography in percutaneous mitral balloon valvuloplasty of rheumatic mitral stenosis is discussed.

Surgical Mitral Valve Replacement and Repair

Historical Overview

Orthotopic replacement of diseased heart valves was first made possible following the advent of heart-lung machines in the 1950s. The development of mechanical and subsequently bioprosthetic valves was made possible through a close collaboration between surgeons and engineers. This is reflected in the naming convention of many prosthetic valves as in Starr-Edwards and Björk-Shiley valve; in each case the former name refers to the cardiac surgeon and the latter refers to the engineer. Historical timeline is outlined in Table 11.1.

Two- and 3DE are essential for in-depth diagnosis of valvular pathology prior to surgical or transcatheter intervention, assessment of success during the procedure and for evaluation of possible complications after the procedure.

Electronic Supplementary Material The online version of this chapter (https://doi.org/10.1007/978-3-030-14032-8_11) contains supplementary material, which is available to authorized users.

M. Saric (✉)
Echocardiography Lab, Leon H. Charney Division of Cardiology, New York University Langone Medical Center, New York, NY, USA
e-mail: muhamed.saric@nyumc.org

G. Perk
Interventional Echocardiography, Mount Sinai School of Medicine, New York, NY, USA
e-mail: gila.perk@mountsinai.org

I. Kronzon
Hofstra University School of Medicine, North Shore LIJ/Lenox Hill Hospital, New York, NY, USA
e-mail: ikronzon@nshs.edu

L. P. Badano et al. (eds.), *Textbook of Three-Dimensional Echocardiography*, https://doi.org/10.1007/978-3-030-14032-8_11

Table 11.1 Historical timeline of mitral valve surgeries and repairs

Mechanical valves	
1960	Starr-Edwards ball-in-cage
1969	Björk-Shiley single tilting disc
1977	Medtronic-Hall single tilting disc
	St. Jude Medical bileaflet tilting disc
1978	Omniscience single tilting disc
1986	CarboMedics bileaflet tilting disc
Bioprosthetic valves	
1975	Carpentier-Edwards porcine
1984	Carpentier-Edwards bovine pericardial
Surgical mitral valve repairs	
1971	Annuloplasty ring
1983	Carpentier's 'French correction'
1995	Annuloplasty band
2001	Edge-to-edge surgical repair (Alfieri stitch)
Percutaneous mitral valve repairs and replacements	
2013	Mitral clip
2015	Valve-in-valve

Transesophageal 3DE Imaging of Prosthetic and Repaired Mitral Valves

At the turn of the twenty-first century, 3DE was revolutionized with the introduction of novel 3D matrix array transducers. Modern transesophageal 3DE probes have 3000 imaging elements while a standard two-dimensional transesophageal probe typically has 64 imaging elements. With this novel transducer technology, real-time 3D echocardiographic imaging became feasible for the first time (see also Chap. 3).

Transesophageal 3DE is capable of producing excellent views of the mitral valve apparatus (native or prosthetic mitral leaflets, annulus, subvalvular structures and various prosthetic materials) including the novel *en face* views [1]. Transesophageal 3DE has become indispensable for the diagnosis of mitral valve pathology, guidance of surgical and percutaneous intervention, and identification of potential complications, such as paravalvular or para-annular leaks, with unprecedented clarity [2].

Native mitral valves, mitral bioprostheses and repairs can easily be visualized from both left atrial and left ventricular perspectives. However, mechanical mitral prostheses are best imaged from the left atrial perspective as left ventricular aspects of mechanical prostheses are often obscured by shadowing and reverberation artifacts.

Transesophageal 3DE images of the mitral valve in this chapter are displayed primarily from the left atrial perspective in the so-called 'surgical' view. In this view, the mitral valve resembling an analog clock face is placed in the center of the image in such a way that the aortic valve is seen at 12 o'clock, the left atrial appendage at 9 o'clock, and the interatrial septum at 3 o'clock.

Alternatives to Echocardiography: Radiography and Fluoroscopy

Despite major advances in 3DE, radiographic imaging plays an important role in evaluating the appearance of prosthetic valves and complements the information obtained by echocardiography. Radiopacity of the prosthetic occluders, sewing rings and other components of prosthetic valves and valve repairs allows for visualization with relative clarity and ease on chest X rays, fluoroscopy or computed tomography. Based on the characteristic radiographic appearance, the type and location of a prosthetic valve or valve repair can be deduced [3]. Furthermore, radiographic imaging is essential for percutaneous mitral valve procedures.

Fluoroscopy is still the preferred modality for real-time assessment of the mobility of mechanical prosthetic valve occluder. Furthermore, on fluoroscopy one can measure the opening and closing angles of the mechanical prosthetic valve leaflet which are defined as the angles between the two leaflets in the fully open and completely closed position, respectively. By measuring these angles one can determine if the prosthesis function is normal or abnormal. The opening and closing are listed in Table 11.2.

In addition to fluoroscopy, computed tomography (CT) and cardiac magnetic resonance (CMR) imaging are playing an ever increasing role in valvular assessment before, during and after surgical and transcatheter interventions.

Mechanical Valves

Starr-Edwards Ball-in-Cage Mechanical Prosthesis

In 1957, Dr. Albert Starr, then a young cardiac surgeon at the University of Oregon, met Miles Lowell Edwards, an already retired engineer. Inspired by the design of a nineteenth century bottle stopper [4], they developed a ball-in-cage mechanical prosthesis which was implanted in 1960 in the first human patient [5].

In 1965, after multiple design adjustments, the standard 6120 mitral valve model was established [6]. This mitral model has a barium-impregnated silastic ball and a 4-strut cobalt-chromium stellite alloy cage. In contrast, the aortic Starr-Edwards prosthesis has three struts [7]. Despite its bulky design and relatively high thrombogenicity, the Starr-Edwards mechanical valve became a cost-effective option for surgical valve replacement in several parts of the world [8].

As it passes through the sewing ring, flow through the Starr-Edwards valve first converges and then deviates circumferentially as it passes around the ball-shaped occluder. Because of a relatively inefficient flow around the ball, the

Table 11.2 Imaging parameters of mechanical mitral valves

Opening angle	Closing angle	Valve size		Peak gradient	Mean gradient	Peak velocity	Pressure half-time	Effective orifice area
degrees	degrees	mm	Valve type	mm Hg	mm Hg	m/s	ms	cm^2
Not applicable	Not applicable	26	Starr-Edwards caged ball		10			1.4
		28			7 ± 2.75			1.9 ± 0.57
		30		12.2 ± 4.6	6.99 ± 2.5	1.7 ± 0.3	125 ± 25	1.65 ± 0.4
		32		11.5 ± 4.2	5.08 ± 2.5	1.7 ± 0.3	110 ± 25	1.98 ± 0.4
		34			5			2.6
60–70	0	23	Björk-Shiley tilting disk			1.7	115	
		25		12 ± 4	6 ± 2	1.75 ± 0.38	99 ± 27	1.72 ± 0.6
		27		10 ± 4	5 ± 2	1.6 ± 0.49	89 ± 28	1.81 ± 0.54
		29		7.83 ± 2.93	2.83 ± 1.27	1.37 ± 0.25	79 ± 17	2.1 ± 0.43
		31		6 ± 3	2 ± 1.9	1.41 ± 0.26	70 ± 14	2.2 ± 0.3
70	0	27	Medtronic Hall tilting disk			1.4	78	
		29				1.57 ± 0.1	69 + 15	
		31				1.45 ± 0.12	77 + 17	
85	25–30	23	St. Jude Medical bileaflet		4	1.5	160	1
		25			2.5 ± 1	1.34 ± 1.12	75 ± 4	1.35 ± 0.17
		27		11 ± 4	5 ± 1.82	1.61 ± 0.29	75 ± 10	1.67 ± 0.17
		29		10 ± 3	4.15 ± 1.8	1.57 ± 0.29	85 ± 10	1.75 ± 0.24
		31		12 ± 6	4.46 ± 2.22	1.59 ± 0.33	74 ± 13	2.03 ± 0.32
78	25	23	CarboMedics bileaflet			1.9 ± 0.1	126 ± 7	
		25		10.3 ± 2.3	3.6 ± 0.6	1.3 ± 0.1	93 ± 8	2.9 ± 0.8
		27		8.79 ± 3.46	3.46 ± 1.03	1.61 ± 0.3	89 ± 20	2.9 ± 0.75
		29		8.78 ± 2.9	3.39 ± 0.97	1.52 ± 0.3	88 ± 17	2.3 ± 0.4
		31		8.87 ± 2.34	3.32 ± 0.87	1.61 ± 0.29	92 ± 24	2.8 ± 1.14
		33		8.8 ± 2.2	4.8 ± 2.5	1.5 ± 0.2	93 ± 12	

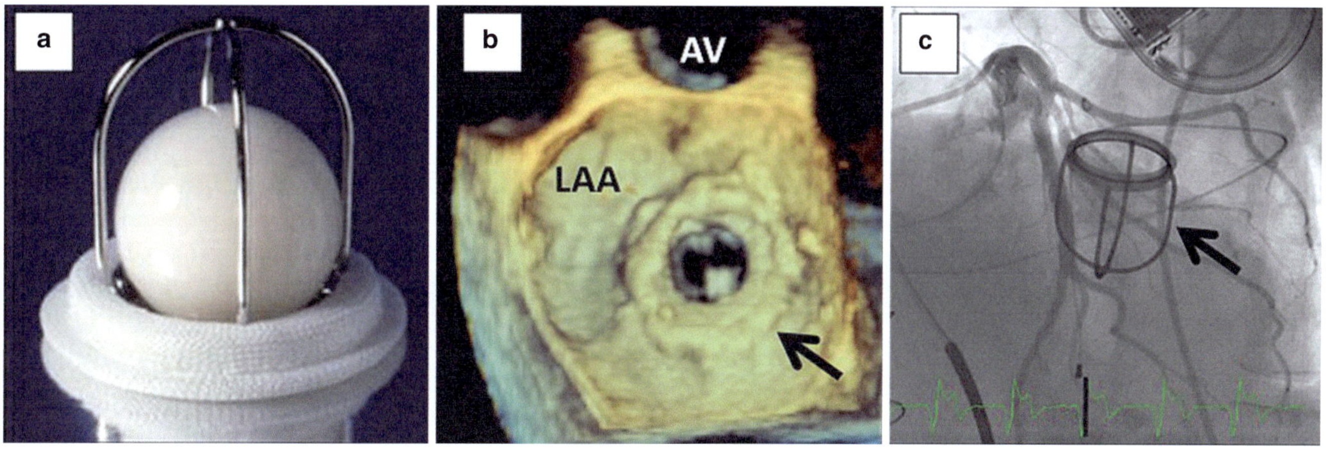

Fig. 11.1 Starr-Edwards mechanical mitral valve. (**a**) Photograph of a mitral Starr-Edwards ball-in-cage valve; note the four struts surrounding the ball. (**b**) Left atrial aspect of a mitral Starr-Edwards valve (arrow). *AV* aortic valve, *LAA* left atrial appendage (Video 11.1). (**c**) Fluoroscopic appearance of a mitral Starr-Edwards valve (arrow)

effective orifice area of a Starr-Edwards valve is smaller and its transvalvular gradients higher compared to more modern mechanical prostheses [9]. Early systolic retrograde flow, which is necessary for normal valve closure, creates a characteristic color Doppler pattern [10].

The Starr-Edwards valve, including its 3DE appearance, is depicted in Fig. 11.1 and Video 11.1.

Björk-Shiley Tilting Disk Mechanical Prosthesis

After the introduction of the Starr-Edwards prosthesis, several single tilting disc valves were developed. Björk-Shiley valve, introduced in 1969, was one of the first commercially successful tilting disc valves. It was invented by the Swedish cardiac surgeon Viking Björk and the American engineer Donald Shiley [11, 12].

A Björk-Shiley mechanical prosthetic valve consists of a single tilting disc held in place by an inlet strut and an outlet strut [7]. The disc is 1 mm thick with a graphite core surrounded by either pyrolytic carbon or low-temperature-isotropic carbon [13]. The closing angle of the Björk-Shiley tilting is 0° while the opening angle varies from 60° to 70° depending on the model. Two holosystolic backflow jets through a small space between the disc and housing are necessary for normal disc closure [14].

In 1986, the United States Food and Drug Administration (FDA) recalled the Björk-Shiley valve after several hundred valves having the convexo-concave design fractured resulting in disc embolization. Although the Björk-Shiley valve is no longer implanted, echocardiographers should be familiar with its appearance and function since patients with this prosthesis can still be encountered in clinical practice.

The Björk-Shiley valve, including its 3DE appearance, is depicted in Fig. 11.2 and Video 11.2.

Medtronic-Hall Single-Tilting Disk Prosthesis

Karl Victor Hall, a Norwegian cardiac surgeon, working with the engineer Robert Kaster developed the Hall-Kaster single-tilting disc valve that served as the blueprint for the subsequent Medtronic-Hall prosthesis [7]. This prosthetic valve consists of radiopaque titanium housing, a radiolucent carbon-coated disc, and a Teflon sewing ring. The disc is mounted on a sigmoid strut with an opening angle of 70° and a closing angle of 0° [15].

When the valve opens, two antegrade jets pass through a major orifice and a minor orifice [16]. The disc design enhances washing of the valve and eliminates regions of low velocity flow [17]. During valve closure, gaps between the disc and the housing create regurgitant jets. The most characteristic is the central regurgitant jet around the sigmoid strut. Additional smaller peripheral regurgitant jets may also occur around the rim of the disc, although not necessarily around the entire circumference [8].

The Medtronic-Hall mechanical valve, including its 3DE appearance, is depicted in Fig. 11.3 and Video 11.3.

Omniscience Single-Leaflet Mechanical Prosthesis

The Omniscience single tilting-disc mechanical prosthesis, which became available in 1978, is an improved version of the Lillehei-Kaster disc valve [10]. Inside a titanium cage, there is a curvilinear disc made of pyrolytic carbon surrounded by a polytetrafluoroethylene sewing ring. The disc pivots to a maximum opening angle of 80° and a closing angle of 12° [7].

The low-profile design of the Omniscience prosthesis enables a central antegrade flow with a trans-prosthetic gradient that is somewhat elevated compared to those of the other mechanical disc valves. Multiple studies have demonstrated decreased opening angles leading to decreased hemodynamic performance and predisposing to clot formation. A revised version of the Omniscience prosthesis was introduced in 1982, resulting in decreased complication rates [18].

During leaflet closure, there is normally minimal regurgitation [19]. The Omniscience mechanical valve is depicted in Fig. 11.4 and Video 11.4.

St. Jude Medical Bileaflet Mechanical Prosthesis

The St. Jude bileaflet mechanical valve was the result of the collaboration between Xinon C. Posis, an engineer, Demetre Nicoloff, an American cardiovascular surgeon, and Manny Villafaña, the founder of Cardiac Pacemakers, Inc. With the introduction of the St. Jude prosthesis in 1977, the notion of unimpeded central flow within mechanical prostheses was pioneered. Since its introduction, there were several modifications. Currently, St. Jude is the most commonly implanted mechanical prosthesis.

The bileaflet tilting-disc design consists of two semicircular leaflets made of pyrolytic carbon; the leaflets are impregnated with tungsten to make them radiopaque. Two pivot housings are also made of pyrolytic carbon and are positioned on the inflow side of the prosthesis (that is on the left atrial side when the prosthesis is implanted in the mitral position). The semicircular discs of the St. Jude prosthesis have an opening angle of 85° and a closing angle of 25–30°.

Upon leaflet opening, three orifices are created which allows for less turbulent and more central forward flow when compared to the mechanical prostheses with a ball-in-cage or single-tilting disc design [20]. The two lateral orifices are significantly larger than the central orifice of a St. Jude prosthesis.

During valve closure, a complicated array of regurgitant jets is created. When viewed in the plane parallel to the leaflet axes, regurgitant jets are seen originating from the valve periphery and converging toward the center of the valve in the shape of an inverted letter V. On the other hand, when viewed in the plane orthogonal to the leaflet axes, regurgitant jets diverge from the central axis toward the periphery of the valve to form an upright letter V. In addition to these peripheral jets, a small regurgitant jet from the central orifice is seen in all planes [8]. The St. Jude valve is depicted in Fig. 11.5 and Video 11.5.

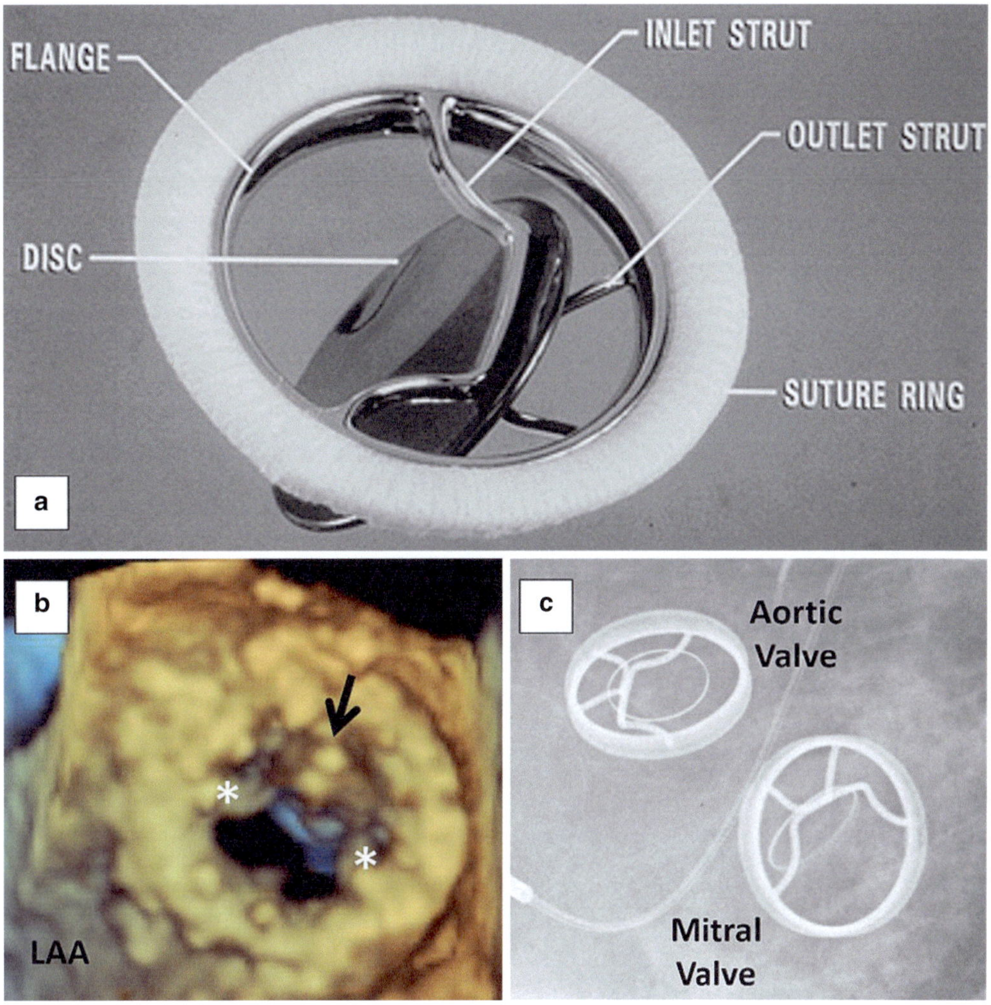

Fig. 11.2 Björk-Shiley mechanical mitral valve. (**a**) Photograph of a Björk-Shiley valve; note the appearance of inlet and outlet strut surrounding the tilting disc. (**b**) Left atrial aspect of a mitral a Björk-Shiley valve. The inlet strut (asterisks) and the tilting disc (arrow) are visible. *LAA* left atrial appendage (Video 11.2). (**c**) Fluoroscopic appearance of a mitral and an aortic Björk-Shiley valve

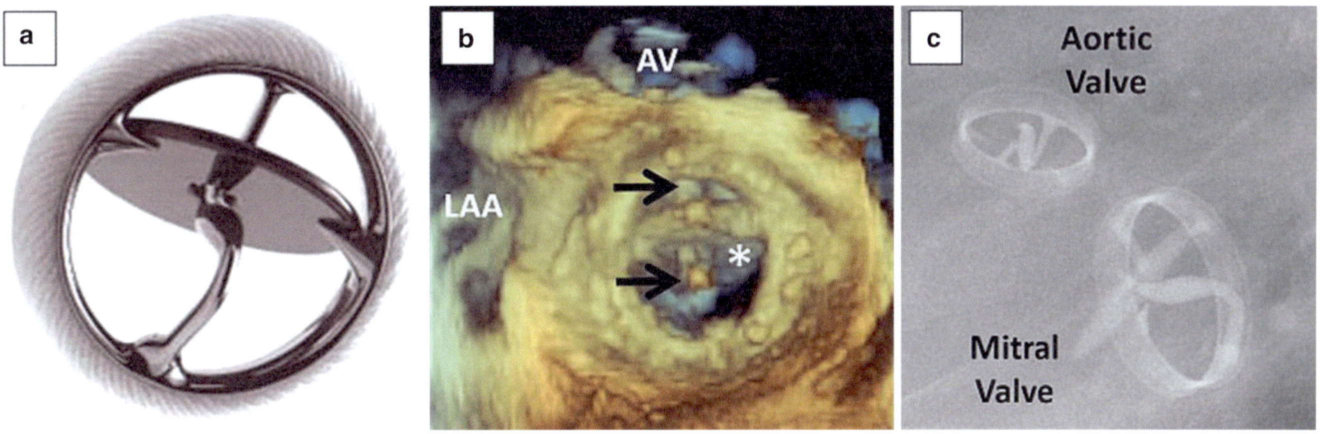

Fig. 11.3 Medtronic Hall mechanical mitral valve. (**a**) Photograph of a Medtronic Hall valve; note the tilting disc mounted on a sigmoid shaped central shaft. (**b**) Left atrial aspect of a mitral Medtronic Hall prosthesis. The tilting disc (asterisk) and the sigmoid shaft (arrows) are clearly delineated. *AV* aortic valve, *LAA* left atrial appendage (Video 11.3). (**c**) Fluoroscopic appearance of a mitral and an aortic Medtronic Hall prosthesis

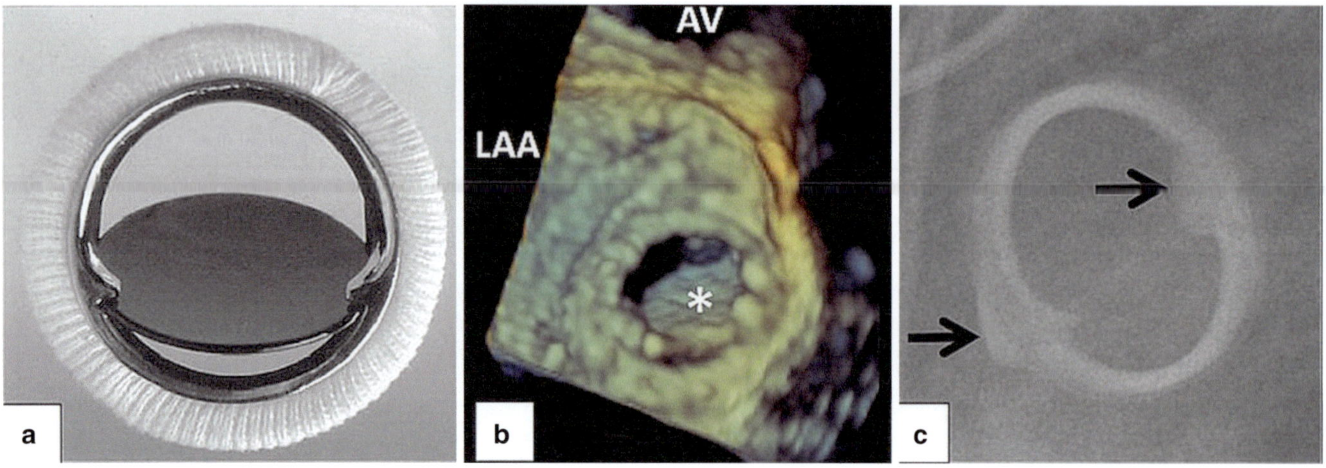

Fig. 11.4 Omniscience mechanical mitral valve. (**a**) Photograph of a Omniscience valve. Note the absence of any central struts or shafts. Instead, the disc's hinge mechanism is located at the disc periphery. (**b**) Left atrial aspect of a mitral Omniscience prosthesis during early diastole. The disc (asterisk) is partly open. *AV* aortic valve, *LAA* left atrial appendage (Video 11.4). (**c**) Fluoroscopic appearance of a mitral Omniscience valve. Arrows point to the peripherally located hinges

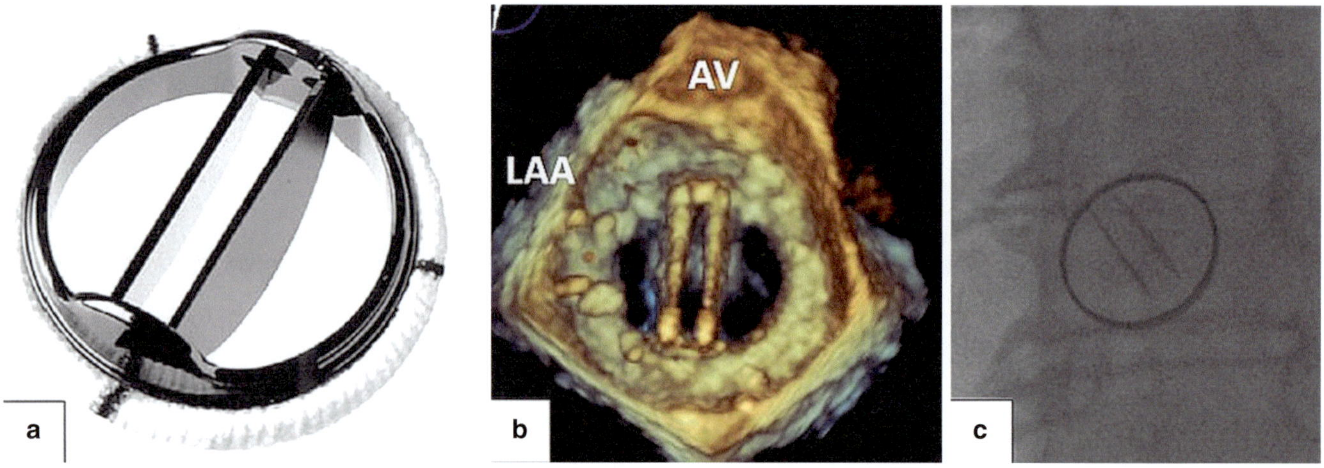

Fig. 11.5 St. Jude mechanical mitral valve. (**a**) Photograph of a St. Jude prosthesis. (**b**) Left atrial aspect of a mitral St. Jude prosthesis in the so-called anti-anatomic orientation with a left disc and a right disc. (This is in contrast to the so-called anatomic orientation in which one disc is anterior and the other is posterior.) Note the smaller central orifice and two larger peripheral orifices. *AV* aortic valve, *LAA* left atrial appendage (Video 11.5). (**c**) Fluoroscopic appearance a mitral St. Jude prosthesis in a fully open position during diastole

CarboMedics

The CarboMedics bileaflet mechanical valve, which was developed by Jack Bokros, was approved in 1993 for commercial use [21]. The design of the CarboMedics valve is very similar to that of the St. Jude Medical mechanical bileaflet prosthesis. The CarboMedics prosthesis consists of two carbon-coated discs having an opening angle of 78° and a closing angle of 25°. The CarboMedics valve housing can rotate within the sewing ring and thus allows for orientation adjustments during implantation. The trans-prosthetic antegrade pressure gradient across the CarboMedics prosthesis is somewhat higher than that of the St. Jude valve [6].

Despite design differences, closing regurgitant volumes and backflow patterns between these two prostheses are similar [22]. The rates of survival, bleeding, thromboembolism, and prosthetic valve dysfunction at 10 years after valve implantation were similar for the two prostheses [21].

Bioprosthetic Mitral Valves

The French cardiovascular surgeon Alain Carpentier was instrumental in the development of bioprosthetic valves. He also coined the term "bioprosthesis". Bioprosthetic valves with characteristics similar to those of Carpentier-Edwards valves are marked by other manufacturers, including Medtronic, St. Jude Medical and LivaNova.

Typically, bioprosthetic valves are either porcine or bovine in origin. The porcine bioprostheses are chemically preserved pig aortic valves while bovine bioprostheses are fashioned from bovine pericardial tissue to resemble the native aortic valve. These original bioprostheses were all stented but some stentless bioprostheses have recently been developed.

The Carpentier-Edwards porcine valve is the prototypical bioprosthesis and has been commercially available since 1975. Carpentier and colleagues, fixed the porcine valves with glutaraldehyde and encased them in an asymmetric wire stent made of elgiloy [23]. The stent, which is radiopaque, is covered with polytetrafluoroethylene cloth to facilitate tissue ingrowth [24]. The Carpentier-Edwards bovine pericardial valve, introduced in 1984, is one of the first biomechanically engineered prostheses. Bovine bioprostheses typically have superior hemodynamics to the porcine ones.

Trans-prosthetic regurgitation may occur with normally functioning bioprostheses, especially the bovine ones. This physiologic regurgitation typically consists of a single, central jet. The stentless prostheses are more likely to exhibit this trans-prosthetic regurgitation than stented valves [25].

A bioprosthetic mitral valve is depicted in Fig. 11.6 and Video 11.6.

Mitral Valve Repairs

Surgical mitral valve repairs can be performed with or without an annuloplasty ring. Ringless annuloplasty for mitral valve repair was first introduced in 1957. Alain Carpentier pioneered the use of an annuloplasty ring 12 years later. Currently there is a variety of mitral annuloplasty rings on the market. Rings may be either complete (D-shaped rings) or partial (C-shaped rings, also referred to as annuloplasty bands). At present, an annuloplasty ring or band is used for most surgical repair of the mitral valve.

A special form of ringless mitral valve repair is known as the edge-to-edge technique and colloquially referred to as the Alfieri stitch [26]. The Alfieri technique requires suturing the anterior and posterior mitral valve leaflets, typically in the central portion of the mitral valve, creating a valve with two orifices [27]. As discussed in the section below, percutaneous mitral valve clipping is a transcatheter procedure emulating the surgical Alfieri procedure.

Complete mitral annuloplasty ring is depicted in Fig.11.7 and Video 11.7. Partial annuloplasty ring (band) is shown in Fig. 11.8 and Video 11.8. A mitral repair using the Alfieri's surgical edge-to-edge technique is depicted in Fig. 11.9 and Video 11.9.

Mitral Valve Clip

It is over 20 years since Alfieri, an Italian surgeon, demonstrated that a stitch suturing the free edges of the middle mitral scallops (A2 and P2) resulted in better approximation of the mitral leaflets and improved results of surgical repair of mitral regurgitation due to flail anterior mitral leaflet [28, 29]. Later, in a series of 260 patients, those who underwent traditional mitral annuloplasty repair, the addition of the now called "Alfieri stitch", had better long term results with lower 5 years need for reoperation [30, 31].

During the last decade, a system capable of transcutaneous implantation of mitral clip for edge-to-edge repair was developed and used. The MitraClip valve repair system (Abbott Laboratories, Abbott Park, IL, USA), delivers a cobalt chrome clip via a large peripheral vein to the right atrium and then across the interatrial septum into the left atrium. Thereafter, the catheter is placed across the mitral valve. The clip is used to grab and connect the free middle edges (A2 and P2) of the ventricular side of the regurgitant mitral valve, thus creating two mitral valve orifices [32].

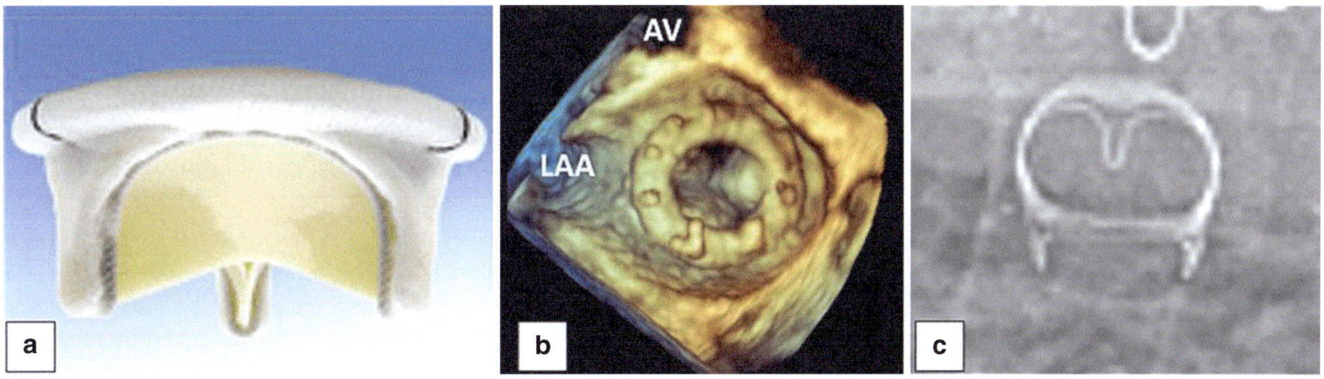

Fig. 11.6 Carpentier-Edwards (CE) bovine pericardial bioprosthetic mitral valve. (**a**) Photograph of a mitral CE bioprosthesis. (**b**) Left atrial aspect of a mitral CE bioprosthesis with three leaflets clearly visible during systole. *AV* aortic valve, *LAA* left atrial appendage (Video 11.6). (**c**) Fluoroscopic appearance of a mitral CE bovine pericardial valve

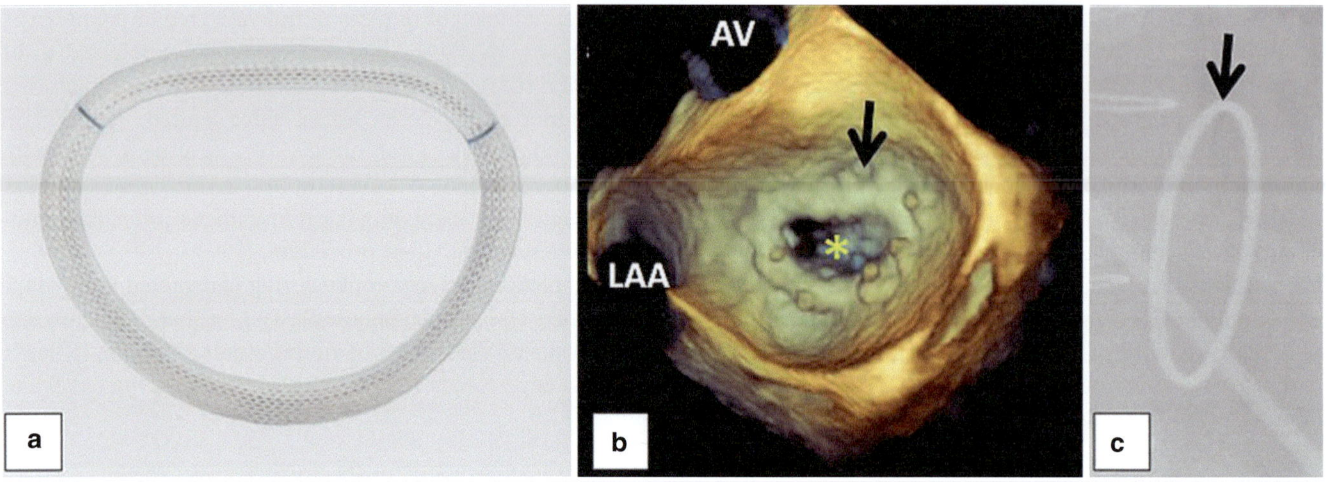

Fig. 11.7 Complete mitral annuloplasty ring. (**a**) Photograph of a complete (D-shaped) mitral annuloplasty ring. (**b**) Left atrial aspect of a complete mitral annuloplasty ring (arrow) during early diastole. Asterisk denotes the partly open anterior mitral leaflet. *AV* aortic valve, *LAA* left atrial appendage (Video 11.7). (**c**) Fluoroscopic appearance of a complete mitral annuloplasty ring (arrow)

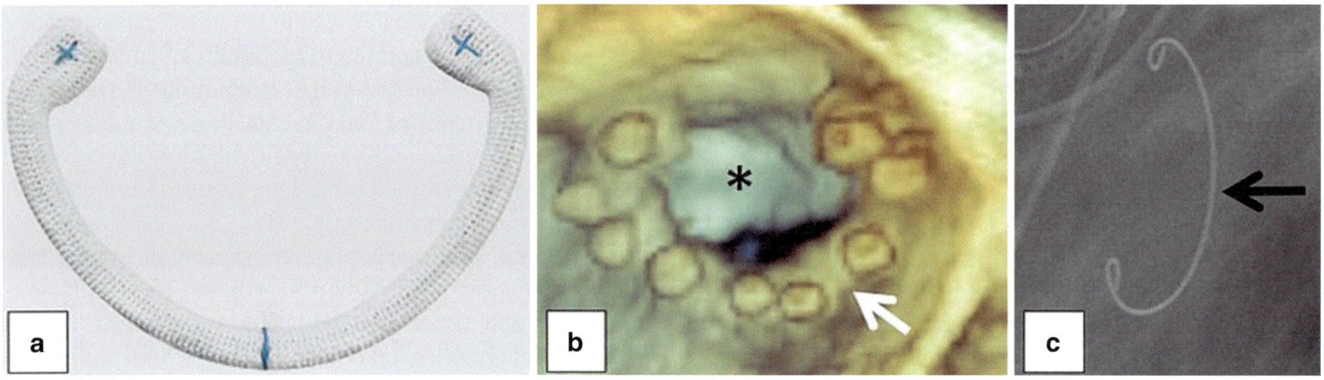

Fig. 11.8 Mitral annuloplasty band. (**a**) Photograph of a partial (C-shaped) annuloplasty ring (band). (**b**) Left atrial aspect of a C-shaped annuloplasty band (arrow) during diastole. Asterisk denotes the partly open anterior mitral leaflet (Video 11.8). (**c**) Fluoroscopic appearance of a mitral C-shaped annuloplasty band

After successful deployment, the degree of mitral regurgitation is expected to decrease or disappear, without new mitral stenosis. By now, this procedure has been performed on nearly 20,000 high risk or inoperable patients worldwide, with very encouraging clinical results. This includes superior safety profile when compared with surgical repair, based mainly on a lower risk of transfusions, decrease of mitral regurgitation, improvement of New York Heart Association functional class and improved quality of life [33–35].

Cardiac imaging is an important part of this procedure. Fluoroscopy and transesophageal echocardiography are routinely used in each patient. Real time 3DE is now available and is used to assess, guide and monitor most stages of the procedure. It has been shown to improve the results, shorten the procedure duration and better identify complications and failure [36].

Transesophageal 3DE is useful in the pre-procedure evaluation. It can better assess the anatomy of the mitral valve and the detailed mechanism of the mitral regurgitation, functional or degenerative [37] (see also Chaps. 9 and 10). Furthermore, it is useful in identifying conditions which may lead to a less successful procedure (e.g. mitral valve area of less than 4 cm^2, or presence of multiple jet of mitral regurgitation).

During the early part of the procedure, 3DE imaging can identify the correct site of the transseptal puncture. This site is generally between 4 and 5 cm above the mitral annulus. However, may be lower in cases of functional mitral regurgitation (where tethering displaces the mitral line of coaptation

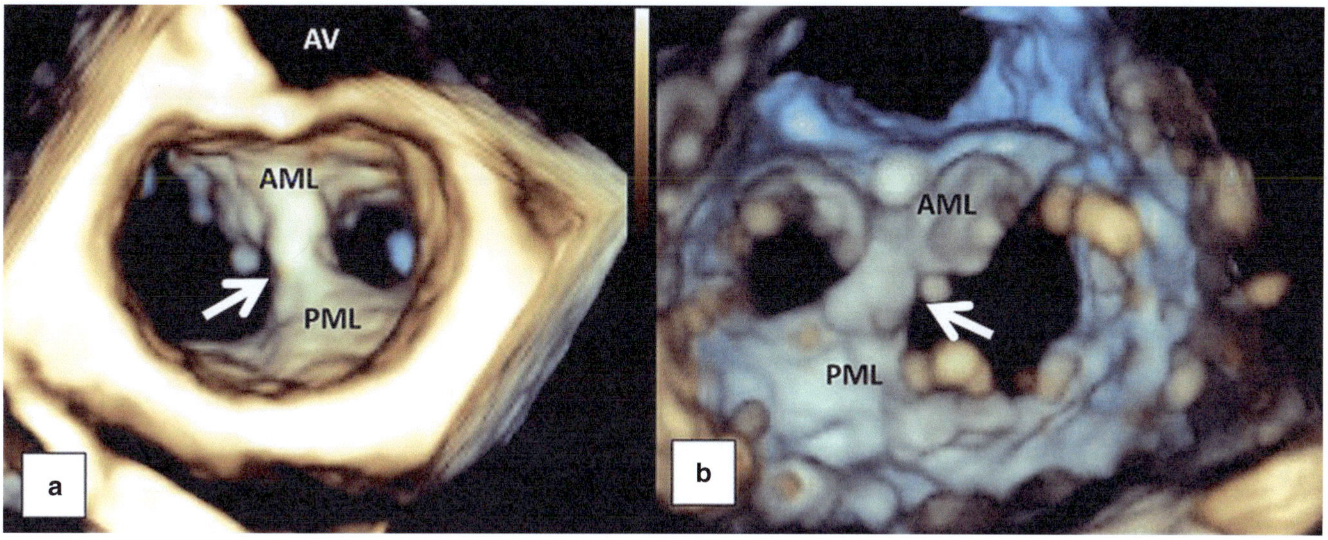

Fig. 11.9 Alfieri edge-to-edge repair. (**a**) Left atrial aspect of a native mitral valve repaired an Alfieri stitch (arrow) (Video 11.9). (**b**) Mitral valve of the same patient seen from the left ventricular perspective. *AML* anterior mitral leaflet, *PML* posterior mitral leaflet

towards the apex) or higher in cases of severe prolapse (where the coaptation line is displaced superiorly).

Transesophageal 3DE is helpful in the identification and the manipulation of the clip delivery system in the left atrium and in the positioning of the MitraClip above the mitral valve. The clip is then opened and oriented perpendicular to the mitral coaptation line and then advanced into the left ventricle, in order to grasp the free edges of the opposing leaflets. The clip position and function are carefully monitored. Possible residual mitral regurgitation, new mitral stenosis and complications are carefully evaluated [38].

The steps of the MitraClip procedure are depicted in Figs. 11.10 and 11.11 and Video 11.10.

Mitral Paravalvular Leak Closure

Mitral paravalvular leaks (PVLs) are not an uncommon complication after mitral valve replacement. PVL is defined as an abnormal communication between the left ventricle and left atrium, occurring outside the prosthetic ring. PVLs can be small and asymptomatic; however, can also present with debilitating symptoms of heart failure or intravascular hemolysis.

Difficulties in estimating the exact prevalence of PVL stem from variability in reported incidence; various techniques can be used to diagnose PVL (transthoracic echo, transesophageal echo, computed tomography), different reports include clinically insignificant PVLs as well as clinically important PVLs, and many reports include all types of valves (aortic, mitral, bioprosthetic, mechanical prosthetic and percutaneous valves). Currently, it is estimated that clinically significant PVLs occur in approximately 3–5% of patients who underwent mitral valve replacement or repair [39–42].

Until recent years, mitral PVLs were treated surgically. As these surgeries are by definition re-operation, the inherent surgical risk is elevated, even for the lowest risk patients. Over the past several years, percutaneous treatment of mitral PVL has become an increasingly acceptable alternative, allowing avoidance of re-operation for a selected group of patients. The developments of the percutaneous treatment options for mitral PVLs were made possible by the concomitant advancements in 3DE imaging.

3DE, and in particular transesophageal 3DE is paramount for the diagnosis, treatment and monitoring of patients with mitral PVL. Transesophageal 3DE is used for the accurate diagnosis of PVL, guidance of the percutaneous closure procedure and short and long-term follow up for procedure success or complications.

The Role of Transesophageal 3DE in the Diagnosis of Mitral PVL

Transthoracic echocardiography with Doppler evaluation is considered the test of choice for initial evaluation of patients suspected to have a mitral PVL. Transthoracic echocardiography can be useful is assessing chamber size and function, gradient across the mitral valve and for evaluation for presence of “rocking motion” of the prosthetic valve. However due to acoustic shadowing and reverbera-

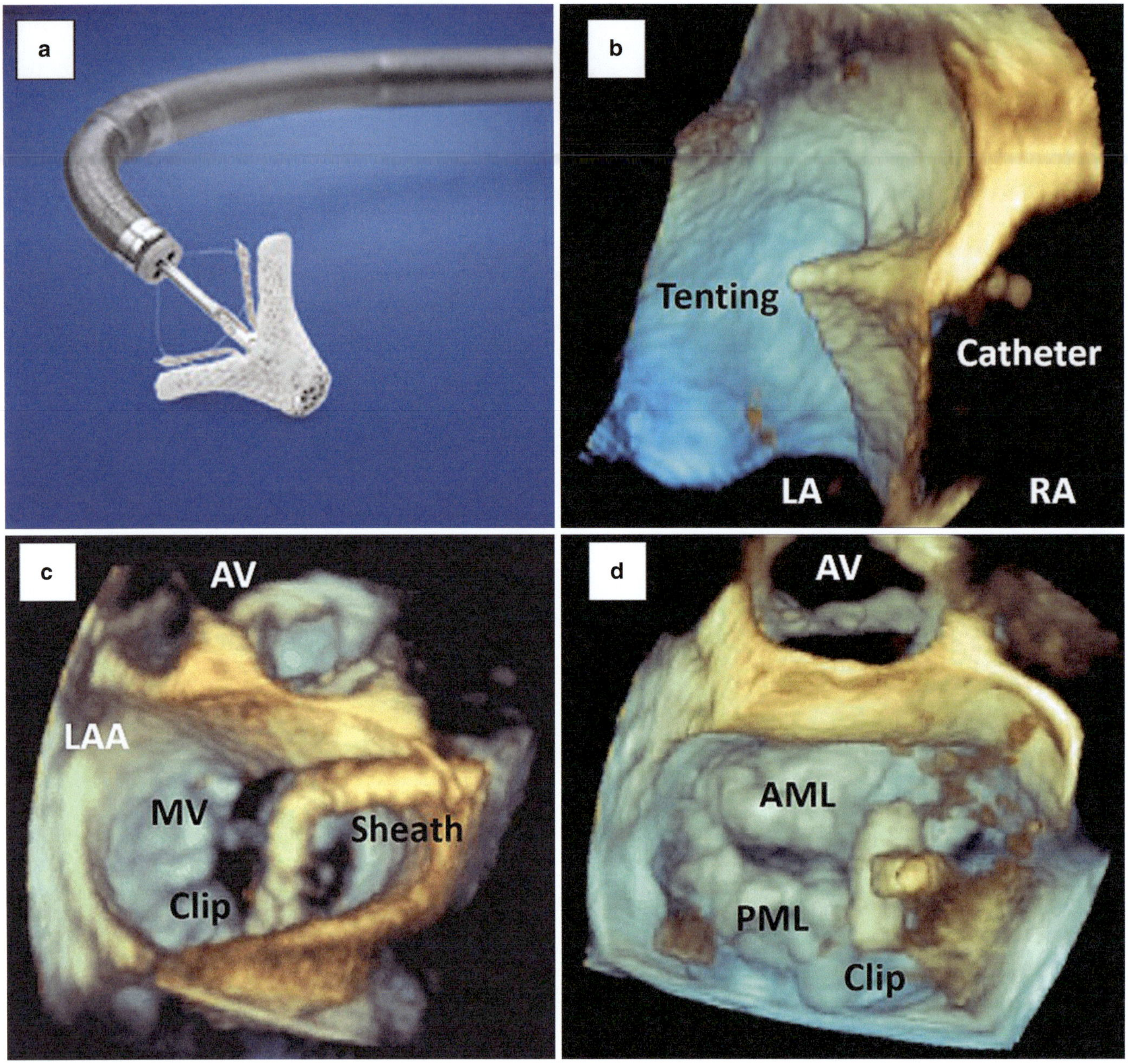

Fig. 11.10 Guidance of mitral clip procedure. (**a**) Photograph of the mitral clip. (**b**) Zoom 3D TEE image during transseptal puncture demonstrates tenting of the interatrial septum. *LA* left atrium, *RA* right atrium. (**c**) Deliver sheath carrying the mitral clip assembly is seen crossing the interatrial septum into the left atrium. *AV* aortic valve, *LAA* left atrial appendage, *MV* mitral valve. (**d**) Mitral clip is open and is being oriented perpendicular to the mitral coaptation line. *AML* anterior mitral leaflet, *AV* aortic valve, *PML* posterior mitral leaflet

tion artifacts, a transesophageal study is invariably required for proper anatomic and functional evaluation of a PVL [43].

When transesophageal echocardiography is used for assessment of mitral PVL it is essential to combine data obtained by all the available modalities; two-dimensional, 3D and Doppler echocardiography. The mitral valve is visualized from multiple angles, and color Doppler interrogation is performed at all angles as well. When visualizing the valve on 3DE, typically it is displayed in a "surgical view"; assuming the mitral annulus is a clock face, the valve is positioned such that the aortic valve is at 12 o'clock position, the left atrial appendage at 9 o'clock, and the interatrial septum is at 3 o'clock (Fig. 11.12). This allows for unified description of PVL location and proper communication between the different heart-team members [44, 45].

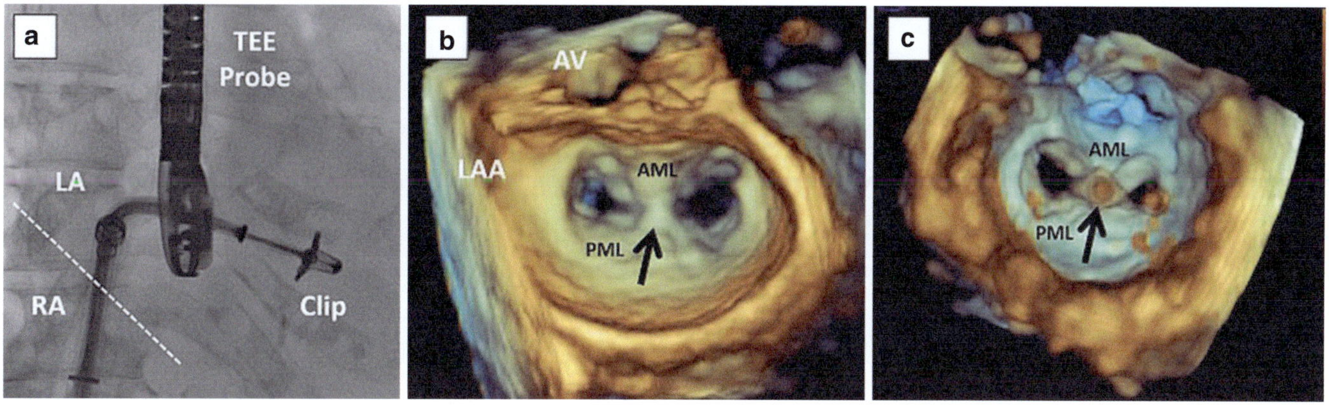

Fig. 11.11 Completion of mitral clip procedure. (**a**) Fluoroscopy during mitral clip procedure. (**b, c**) Demonstrate completely deployed mitral clip across the A2/P2 coaptation line from the left atrial (**b**) and left ventricular side (**c**). *AML* anterior mitral leaflet, *AV* aortic valve, *LAA* left atrial appendage, *PML* posterior mitral leaflet (Video 11.10)

Transesophageal 3DE is necessary for defining the anatomic characteristics of all PVLs identified [46–48]. The number, location and size of all PVLs can be accurately assessed (Figs. 11.13 and 11.14). It is crucial to combine the anatomical data with Doppler data, in order to avoid diagnosing a drop out artifact as a PVL. Presence of color flow through a defect positively establishes the diagnosis of a PVL. 3DE color Doppler imaging can further be used to accurately quantify the severity of a mitral PVL, for example by measuring the paravalvular effective regurgitant orifice area based on transesophageal 3DE color Doppler.

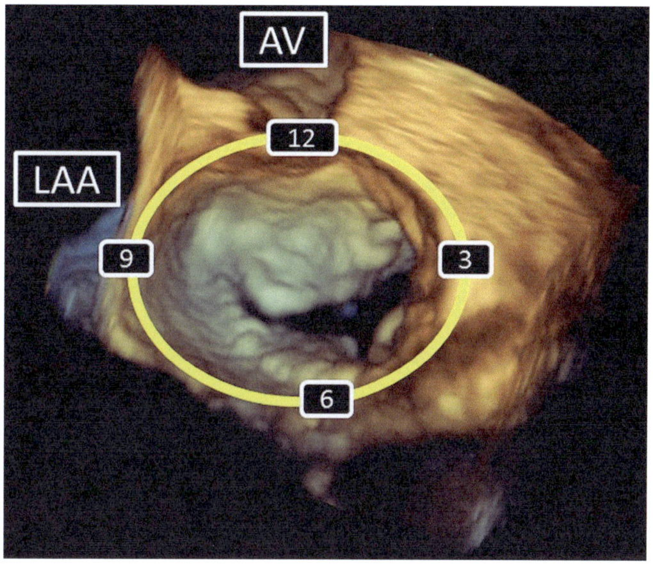

Fig. 11.12 Surgical view of the mitral valve. By convention, the mitral valve is rotated on the Z axis until the aortic valve (AV) is at 12 o'clock, the left atrial appendage (LAA) is at 9 o'clock

The Role of Transesophageal 3DE During Percutaneous Closure of Mitral PVL

Percutaneous closure procedures are always performed under transesophageal 3DE surveillance and guidance. While other imaging modalities are used as well during these complex trans-catheter procedures, only transesophageal 3DE allows for real time monitoring of all catheters, wires and devices with appropriate spatial resolution. Transesophageal 3DE guidance is paramount at every stage of the procedure [49, 50].

Access

There are several methods by which a mitral PVL can be accessed: antegrade transvenous access and a trans-septal puncture, retrograde approach through a femoral artery puncture, and a trans-apical puncture. Which approach is utilized is determined based on the location of the PVL treated, as well as underlying anatomical considerations (e.g. course of the left anterior descending coronary artery or presence of concomitant other valve disease).

Initial evaluation for trans-septal puncture requires echocardiographic assessment of the interatrial septum for suitability. In many instances the interatrial septum may be thickened, patched, or scarred from prior manipulation, which must be taken into account when planning the trans-septal access. Next, the appropriate location for the puncture must be determined. Depending on the PVL site, a proper puncture site needs to be chosen (e.g. a more posterior-inferior site for medially located PVLs to allow for catheter steering and manipulation in the left atrium).

While the interventionalist pulls down the trans-septal needle against the septum, the septum is visualized simultaneously in two planes, utilizing the echocardiographic biplane mode. Pushing the needle against the septum will first result in tenting of the septum, which can be visualized echocardiographically. Having the biplane view allows immediate assessment of the position of the

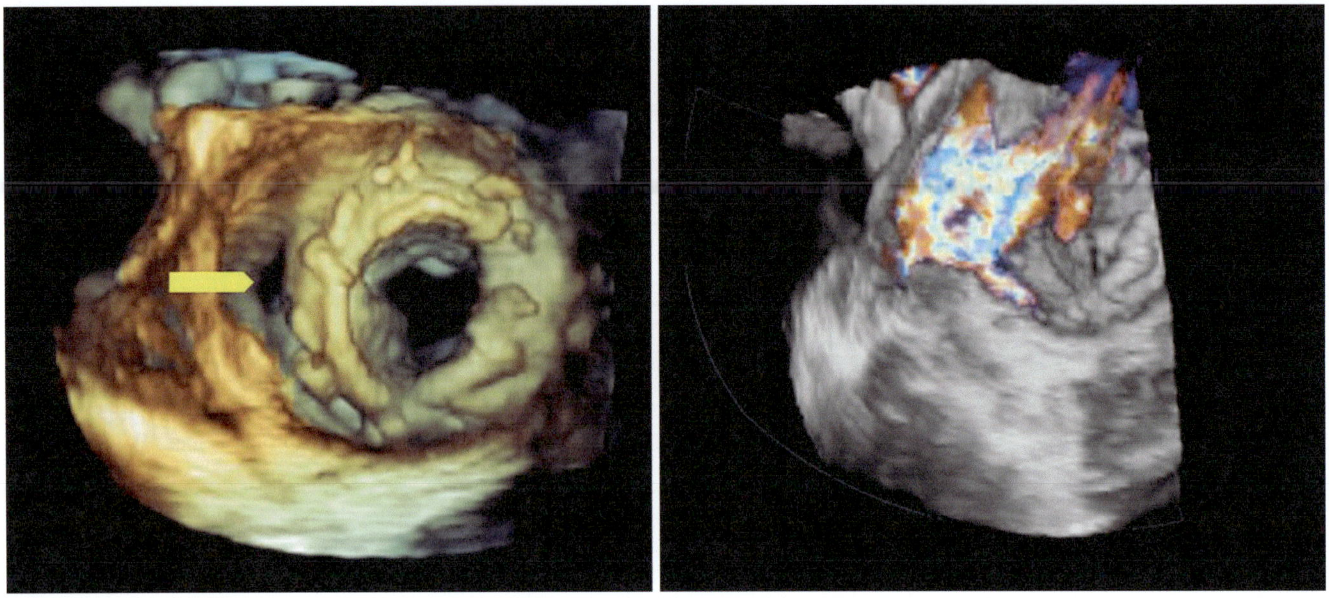

Fig. 11.13 PVL in a bioprosthetic valve. A large, lateral PVL (arrow) in a patient with a bioprosthetic valve. Left panel shows the anatomic depiction of the defect on a 3D zoom mode, right panel shows severe mitral regurgitation through the defect

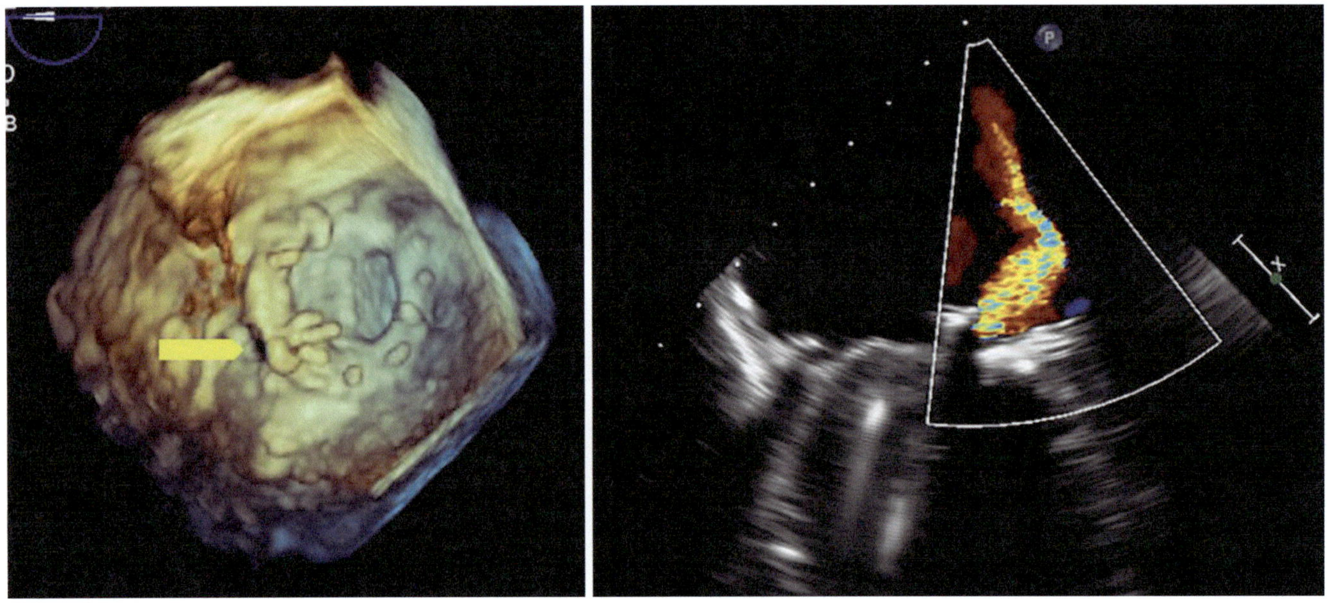

Fig. 11.14 PVL in a mechanical valve. A lateral PVL (arrow) in a patient with a mechanical valve. Left panel shows the anatomic depiction of the defect on a 3D zoom mode, right panel shows severe mitral regurgitation through the defect

needle both in the anteroposterior axis, as well as the superior-inferior axis (Fig. 11.15). Once the tenting is observed in a satisfactory location, puncture is performed. Occasionally radiofrequency or electrocautery may be used to facilitate puncture of a thicker, scarred septum.

During a trans-apical or retrograde aortic approach transesophageal echocardiography is utilized to monitor catheter location and manipulation within the heart.

Crossing the PVL

Once the access to the left heart has been established, the PVL has to be crossed. A wire is manipulated within the heart (either via an antegrade or retrograde approach to the mitral valve) and directed towards the PVL. Transesophageal 3DE imaging is crucial at this point. It is the only imaging modality that can reliably determine whether the wire has been passed through the PVL, through the prosthetic valve,

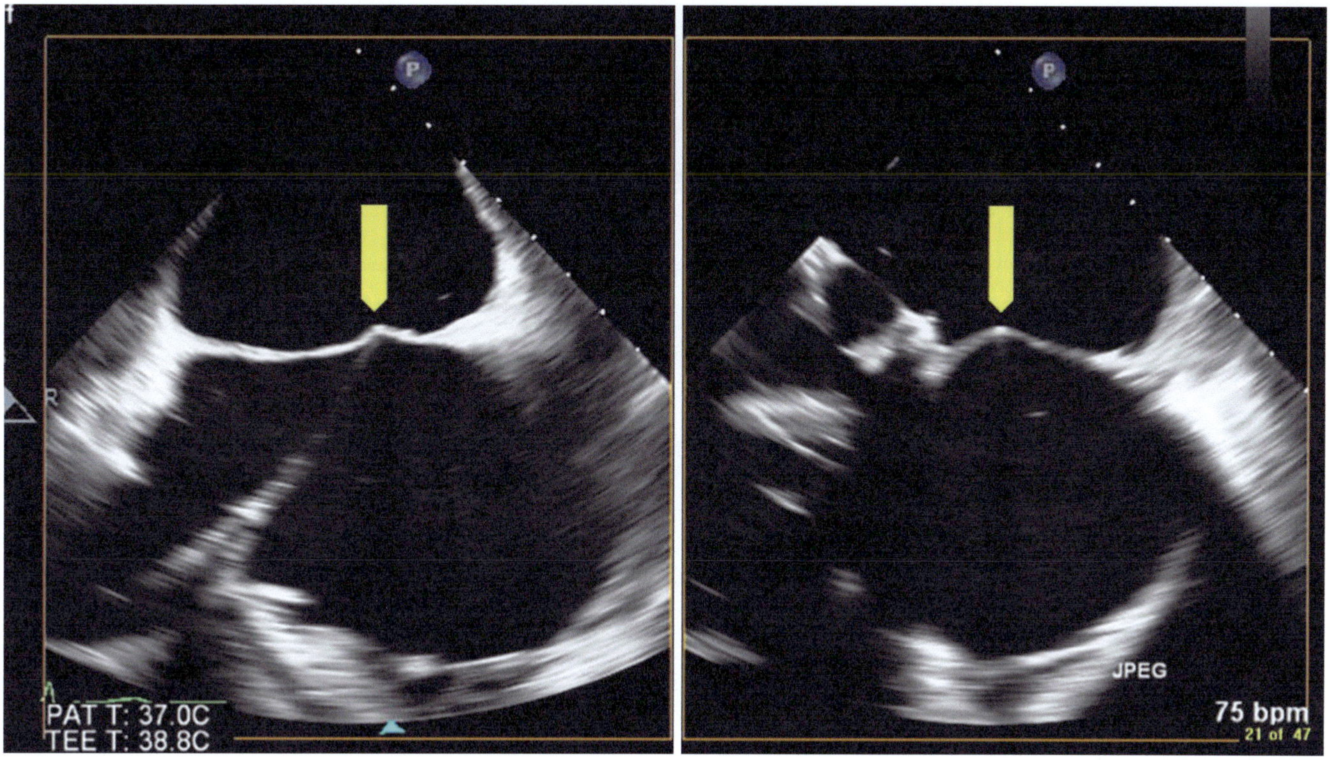

Fig. 11.15 Tenting of the interatrial septum. Biplane view showing trans-septal needle causing tenting of the interatrial septum (arrow). The biplane views allow for simultaneous depiction of the location of the tenting both in the superior-inferior axis (left panel) and the anterior posterior axis (right panel)

or into other structures (e.g., pulmonary vein, left atrial appendage).

The *en face* view of the mitral valve is particularly useful for this assessment, allowing for direct visualization of the wire and its course (Fig. 11.16). If there is any doubt, two-dimensional color Doppler may be utilized; if a wire is passed through the mitral valve, significant mitral regurgitation can nearly always be seen, confirming the need to re-adjust wire positioning. In many instances, once the PVL is crossed snaring of the wire is done (e.g. via a retrograde aortic approach) such that a rail is created. This further secures wire positioning and allows for safer catheter and device manipulations (Fig. 11.17).

Guide catheters are then advanced through the defect and occlusion devices are introduced via these catheters. Currently there is no FDA approved device for PVL closure; the ones used, are utilized by off-label manner. The choice of which device to use is based on the size and shape of the PVL, as assessed by 3DE and often by pre-procedure computed tomography scan. After the closure device is advanced into the PVL, echocardiographic interrogation is performed while the device is still connected to the delivery system. The anatomical position of the device is checked both by 3DE imaging and two-dimensional imaging. The device should fit securely into the PVL, however without compromising the leaflets or discs motion (Fig. 11.18).

Color Doppler interrogation from multiple angles is performed to evaluate the success of the closure. If the regurgitation is adequately decreased and no valve dysfunction is identified, the device can be deployed. Repeat interrogation of the device should be performed again, to ascertain that no movement has occurred, the device is secure and the result is satisfactory. In many cases the PVL may be large, however not continuous (likely separated by sutures). In these cases, the PVL needs to be re-crossed after placing the closure devices. Guidance is similar for every crossing attempt.

Depending on clinical characteristics and other co-morbidities (e.g. presence of severe tricuspid regurgitation or severe pulmonary hypertension), closure of the trans-septal puncture may be desired. RT3D guidance is performed similarly to atrial septal defect closure procedures described elsewhere in this book. Closure of trans-apical puncture site can be done surgically (if surgical cut down was utilized for the access), or utilizing a closure device. When device closure is performed, echocardiography is used to confirm positioning of the plug within the myocardium and proper seal of the puncture site.

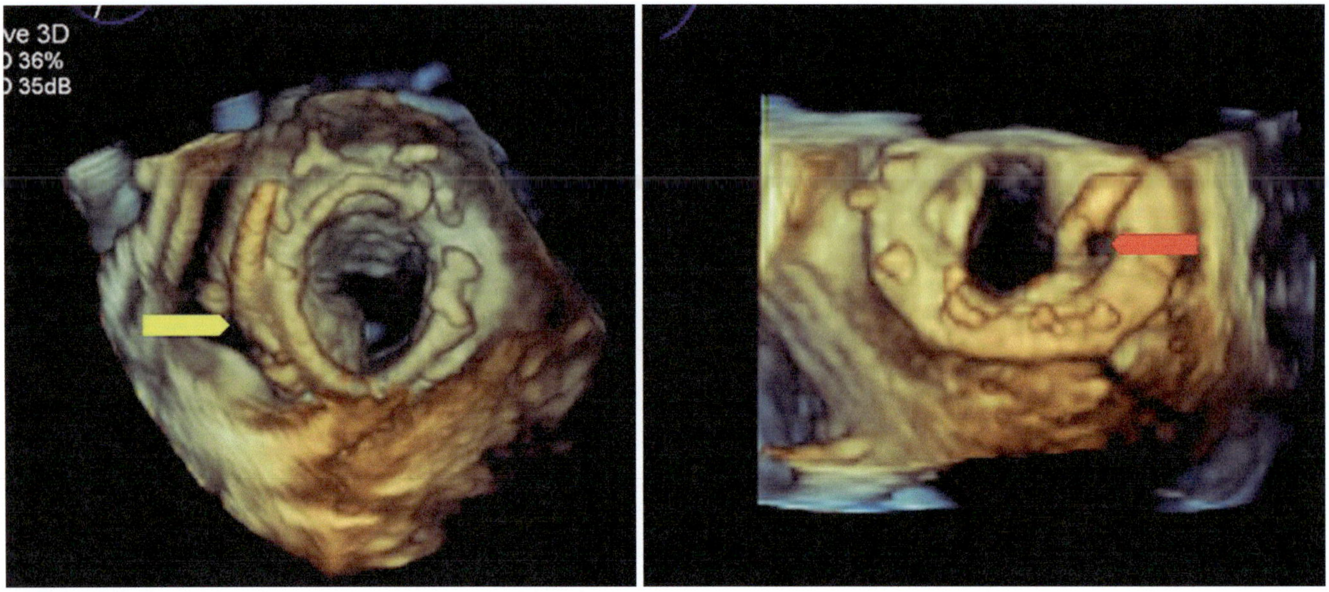

Fig. 11.16 Guidance of wire across PVL. 3D zoom mode showing clear depiction of the position of the wire as attempts to cross the PVL are in place. Left panel shows the wire crossing the PVL as desired (yellow arrow). Right panel shows the wire through the mitral valve (red arrow)

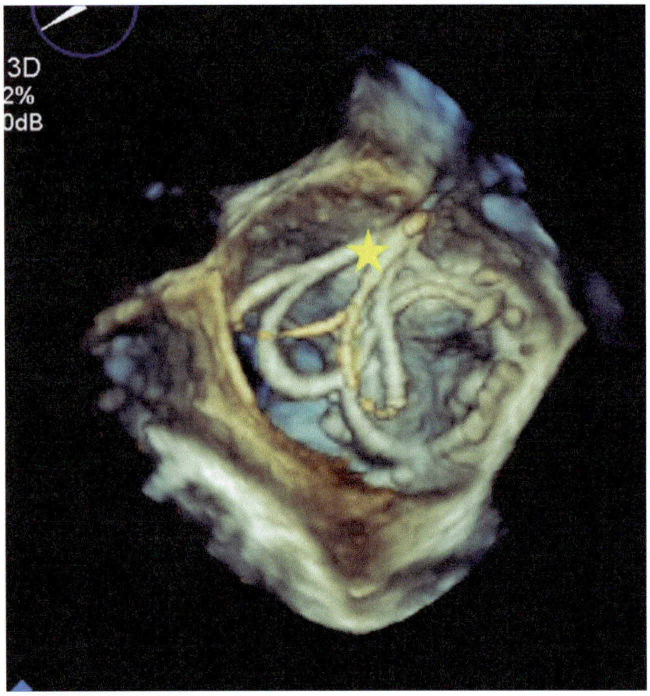

Fig. 11.17 Snaring and creation of a rail. After crossing the PVL (utilizing a trans-apical puncture) the wire is snared by a lasso catheter (asterisk) that is brought into the left atrium via a trans-septal approach

Echocardiographic monitoring during the procedure is also paramount for rapid assessment of any possible intra-procedural complications. Immediately following device deployment, the device may move or shift and may need to be recaptured and repositioned. Echocardiographic surveillance after device deployment, as described above, is essential for confirming proper device positioning after it has been released from the delivery system.

Device embolization is an infrequent complication that may occur if the device was undersized. This can be seen by echocardiography. However, if the device embolizes distally, it will be located utilizing fluoroscopy. Pericardial tamponade can occur at any stage of the procedure; real time echocardiographic monitoring allows for the rapid identification of pericardial fluid and cardiac compression such that immediate pericardiocentesis can be performed.

The Role of Transesophageal 3DE After Percutaneous Closure of Mitral PVL

Data regarding long term follow up after percutaneous closure of mitral PVL are somewhat limited as the technique is relatively new [51–53]. It appears that there is no significant progression of the treated PVL at a mid-term follow up of 90 days to a year. However, as data are still incomplete, patients who develop recurrent symptoms after a PVL percutaneous closure procedure should undergo thorough evaluation, including transesophageal 3DE. All devices previously placed should be identified, assessment of any interference between the devices and the prosthetic valve leaflets should be performed, and color Doppler interrogation looking for recurrent PVL at the same site or a new site should be meticulously carried out.

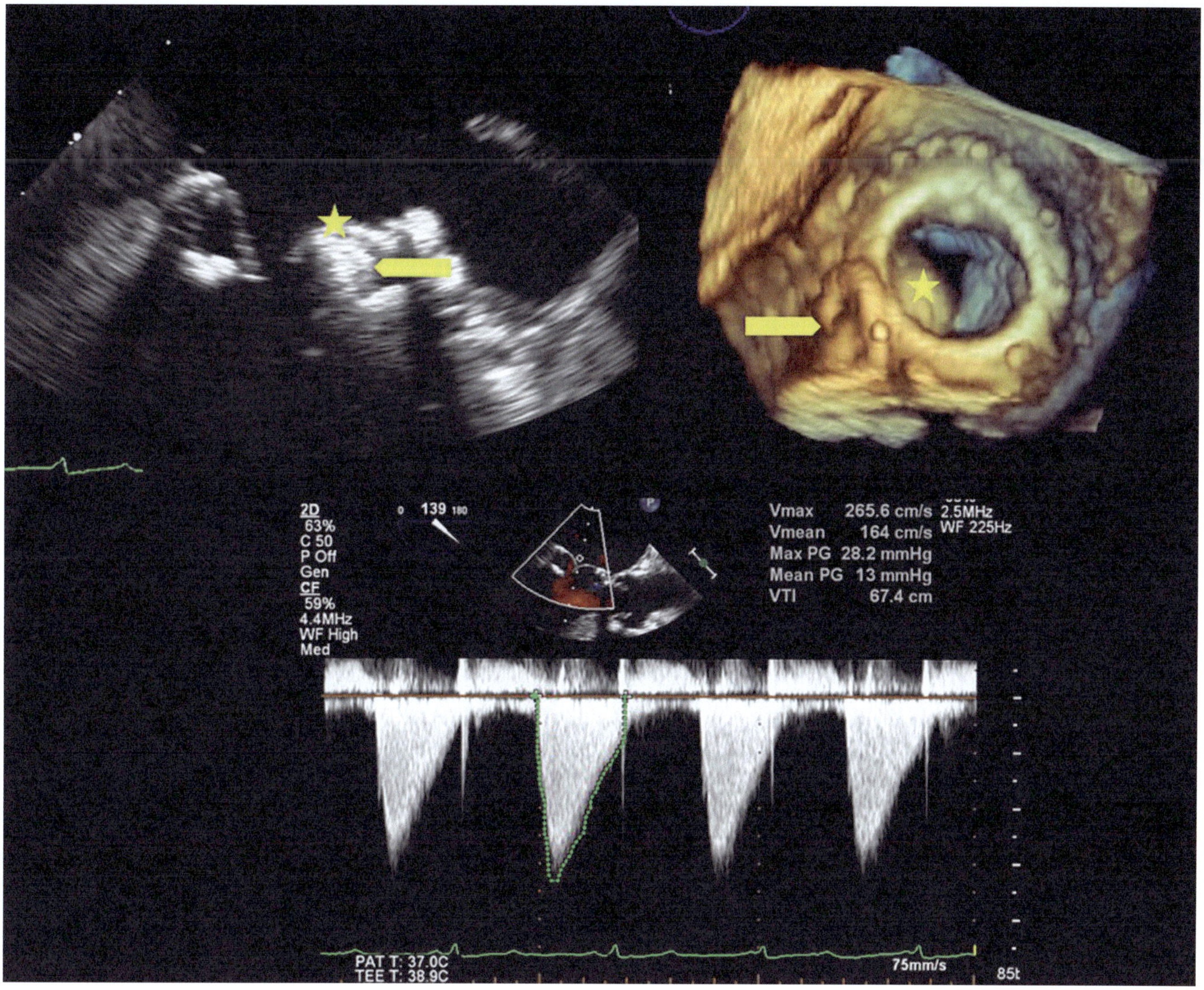

Fig. 11.18 Complication of device closure of PVL. A device was placed in a lateral PVL (arrow). However, the ventricular portion of the device was angulated in such a way that it interfered with the motion of one of the bioprosthetic leaflets (asterisk). This resulted in a significant gradient across the mitral valve (mean 13 mmHg) so the device had to be removed

Valve-in-Valve Procedure

Mitral valve replacement is considered the treatment of choice for selected patients with severe, symptomatic mitral valve disease which cannot be treated by mitral valve surgical repair or by balloon mitral valvuloplasty as discussed earlier in this chapter. Surgical valve replacement or repair usually requires open heart surgery.

The prosthetic valves used are less than optimal. There are two types of prosthetic mitral valves, namely, mechanical prosthetic valves and tissue (biological) prosthetic valves. The mechanical valves are durable and can potentially last for a lifetime. However, they are associated with clot formation and therefore require full, lifelong anticoagulation. The tissue valves may not require anticoagulation, however, tissue valves may degenerate over time. Over time, tissue prostheses can develop prosthetic valve dysfunction, which includes prosthesis stenosis, insufficiency or both. Interestingly, the degeneration rate is faster in children and young patients compared to adults [54, 55].

In today's practice, the tissue prostheses are used for patients in whom the use of anticoagulation is not desired and in those who have relatively short life expectancy (and therefore will be less likely to be exposed to valve degeneration and the need for another valve replacement). In these patients, the repeated valve replacement by open heart surgery is associated with high mortality and morbidity [56].

Mitral valve-in-valve implantation is a new transcatheter procedure that has been recently used in patients with degenerated tissue valve with significant stenosis and/or insufficiency [57, 58]. In selected patients this procedure may be an alternative to surgical valve re-replacement. At present, this procedure requires the presence of previously installed prosthetic mitral ring (either the ring of a prosthetic tissue valve or even a mitral annuloplasty ring [59]. This rigid ring will help maintain the deployment of the new prosthetic implanted valve. The procedure should be distinguished from transcatheter aortic valve replacement, in which the implanted prosthetic valve is deployed in the native aortic ring, and previous rigid ring installation is not required.

Mitral valve-in-valve procedure is no longer an investigational procedure. The percutaneous Sapien 3 valve (Edwards, Irvine, CA, USA), and the CoreValve Evolut R valve (Medtronic, Minneapolis, MN, USA) are now approved for valve-in-valve implantation to treat patients with malfunctioning prosthetic mitral tissue valves who are considered high risk for surgical mitral valve replacement.

Imaging During Valve-in-Valve Procedure

Cardiac imaging is critical in the pre-procedural evaluation, during the procedure and in the follow up after the procedure. Two-dimensional and 3DE are essential, and provide important information about the mitral valve anatomic pathology. Information about the size, shape and perimeter of the mitral annulus and the mitral orifice is crucial for the prosthesis selection. The leaflets thickness, motion, and the degree of mitral stenosis (including mitral valve area by planimetry and assessment of transmitral diastolic gradient) are all carefully measured.

The degree of mitral regurgitation, the magnitude, shape and location of the regurgitant orifice and the presence of paravalvular leak in addition to valvular regurgitation are checked. The degree of regurgitation is assessed by echocardiographic and Doppler techniques as suggested by the American Society of Echocardiography [60]. The echocardiographic examination also includes comprehensive evaluation of the other valves, the cardiac chambers and the great vessels. Finding of left atrial thrombus or other intracardiac masses may be a contraindication for the procedure, because of the risk of systemic embolism.

Cardiac computed tomography (CCT) can also provide high resolution imaging of the heart and other intrathoracic structures. Fusion imaging techniques are quite helpful. These sophisticated technologies are able to superimpose different imaging modalities and provide a simultaneous fluoroscopy and echocardiography (Echo Navigator), or Fluoroscopy and CCT (Cardiac Navigator; both by Philips, Best, The Netherlands). These technologies provide better orientation with accurate localization of cardiac structures, catheter and devices [61].

Procedural Guidance

The dysfunctional mitral tissue valve can be approached in an antegrade fashion. This is done after femoral vein cannulation, and transseptal puncture which is frequently performed under two- or 3DE surveillance. In cases of tissue mitral stenosis balloon dilatation may be performed.

Another approach utilizes transcutaneous left ventricular apical needle puncture with retrograde crossing of the dysfunctional bioprosthetic mitral valve.

Under fluoroscopic and transesophageal echocardiographic surveillance, the dysfunctional valve is crossed. A catheter with a collapsed new valve on a deflated balloon is then advanced and deployed across the dysfunctional mitral orifice. After echocardiography and fluoroscopy suggest proper positioning, the balloon is inflated, to expand the new valve. The new valve is thus supported in place by the dysfunctional prosthetic valve, which keeps it in a secure, stable position. Doppler echocardiography is used to evaluate the function of the newly implanted valve, and to ascertain no residual mitral regurgitation and no significant mitral stenosis.

A combined approach utilizing both transseptal and transapical access can also be used. The apical wire is used to snare the transseptal wire, creating a continuous rail from the left to the right heart. With the catheters across this rail, the apical wire helps to maintain the new valve in place. At the end of the procedure the iatrogenic puncture-holes are obliterated by closure devices. This includes closure of the interatrial septal puncture as well as the apical puncture. Echocardiography is used to confirm closure and rule out bleeding and new pericardial effusion.

Complications

Occasionally, mitral paravalvular leaks may be present. When present, they are obliterated by a closure device as outlined previously [62]. Complications include dehiscence of the new valve, which rarely may be completely detached such that it can move freely within the left atrium. Cardiac punctures or tears may result in cardiac tamponade. Large iatrogenic atrial septal defect may require device closure.

The steps of the valve-in-valve procedure are depicted in Figs. 11.19 and 11.20 and Video 11.11.

Percutaneous Mitral Balloon Valvuloplasty

Rheumatic mitral valve disease is a progressive life-long autoimmune-like disorder triggered by and further exacerbated by recurrent group A streptococcal infections (typically pharyngitis). Rheumatic mitral stenosis is the most common form of valvular disease in developing parts of the world. This is in contrast to, North America, Japan and Northern and Western Europe where rheumatic mitral stenosis is typically seen only among immigrants from countries where the disease is endemic. Percutaneous mitral balloon valvuloplasty is the preferred means of treating

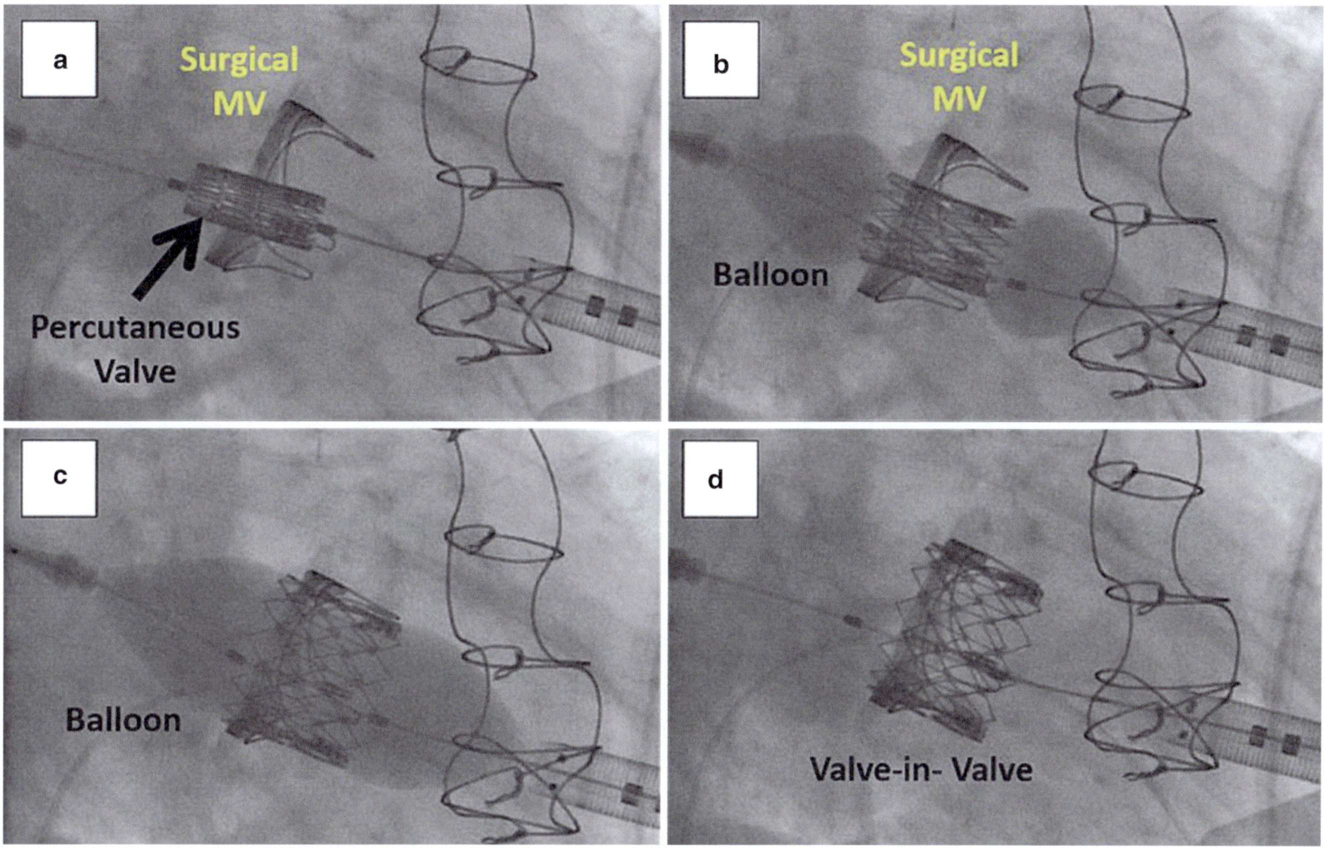

Fig. 11.19 Fluoroscopy of valve-in-valve procedure. (**a**–**d**) Demonstrate deployment steps of a percutaneous valve inside a failed surgical mitral bioprosthesis. *MV* mitral valve. Courtesy of Dr. Mathew Williams, NYU Langone Medical Center

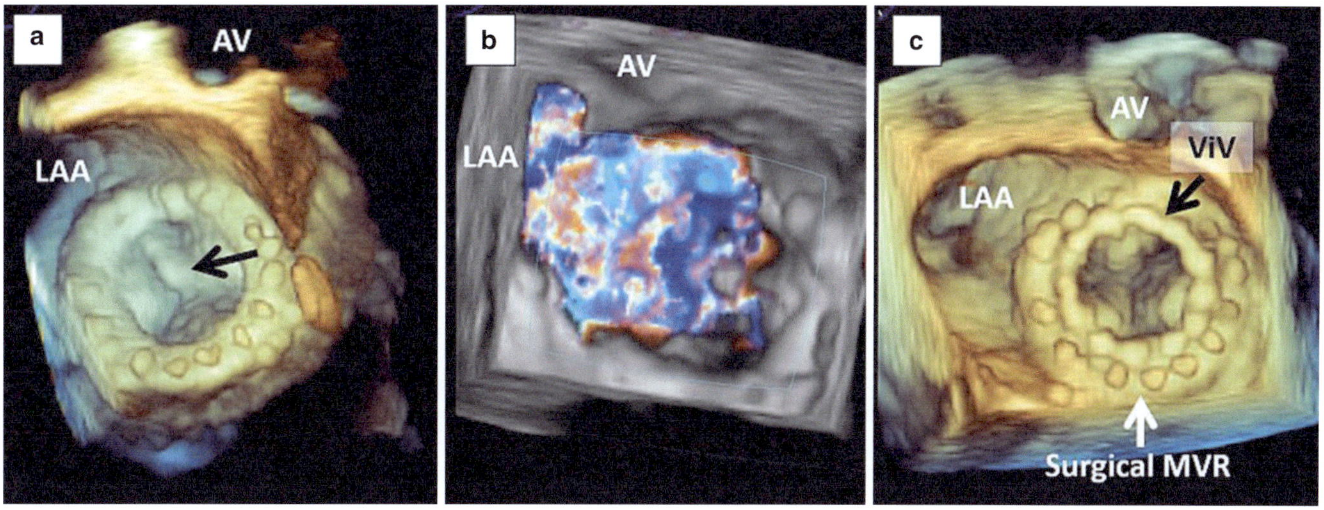

Fig. 11.20 3D TEE of valve-in-valve procedure. (**a**) Prior to valve-in-valve procedure, the left atrial aspect of a surgical bioprosthesis demonstrates a flail prosthetic leaflet (arrow). *AV* aortic valve, *LAA* left atrial appendage. (**b**) 3D TEE color Doppler demonstrates severe mitral regurgitation of the failed mitral bioprosthesis (seen in Panel **a**) from the left atrial perspective. (**c**) Post valve-in-valve (ViV) procedure, a well-positioned percutaneous valve (black arrow) is seen inside the surgical mitral valve prosthesis (MVR) (Video 11.11)

mitral stenosis in patients with suitable mitral valve anatomy [63].

Rheumatic mitral stenosis is notable for several 'firsts': it was the first valvular heart disease to be treated surgically (using initially commissurotomy and subsequently valve replacement with a prosthesis); it was the first heart disease to be diagnosed by echocardiography and it was the first acquired valvular disease to be treated with a percutaneous procedure.

In the 1980s, Kanji Inoue of Japan developed the ingenious balloon (Inoue balloon, Toray Industries (America) Inc., San Mateo, CA, USA) and the technique of percutaneous mitral balloon valvuloplasty (PMBV) which remains the preferred treatment for the relief of rheumatic mitral stenosis in eligible patients.

In the absence of contraindications, PMBV is recommended in following clinical scenarios:

1. Symptomatic patients with moderate or severe mitral stenosis.
2. In asymptomatic patients with moderate or severe mitral stenosis, PMBV is indicated when there is pulmonary artery systolic pressure is >50 mmHg at rest or >60 mmHg with exercise, or when there is new onset atrial fibrillation.
3. PMBV may also be considered in symptomatic patient with less than severe mitral stenosis (valve area >1.5 cm^2) when pulmonary artery systolic pressure greater >60 mmHg, pulmonary artery wedge pressure >25 mmHg, or mean mitral valve gradient >15 mmHg during exercise.

Contraindication for PMBV include: the presence of an intracardiac thrombus, a high mitral valve Wilkins score (greater than or equal to 10; see below) and more than moderate mitral regurgitation.

Two- and 3DE imaging is important for the following: confirmation of the diagnosis of mitral stenosis, possible refinement of the mitral valve Wilkins score and guidance of the PMBV procedure itself.

Diagnosis of Mitral Stenosis

Mitral valve planimetry by 3D transthoracic or transesophageal echocardiography may be considered the gold standard for calculating the mitral valve area. The mitral valve has a funnel shape; its narrowest portion is located in the left ventricle in a plane that is not typically parallel with standard imaging planes of two-dimensional echocardiography. Using multiplane reconstructions techniques of 3DE data sets, one can measure the area of at the very tip of the mitral valve funnel. Additionally, the mitral valve area can be measured on zoomed *en face* views of the mitral valve either semi-quantitatively using either calibrated grids or direct on-image planimetry (Fig. 11.21 and Video 11.12).

Furthermore, transesophageal 3DE may also refine the mitral valve Wilkins score, an essential prerequisite for PMBV. The Wilkins score was originally developed in the late 1980s using two-dimensional transthoracic echocardiography; the score takes into account mitral leaflet thickness, calcifications and mobility as well as the thickness of the subvalvular apparatus. Each of the four categories is graded on a scale ranging from 0 (normal) to 4 (severely abnormal). A normal mitral valve has a score of 0. The most diseased valve has a score is 16.

Typically, PMBV is contraindicated when mitral score is >10. High Wilkins scores are characterized by marked thickening, calcifications and immobility of mitral valve leaflets and well as significant thickening of the mitral subvalvular apparatus. The higher the Wilkins scores, the higher the risk of mitral valve leaflet tear during PMBV; a tear may lead to significant de novo mitral regurgitation. Transesophageal 3DE may enhance the Wilkins scoring through better visualization of leaflet mobility and the details of the subvalvular mitral apparatus compared to two-dimensional echocardiography.

Transesophageal 3DE may also be used to guide PMBV procedure. After venous access is obtained (typically using the femoral vein), transseptal puncture of the interatrial septum is performed under echocardiographic guidance. Thereafter, a deflated Inoue valvuloplasty balloon is threaded into the left atrium through the transseptal puncture. Using 3DE *en face* views of the mitral valve, precisely guide positioning of the valvuloplasty balloon across the mitral valve can be achieved. Once placed across the mitral valve, the balloon is inflated under 3D TEE and fluoroscopy guidance in order to separate the mitral valve leaflets along the commissures (Fig. 11.22 and Video 11.13).

PMBV outcomes are assessed in real time by transesophageal 3DE; *en face* views of the left ventricular side of the mitral valve are particularly important. A controlled commissural tear which enlarges the mitral valve orifice and does not create de novo or worsens pre-existing mitral regurgitation is the preferred outcome. Complications of the procedure, namely a non-commissural leaflet tear often leading to significant de novo acute mitral regurgitation, can also be well visualized by transesophageal 3DE (Fig. 11.23 and Video 11.14).

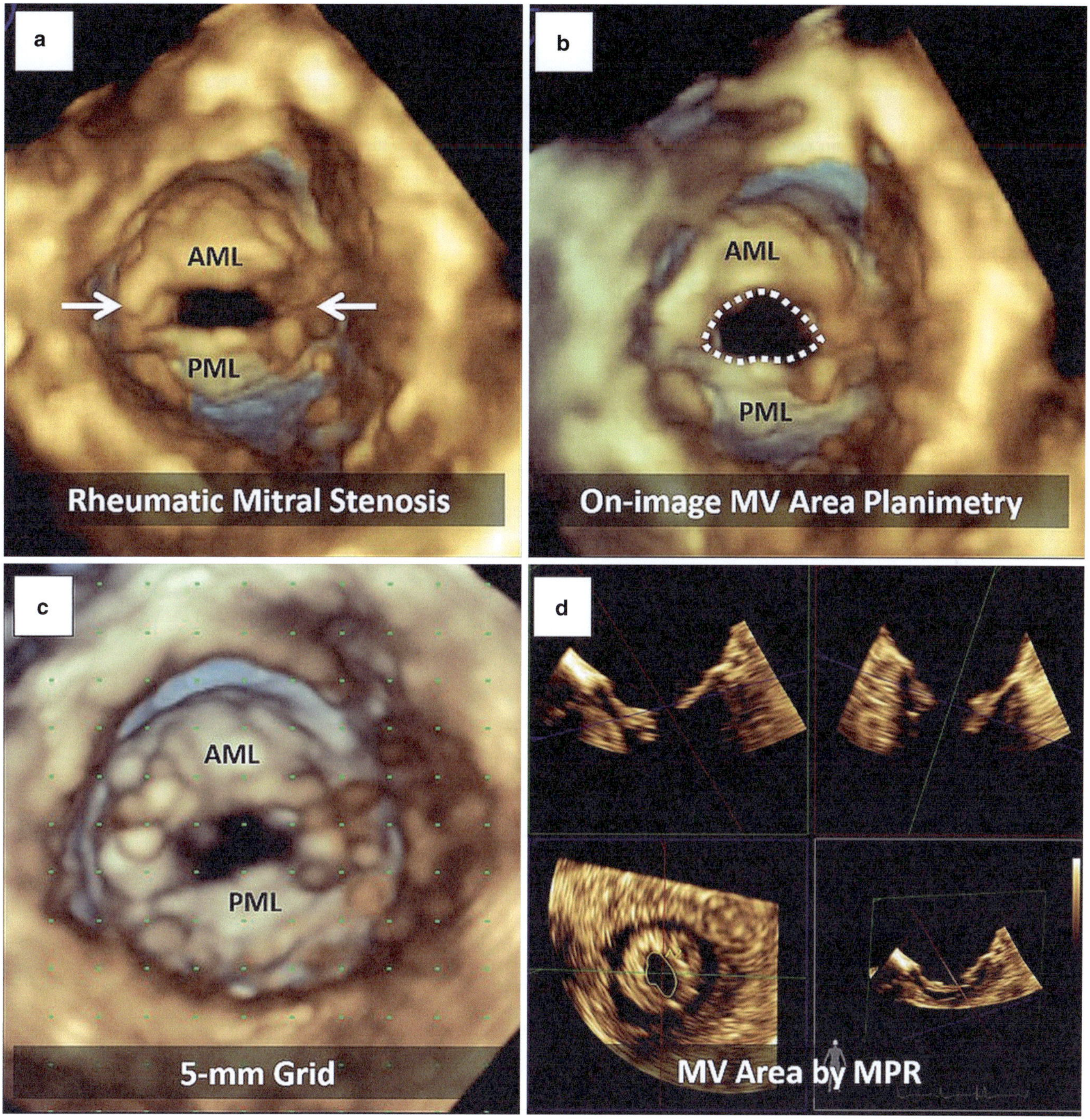

Fig. 11.21 Mitral valve area by 3D echocardiography in rheumatic mitral stenosis. (**a**) Left ventricular appearance of commissural fusions (arrows) in a patient with severe rheumatic mitral stenosis (Video 11.12). (**b–d**) Demonstrates various 3D echocardiographic methods of calculating anatomic mitral valve area. *MPR* multi-plane reconstruction, *MV* mitral valve

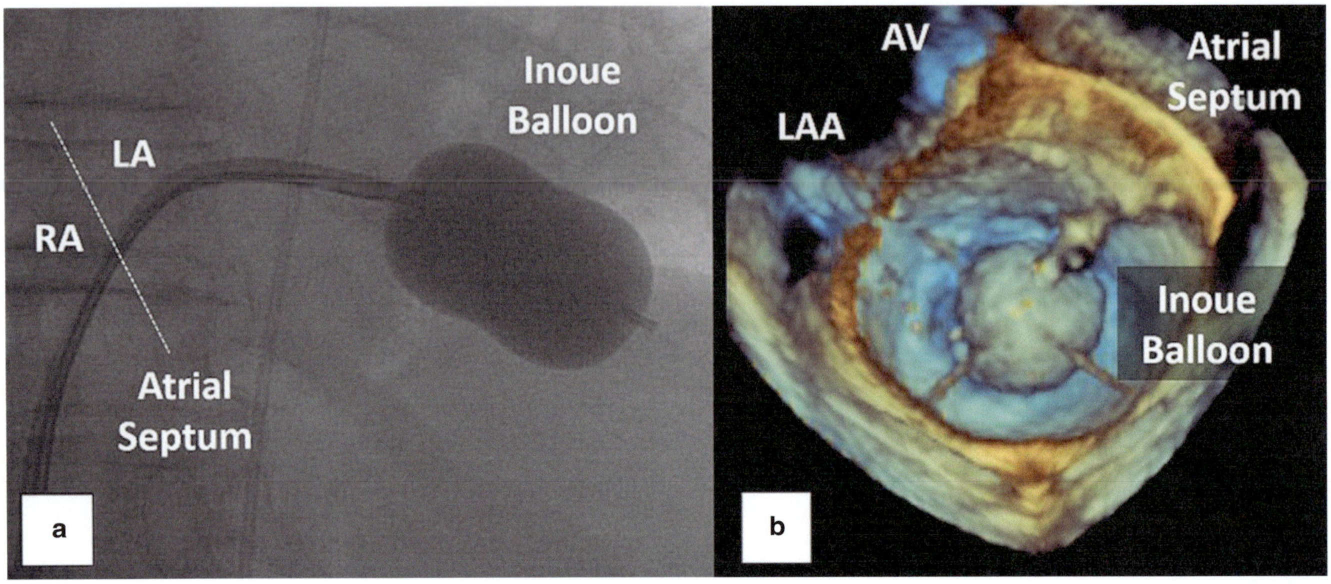

Fig. 11.22 Percutaneous mitral balloon valvuloplasty (PMBV) procedure. (**a**) A fully inflated Inoue balloon is seen across the mitral valve on fluoroscopy during PMBV. *LA* left atrium, *RA* right atrium. (**b**) 3D TEE from the left atrial perspective is used to guide placement of the Inoue balloon inside the stenotic mitral valve. *AV* aortic valve, *LAA* left atrial appendage (Video 11.13)

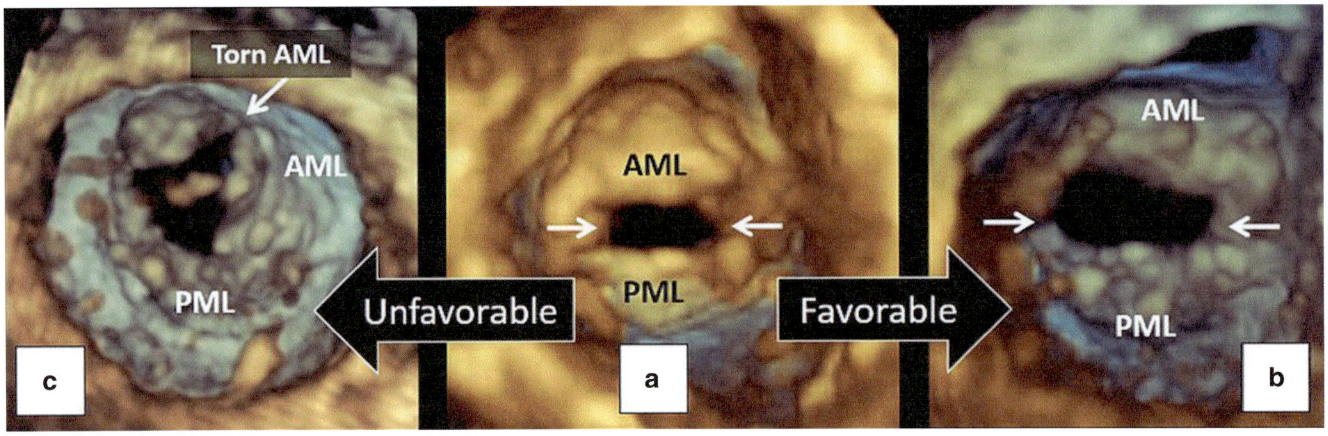

Fig. 11.23 Outcomes of PMBV procedure. (**a**) Left ventricular aspect of a severely stenotic rheumatic mitral valve prior to PMBV. (**b**) Favorable outcome of PMBV is characterized by an increase in mitral valve area due to commissural separation. (**c**) Torn mitral leaflets is a potential complication of PMBV which may lead to severe mitral regurgitation (Video 11.14)

References

1. Lang RM, Tsang W, Weinert L, Mor-Avi V, Chandra S. Valvular heart disease. The value of 3-dimensional echocardiography. J Am Coll Cardiol. 2011;58(19):1933–44.
2. Benenstein R, Saric M. Mitral valve prolapse: role of 3D echocardiography in diagnosis. Curr Opin Cardiol. 2012;27:465–76.
3. Piazza N, Bleiziffer S, Brockmann G, Hendrick R, Deutsch MA, Opitz A, et al. Transcatheter aortic valve implantation for failing surgical aortic bioprosthetic valve: from concept to clinical application and evaluation (part 1). JACC Cardiovasc Interv. 2011;4(7):721–32.
4. Williams, JB. Improved bottle stopper. US patent 19,323; 1858.
5. Alton ME, Pasierski TJ, Orsinelli DA, Eaton GM, Pearson AC. Comparison of transthoracic and transesophageal echocardiography in evaluation of 47 Starr-Edwards prosthetic valves. J Am Coll Cardiol. 1992;20(7):1503–11.
6. Wernly JA, Crawford MH. Choosing a prosthetic heart valve. Cardiol Clin. 1991;9(2):329–38.
7. Gott VL, Alejo DE, Cameron DE. Mechanical heart valves: 50 years of evolution. Ann Thorac Surg. 2003;76(6):S2230–9.
8. Flachskampf FA, O'Shea JP, Griffin BP, Guerrero L, Weyman AE, Thomas JD. Patterns of normal transvalvular regurgitation in mechanical valve prostheses. J Am Coll Cardiol. 1991;18(6):1493–8.
9. Zilla P, Brink J, Human P, Bezuidenhout D. Prosthetic heart valves: catering for the few. Biomaterials. 2008;29(4):385–406.
10. van den Brink RB, Visser CA, Basart DC, Düren DR, de Jong AP, Dunning AJ. Comparison of transthoracic and transesophageal color Doppler flow imaging in patients with mechanical prostheses in the mitral valve position. Am J Cardiol. 1989;63(20):1471–4.

11. DeWall RA, Qasim N, Carr L. Evolution of mechanical heart valves. Ann Thorac Surg. 2000;69(5):1612–21.
12. Vongpatanasin W, Hillis LD, Lange RA. Prosthetic heart valves. N Engl J Med. 1996;335(6):407–16.
13. jörk VO. The pyrolytic carbon occluder for the Björk-Shiley tilting disc valve prosthesis. Scand J Thorac Cardiovasc Surg. 1972;6:109–13.
14. Taams MA, Gussenhoven EJ, Cahalan MK, Roelandt JR, van Herwerden LA, The HK, et al. Transesophageal Doppler color flow imaging in the detection of native and Björk-Shiley mitral valve regurgitation. J Am Coll Cardiol. 1989;13(1):95–9.
15. Butany J, Ahluwalia MS, Munroe C, Fayet C, Ahn C, Blit P, et al. Mechanical heart valve prostheses: identification and evaluation. Cardiovasc Pathol. 2003;12(1):1–22.
16. Yoganathan AP, He Z, Casey Jones S. Fluid mechanics of heart valves. Annu Rev Biomed Eng. 2004;6:331–62.
17. Butchart EG, Li HH, Payne N, Buchan K, Grunkemeier GL. Twenty years' experience with the Medtronic Hall valve. J Thorac Cardiovasc Surg. 2001;121(6):1090–100.
18. Edwards MS, Russell GB, Edwards AF, Hammon JW Jr, Cordell AR, Kon ND. Results of valve replacement with Omniscience mechanical prostheses. Ann Thorac Surg. 2002;74(3):665–70.
19. Misawa Y, Taguchi M, Aizawa K, Takahashi H, Sakano Y, Kaminishi Y, et al. Twenty-two year experience with the Omniscience prosthetic heart valve. ASAIO J. 2004;50(6):606–10.
20. Czer L, Matloff J, Chaux A, Derobertis M, Yoganathan A, Gray RJ. A 6-year experience with the St. Jude Medical valve: hemodynamic performance, surgical results, biocompatibility, and follow-up. J Am Coll Cardiol. 1985;6(4):904–12.
21. Bryan AJ, Rogers CA, Bayliss K, Wild J, Angelini GD. Prospective randomized comparison of CarboMedics and St. Jude Medical bileaflet mechanical heart valve prostheses: ten-year follow-up. J Thorac Cardiovasc Surg. 2007;133(3):614–22.
22. Johnston RT, Weerasena NA, Butterfield M, Fisher J, Spyt TJ. Carbomedics and St. Jude Medical bileaflet valves: an in vitro and in vivo comparison. Eur J Cardiothorac Surg. 1992;6(5):267–71.
23. Harrison EC, Rashtian MY, Allen DT, Yoganathan AP, Rahimtoola SH. An emergency physician's guide to prosthetic heart valves: identification and hemodynamic function. Ann Emerg Med. 1988;17(3):194–200.
24. Jamieson WR, Munro AI, Miyagishima RT, Allen P, Burr LH, Tyers GF. Carpentier-Edwards standard porcine bioprosthesis: clinical performance to seventeen years. Ann Thorac Surg. 1995;60(4):999–1006; discussion 1007.
25. Pibarot P, Dumesnil JG. Doppler echocardiographic evaluation of prosthetic valve function. Heart. 2012;98(1):69–78.
26. Maisano F, Caldarola A, Blasio A, De Bonis M, La Canna G, Alfieri O. Midterm results of edge-to-edge mitral valve repair without annuloplasty. J Thorac Cardiovasc Surg. 2003;126(6):1987–97.
27. Fedak PW, McCarthy PM, Bonow RO. Evolving concepts and technologies in mitral valve repair. Circulation. 2008;117(7):963–74.
28. Maisano F, Redaelli A, Pennati G, Fumero R, Torracca L, Alfieri O. The effects of double orifice valve repair for mitral regurgitation: a 3D computational model. Eur J Cardiothorac Surg. 1999;15(4):419–25.
29. Alfieri O, Denni P. Alfieri stitch and its impact on mitral clip. Eur J Cardiothorac Surg. 2011;39:807–8.
30. Maisano F, La Canna G, Colombo A, Alfieri O. The evolution from surgery to percutaneous mitral valve interventions: the role of edge to edge technique. J Am Coll Cardiol. 2011;58:2174–82.
31. Alfieri O, Maisano F, De Bonis M, Stefano PL, Torracca L, Oppizzi M, et al. The double orifice technique in mitral valve repair: a simple solution for complex problem. J Thorac Cardiovasc Surg. 2001;122:674–81.
32. Feldman T, Foster E, Glower DD, Kar S, Rinaldi MJ, Fail PS, et al. for the EVEREST II investigators. Percutaneous repair or surgery for mitral regurgitation. N Engl J Med. 2011;364:1395–406.
33. Maisano F, Franzen O, Baldus S, Schäfer U, Hausleiter J, Butter C, et al. Percutaneous mitral valve interventions in the real world: early and 1-year results from the ACCESS EU, a prospective multicenter, non-randomized post approval study of the MitraClip therapy in Europe. J Am Coll Cardiol. 2013;62(12):1052–61.
34. Wiebe J, Franke J, Lubos E, Boekstegers P, Schillinger W, Ouarrak T, et al. German transcatheter mitral valve interventions (TRAMI) investigators. Percutaneous mitral valve repair with the MitraClip system according to the predicted risk by the logistic EuroSCORE: preliminary results from the German Transcatheter Mitral Valve Interventions (TRAMI) registry. Catheter Cadiovasc Interv. 2014;84:591–8.
35. Biner S, Perk G, Kar S, Rafique AM, Slater J, Shiota T, et al. Utility of combined two-dimensional and three-dimensional transesophageal imaging for catheter based mitral valve clip repair of mitral regurgitation. J Am Soc Echocardiogr. 2011;24:611–7.
36. Faletra F, Grimaldi A, Pasotti E, Klimusina J, Evangelista A, Alfieri O, et al. Real time 3-dimenasional transesophageal echocardiography during double percutaneous mitral edge-to-edge procedure. JACC Cardiovasc Imaging. 2009;2:1031–3.
37. Altiok E, Hamada S, Brehmer K, Kuhr K, Reith S, Becker M, et al. Analysis of procedural effect of percutaneous edge-to-edge mitral valve repair by 2D and 3D echocardiography. Circ Cardiovasc Imaging. 2012;5(6):748–55.
38. Ruiz CE, Kliger C, Perk G, Maisano F, Cabalka AK, Landzberg M, et al. Transcatheter therapies for the treatment of valvular and paravalvular regurgitation in acquired and congenital valvular heart disease. J Am Coll Cardiol. 2015;66:169–83.
39. Duncan BF, McCarthy PM, Kruse J, Andrei AC, Li Z, Russell HM, et al. Paravalvular regurgitation after conventional aortic and mitral valve replacement: a benchmark for alternative approaches. J Thorac Cardiovasc Surg. 2015;150(4):860–8.
40. Ionescu A, Fraser AG, Butchart EG. Prevalence and clinical significance of incidental paraprosthetic valvar regurgitation: a prospective study using transoesophageal echocardiography. Heart. 2003;89:1316–21.
41. Shimokawa T, Kasegawa H, Katayama Y, Matsuyama S, Manabe S, Tabata M, et al. Mechanism of recurrent regurgitation after valve repair for prolapsed mitral valve disease. Ann Thorac Surg. 2011;91:1433–8.
42. Hwang HY, Choi JW, Kim HK, Kim KH, Kim KB, Ahn H. Paravalvular leak after mitral valve replacement: 20-year follow-up. Ann Thorac Surg. 2015;100(4):1347–52.
43. Zoghbi WA, Chambers JB, Dumesnil JG, Foster E, Gottdiener JS, Grayburn PA, et al. Recommendations for evaluation of prosthetic valves with echocardiography and Doppler ultrasound: a report from the American Society of Echocardiography's Guidelines and Standards Committee and the Task Force on Prosthetic Valves. J Am Soc Echocardiogr. 2009;22(9):975–1014; quiz 1082–4.
44. Kronzon I, Sugeng L, Perk G, Hirsh D, Weinert L, Garcia Fernandez MA, et al. Real-time 3-dimensional transesophageal echocardiography in the evaluation of post-operative mitral annuloplasty ring and prosthetic valve dehiscence. J Am Coll Cardiol. 2009;53(17):1543–7.
45. Spoon DB, Malouf JF, Spoon JN, Nkomo VT, Sorajja P, Mankad SV, et al. Mitral paravalvular leak: description and assessment of a novel anatomical method of localization. JACC Cardiovasc Imaging. 2013;6(11):1212–4.
46. Singh P, Manda J, Hsiung MC, Mehta A, Kesanolla SK, Nanda NC, et al. Live/real time three-dimensional transesophageal echocardiographic evaluation of mitral and aortic valve prosthetic paravalvular regurgitation. Echocardiography. 2009;26(8):980–7.
47. Franco E, Almería C, de Agustín JA, Arreo Del Val V, Gómez de Diego JJ, García Fernández MÁ, et al. Three-dimensional color Doppler transesophageal echocardiography for mitral paravalvular leak quantification and evaluation of percutaneous closure success. J Am Soc Echocardiogr. 2014;27(11):1153–63.

48. Biner S, Kar S, Siegel RJ, Rafique A, Shiota T. Value of color Doppler three-dimensional transesophageal echocardiography in the percutaneous closure of mitral prosthesis paravalvular leak. Am J Cardiol. 2010;105(7):984–9.
49. Eleid MF, Cabalka AK, Malouf JF, Sanon S, Hagler DJ, Rihal CS. Techniques and outcomes for the treatment of paravalvular leak. Circ Cardiovasc Interv. 2015;8(8):e001945.
50. Kumar R, Jelnin V, Kliger C, Ruiz CE. Percutaneous paravalvular leak closure. Cardiol Clin. 2013;31(3):431–40.
51. Smolka G, Pysz P, Jasiński M, Roleder T, Peszek-Przybyła E, Ochała A, et al. Multiplug paravalvular leak closure using Amplatzer Vascular Plugs III: a prospective registry. Catheter Cardiovasc Interv. 2016;87(3):478–87.
52. Taramasso M, Maisano F, Latib A, Denti P, Guidotti A, Sticchi A, et al. Conventional surgery and transcatheter closure via surgical transapical approach for paravalvular leak repair in high-risk patients: results from a single-centre experience. Eur Heart J Cardiovasc Imaging. 2014;15(10):1161–7.
53. Cruz-Gonzalez I, Rama-Merchan JC, Arribas-Jimenez A, Rodriguez-Collado J, Martin-Moreiras J, Cascon-Bueno M, et al. Paravalvular leak closure with the Amplatzer Vascular Plug III device: immediate and short-term results. Rev Esp Cardiol (Engl Ed). 2014;67(8):608–14.
54. Hartz RS, Fisher EB, Finkelmeier B, DeBoer A, Sanders JH Jr, Moran JM, et al. An eight-year experience with porcine bioprosthetic cardiac valves. J Thorac Cardiovasc Surg. 1986;91:910–7.
55. Holper K, Wottke M, Lewe T, Baumer L, Meisner H, Paek SU, et al. Bioprosthetic and mechanical valves in the elderly: benefits and risks. Ann Thorac Surg. 1995;60(2 Suppl):S443–6.
56. Echevarria JR, Bernal JM, Rabasa JM, Morales D, Revilla Y, Revuelta JM, et al. Reoperation for bioprosthesis valve dysfunction. A decade of clinical experience. Eur J Cardiothorac Surg. 1991;5:523–6.
57. Webb JG, Wood DA, Ye J, Gurvitch R, Masson JB, Rodés-Cabau J, et al. Transcatheter valve-in-valve implantation for failed bioprosthesis heart valves. Circulation. 2010;121:1848–57.
58. Cheung AW, Gurvitch R, Ye J, Wood D, Lichtenstein SV, Thompson C, et al. Transcatheter transapical mitral valve-in-valve implantation for failed surgical prosthetic valve. J Thorac Cardiovasc Surg. 2011;141(3):711–5.
59. Shuto T, Kondo N, Dori Y, Koomalsingh KJ, Glatz AC, Rome JJ, et al. Percutaneous, transvenous Melody valve-in-valve in ring procedure for mitral valve replacement. J Am Coll Cardiol. 2011;58:2475–80.
60. Zoghbi WA, Chambers JB, Dumesnil JG, Foster E, Gottdiener JS, Grayburn PA, et al. Recommendations for evaluation of prosthetic valves with echocardiography and doppler ultrasound: a report From the American Society of Echocardiography's Guidelines and Standards Committee and the Task Force on Prosthetic Valves, developed in conjunction with the American College of Cardiology Cardiovascular Imaging Committee, Cardiac Imaging Committee of the American Heart Association, the European Association of Echocardiography, a registered branch of the European Society of Cardiology, the Japanese Society of Echocardiography and the Canadian Society of Echocardiography, endorsed by the American College of Cardiology Foundation, American Heart Association, European Association of Echocardiography, a registered branch of the European Society of Cardiology, the Japanese Society of Echocardiography, and Canadian Society of Echocardiography. J Am Soc Echocardiogr. 2009;22:975–1014.
61. Kliger C, Angulo R, Maranan L, Kumar R, Jelnin V, Kronzon I, et al. Percutaneous repair of failed mitral valve prosthesis: simultaneous closure of mitral paravalvular leaks and transcatheter mitral valve implantation—single-centre experience. EuroIntervention. 2015;10(11):1336–45.
62. Kliger C, Jelnin V, Sharma S, Panagopoulos G, Einhorn BN, Kumar R, et al. Angiography-fluoroscopy fusion imaging for percutaneous transapical access. JACC Cardiovasc Imaging. 2014;7(2):169–77.
63. Saric M, Benenstein R. Chapter 28: Three-dimensional echocardiographic guidance of percutaneous procedures. In: Nanda N, editor. Comprehensive textbook of echocardiography. 1st ed. New Delhi: Jaypee Brothers Medical Publisher; 2013.

The Normal Aortic Valve Complex

12

Rebecca T. Hahn

Abstract

The aortic valve (AV) complex involves the left ventricular outflow tract (LVOT), aortic annulus, AV leaflets, and the aortic root (to the sinotubular junction). Three-dimensional imaging studies have advanced our current understanding of the AV anatomy. Acquisition protocols and standardized imaging planes allow for more accurate descriptions of anatomy.

Keywords

Left ventricular outflow tract · Aortic valve
Aortic annulus · Three-dimensional imaging

Introduction

The aortic valve (AV) complex involves the left ventricular outflow tract (LVOT), aortic annulus, AV leaflets, and the aortic root (to the sinotubular junction). Knowledge of normal anatomy is essential to the understanding of both congenital and pathologic states. Three-dimensional echocardiography (3DE) has been integral to our understanding of the normal AV anatomy. Recent imaging studies have advanced our current understanding of the AV complex anatomy: the shape of the left ventricular outflow tract (LVOT) and annulus [1–7], aortic root [8, 9] and AV leaflets [10, 11]. Planimetry of the AV and LVOT area by 3DE methods has been shown to be accurate and reproducible [12–14] and compare favorably to multislice computed tomography [15, 16]. This chapter will describe 3DE acquisition protocols and imaging displays for the AV complex as well as describe the normal anatomy of this cardiac structure.

Electronic Supplementary Material The online version of this chapter (https://doi.org/10.1007/978-3-030-14032-8_12) contains supplementary material, which is available to authorized users.

R. T. Hahn (✉)
Department of Cardiology/Structural Heart and Valve Center, Columbia University Medical Center, New York, NY, USA
e-mail: rth2@columbia.edu

Aortic Valve Complex Functional Anatomy

The AV is a more complex functional unit than just its three semilunar cusps may suggest. The aortic root, including the Valsalva sinuses and the fibrous interleaflet triangles, provides support for the three leaflets that are semilunar in shape (also called cusps). The cusps are inserted into a fibrous connective sleeve attached to the aorta media above the Valsalva sinuses (the sinotubular junction). Therefore, both the Valsalva sinuses and the sino-tubular junction are integral part of the AV complex and any significant dilatation of these anatomical structure will result in AV regurgitation. The cusps are named left coronary, right coronary and non-coronary according to the location of coronary artery ostia. They are thicker towards the free margin and meet at three commissures that are equally spaced along the circumference of the sleeve at the supra-aortic ridge. In normal AV, the cusps are symmetrical, mobile, and free at the commissures, with equal overlap on closure. The basal attachments of the aortic cusps extend within the LV, below the anatomic ventriculo-aortic junction. Therefore, the actual anatomic aortic annulus is not the ring projected at the most basal leaflet insertion—as conventionally defined and measured by the various imaging modalities—but a crown-like 3D structure [17].

The aortic root is centrally located within the heart and it has complex spatial relationships with the surrounding cardiac structures. The aortic root lies on the right and posterior to the sub-pulmonary infundibulum. Approximately, one third of the ventriculo-anatomic junction (in correspondence to the non-coronary and left cusps) is in continuity with the anterior mitral leaflet via a fibrous structure (aortic-mitral curtain). The remaining two thirds of its circumference are muscular and correspond the interventricular septum [18].

L. P. Badano et al. (eds.), *Textbook of Three-Dimensional Echocardiography*, https://doi.org/10.1007/978-3-030-14032-8_12

The size of aortic annulus and root is influenced by inner pressure and changes dynamically during the cardiac cycle by 12% and 16%, respectively [7, 19, 20]. Therefore, timing of measurements will be highly relevant to compare measurements performed with different imaging techniques.

3DE Aortic Complex Acquisition Modes

Qualitatively adequate 3DE data sets of the AV using transthoracic approaches are more difficult to obtain than of the atrio-ventricular valves. Particularly in healthy subjects and in patients with functional aortic regurgitation, because, due to suboptimal spatial resolution of current transthoracic 3DE technology, the thin AV cusps result in frequent drop-out artifacts. On the other end, heavily calcified aortic annuli and/or cusps can also present drop-outs artifacts because of shadowing. However, the continuous improvement of 3DE transducer technology and of the acquisition techniques have greatly increased the feasibility of good quality 3DE rendering of the AV using the transthoracic approaches. As with any other cardiac structure, there is no *a priori* preferred transthoracic approach from which to acquire the data sets of the AV. The acoustic window (either parasternal, apical or subcostal) which provides the best definition of the AV throughout the cardiac cycle in that particular patient is usually taken. The acquisition volume should be the smallest able to encompass the AV and, at least partially, some surrounding structures (e.g. the anterior leaflet of the mitral valve and the interatrial septum) in order to allow proper anatomical orientation of the AV. To properly size the acquisition volume, two orthogonal tomographic planes (one showing the axial and azimuthal dimensions and the other one showing the elevations) are conventionally used (Fig. 12.1, Video 12.1). For the morphological analysis of AV, the acquisition modes may be real-time or multi-beat (either full-volume or zoom modes) (see also Chap. 2) and the temporal resolution should be between 10 and 15 vps.

Transesophageal 3DE acquisition from mid-esophageal probe position provides superior spatial resolution and image quality for AV and LVOT assessment and should be used when a definite diagnosis cannot be made by transthoracic 3DE. Inter-commissural distance and free leaflet edge lengths, which can be measured by 3DE, are used to choose the tube graft size in valve-sparing root operations [19, 20].

The superior spatial and temporal resolution of real-time 3DE narrow sector acquisitions permits accurate diagnoses of complex pathologies while preserving optimal temporal resolution. This acquisition mode is typically most useful for intra-procedural monitoring since the easy display method and high temporal resolution is ideal for accurate and rapid decision-making in this setting. However, the narrow volume of acquisition rarely captures the entire aortic valve complex and thus limits its use for comprehensive evaluation of AV and aortic root morphology. Depending on the anatomy of interest, the initial 2D image of the aortic valve at the 60° mid-esophageal, short-axis AV view or the 120° mid-esophageal, long-axis AV view can be used (Figs. 12.1 and

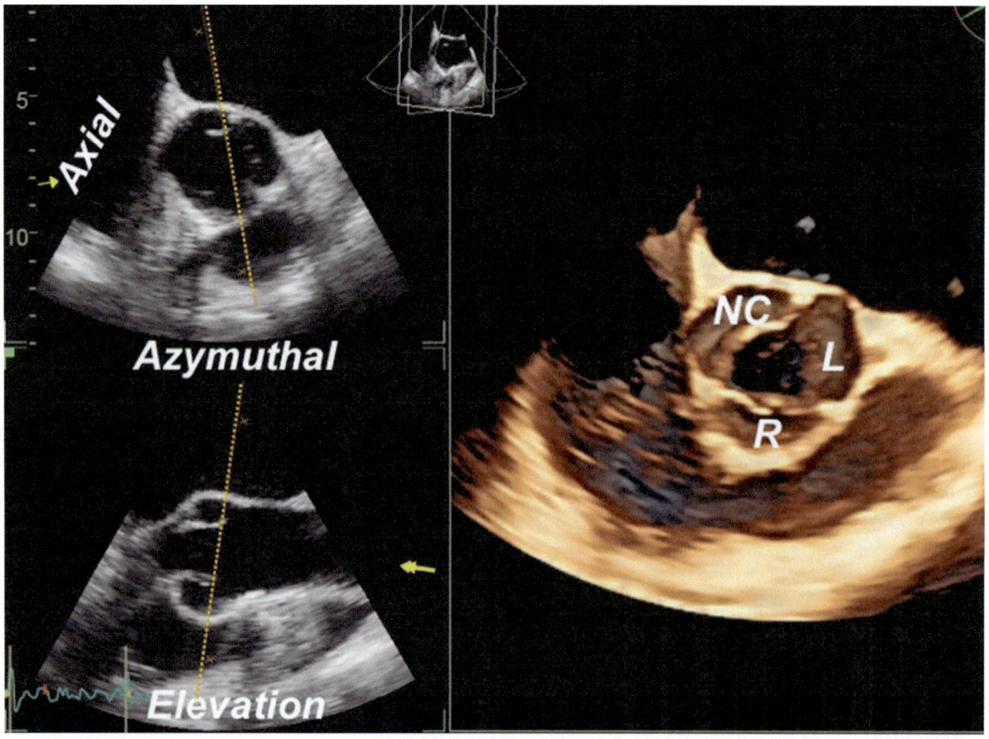

Fig. 12.1 Zoom acquisition of the aortic valve by transesophageal three-dimensional echocardiography (Video 12.1). Using two orthogonal two-dimensional views (upper and lower left panels), the region of interest is positioned in order to include the whole aortic valve in the data set. The volume renderd aortic valve (right panel) is shown from the aortic perspective as indicated by the position of the cropping plane (dotted orange line) and the yellow arrow in the left lower panel. *L* left coronary cusp, *NC* non-coronary cusp, *R* right coronary cusp

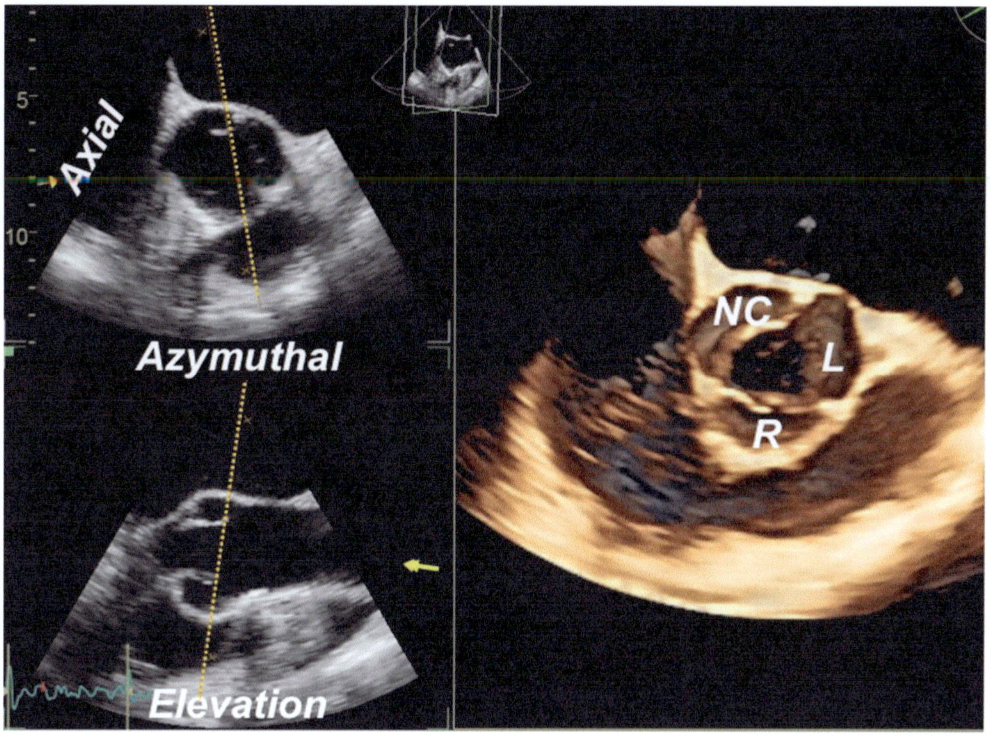

Fig. 12.2 Zoom acquisition of the aortic valve by transesophageal three-dimensional echocardiography using the long-axis view as reference plane (upper left panel). *L* left coronary cusp, *NC* non-coronary cusp, *R* right coronary cusp

12.2). After the two-dimensional image is optimized, the size of the acquisition volume itself can be changed; narrowing the volume will increase both temporal and spatial resolution while increasing the volume will reduce them. In general, the primary use of the real-time acquisition is to acquire 3DE data sets in patients in whom the multibeat acquisition is not possible (arrhythmias, non-cooperative patients, etc.) and to monitor interventional procedures.

The "zoom" mode allows acquisition of a focused, wide sector view of the AV complex. To optimize the acquisition volume, simultaneous biplane imaging should be used to center the AV complex in both the reference view and elevation planes. The user-defined ROI for the 3D acquisition should cover the regions of interest in both planes and throughout the cardiac cycle (Figs. 12.1 and 12.2). Prior to acquisition, the AV can be viewed either just as a volume rendered display, as simultaneous volume rendering with multiple orthogonal two-dimensional imaging planes. The latter is particularly useful to check the image quality of the entire data set, to check for the absence of artifacts and to ensure that all the structures of interest have been imaged. 3DE data sets in zoom mode can be obtained either in single- or multi-beat. Because the volume of acquisition is typically larger than the real-time mode, the volume rate and temporal resolution may be lower when the zoom mode data set is acquired in single-beat. In general (but depending on the heart rate), a minimum volume rate of 10 volume per second (Hz) is desirable in order to clearly distinguish systolic and diastolic components of the cardiac cycle. If area or perimeter measurements of the annulus or LVOT are being performed, it is of upmost importance that the 3DE data set is free of stiching artifacts since even small artifacts could significantly affect the measurements (see also Chap. 2).

Once a wide-angle acquisition 3DE dataset of the AV complex is obtained the AV is displayed in the surgical view with the right coronary cusp located inferiorly (far field), regardless of whether the aortic or the LV outflow tract perspective is presented (Fig. 12.3). To manipulate the volume for measurements, vendor-specific tools may be used to crop the volume in any plane. Measurements directly on the 3DE volume can be performed, but should always be verified using reconstructed tomographic cut planes to be sure that structures at a different depth are not mistakenly measured.

Full Volume, gated 3DE acquisition yields the largest 3DE data sets. However, to obtain adequate temporal resolution a gated, multi-beat acquisition is required. This acquisition modality is typically used to obtain larger data sets that allow measurement of additional parameters of the AV complex such as the distance of the coronary ostia from the hinge points of the aortic cusps, size and geometry of the Valsalva sinuses etc. (Fig. 12.4, Video 12.2).

Transesophgeal color Doppler 3DE imaging may be useful for quantifying the severity of aortic regurgitation. High volume rates (15–25 Hz) are even more important for these measurements. Although 3DE color flow Doppler ideally should be acquired with a single beat acquisition, now

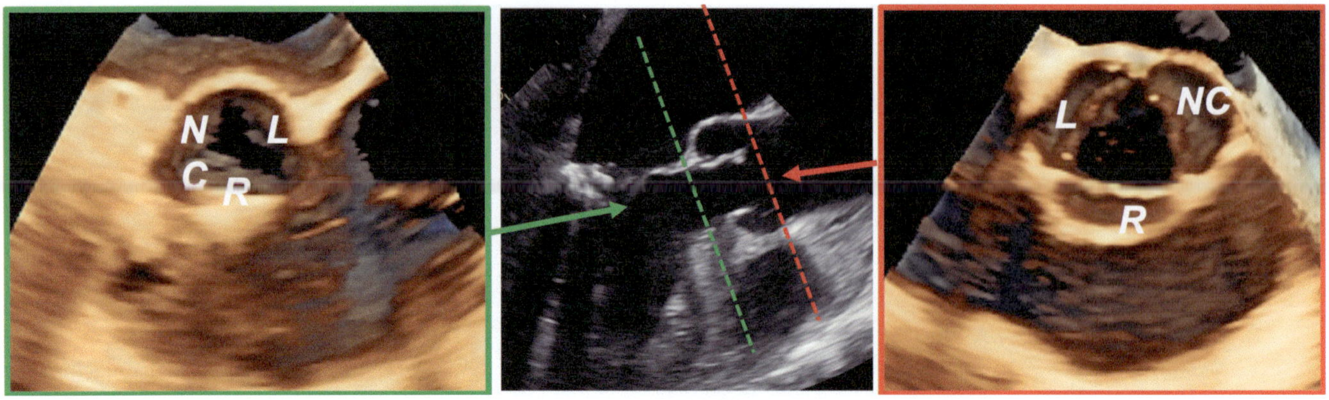

Fig. 12.3 Volume rendering of the aortic valve acquired using the transesophageal approach. *En face* views from the ventricular (left panel) and aortic perspective (right panel). The position of the corresponding cropping planes (dotted colored lines) and view directions (coored arrows) are shown on the two-dimensional view (central panel). *L* left coronary cusp, *NC* non-coronary cusp, *R* right coronary cusp

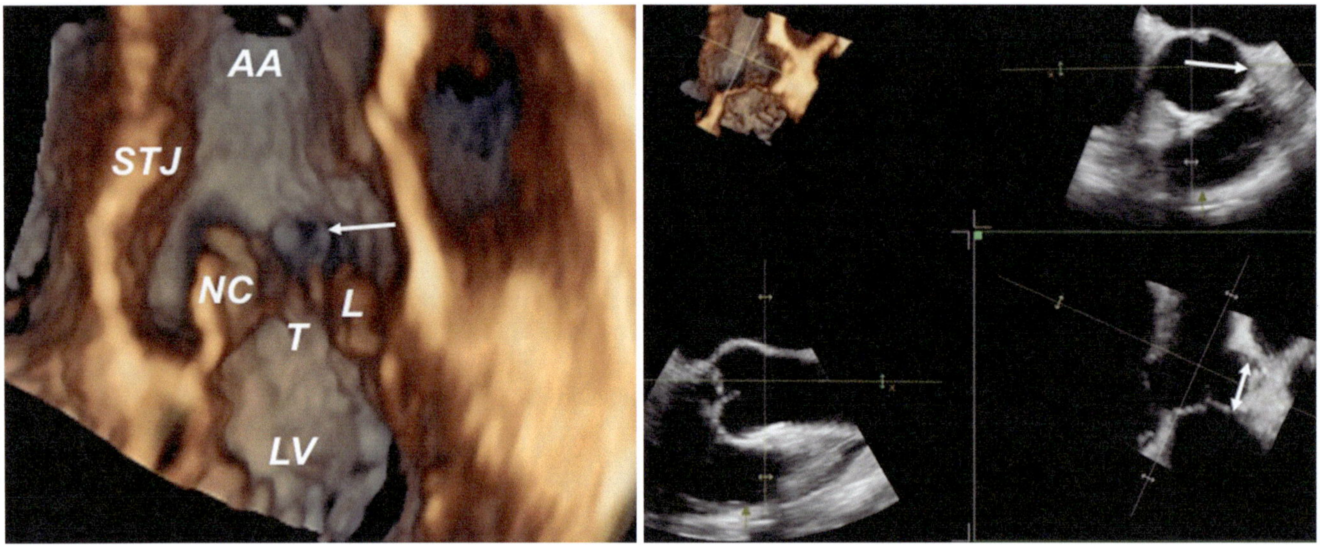

Fig. 12.4 Anatomical study of the aortic complex and measurement of the aortic cusp hinge point to coronary ostia distance using a data set acquired using the transesophageal approach. Left panel (Video 12.2), volume rendering of the aortic complex with the left main coronary ostia (white arrow). Right panel, the data set is sliced at the level of the left main coronary ostial (green line in the right upper quadrant) shown by the white arrow in order to obtain a longitudinal cut plane showing the left main and the aortic cusps. The linear distance is shown by the white double arrow line. *AA* ascending aorta, *L* left coronary cusp, *LV* left ventricle, *NC* non-coronary cusp, *STJ* sino-tubular junction, *T* intercusp triangle

possible with some ultrasound vendors, other vendors require multi-beat, gated acquisitions. Cropping of 3DE color Doppler data sets is determined mainly by the analysis required. For regurgitant jets, planimetry of short-axis view of the jet at the level of the vena contracta are feasible for native regurgitant valve disease [21–24] as well as following surgical [25] or transcatheter interventions [26]. Identification of the vena contracta of the regurgitant jet can be obtained using either a selective slicing of the jet or using the multislice display modality. The former method requires using two orthogonal long-axis views of the jet to identify its neck that will be sliced by a third, transversal cut plane to display the cross sectional area, of the vena contracta. The vena contracta is then directly planimetered from this short-axis view (Fig. 12.5).

Calculation of regurgitant volume in native valvular disease using the proximal isovelocity surface area (PISA) method [27] has known technical limitations, primarily the geometric assumptions of PISA shape required to calculate effective regurgitant orifice area. Multiple studies have vali-

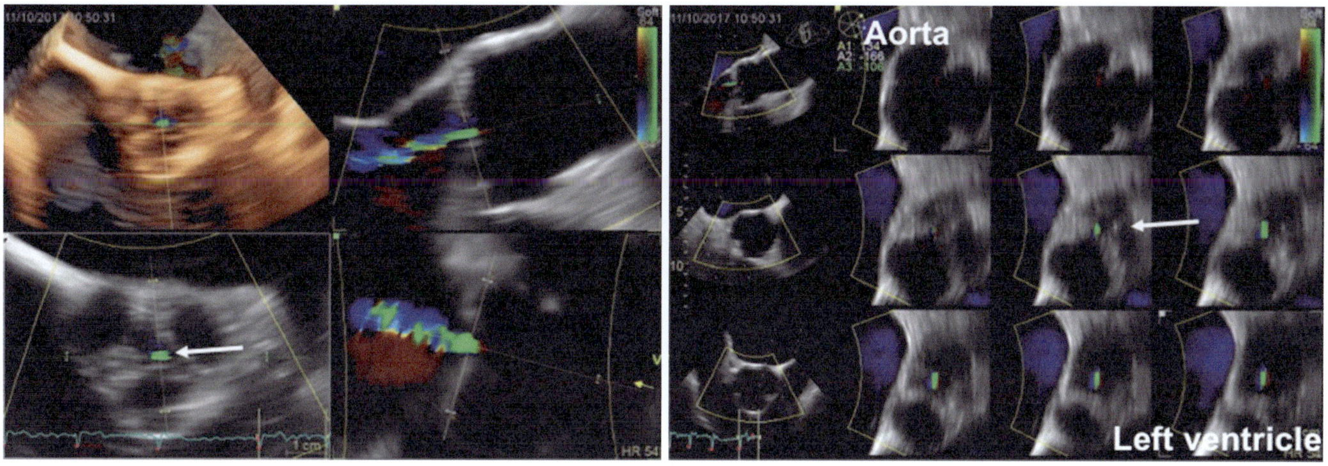

Fig. 12.5 Planimetry of the area of the vena contracta using 3DE color Doppler data set. Left panel, the longitudinal (upper, right quadrant) and coronal (lower, right quadrant) planes are placed in the center of the jet, oriented parallel to the jet direction. A trasversal cut plane (lower, left quadrant) has been positioned at the level of the vena contracta, perpendicular to longitudinal and coronal planes. The area of the vena contracta can be planimeterd on the transversal cut plane. Right panel, multislice display of the proximal portion of the regurgitant jet obtained by placing the most proximal cut plane (Aorta) in the aortic root at the lel of the PISA and the most distal (Left ventricle) in the outflow tract, immediately below the vena contracta. Both planes are oriented perpendicular to the direction of the jet in order to obtain a series of transversal cut planes of the proximal part of the jet. The one with the smallest color Dopple area will be the actual vena contracta

dated the use of single-beat 3DE color Doppler imaging allows the direct measurement of PISA without geometric assumptions for aortic, mitral and tricuspid regurgitation assessment [28–31].

Newer methods of determining relative flows within the heart make use of the velocity and direction of flow information inherent in color Doppler. Off-line software has been developed which uses two-dimensional color Doppler images to determine the velocity, flow rate and flow volume in any given region of the heart [32]. Extension of this technology to 3DE color Doppler volume sets is now possible and allows rapid, accurate and reproducible quantitation of relative stroke volumes [33, 34]. Thavendiranathan et al. [34] used the velocity information encoded in the volume color Doppler data, targeting the appropriate region of interest by using the simultaneous 3DE imaging of the mitral annulus and LVOT. Color Doppler velocity is multiplied by a known area of this cross-section (a voxel area) and the resulting spatially averaged flow rates used to generate flow-time curves that resemble those obtained by magnetic resonance imaging. The temporal integration of the flow-time curve generates the stroke volume. There was excellent correlation between the automated measured mitral inflow and aortic stroke volumes, and magnetic resonance imaging stroke volume ($r = 0.91$, 95% CI, 0.83–0.95, and $r = 0.93$, 95% CI, 0.87–0.96, respectively, $P < 0.001$) and very low interobserver variability. Automation of the measurement process allowed calculations of mitral inflow and aortic stroke volumes to be performed very rapidly. This methodology will likely become the standard for measurement of regurgitant volumes in the future (Fig. 12.6).

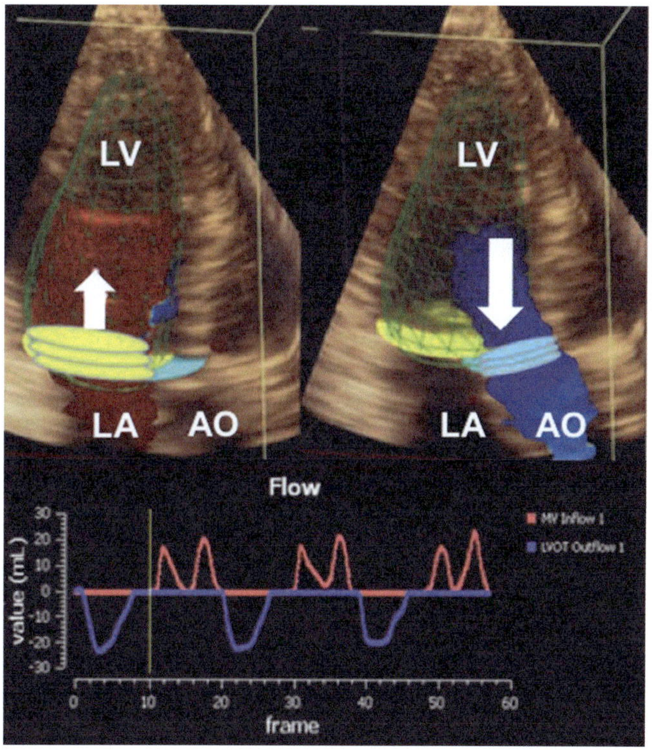

Fig. 12.6 Three-dimensional echocardiography color Doppler measurement of aortic regurgitant volume using the automated cardiac flow measurement. Left panel, measurement of the mitral inflow volume during the diastolic period. Right panel, measurmeent of the left ventricular outflow volume during the systolic period. The regions of interest are shown in yellow (mitral annulus) and blue (aortic annulus). Flow volume is obtained by the temporal integration of the flow volume rate obtained by spatial profile integration of the velocity profile. *AO* aorta, *LA* left atrium, *LV* left ventricle

Anatomy of the Normal Aortic Valve Complex

Left Ventricular Outflow Tract

Although echocardiographic guidelines recommend a single diameter measurement of the LVOT to calculate aortic valve area [35], 3DE measurements of the LVOT area and perimeter may be more reproducible and accurate [5, 36]. Numerous studies have shown that the LVOT is often elliptical [13, 36, 37] and the long-axis (sagittal) plane diameter derived from two-dimensional echocardiography may underestimate the true LVOT dimensions (Fig. 12.7, Right panel). Compared to computed tomography, two-dimensional echocardiography may underestimate LVOT area and thus aortic valve area [38, 39]. Studies comparing conventional two-dimensional linear measurements to 3DE planimetry of LVOT area show a 10–23% underestimation of cardiac output [40] or effective aortic orifice area using both transthoracic and transesophageal two-dimensional echocardiography modalities [5, 6] On the other hand, other studies suggest that computed tomography overestimates LVOT area compared to magnetic resonance imaging or 3DE [41]. Thresholds for excess mortality differ however between imaging modalities: aortic valve area ≤1.0 cm^2 for echocardiographic methods versus ≤1.2 cm^2 for computed tomography methods [42]. Thus in the presence of strong outcomes data using conventional two-dimensional methods of measuring LVOT and calculating AVA [42, 43], we may continue to use a single sagittal plane LVOT dimension to calculate AVA as per the recent AHA/ACC guidelines [44].

Aortic Annulus

The aortic annulus is the plane at the level of the hinge-point (lowest attachment site) of the three cusps [18]. There is no anatomic demarcation between the LVOT and the annulus which is why it is referred to as a virtual annulus. Between these leaflet hingepoints and scalloped aortic leaflets, is the fibrous tissue of the interleaflet triangles (Fig. 12.4, Left panel). Measurement of the diameter of this virtual ring is thus difficult because: (1) with a tricuspid aortic valve, any long-axis plane bisecting a cusp hinge-point on one side, will not image a hinge-point on the other side but rather a region of fibrous tissue between the scalloped cusps; (2) the annulus is often asymmetric and oval with annular diameters largest in the coronal plane and shortest in the sagittal plane [2, 4, 45] (Fig. 12.7, Right panel).

The traditional measurement for sizing the annulus has been the systolic diameter in the long-axis (sagittal) plane. Multiple imaging studies however have documented not only the oval shape, but the dynamic anatomy of the aortic annulus [2, 7, 45, 46]. Because of the dynamic nature of the annular shape which becomes less elliptical (i.e. more round) in systole [7, 46] measurements in the long-axis plane in this part of the cardiac cycle typically yield a larger measurement than in diastole. The correct long-axis imaging window should bisect the maximum diameter of the aorta and simultaneous multiplane imaging using 3D technology allows imaging of both the short-axis and long-axis planes to ensure imaging of the correct plane (Fig. 12.7). The right coronary cusp hinge-point is imaged anteriorly, and the fibrous interleaflet trigone posteriorly. Because there is no anatomic

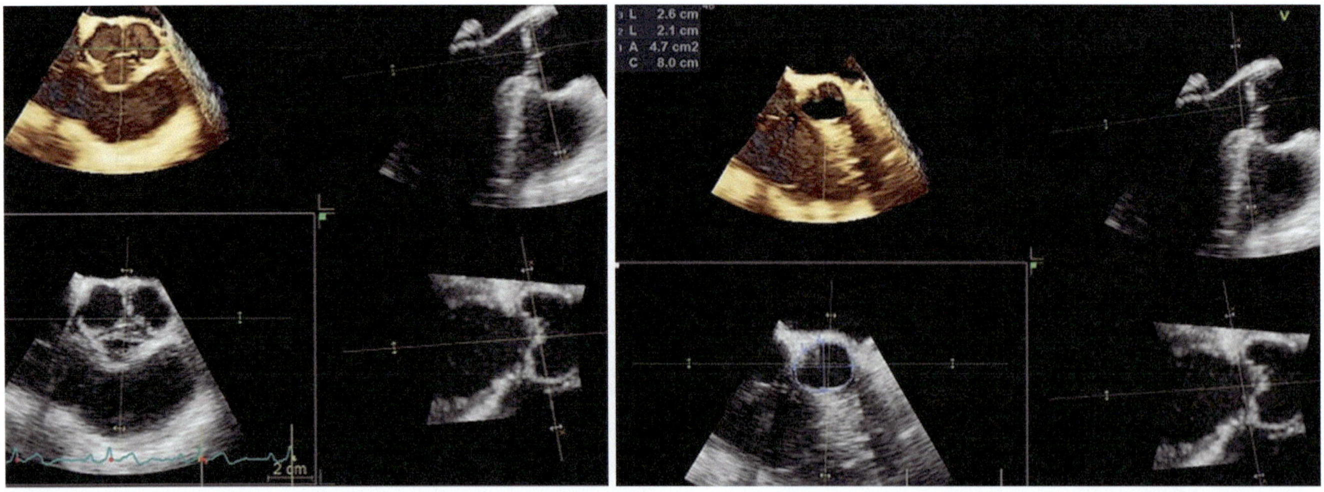

Fig. 12.7 Direct planimetry of aortic annulus. Left panel, after having selected the correct frame, the sagittal (right, upper box) and the coronal (left, lower box) axes are aligned in the center of the aortic valve, parallel to the long axis of the aorta. The transversal cut plane is at the level of the aortic cusps to allow to rotate the data set in order to aling it in the center of the right coronary aortic cusp and in the commissure between the left and the non-coronary cusps. Right panel, The transversal cut plane is moved towards the left ventricle at the level of the hinge point of insertion of the cusps to see the aortic annulus en-face and planimeter its contour. Notice that, even in normal subjects, the shape of the aortic annulus is oval and the anterior-posterior diameter (L2) is significantly shorter than the transverse one (L1)

marker for the virtual annular plane within the interleaflet trigone, the correct annular diameter is measured by assuming the virtual annulus is perpendicular to the long-axis of the aorta. Calcification of the scalloped lines of leaflet attachment within the sinuses (and defining the borders of the interleaflet trigone) should not be mistaken for the hinge-point of the aortic cusps.

Multi-slice computed tomography (MSCT) annular perimeter or area measurements have repeatedly been shown to improve the accuracy of transcatheter aortic valve implant (TAVI) sizing algorithms, [2–4, 7, 45, 47, 48] and has become the standard imaging modality to measure the aortic annulus and characterize the landing zone. 3DE however can also accurately measure the annular aortic annulus [41, 49–53]. 3DE measurements of aortic annulus geometry are highly reproducible and compare favorably to MSCT [16, 49]. Altiok et al showed high agreement between transesophageal 3DE and MSCT for coronal diameters (23.60 ± 1.89 vs. 23.46 ± 2.07 mm) and sagittal diameters (22.19 ± 1.96 vs. 22.27 ± 2.01 mm) with high correlation [2]. Khalique et al. showed similar high agreement and correlation with transesophageal 3DE and MSCT measurements of annulus perimeter (74.8 ± 7.0 vs. 75.8 ± 6.6 mm) and area (434.9 ± 81.3 vs. 442.8 ± 78.9) [16]. Advantages of the 3DE technique include real time imaging of the hinge-points and elimination of hand-tracing errors of direct planimetry, and averaging measurements from multiple cardiac cycles. Although echocardiographic imaging (whether two- or 3DE) may be limited by blooming and side-lobe artifacts as well as acoustic drop-out, MSCT also suffers from artifacts generated by annular and valve calcification. Consequently, these techniques require expertise and practice. Advances in software packages are currently being developed which should automate many of the steps outlined above and reduce interobserver variability of echocardiographic measurement of the aortic annulus.

Currently two manual methods can be used; direct planimetry of the annulus, and indirect planimetry. In the setting of a non-calcified valve with minimal acoustic shadowing or noise, either can be used, however in the setting of a calcified aortic valve apparatus, direct planimetry has its limitations. The first uses commercially available software packages which manipulates the 3D volume using a multi-planar approach (Fig. 12.7). The short-axis (transverse) annular plane is obtained using the orthogonal long-axis views (sagittal and coronal) as a guide and the annulus is directly planimetered for area, or the minimum and maximum diameters can be measured [54]. Using this method, Jilaihawi et al showed that transesophageal 3DE significantly underestimated MSCT measurements of the aortic annulus but was better than 2D TEE in predicting significant paravalvular regurgitation [15]. The second method of measuring the annulus avoids direct planimetry of the transverse plane thus eliminating hand-tracing errors and allowing the use of anatomic structures in the long-axis planes to identify the annulus. This indirect planimetry method uses vendor-specific software originally designed for the mitral valve (Fig. 12.8), and "tricks" the program into measuring the aortic annulus instead of the mitral annulus [49]. This method has inherent advantages over direct planimetry: using the long-axis planes allows the use of anatomic structures such as the mitral leaflet, aortic root and septum, to help define the annulus; acoustic noise (side-lobes) are identifiable on the long-axis images and not mistaken for the annulus; acoustic shadowing can be managed using the short-axis annular plane as a reference and making sure to keep the annular points consistent with their neighboring points and reflective of the shape of the "virtual" annulus. Validation of this method has been described above with no significant difference in area and perimeter measurements compared to MSCT [16].

Current automated measurements of the annulus are in development but require further validation (Fig. 12.9). These automated packages should help reduce variability and improve accuracy for annular measurements.

Aortic Valve Leaflets

The AV is a semilunar valve with three cusps located close to the center of the heart. The aortic cusps are identified by the presence or absence of the coronary arteries arising from the corresponding sinuses of Valsalva (left coronary, right coronary and non-coronary cusps). These three semilunar cusps form part of the sinuses of Valsalva, and the fibrous interleaflet triangles. Each semilunar cusp is attached to the aortic wall in a curved manner, with the basal attachment located in the left ventricle below the anatomic ventriculo-aortic junction and the distal attachment at the sinotubular junction [17]. The sinuses of Valsalva and the sinotubular junction are integral parts of the valvular mechanism, such that any significant dilatation of these structures will result in aortic valve incompetence. Overall, when tracking the curved path of the aortic leaflet insertion points, the 3D spatial configuration of the AV resembles a crown [18]

The primary pitfall of 3D imaging the aortic valve and the aortic valve complex is the orientation of this structure relative to the insonation beam. From the mid-esophageal views, portions of the AV complex in the sagittal plane are perpendicular to the insonation beam and thus have good axial resolution. However, the coronal plane is parallel to the insonation beam and thus, the inferior lateral resolution of this plane are difficult to overcome. This issue is even more prominent for the AV leaflets which are not only thinner and more mobile than other AV complex structures, but large portions of the leaflets are again parallel to the insonation beam particularly in diastole, resulting in large areas of echo-dropout

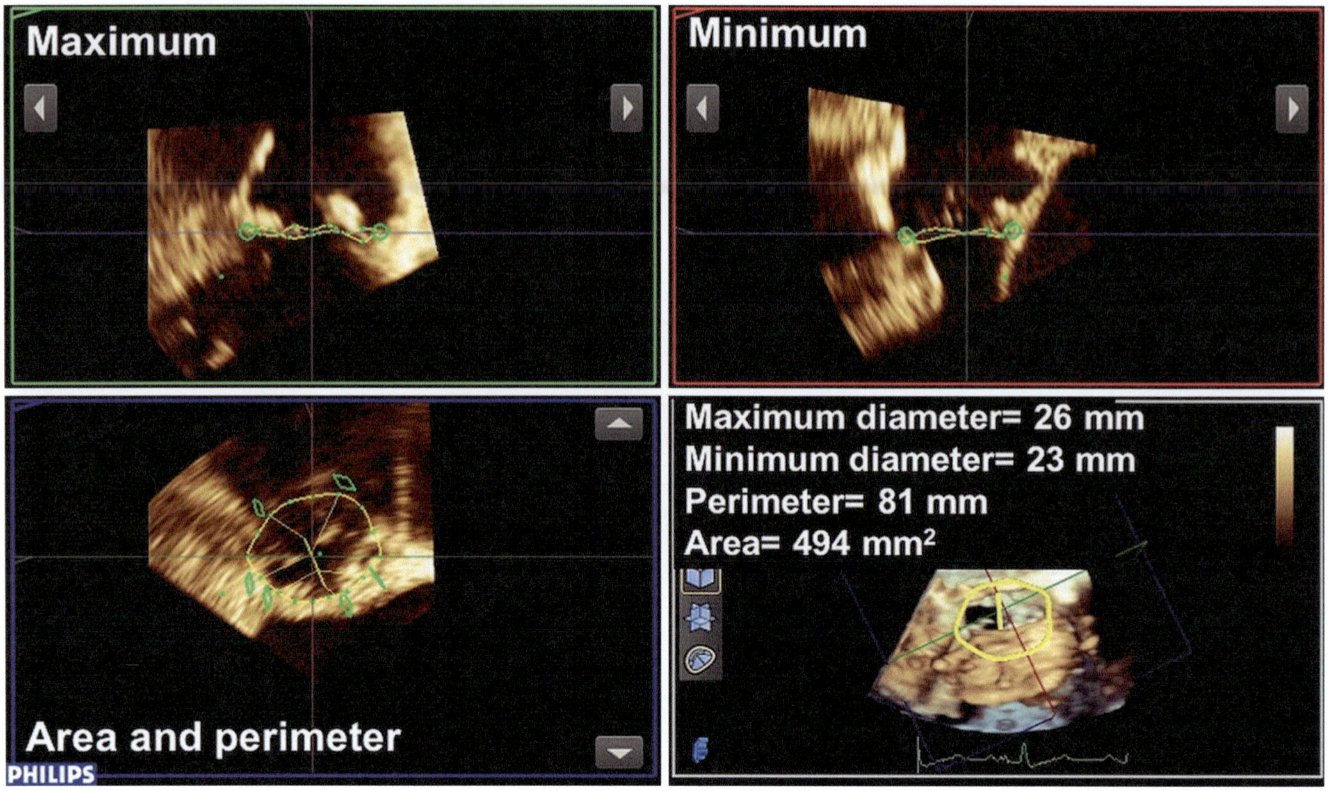

Fig. 12.8 Multiplanar reconstruction with off-label use of Q-Lab 10 (Philips Healthcare, Andover, MA) for assessment of annular dimensions and area using transesophageal 3DE data set of the aortic valve according to Hahn RT et al. [49]. A step-by-step approach will require to: (1) position of a short-axis view of the annulus in the "blue" plane (right lower box) using a double oblique technique; (2) select an early systolic frame; (3) use the blue plane to center the orthogonal green and red long-axis planes on the annulus; (4) use the green and red planes as references to move the blue plane at the most caudal attachments of the aortic valve leaflets (hinge points); (5) rotate the green and red orthogonal planes in the blue plane to confirm it is at the level of the annulus; (6) return the green and red planes to position on the blue plane in order to bisect the minimal diameter (Minimum) and maximal (Maximal) diameters, respectively. (7) Initialize the the MVQ package by selecting four orthogonal points on the red and green planes and the software package will automatically approximate the annulus; (8) edit the contour of the annulus using the eight-slice protocol by which the annular plane contour is confirmed for eight pairs of orthogonal segments in the green and red planes; (9) exclude ectopic calcifications, with the points measured outside the calcifications so as not to underestimate the annular area

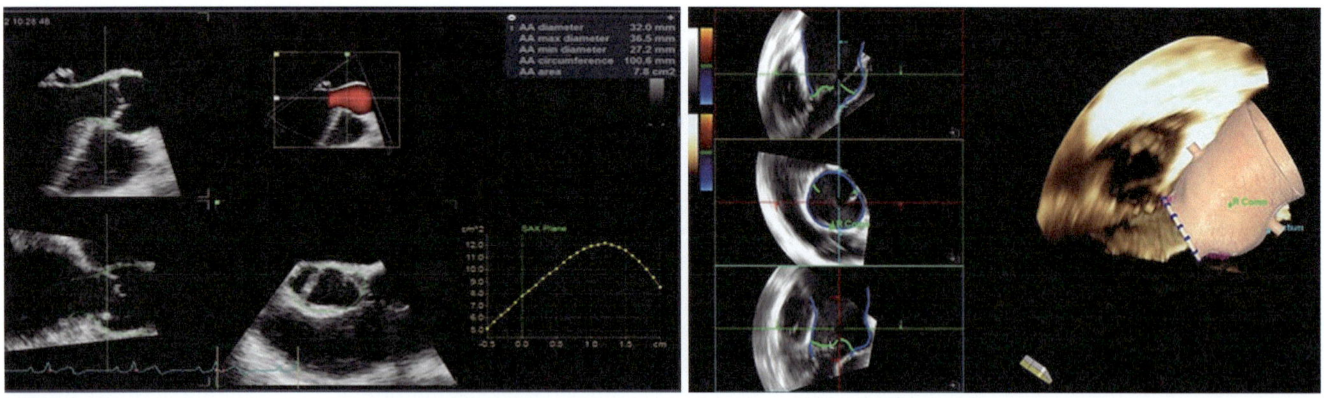

Fig. 12.9 Automated quantitation of aortic annulus (left panel: 4DAuto AVQ, EchoPac, GE Vingmed, Horten, N) and aortic root geometry (Auto Valve Analysis, Siemens Healthineer, CA) using 3DE data set of the aortic root acquired from the transesophageal approach

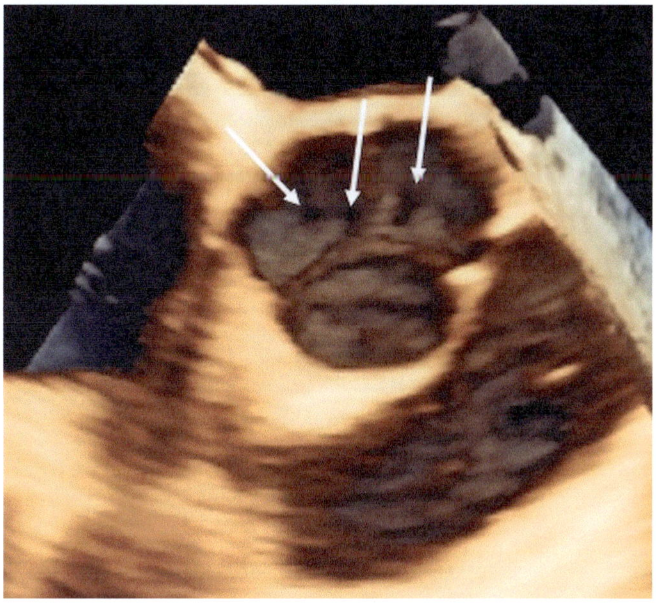

Fig. 12.10 En face view of the aortic valve from the aortic perspective in a normal subject. Several little holes (due to drop-out artifacts) can be visualized (Video 12.3) in the left and non-coronary cusps (white arrows)

(Fig. 12.10, Video 12.3). Understanding this ultrasound pitfall is essential to correct interpretation; not infrequently changing the orientation of the valve by utilizing the deep transgastric view, will help define pathologic from normal dropout.

References

1. Messika-Zeitoun D, Serfaty JM, Brochet E, Ducrocq G, Lepage L, Detaint D, et al. Multimodal assessment of the aortic annulus diameter: implications for transcatheter aortic valve implantation. J Am Coll Cardiol. 2010;55(3):186–94.
2. Altiok E, Koos R, Schroder J, Brehmer K, Hamada S, Becker M, et al. Comparison of two-dimensional and three-dimensional imaging techniques for measurement of aortic annulus diameters before transcatheter aortic valve implantation. Heart. 2011;97(19):1578–84.
3. Gurvitch R, Webb JG, Yuan R, Johnson M, Hague C, Willson AB, et al. Aortic annulus diameter determination by multidetector computed tomography: reproducibility, applicability, and implications for transcatheter aortic valve implantation. JACC Cardiovasc Interv. 2011;4(11):1235–45.
4. Tzikas A, Schultz CJ, Piazza N, Moelker A, Van Mieghem NM, Nuis RJ, et al. Assessment of the aortic annulus by multislice computed tomography, contrast aortography, and trans-thoracic echocardiography in patients referred for transcatheter aortic valve implantation. Catheter Cardiovasc Interv. 2011;77(6):868–75.
5. Gaspar T, Adawi S, Sachner R, Asmer I, Ganaeem M, Rubinshtein R, et al. Three-dimensional imaging of the left ventricular outflow tract: impact on aortic valve area estimation by the continuity equation. J Am Soc Echocardiogr. 2012;25(7):749–57.
6. Saitoh T, Shiota M, Izumo M, Gurudevan SV, Tolstrup K, Siegel RJ, et al. Comparison of left ventricular outflow geometry and aortic valve area in patients with aortic stenosis by 2-dimensional versus 3-dimensional echocardiography. Am J Cardiol. 2012;109(11):1626–31.
7. Hamdan A, Guetta V, Konen E, Goitein O, Segev A, Raanani E, et al. Deformation dynamics and mechanical properties of the aortic annulus by 4-dimensional computed tomography insights into the functional anatomy of the aortic valve complex and implications for transcatheter aortic valve therapy. J Am Coll Cardiol. 2012;59(2):119–27.
8. Akhtar M, Tuzcu EM, Kapadia SR, Svensson LG, Greenberg RK, Roselli EE, et al. Aortic root morphology in patients undergoing percutaneous aortic valve replacement: evidence of aortic root remodeling. J Thorac Cardiovasc Surg. 2009;137(4):950–6.
9. Buellesfeld L, Stortecky S, Kalesan B, Gloekler S, Khattab AA, Nietlispach F, et al. Aortic root dimensions among patients with severe aortic stenosis undergoing transcatheter aortic valve replacement. JACC Cardiovasc Interv. 2013;6(1):72–83.
10. Ewe SH, Ng AC, Schuijf JD, van der Kley F, Colli A, Palmen M, et al. Location and severity of aortic valve calcium and implications for aortic regurgitation after transcatheter aortic valve implantation. Am J Cardiol. 2011;108(10):1470–7.
11. Colli A, D'Amico R, Kempfert J, Borger MA, Mohr FW, Walther T. Transesophageal echocardiographic scoring for transcatheter aortic valve implantation: impact of aortic cusp calcification on postoperative aortic regurgitation. J Thorac Cardiovasc Surg. 2011;142(5):1229–35.
12. Goland S, Trento A, Iida K, Czer LS, De Robertis M, Naqvi TZ, et al. Assessment of aortic stenosis by three-dimensional echocardiography: an accurate and novel approach. Heart. 2007;93(7):801–7.
13. Doddamani S, Bello R, Friedman MA, Banerjee A, Bowers JH Jr, Kim B, et al. Demonstration of left ventricular outflow tract eccentricity by real time 3D echocardiography: implications for the determination of aortic valve area. Echocardiography. 2007;24(8):860–6.
14. Shahgaldi K, Manouras A, Brodin LA, Winter R. Direct measurement of left ventricular outflow tract area using three-dimensional echocardiography in biplane mode improves accuracy of stroke volume assessment. Echocardiography. 2010;27(9):1078–85.
15. Jilaihawi H, Doctor N, Kashif M, Chakravarty T, Rafique A, Makar M, et al. Aortic annular sizing for transcatheter aortic valve replacement using cross-sectional 3-dimensional transesophageal echocardiography. J Am Coll Cardiol. 2013;61(9):908–16.
16. Khalique OK, Kodali SK, Paradis JM, Nazif TM, Williams MR, Einstein AJ, et al. Aortic annular sizing using a novel 3-dimensional echocardiographic method: use and comparison with cardiac computed tomography. Circ Cardiovasc Imaging. 2014;7(1):155–63.
17. Anderson RH. Clinical anatomy of the aortic root. Heart. 2000;84(6):670–3.
18. Piazza N, de Jaegere P, Schultz C, Becker AE, Serruys PW, Anderson RH. Anatomy of the aortic valvar complex and its implications for transcatheter implantation of the aortic valve. Circ Cardiovasc Interv. 2008;1(1):74–81.
19. Brewer RJ, Deck JD, Capati B, Nolan SP. The dynamic aortic root. Its role in aortic valve functon. J Thorac Cardiovasc Surg. 1976;72:413–7.
20. Otani K, Takeuchi M, Kaku K, Sugeng L, Yoshitani H, Haruki N, et al. Assessment of the aortic root using real-time 3D transesophageal echocardiography. Circ J. 2010;74(12):2649–57.
21. Mori Y, Shiota T, Jones M, Wanitkun S, Irvine T, Li X, et al. Three-dimensional reconstruction of the color Doppler-imaged vena contracta for quantifying aortic regurgitation: studies in a chronic animal model. Circulation. 1999;99(12):1611–7.
22. Fang L, Hsiung MC, Miller AP, Nanda NC, Yin WH, Young MS, et al. Assessment of aortic regurgitation by live three-dimensional transthoracic echocardiographic measurements of vena contracta area: usefulness and validation. Echocardiography. 2005;22(9):775–81.

23. Perez de Isla L, Zamorano J, Fernandez-Golfin C, Ciocarelli S, Corros C, Sanchez T, et al. 3D color-Doppler echocardiography and chronic aortic regurgitation: a novel approach for severity assessment. Int J Cardiol. 2013;166(3):640–5.
24. Chen TE, Kwon SH, Enriquez-Sarano M, Wong BF, Mankad SV. Three-dimensional color Doppler echocardiographic quantification of tricuspid regurgitation orifice area: comparison with conventional two-dimensional measures. J Am Soc Echocardiogr. 2013;26(10):1143–52.
25. Franco E, Almeria C, de Agustin JA, Arreo Del Val V, Gomez de Diego JJ, Garcia Fernandez MA, et al. Three-dimensional color Doppler transesophageal echocardiography for mitral paravalvular leak quantification and evaluation of percutaneous closure success. J Am Soc Echocardiogr. 2014;27(11):1153–63.
26. Altiok E, Hamada S, Brehmer K, Kuhr K, Reith S, Becker M, et al. Analysis of procedural effects of percutaneous edge-to-edge mitral valve repair by 2D and 3D echocardiography. Circ Cardiovasc Imaging. 2012;5(6):748–55.
27. Zoghbi WA, Enriquez-Sarano M, Foster E, Grayburn PA, Kraft CD, Levine RA, et al. Recommendations for evaluation of the severity of native valvular regurgitation with two-dimensional and Doppler echocardiography. J Am Soc Echocardiogr. 2003;16(7):777–802.
28. Pirat B, Little SH, Igo SR, McCulloch M, Nose Y, Hartley CJ, et al. Direct measurement of proximal isovelocity surface area by real-time three-dimensional color Doppler for quantitation of aortic regurgitant volume: an in vitro validation. J Am Soc Echocardiogr. 2009;22(3):306–13.
29. Little SH, Igo SR, Pirat B, McCulloch M, Hartley CJ, Nose Y, et al. In vitro validation of real-time three-dimensional color Doppler echocardiography for direct measurement of proximal isovelocity surface area in mitral regurgitation. Am J Cardiol. 2007;99(10):1440–7.
30. de Agustin JA, Marcos-Alberca P, Fernandez-Golfin C, Goncalves A, Feltes G, Nunez-Gil IJ, et al. Direct measurement of proximal isovelocity surface area by single-beat three-dimensional color Doppler echocardiography in mitral regurgitation: a validation study. J Am Soc Echocardiogr. 2012;25(8):815–23.
31. de Agustin JA, Viliani D, Vieira C, Islas F, Marcos-Alberca P, Gomez de Diego JJ, et al. Proximal isovelocity surface area by single-beat three-dimensional color Doppler echocardiography applied for tricuspid regurgitation quantification. J Am Soc Echocardiogr. 2013;26(9):1063–72.
32. Li C, Zhang J, Li X, Zhou C, Li H, Tang H, et al. Quantification of chronic aortic regurgitation by vector flow mapping: a novel echocardiographic method. Eur J Echocardiogr. 2010;11(2):119–24.
33. Little SH, Igo SR, McCulloch M, Hartley CJ, Nose Y, Zoghbi WA. Three-dimensional ultrasound imaging model of mitral valve regurgitation: design and evaluation. Ultrasound Med Biol. 2008;34(4):647–54.
34. Thavendiranathan P, Liu S, Datta S, Walls M, Nitinunu A, Van Houten T, et al. Automated quantification of mitral inflow and aortic outflow stroke volumes by three-dimensional real-time volume color-flow Doppler transthoracic echocardiography: comparison with pulsed-wave Doppler and cardiac magnetic resonance imaging. J Am Soc Echocardiogr. 2012;25(1):56–65.
35. Baumgartner H, Hung J, Bermejo J, Chambers JB, Evangelista A, Griffin BP, et al. Echocardiographic assessment of valve stenosis: EAE/ASE recommendations for clinical practice. J Am Soc Echocardiogr. 2009;22(1):1–23; quiz 101–2.
36. De Vecchi C, Caudron J, Dubourg B, Pirot N, Lefebvre V, Bauer F, et al. Effect of the ellipsoid shape of the left ventricular outflow tract on the echocardiographic assessment of aortic valve area in aortic stenosis. J Cardiovasc Comput Tomogr. 2014;8(1):52–7.
37. Burgstahler C, Kunze M, Loffler C, Gawaz MP, Hombach V, Merkle N. Assessment of left ventricular outflow tract geometry in non-stenotic and stenotic aortic valves by cardiovascular magnetic resonance. J Cardiovasc Magn Reson. 2006;8(6):825–9.
38. Halpern EJ, Mallya R, Sewell M, Shulman M, Zwas DR. Differences in aortic valve area measured with CT planimetry and echocardiography (continuity equation) are related to divergent estimates of left ventricular outflow tract area. AJR Am J Roentgenol. 2009;192(6):1668–73.
39. O'Brien B, Schoenhagen P, Kapadia SR, Svensson LG, Rodriguez L, Griffin BP, et al. Integration of 3D imaging data in the assessment of aortic stenosis: impact on classification of disease severity. Circ Cardiovasc Imaging. 2011;4(5):566–73.
40. Montealegre-Gallegos M, Mahmood F, Owais K, Hess P, Jainandunsing JS, Matyal R. Cardiac output calculation and three-dimensional echocardiography. J Cardiothorac Vasc Anesth. 2014;28(3):547–50.
41. Tsang W, Bateman MG, Weinert L, Pellegrini G, Mor-Avi V, Sugeng L, et al. Accuracy of aortic annular measurements obtained from three-dimensional echocardiography, CT and MRI: human in vitro and in vivo studies. Heart. 2012;98(15):1146–52.
42. Clavel MA, Malouf J, Messika-Zeitoun D, Araoz PA, Michelena HI, Enriquez-Sarano M. Aortic valve area calculation in aortic stenosis by CT and Doppler echocardiography. JACC Cardiovasc Imaging. 2015;8(3):248–57.
43. Malouf J, Le Tourneau T, Pellikka P, Sundt TM, Scott C, Schaff HV, et al. Aortic valve stenosis in community medical practice: determinants of outcome and implications for aortic valve replacement. J Thorac Cardiovasc Surg. 2012;144(6):1421–7.
44. Nishimura RA, Otto C. 2014 ACC/AHA valve guidelines: earlier intervention for chronic mitral regurgitation. Heart. 2014;100(12):905–7.
45. Koos R, Altiok E, Mahnken AH, Neizel M, Dohmen G, Marx N, et al. Evaluation of aortic root for definition of prosthesis size by magnetic resonance imaging and cardiac computed tomography: implications for transcatheter aortic valve implantation. Int J Cardiol. 2012;158(3):353–8.
46. Murphy DT, Blanke P, Alaamri S, Naoum C, Rubinshtein R, Pache G, et al. Dynamism of the aortic annulus: effect of diastolic versus systolic CT annular measurements on device selection in transcatheter aortic valve replacement (TAVR). J Cardiovasc Comput Tomogr. 2016;10(1):37–43.
47. Willson AB, Webb JG, Labounty TM, Achenbach S, Moss R, Wheeler M, et al. 3-dimensional aortic annular assessment by multidetector computed tomography predicts moderate or severe paravalvular regurgitation after transcatheter aortic valve replacement: a multicenter retrospective analysis. J Am Coll Cardiol. 2012;59(14):1287–94.
48. Jilaihawi H, Kashif M, Fontana G, Furugen A, Shiota T, Friede G, et al. Cross-sectional computed tomographic assessment improves accuracy of aortic annular sizing for transcatheter aortic valve replacement and reduces the incidence of paravalvular aortic regurgitation. J Am Coll Cardiol. 2012;59(14):1275–86.
49. Hahn RT, Khalique O, Williams MR, Koss E, Paradis JM, Daneault B, et al. Predicting paravalvular regurgitation following transcatheter valve replacement: utility of a novel method for three-dimensional echocardiographic measurements of the aortic annulus. J Am Soc Echocardiogr. 2013;26(9):1043–52.
50. Santos N, de Agustin JA, Almeria C, Goncalves A, Marcos-Alberca P, Fernandez-Golfin C, et al. Prosthesis/annulus discongruence assessed by three-dimensional transoesophageal echocardiography: a predictor of significant paravalvular aortic regurgitation after

transcatheter aortic valve implantation. Eur Heart J Cardiovasc Imaging. 2012;13(11):931–7.
51. Janosi RA, Kahlert P, Plicht B, Wendt D, Eggebrecht H, Erbel R, et al. Measurement of the aortic annulus size by real-time three-dimensional transesophageal echocardiography. Minim Invasive Ther Allied Technol. 2011;20(2):85–94.
52. Gripari P, Ewe SH, Fusini L, Muratori M, Ng AC, Cefalu C, et al. Intraoperative 2D and 3D transoesophageal echocardiographic predictors of aortic regurgitation after transcatheter aortic valve implantation. Heart. 2012;98(16):1229–36.
53. Smith LA, Dworakowski R, Bhan A, Delithanasis I, Hancock J, Maccarthy PA, et al. Real-time three-dimensional transesophageal echocardiography adds value to transcatheter aortic valve implantation. J Am Soc Echocardiogr. 2013;26(4):359–69.
54. Kasel AM, Cassese S, Bleiziffer S, Amaki M, Hahn RT, Kastrati A, et al. Standardized imaging for aortic annular sizing: implications for transcatheter valve selection. JACC Cardiovasc Imaging. 2013;6(2):249–62.

Aortic Valve Congenital Abnormalities and Stenosis

13

Rebecca T. Hahn and Alex S. Felix

Abstract

The spectrum of congenital anomalies of the aortic valve, which typically result in significant outflow obstruction, include subaortic stenosis, aortic valve anomalies (most commonly a bicuspid aortic valve) and supravalvular aortic stenosis. Although the latter is typically seen in the pediatric population, both congenital subaortic and aortic valvular abnormalities will commonly be seen in adults. This chapter will review the congenital anomalies leading to left ventricular outflow obstruction at the level of outflow tract and aortic root.

Keywords

Aortic stenosis · Subaortic stenosis · Bicuspid aortic valve · Supravalvular stenosis

Introduction

Congenital obstruction of left ventricular outflow in the adult can occur at any level within the aortic valve (AV) complex; the left ventricular outflow tract (subvalvular stenosis), AV leaflets (valvular stenosis) and aorta (supravalvular stenosis) [1]. In the pediatric population, supra-valvular stenosis typically in association with Williams-Beuren syndrome, may also result in significant outflow obstruction [2]. This chapter will review the echocardiographic diagnosis of congenital anomalies involving subaortic, aortic valve and supravalvular stenosis.

Electronic Supplementary Material The online version of this chapter (https://doi.org/10.1007/978-3-030-14032-8_13) contains supplementary material, which is available to authorized users.

R. T. Hahn (✉)
Department of Cardiology/Structural Heart and Valve Center, Columbia University Medical Center, New York, NY, USA
e-mail: rth2@columbia.edu

A. S. Felix
Department of Echocardiography, National Institute of Cardiology, Rio de Janeiro, Brazil

Subaortic Stenosis

Fixed subaortic stenosis may occur in the setting of a discrete, thin fibrous membrane, a discrete fibromuscular collar, or a tunnel-type muscular narrowing of the left ventricular outflow tract (LVOT) [3]. The prevalence of subaortic stenosis in adults with congenital heart disease is estimated to be about 6.5%, with a male-to-female ratio of 2:1 [4]. The fibromuscular collar is most common and is caused by a crescent shaped or circumferential ridge of fibromuscular band in the LVOT (Fig. 13.1, Videos 13.1a and 13.1b). However, the tunnel-type narrowing of the LVOT has been associated with a greater degree of stenosis [1, 5]. Not infrequently these congenital abnormalities may be associated with other congenital abnormalities such as ventricular septal defect and coarctation of the aorta, as well as with a series of lesions such as in Shone's complex (parachute mitral valve, mitral stenosis, bicuspid aortic valve, and coarctation of the aorta) [1, 6]. Tunnel-type stenosis has been associated with small aortic annulus, small mitral orifice, and asymmetric septal hypertrophy [7]. There has been some controversy over whether this entity is a true congenital disease or an acquired disease. Many studies have suggested that in the setting of the right anatomic and hemodynamic substrate, alterations in basal septal shear stress may stimulate cellular proliferation [6, 8–10]. These theories may explain the recurrence of obstruction in patients who have undergone prior surgical resection [11–13]. Higher recurrence rates have been reported in patients with tunnel-type stenosis, higher resting pre-operative gradients (>40 mmHg) and a residual post-operative gradient of >10 mmHg.

In the setting turbulent systolic flow, trauma to the aortic valve may result in aortic stenosis [14] or aortic regurgitation

L. P. Badano et al. (eds.), *Textbook of Three-Dimensional Echocardiography*, https://doi.org/10.1007/978-3-030-14032-8_13

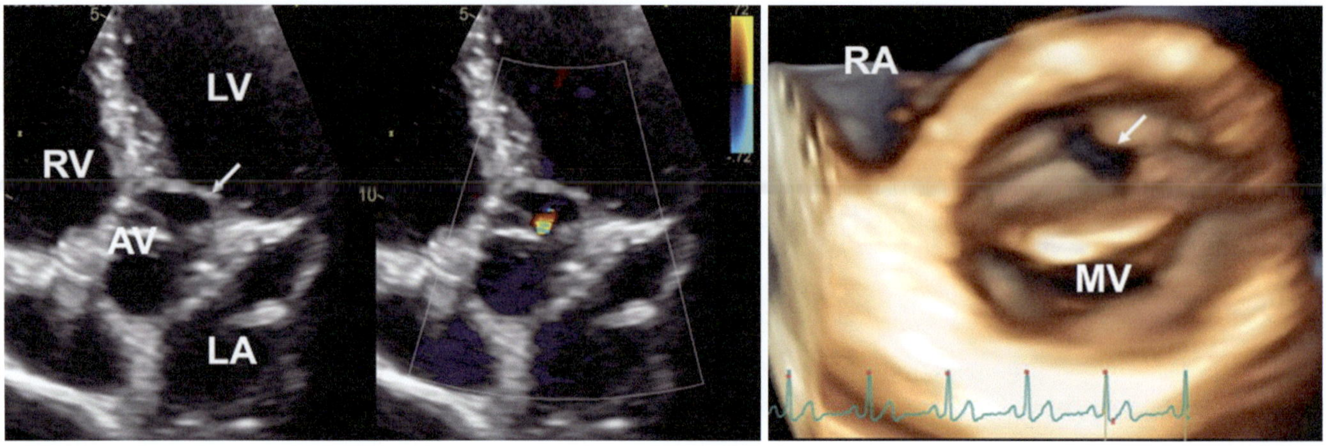

Fig. 13.1 Fixed subaortic stenosis. Left panel. A discrete fibromuscular collar (white arrow) is visualized in the left ventricular outflow tract by tow-dimensional echocardiography. The aortic valve shows a mild regurgitation (Video 13.1a/left). Right panel: volume rendering of a 3DE data set of the left ventricular outflow tract and aortic root allowing an en-face view of the membrane and its orifice (white arrow) from the ventricular perspective (Video 13.1b/right). *AV* aortic valve, *LA* left atrium, *LV* left ventricle, *MV* mitral valve, *RA* right atrium, *RV* right ventricle

[4, 12, 15, 16]. LVOT gradients ≥50 mmHg are associated with a higher risk of developing aortic regurgitation [17]. Despite surgical repair, some patients may continue to develop aortic regurgitation. This may be related to a persistent LVOT gradient.

Congenital Aortic Stenosis (AS)

Congenital AS occurs as a unicuspid aortic valve (Fig. 13.2a, Video 13.2a), bicuspid aortic valve (Fig. 13.2b, c, Videos 13.2b and 13.2c), or aortic annular hypoplasia. Rarely, a quadricuspid valve may develop stenosis (Fig. 13.2d, Video 13.2d). The bicuspid aortic valve (BAV) anomaly occurring is 1–2% of the population [18] with male:female prevalence ratio is 3.7:1 [19]. Although BAV is a congenital anomaly, complications associated with this anomaly develop in adulthood making early diagnosis important. A number of different classification systems have been used in the past, most based on the fusion of cusps and orientation or number of the raphe [20–22]. Some of these classification systems then identified patients with no raphe as "pure" BAV or type 0 [22] (Fig. 13.2b). A recent classification system identifies just two BAV phenotypes: fusion of the right and left coronary cusps (BAV-AP) (Fig. 13.3, Video 13.3) and fusion of the right or left coronary cusp and non-coronary cusp (BAV-RL, Fig. 13.2c) [23]. These two phenotypes have some support in recent animal studies identifying defective development of different embryological structures [24]. Morphology may provide valuable data regarding risk stratification of BAV patients [23, 25, 26]. Kang et al. showed in a small population of 167 patients, that moderate-to-severe aortic stenosis is more prevalent in patients with BAV-RL (66.2% vs. 46.2% in BAV-AP; p = 0.01), and moderate-to-severe aortic regurgitation in BAV-AP (32.3% vs. 6.8% in BAV-RL; p < 0.0001).

In addition, the association with BAV and dilatation of the ascending aorta has been well-established [27–29]. Aortopathy type (0–3), type 0, normal aorta; type 1, dilated aortic root; type 2, aortic enlargement involving the tubular portion of the ascending aorta; and type 3, diffuse involvement of both the entire ascending aorta and the transverse aortic arch. Some authors have suggested that the aortic abnormality is unrelated to the valvular pathology [27, 29] and thus a primary anomaly associated with this entity. More recent studies using advanced imaging techniques have suggested that regional wall stress in the setting of eccentric outflow patterns contributes to the pattern of aortic dilatation [30–33]. Overall outcomes for BAV are related not only to valvular pathology (stenosis or regurgitation) but also to aortopathy. Tzemos et al. [25] identified the following cardiac event risk factors: age >30 years, moderate or severe aortic stenosis, and moderate or severe aortic incompetence. Although fatal events are rare, surgical intervention is not uncommon. Most surgical procedures involve aortic valve and aortic root replacements with the 25-year rate of aortic surgery as high as 25% [25, 34, 35].

Although valvular disease may present in the fourth and fifth decades, in a series of operatively excised, stenotic aortic valves (isolated aortic valve surgery) from 932 patients (mean age of 70 ± 12 years) 54% of patients had congenital abnormalities commonly BAV, with the median age at surgery of 67 years [36]. Another series of excised aortic stenosis valves in patients greater than 80 years of age showed a prevalence of bicuspid aortic valve in 22% [37]. Importantly, although current transcatheter aortic valve devices are designed for use in tricuspid aortic valves, numerous case

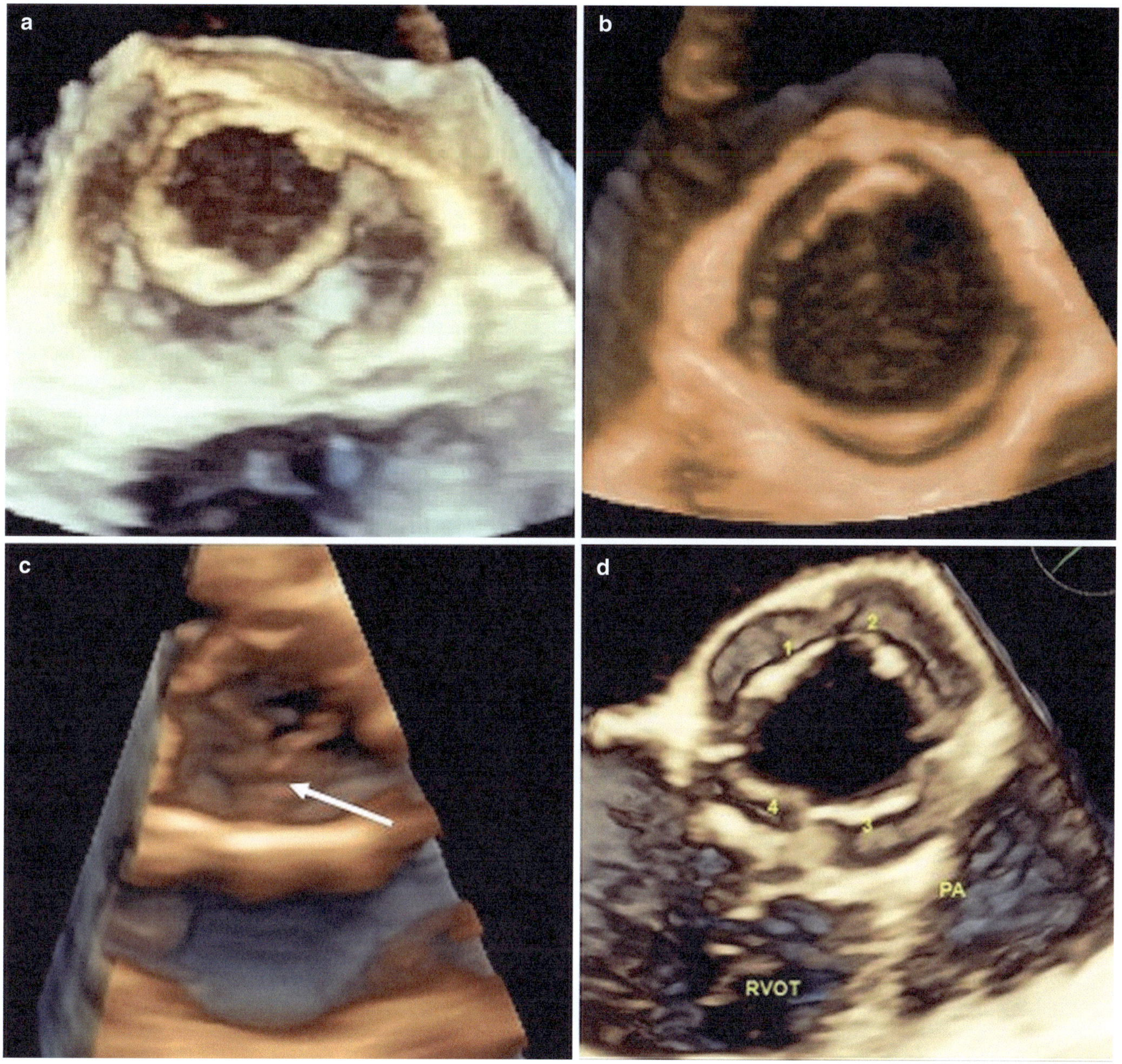

Fig. 13.2 Congenital abnormalities of the aortic valve. Volume rendered *en face* views of the valve from the aortic perspective. (**a**) Transesophageal 3DE acquisition of unicuspid aortic valve (Video 13.2a); (**b**) transthoracic 3DE acquisition of a pure bicuspid aortic valve with typical fish mouth opening appearance (Video 13.2b); (**c**) transthoracic 3DE acquisition of a bicuspid aortic valve with calcified rafe between the left and the non-coronary cusps (Video 13.2c); (**d**) transesophageal acquisition of a quadricuspid aortic valve (Video 13.2d)

reports and two reports of transcatheter aortic valve (TAVR) in a series of BAV patients have shown that, compared to matched trileaflet aortic valve patients, there was no difference in acute procedural success, valve hemodynamics, or short-term survival [38, 39].

Echocardiography remains the most validated imaging modality for the diagnosis, phenotyping, and hemodynamic assessment of BAV dysfunction and the initial assessment of the thoracic aorta. With conventional echocardiography, the diagnosis is typically made using the short-axis views of the valve. Although in diastole, the raphe may be mistaken for a commissure, particularly in calcified valves, in systole in the short-axis view there is a typical “fish-mouth” appearance of valve opening and absence of opening at the raphe. In patients with good-quality transthoracic images who do not have dense BAV calcification, diagnostic sensitivity and specificity are >70% and >90%, respectively [40, 41]. However, diagnostic uncertainty may remain in 10–15% of patients after echocardiogram [35]. Particularly in the setting of calcification, color Doppler in systole may be helpful in distinguishing immobile trileaflet aortic valves without commissural fusion from bicuspid valves with fusion. Diagnostic and phenotyping accuracy can be significantly improved with the use of higher-resolution imaging techniques such as transesophageal echocardiography (TEE) and 3DE imaging [42–45]. Using longitudinal cut planes of 3DE data sets of the aortic root, the presence or absence of interleaflet triangles (the anatomical landmark for the diagnosis of BAV) can be diagnosed (Fig. 13.4, Videos 13.4a and 13.4b). 3DE has also been utilized to quantify BAV function. For stenotic valves, direct planimetry of the orifice [46–49] has been validated. Machida et al. in fact showed that in the bicuspid AS group, the planimetered aortic valve area (AVA) by 3D TEE significantly correlated with AVA calculated by the Doppler continuity equation ($r = 0.83$, mean difference 0.10 ± 0.18 cm^2, $P < 0.001$), whereas AVA by two-dimensional TEE did not ($r = 0.42$, mean difference 0.48 ± 0.32 cm^2, $P = 0.066$) [49].

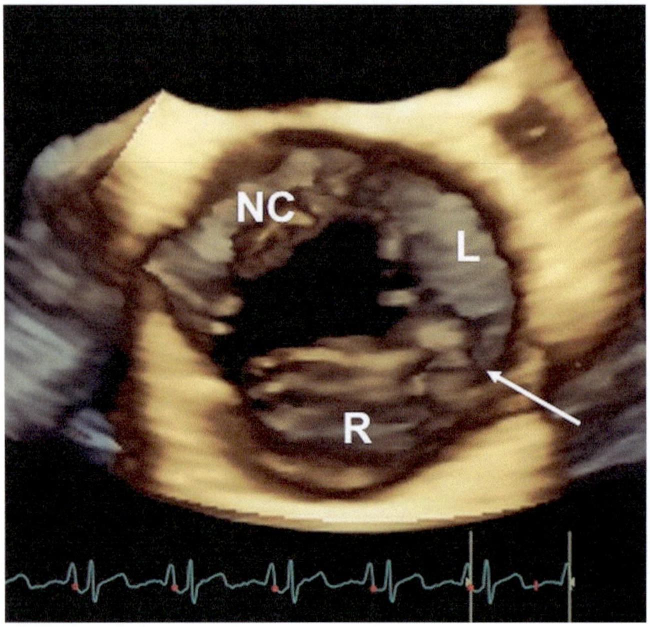

Fig. 13.3 Volume rendered image of a bicuspid valve with rafe (white arrow) between the right and left coronary cusps. The 3DE data set has been acquired from transesophageal approach and the valve is seen *en face* from the aorta perspective (Video 13.3). *L* left coronary cusp, *NC* non-coronary cusp, *R* right coronary cusp

Particularly in the setting of concomitant subvalvular stenosis when the continuity equation may be erroneous, direct planimetry of the AVA may be the primary means of quantifying valvular stenosis. Acquisition of the 3D volume to accurately assess valvular morphology and function requires using the higher volume rate, thus smallest volume that images the entire aortic valve and proximal aortic root (Fig. 13.5, Videos 13.5a and 13.5b). The orientation of the valve may vary significantly depending on the number of cusps and the size, shape and orientation of the aortic root which is the main advantage of using 3D imaging to assess the aortic valve. Because longitudinal, lateral and elevational resolution are different, structures most perpendicular to the insonation beam will have the best linear definition. Thus acquiring 3DE volumes from multiple imaging planes is always recommended. For transthoracic imaging, acquire a user-defined volume from both parasternal long-axis and short-axis views as well as from both apical 5-chamber and 3-chamber views. Similarly, mid-esophageal TEE volumes should be acquired from short-axis view (~60°) and long-axis (~120°) views as well as transgastric 5-chamber (~0°) and 3-chamber views (~120°).

Once the 3D volume has been acquired, the standard orientation of the aortic valve on TTE is with the right coronary

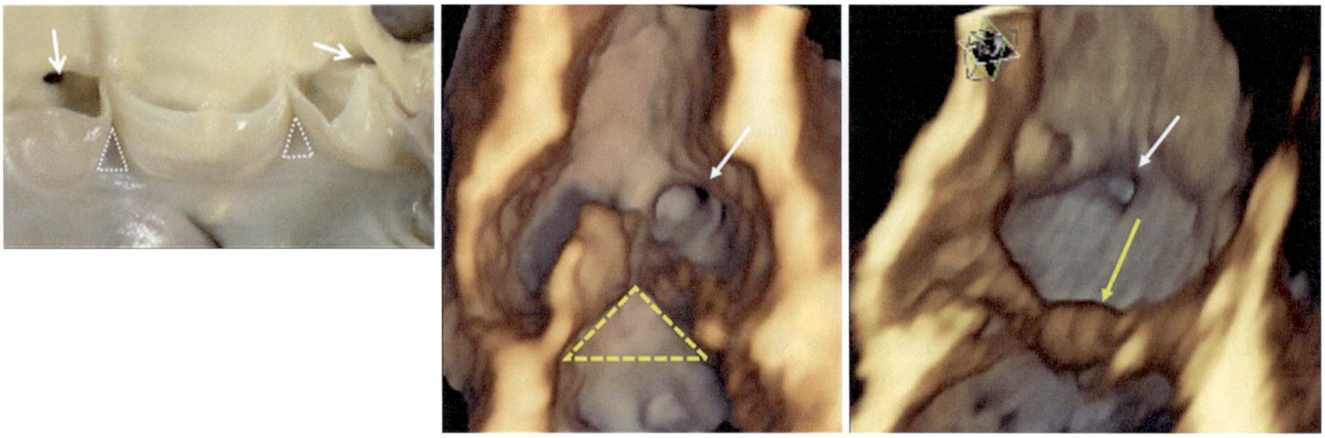

Fig. 13.4 Anatomical diagnosis of bicuspid aortic valve. Left panel, anatomical specimen of the aortic root showing the aortic cusps, coronary ostia (white arrows) and interleaflet triangles (white dashed triangles). Central panel, volume rendered 3DE cut plane of the aortic root showing the left main ostia (white arrow) and the interleaflet triangle between the left and non-coronary cusps (Video 13.4a). Right panel, volume rendered 3DE cut plane of the aortic root showing the right coronary ostia (white arrow) and the rafe (yellow arrow) between the left and the right coronary cusps (Video 13.4b)

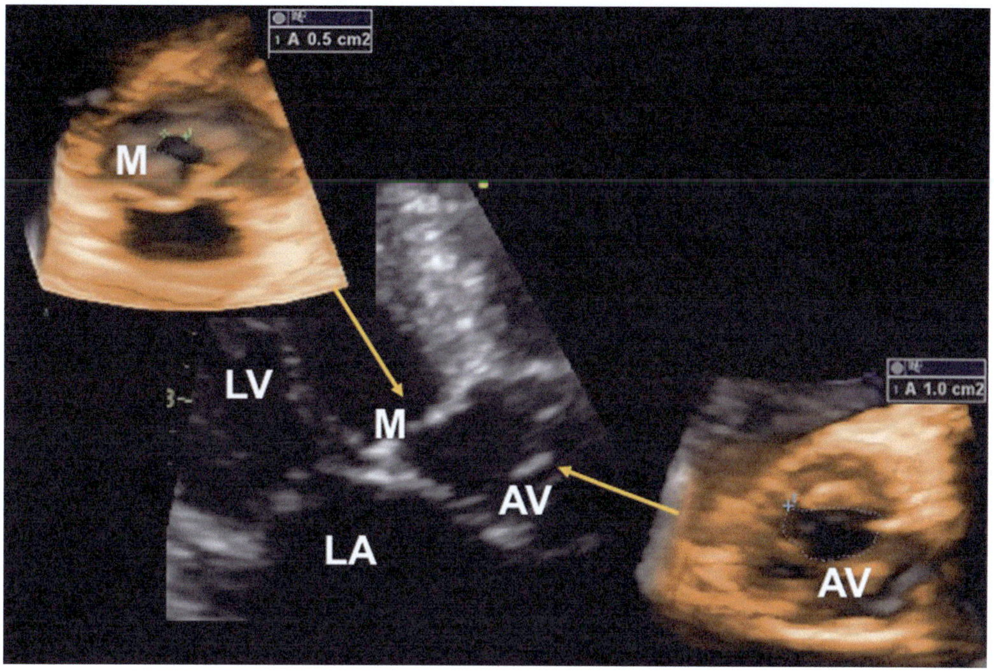

Fig 13.5 Assessment of the relative stenosis severity of subaortic (M) and aortic (AV) stenosis using transthoracic 3DE. By proper cropping of the 3E data set both the subaortic membrane (M, Video 13.5a/M) and the aortic valve (Video 13.5b/A) can be seen *en face* and the residual anatomical orifice area of both subaortic (M) and aortic (AV) stenoses can be planimetered. *LA* left atrium, *LV* left ventricle

cusp in the near field. From the aortic side, the left coronary cusp is in the far field and to the right with the noncoronary cusp in the far field and to the left. From the ventricular side, the left coronary cusp is in the far field and to the left with the noncoronary cusp in the far field and to the right (see also Chap. 12). On TEE however the image is flipped with the right coronary cusp in the far field. From the aortic side, the left coronary cusp is in the near field and to the right with the noncoronary cusp in the near field and to the left. From the ventricular side, the left coronary cusp is in the near field and to the left with the noncoronary cusp in the near field and to the right. Planimetry of the orifice may be performed either on volume rendered images or using multi-planar reconstruction, first ensuring that the cropping plane is positioned at the level of the smallest orifice (Fig. 13.5).

Supravalvular Aortic Stenosis

Supravalvular aortic stenosis is the most common cardiac finding associated with Williams-Beuren syndrome (also known simply as Williams syndrome), and is rarely seen outside of this patient population [2]. This syndrome is a result of a deletion on the long arm of chromosome 7 and affects the encoding of the elastin protein and causing major systemic arteries to become rigid. It typically presents in childhood with a number of phenotypic abnormalities, including a distinct facial appearance, developmental delay, behavioral changes, and hypercalcemia. Other common cardiac anomalies include hypoplasia of the aortic arch and pulmonary artery stenosis. Less common associated cardiac anomalies include: coarctation of the aorta, ventricular septal defect, patent ductus, subaortic stenosis, and hypertrophic cardiomyopathy. The stenosis occurs at the sinotubular junction, distal to the coronary ostia, resulting in abnormal flow within the coronaries. In the setting of significant outflow obstruction severe left ventricular hypertrophy may occur. These patients are at high risk for sudden death and surgical intervention is usually required. Echocardiography remains the initial diagnostic modality for supravalvular stenosis [50] however the constellation of cardiac anomalies may be best evaluated by computed tomography [51]. Newborns with supravalvular aortic stenosis should be followed for rapid progression. Although right ventricular outflow obstruction may regress in some patients, supravalvular aortic stenosis may develop in others with right ventricular outflow obstruction. Patients with right ventricular outflow obstruction (at the valvular, supravalvular, or peripheral pulmonary arterial level) should be evaluated carefully for development of supravalvular aortic stenosis at follow-up [52].

References

1. Aboulhosn J, Child JS. Left ventricular outflow obstruction: subaortic stenosis, bicuspid aortic valve, supravalvar aortic stenosis, and coarctation of the aorta. Circulation. 2006;114(22):2412–22.
2. Gray JC 3rd, Krazinski AW, Schoepf UJ, Meinel FG, Pietris NP, Suranyi P, Hlavacek AM. Cardiovascular manifestations of Williams syndrome: imaging findings. J Cardiovasc Comput Tomogr. 2013;7(6):400–7.
3. Newfeld EA, Muster AJ, Paul MH, Idriss FS, Riker WL. Discrete subvalvular aortic stenosis in childhood. Study of 51 patients. Am J Cardiol. 1976;38(1):53–61.

4. Oliver JM, Gonzalez A, Gallego P, Sanchez-Recalde A, Benito F, Mesa JM. Discrete subaortic stenosis in adults: increased prevalence and slow rate of progression of the obstruction and aortic regurgitation. J Am Coll Cardiol Sep. 2001;38(3):835–42.
5. Brauner R, Laks H, Drinkwater DC Jr, Shvarts O, Eghbali K, Galindo A. Benefits of early surgical repair in fixed subaortic stenosis. J Am Coll Cardiol. 1997;30(7):1835–42.
6. Cilliers AM, Gewillig M. Rheology of discrete subaortic stenosis. Heart. 2002;88(4):335–6.
7. Maron BJ, Redwood DR, Roberts WC, Henry WL, Morrow AG, Epstein SE. Tunnel subaortic stenosis: left ventricular outflow tract obstruction produced by fibromuscular tubular narrowing. Circulation. 1976;54(3):404–16.
8. Choi JY, Sullivan ID. Fixed subaortic stenosis: anatomical spectrum and nature of progression. Br Heart J. 1991;65(5):280–6.
9. Cape EG, Vanauker MD, Sigfusson G, Tacy TA, del Nido PJ. Potential role of mechanical stress in the etiology of pediatric heart disease: septal shear stress in subaortic stenosis. J Am Coll Cardiol. 1997;30(1):247–54.
10. Rosenquist GC, Clark EB, McAllister HA, Bharati S, Edwards JE. Increased mitral-aortic separation in discrete subaortic stenosis. Circulation. 1979;60(1):70–4.
11. Barboza LA, Garcia Fde M, Barnoya J, Leon-Wyss JR, Castaneda AR. Subaortic membrane and aorto-septal angle: an echocardiographic assessment and surgical outcome. World J Pediatr Congenit Heart Surg. 2013;4(3):253–61.
12. Gersony WM. Natural history of discrete subvalvar aortic stenosis: management implications. J Am Coll Cardiol. 2001;38(3):843–5.
13. Leichter DA, Sullivan I, Gersony WM. "Acquired" discrete subvalvular aortic stenosis: natural history and hemodynamics. J Am Coll Cardiol. 1989;14(6):1539–44.
14. Laksman ZW, Silversides CK, Sedlak T, Samman AM, Williams WG, Webb GD, Liu PP. Valvular aortic stenosis as a major sequelae in patients with pre-existing subaortic stenosis changing spectrum of outcomes. J Am Coll Cardiol. 2011;58(9):962–5.
15. Sung CS, Price EC, Cooley DA. Discrete subaortic stenosis in adults. Am J Cardiol. 1978;42(2):283–90.
16. Wright GB, Keane JF, Nadas AS, Bernhard WF, Castaneda AR. Fixed subaortic stenosis in the young: medical and surgical course in 83 patients. Am J Cardiol. 1983;52(7):830–5.
17. McMahon CJ, Gauvreau K, Edwards JC, Geva T. Risk factors for aortic valve dysfunction in children with discrete subvalvar aortic stenosis. Am J Cardiol. 2004;94(4):459–64.
18. Fedak PW, Verma S, David TE, Leask RL, Weisel RD, Butany J. Clinical and pathophysiological implications of a bicuspid aortic valve. Circulation. 2002;106(8):900–4.
19. Tutar E, Ekici F, Atalay S, Nacar N. The prevalence of bicuspid aortic valve in newborns by echocardiographic screening. Am Heart J. 2005;150(3):513–5.
20. Schaefer BM, Lewin MB, Stout KK, Gill E, Prueitt A, Byers PH, Otto CM. The bicuspid aortic valve: an integrated phenotypic classification of leaflet morphology and aortic root shape. Heart. 2008;94(12):1634–8.
21. Buchner S, Hülsmann M, Poschenrieder F, Hamer OW, Fellner C, Kobuch R, et al. Variable phenotypes of bicuspid aortic valve disease: classification by cardiovascular magnetic resonance. Heart. 2010;96(15):1233–40.
22. Sievers HH, Schmidtke C. A classification system for the bicuspid aortic valve from 304 surgical specimens. J Thorac Cardiovasc Surg. 2007;133(5):1226–33.
23. Kang JW, Song HG, Yang DH, Baek S, Kim DH, Song JM, et al. Association between bicuspid aortic valve phenotype and patterns of valvular dysfunction and bicuspid aortopathy: comprehensive evaluation using MDCT and echocardiography. JACC Cardiovasc Imaging. 2013;6(2):150–61.
24. Fernández B, Durán AC, Fernández-Gallego T, Fernández MC, Such M, Arqué JM, Sans-Coma V. Bicuspid aortic valves with different spatial orientations of the leaflets are distinct etiological entities. J Am Coll Cardiol. 2009;54(24):2312–8.
25. Tzemos N, Therrien J, Yip J, Thanassoulis G, Tremblay S, Jamorski MT, et al. Outcomes in adults with bicuspid aortic valves. JAMA. 2008;300(11):1317–25.
26. Michelena HI, Prakash SK, Della Corte A, Bissell MM, Anavekar N, Mathieu P, BAVCon Investigators, et al. Bicuspid aortic valve: identifying knowledge gaps and rising to the challenge from the International Bicuspid Aortic Valve Consortium (BAVCon). Circulation. 2014;129(25):2691–704.
27. Hahn RT, Roman MJ, Mogtader AH, Devereux RB. Association of aortic dilation with regurgitant, stenotic and functionally normal bicuspid aortic valves. J Am Coll Cardiol. 1992;19(2):283–8.
28. Keane MG, Wiegers SE, Plappert T, Pochettino A, Bavaria JE, Sutton MG. Bicuspid aortic valves are associated with aortic dilatation out of proportion to coexistent valvular lesions. Circulation Nov. 2000;102(19 Suppl 3):III35–9.
29. Beroukhim RS, Kruzick TL, Taylor AL, Gao D, Yetman AT. Progression of aortic dilation in children with a functionally normal bicuspid aortic valve. Am J Cardiol. 2006;98(6):828–30.
30. Bissell MM, Hess AT, Biasiolli L, Glaze SJ, Loudon M, Pitcher A, et al. Aortic dilation in bicuspid aortic valve disease: flow pattern is a major contributor and differs with valve fusion type. Circ Cardiovasc Imaging. 2013;6(4):499–507.
31. Hope MD, Hope TA, Crook SE, Ordovas KG, Urbania TH, Alley MT, Higgins CB. 4D flow CMR in assessment of valve-related ascending aortic disease. JACC Cardiovasc Imaging. 2011;4(7):781–7.
32. Meierhofer C, Schneider EP, Lyko C, Hutter A, Martinoff S, Markl M, et al. Wall shear stress and flow patterns in the ascending aorta in patients with bicuspid aortic valves differ significantly from tricuspid aortic valves: a prospective study. Eur Heart J Cardiovasc Imaging. 2013;14(8):797–804.
33. Mahadevia R, Barker AJ, Schnell S, Entezari P, Kansal P, Fedak PW, et al. Bicuspid aortic cusp fusion morphology alters aortic three-dimensional outflow patterns, wall shear stress, and expression of aortopathy. Circulation. 2014;129(6):673–82.
34. Michelena HI, Desjardins VA, Avierinos JF, Russo A, Nkomo VT, Sundt TM, et al. Natural history of asymptomatic patients with normally functioning or minimally dysfunctional bicuspid aortic valve in the community. Circulation. 2008;117(21):2776–84.
35. Michelena HI, Khanna AD, Mahoney D, Margaryan E, Topilsky Y, Suri RM, et al. Incidence of aortic complications in patients with bicuspid aortic valves. JAMA. 2011;306(10):1104–12.
36. Roberts WC, Ko JM. Frequency by decades of unicuspid, bicuspid, and tricuspid aortic valves in adults having isolated aortic valve replacement for aortic stenosis, with or without associated aortic regurgitation. Circulation. 2005;111(7):920–5.
37. Roberts WC, Janning KG, Ko JM, Filardo G, Matter GJ. Frequency of congenitally bicuspid aortic valves in patients >/=80 years of age undergoing aortic valve replacement for aortic stenosis (with or without aortic regurgitation) and implications for transcatheter aortic valve implantation. Am J Cardiol. 2012;109(11):1632–6.
38. Hayashida K, Bouvier E, Lefèvre T, Chevalier B, Hovasse T, Romano M, et al. Transcatheter aortic valve implantation for patients with severe bicuspid aortic valve stenosis. Circ Cardiovasc Interv. 2013;6(3):284–91.
39. Kochman J, Huczek Z, Scisło P, Dabrowski M, Chmielak Z, Szymański P, et al. Comparison of one- and 12-month outcomes of transcatheter aortic valve replacement in patients with severely stenotic bicuspid versus tricuspid aortic valves (results from a multicenter registry). Am J Cardiol. 2014;114(5):757–62.

40. Ocak I, Lacomis JM, Deible CR, Pealer K, Parag Y, Knollmann F. The aortic root: comparison of measurements from ECG-gated CT angiography with transthoracic echocardiography. J Thorac Imaging. 2009;24(3):223–6.
41. Brandenburg RO Jr, Tajik AJ, Edwards WD, Reeder GS, Shub C, Seward JB. Accuracy of 2-dimensional echocardiographic diagnosis of congenitally bicuspid aortic valve: echocardiographic-anatomic correlation in 115 patients. Am J Cardiol. 1983;51(9):1469–73.
42. Malagoli A, Barbieri A, Modena MG. Bicuspid aortic valve regurgitation: quantification of anatomic regurgitant orifice area by 3D transesophageal echocardiography reconstruction. Echocardiography. 2008;25(7):797–8.
43. Koh TW. Diagnosis of bicuspid aortic valve: role of three-dimensional transesophageal echocardiography and multiplane review analysis. Echocardiography. 2013;30(3):360–3.
44. Unsworth B, Malik I, Mikhail GW. Recognising bicuspid aortic stenosis in patients referred for transcatheter aortic valve implantation: routine screening with three-dimensional transoesophageal echocardiography. Heart. 2010;96(8):645.
45. Shibayama K, Harada K, Berdejo J, Tanaka J, Mihara H, Itabashi Y, Shiota T. Comparison of aortic root geometry with bicuspid versus tricuspid aortic valve: real-time three-dimensional transesophageal echocardiographic study. J Am Soc Echocardiogr. 2014;27(11):1143–52.
46. Blot-Souletie N, Hebrard A, Acar P, Carrie D, Puel J. Comparison of accuracy of aortic valve area assessment in aortic stenosis by real time three-dimensional echocardiography in biplane mode versus two-dimensional transthoracic and transesophageal echocardiography. Echocardiography. 2007;24(10):1065–72.
47. Nakai H, Takeuchi M, Yoshitani H, Kaku K, Haruki N, Otsuji Y. Pitfalls of anatomical aortic valve area measurements using two-dimensional transoesophageal echocardiography and the potential of three-dimensional transoesophageal echocardiography. Eur J Echocardiogr. 2010;11(4):369–76.
48. Goland S, Trento A, Iida K, Czer LS, De Robertis M, Naqvi TZ, et al. Assessment of aortic stenosis by three-dimensional echocardiography: an accurate and novel approach. Heart. 2007;93(7):801–7.
49. Machida T, Izumo M, Suzuki K, Yoneyama K, Kamijima R, Mizukoshi K, et al. Value of anatomical aortic valve area using real-time three-dimensional transoesophageal echocardiography in patients with aortic stenosis: a comparison between tricuspid and bicuspid aortic valves. Eur Heart J Cardiovasc Imaging. 2015;16(10):1120–8.
50. Dall'Agata A, Cromme-Dijkhuis AH, Meijboom FJ, Spitaels SE, McGhie JS, Roelandt JR, Bogers AJ. Use of three-dimensional echocardiography for analysis of outflow obstruction in congenital heart disease. Am J Cardiol. 1999;83(6):921–5.
51. Das KM, Momenah TS, Larsson SG, Jadoon S, Aldosary AS, Lee EY. Williams-Beuren syndrome: computed tomography imaging review. Pediatr Cardiol. 2014;35(8):1309–20.
52. Eroglu AG, Babaoglu K, Oztunc F, Saltik L, Demir T, Ahunbay G, et al. Echocardiographic follow-up of children with supravalvular aortic stenosis. Pediatr Cardiol. 2006;27(6):707–12.

14 Aortic Regurgitation

Sorina Mihaila Baldea, Dragos Vinereanu, and Luigi P. Badano

Abstract

Conventional two-dimensional and Doppler echocardiography (2DE) are widely used to establish the pathophysiology and to assess the severity of aortic regurgitation. However, due to its tomographic nature, 2DE has important limitations to appreciate the geometry and the dynamics of the aortic valve complex. Conversely, three-dimensional echocardiography (3DE) can assess the aortic valve complex without geometrical assumptions about the shape of its different components and offer unprecedented, anatomically sound, images of the aortic valve.

The different components of the aortic valve complex can be visualized from any perspective using a single acquired full-volume data set allowing a complete understanding of their anatomy and function. The following chapter describes the additional value of 3DE over 2DE for the assessment of patients with aortic valve regurgitation, with respect to etiology, mechanisms and severity of the disease, as well as planning of future procedures.

Keywords

Aortic regurgitation · Three-dimensional echocardiography · Transesophageal · Transthoracic · Aortic valve morphology · Aortic regurgitation severity

S. M. Baldea (✉) · D. Vinereanu
The University of Medicine and Pharmacy Carol Davila, Bucharest, Romania

Department of Cardiology, Emergency University Hospital Bucharest, Bucharest, Romania

L. P. Badano
University of Milano-Bicocca, and Istituto Auxologico Italiano, IRCCS, San Luca Hospital, Milano, Italy
e-mail: luigi.badano@unimib.it

Introduction

Two-dimensional and Doppler echocardiography is the most widely used imaging technique to perform a non-invasive assessment of the aortic valve morphology and function in humans. Echocardiography is essential to establish the etiology, to assess the mechanisms and to quantify the severity of the aortic regurgitation (AR). However, the inherent tomographic nature of two-dimensional echocardiography poses some limitations to appreciate the anatomy and function of the different components of the aortic valve complex [1]. Conversely, recent advances in three-dimensional echocardiography (3DE) combined with the use of dedicated software packages allow a more accurate assessment of the aortic valve complex in the beating heart. Important advantages of 3DE derive from the possibility to visualize the various components of the aortic valve complex from any perspective and to perform measurements independent on geometric assumptions about the shape of the cardiac structures [2]. Moreover, the use of transesophageal 3DE has provided images of the aortic valve in motion of unprecedented quality [3].

This chapter describes the additional role of 3DE to assess morphology and function of the aortic valve complex in patient aortic regurgitation, to establish the mechanisms and to quantify the severity of the regurgitation.

Aortic Valve Morphology

To understand the pathophysiology of AR we should consider anatomical and functional changes occurring in all the components of the so-called aortic root complex. The aortic root complex is composed of the sinuses of Valsalva, the fibrous inter-leaflet triangles and the aortic valve leaflets [3]. A normal function of the aortic root complex complex requires normal geometry and dimensions of all its components, and a proper coupling of the aortic and mitral valve function [4, 5] (see also Chap. 12).

L. P. Badano et al. (eds.), *Textbook of Three-Dimensional Echocardiography*, https://doi.org/10.1007/978-3-030-14032-8_14

AR may be caused by primary disease of the cusps, congenital abnormalities of aortic valve, or by distortions of the aortic root [6], which lead to insufficient closure of the cusps. Two-dimensional echocardiography is the primary technique used to orientate the etiology and to establish the mechanisms and severity of the aortic regurgitation. However, two-dimensional echocardiography is a tomographic technique and a parallel alignment of the cut-plane to the aortic valve to visualize the valve *en-face* is sometimes impossible in hearts with enlarged aortic roots or a horizontal position [3]. Moreover, the through-plane motion of the aortic annulus due to the longitudinal shortening of the left ventricle during the cardiac cycle often hampers adequate visualization of the aortic valve orifice opening. Conversely, 3DE allows infinite cut-planes inside the acquired full-volumes. An *en face* alignment of the cut-plane with the aortic annulus can be easily obtained, irrespective of the aortic root spatial orientation, and a comprehensive evaluation of the aortic valve complex can be performed in the beating heart [3].

3DE evaluates all aspects of the aortic valve leaflets, including height, width, surface area, and volume of the sinuses of Valsalva [7]. 3DE cut-planes positioned above and below the aortic cusps and longitudinal planes at the level of the aortic valve and left ventricular outflow tract allow the identification of the different lesions leading to aortic regurgitation: bicuspid valve [8, 9] (Fig. 14.1), quadricuspid valve [10] (Fig. 14.2),

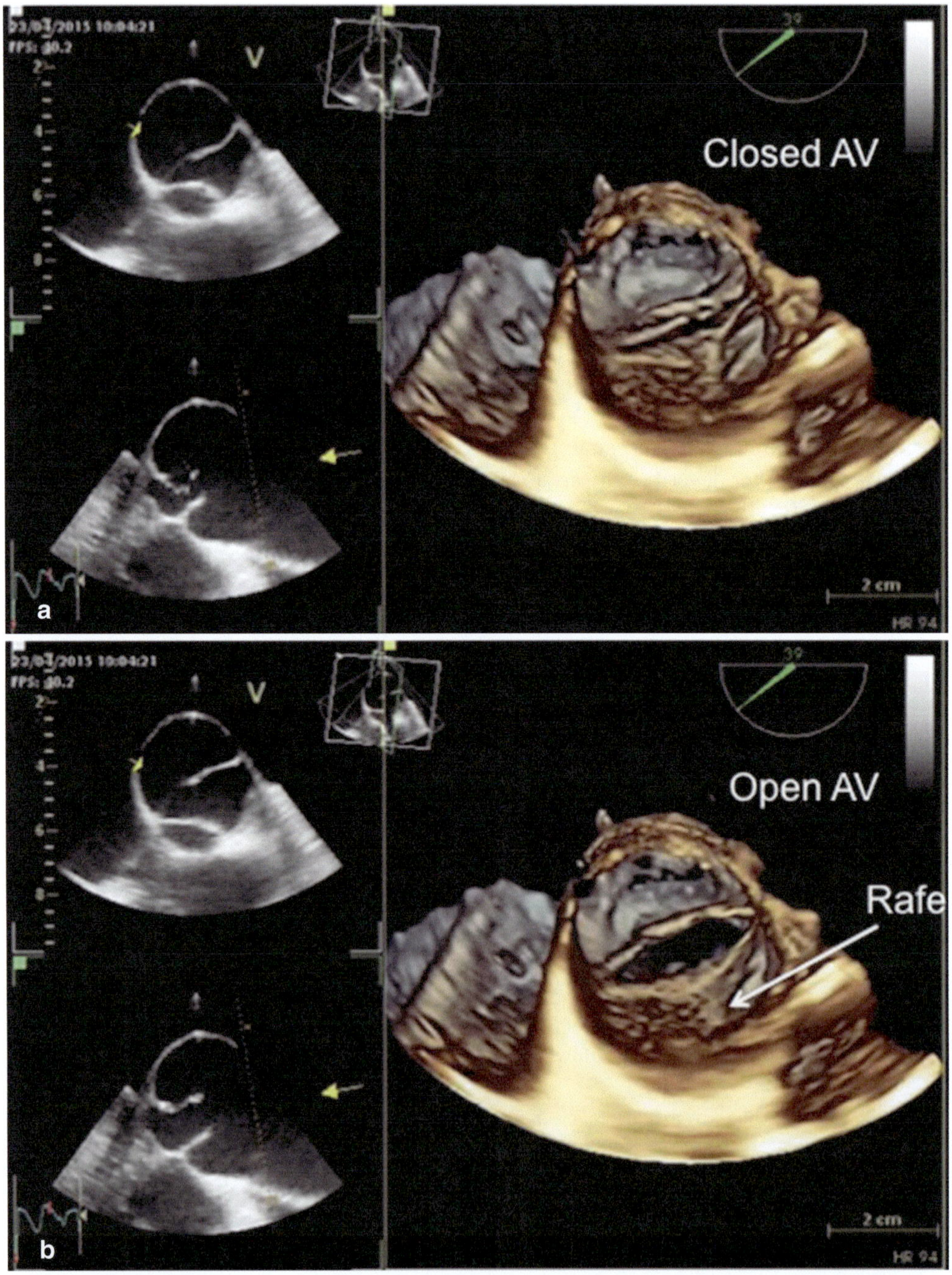

Fig. 14.1 Bicuspid aortic valve by three-dimensional transoeshophageal echocardiography. The aortic valve is visualized from the aortic perspective. This cut-plane is used to analyze the number and the morphology of the leaflets. (**a**) Shows the aortic valve closed, when it might seem tricuspid due to the median rafe; (**b**) shows the aortic valve opened in a "fish mouth" orifice, typical for the bicuspid morphology. *AV* aortic valve

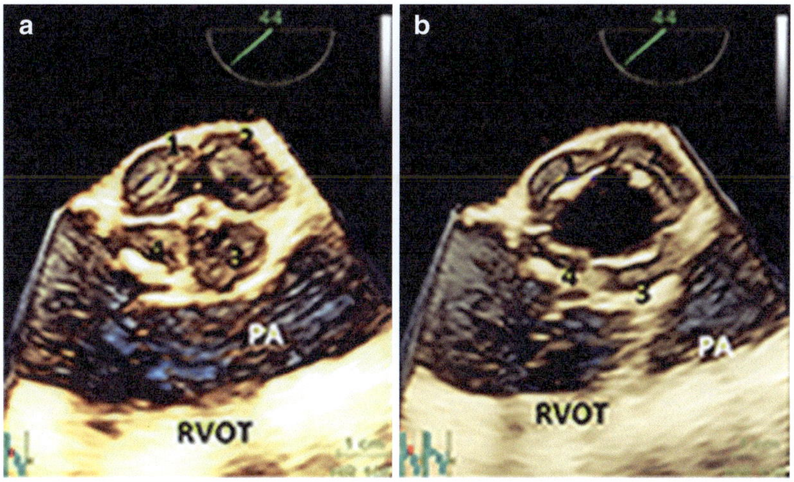

Fig. 14.2 Quadricuspid aortic valve. Three-dimensional echocardiography reveals quadricuspid aortic valve in a young patient with moderate aortic regurgitation. (**a**) Shows the closed aortic valve with four cusps (1, 2, 3, and 4), the pulmonary artery and the right ventricle outflow tract in a short axis view. (**b**) Shows the aortic valve when opened. *PA* pulmonary artery, *RVOT* right ventricular outflow tract

degeneration, vegetations (Fig. 14.3), tumors (Fig. 14.4), perforation [11] (Fig. 14.5), or prolapse [12] (Fig. 14.6).

Bicuspid aortic valve, one of the most important causes of AR, is better identified with 3DE than with two-dimensional echocardiography [8, 9] (Fig. 14.1), 3DE allows discriminating between bicuspid and tricuspid valve by avoiding the confusion created by the raphe between two aortic valve leaflets associated with inadequate aortic valve cross-section by using two-dimensional echocardiography [3]. In addition, transesophageal 3DE provides images of unprecedented quality, allowing a detailed analysis of the congenital abnormalities and the "fish-mouth" opening of the bicuspid aortic valve [7] (Fig. 14.1). Transthoracic 3DE has been validated against anatomic examination of autopsy specimens, demonstrating a reliable morphological characterization of the aortic valve [9].

For the assessment of aortic valve endocarditis, 3DE is capable of defining the size and shape of vegetations, their mobility, and insertion [3] (Fig. 14.3). Moreover, the use of 3DE helps to assess the presence of complications in patients with aortic valve endocarditis, such as perforations, aneurisms, and abscesses [13]. Complications after interventional procedures, such as perforation of one of the aortic valve cusps, can be best visualized with 3DE (Fig. 14.5).

Visualization of the normal thin or heavily calcified aortic cusps is usually difficult when using 3DE transthoracic approach. Therefore, transesophageal 3DE from upper esophageal views provides superior spatial resolution and image quality [3, 14], which allows a more accurate analysis of the aortic cusps morphology, and the aortic valve opening and closure. This applies also for AR of rheumatic etiology, where the commissures are thickened and fused, with restricted opening and closure (Fig. 14.7a, b). Moreover, color transesophageal 3DE has a complementary role to assess the size, shape, and location of the AR jet (Fig. 14.7d). By acquiring the mitral and the aortic valves in the same full-volume dataset, associated with the use of

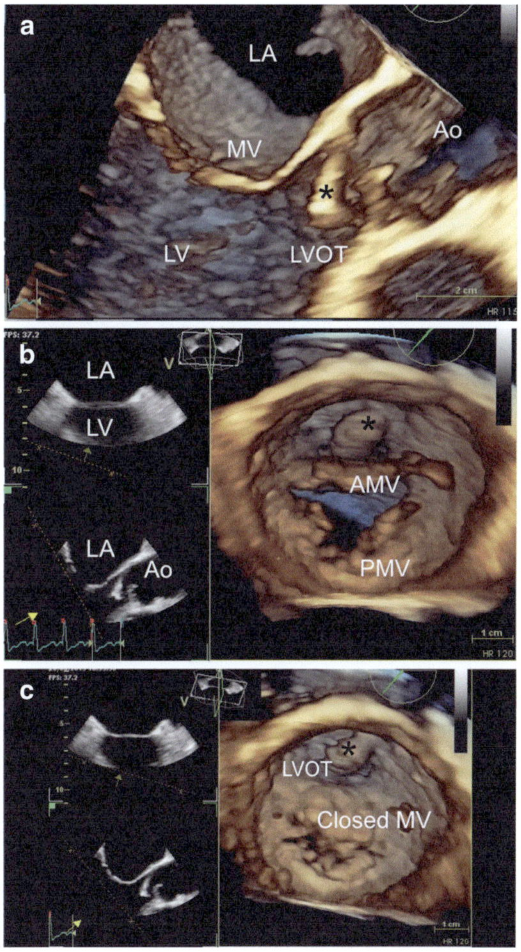

Fig. 14.3 Endocarditis at the level of the aortic valve with flail of a leaflet. The patient had a history of Ross procedure, with the pulmonic valve implanted in the aortic position. Three years after the procedure he developed fatigue and anemia. Two-dimensional echocardiography revealed severe aortic regurgitation and a mobile mass at the level of the left ventricular outflow tract. Three-dimensional echocardiography showed the voluminous mobile mass in both long axis and short axis view, at the level of the left ventricular outflow tract, at the top of the anterior mitral valve. *AMV* anterior mitral valve, *Ao* aorta, *LA* left atrium, *LV* left ventricle, *LVOT* left ventricular outflow tract, *MV* mitral valve, *RV* right atrium, the vegetation on both 2D and 3D images is marked with asterisk

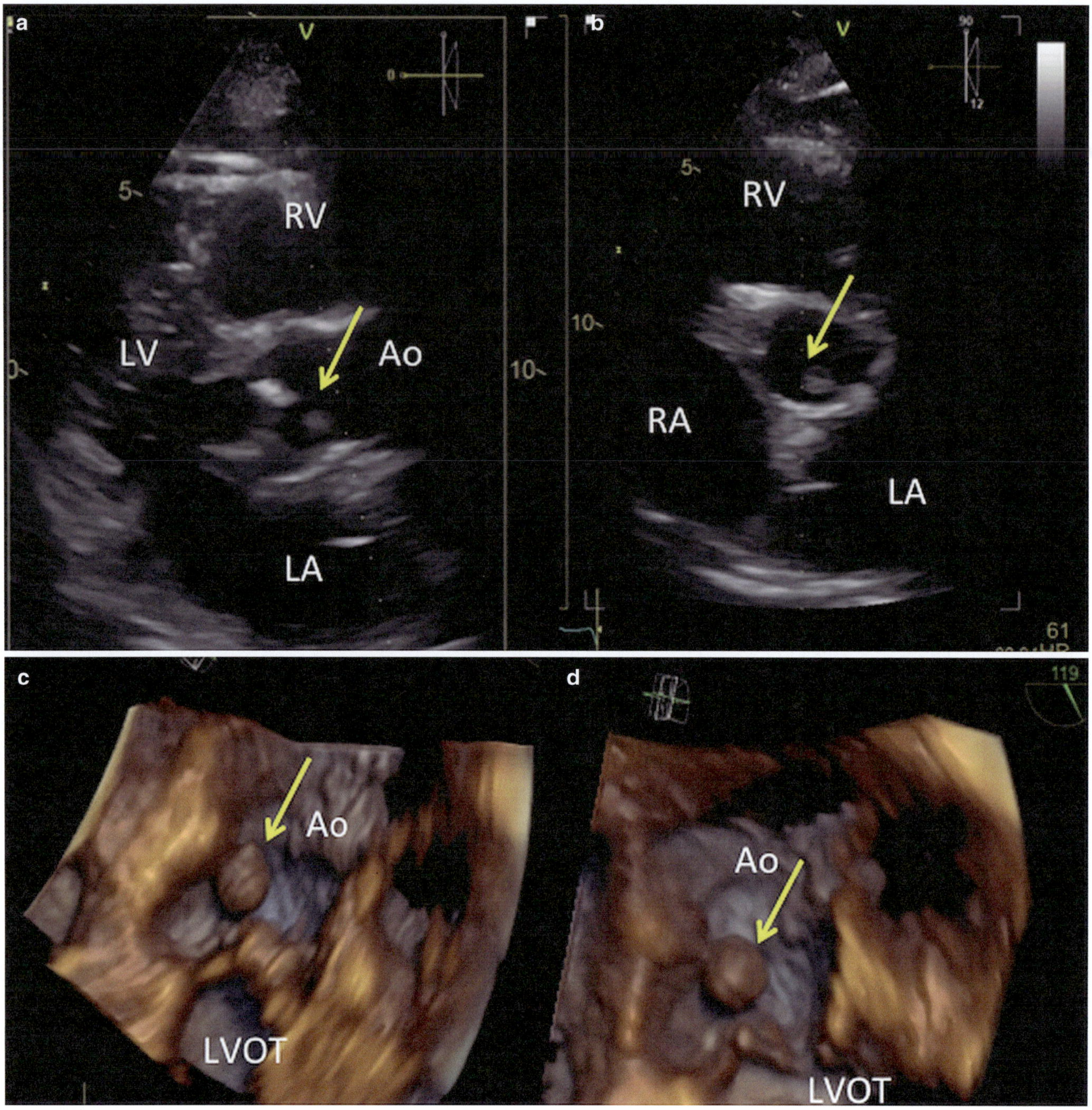

Fig. 14.4 Fibro-elastoma attached to the sinus of Valsalva in a patient with moderate aortic regurgitation. Two-dimensional echocardiography (**a**, **b**) reveals a small mass (yellow arrow), highly mobile through the left ventricular outflow tract with the opening of the aortic valve. Three-dimensional echocardiography (**c**, **d**) shows the real shape and size of the mass and its insertion inside the aorta, at the level of Sinus of Valsalva. *Ao* aorta, *LA* left atrium, *LV* left ventricle, *LVOT* left ventricular outflow tract, *RA* right atrium, *RV* right ventricle

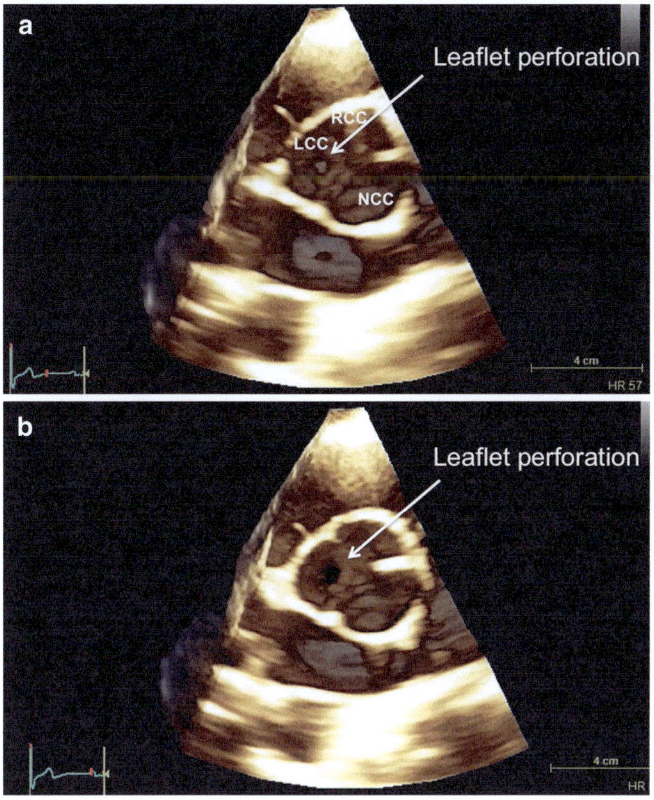

Fig. 14.5 Perforation at the level of the aortic left coronary cusp after angioplasty in a patient presented with unstable angina. The aortic valve is visualized in a short axis view, in which a round orifice is seen during diastole (both in **a**, **b**), when the valve is closed. *LCC* left coronary cusp, *NCC* non-coronary cusp, *RCC* right coronary cusp

dedicated software package, one can analyze the coupling between the aortic and the mitral valve during the cardiac cycle [14] (Fig. 14.7). After aortic valve replacement, a decrease in mitral regurgitation is noted [15], while the motion of the mitral annulus is affected by prosthesis implanted in the aortic position [4].

In patients with AR, aortic valve repair is a desired alternative to replacement, due to lower risks for endocarditis and complications related to prostheses [3]. In this setting, echocardiography is essential for patient selection and procedure planning, which is technically more challenging than aortic valve replacement. 3DE allows the reconstruction of the aortic valve complex into realistic models, visualized in both static and dynamic fashion, on which measurements of different parameters important for the surgeon can be performed and used to ensure a successful procedure (Fig. 14.8).

Severity Assessment of Aortic Regurgitation

Two-dimensional and Doppler echocardiography assessment of valvular regurgitations is based on PISA measurements, which is assumed to have a perfect hemispherical shape, due to a planar and circular regurgitant orifice. This assumption is seldom met into real life [16], where the regurgitant orifice has an irregular, three-dimensional, and dynamic shape. Complementary use of color 3DE allows a more accurate assessment of the vena contracta dimension and shape by cropping the AR jet in a perpendicular fashion at multiple levels, in order to identify and measure the smallest color jet area [17] (Fig. 14.7). This method showed good accuracy in animal models [18, 19] and in patients [17, 20] when compared with angiography, cardiac magnetic resonance and conventional two-dimensional echocardiography and Doppler measurements.

Other 3DE methods to quantify the AR severity, such as deriving regurgitant volume from the difference of the left and right stroke volumes [19] are still experimental and further studies are needed in this direction. Recently, dedicated software package has been developed to measure the true volume of PISA and to offer a more accurate estimation of the regurgitant volume, but at present, it has been validated only for the mitral and tricuspid regurgitation [21]. Similar software might be accustomed also for the AR jet quantification, but this remains to be to be validated.

Clinical Cases

Case 14.1

Thirty-eight-year-old woman presenting for routine two-dimensional echocardiography. Conventional two-dimensional echocardiography reveals dilated ascending aorta and asymmetrical closure of the aortic valve in a parasternal long axis view. Mild AR is visualized. In a short axis view, the aortic valve seems tricuspid when closed, but with an apparent "fish-mouth" orifice when opened. Dilation of the ascending aorta prevented from obtaining a clear cut-plane of the aortic cusps, in order to identify bicuspid aortic valve. Conversely, a full-volume of the aortic valve was acquired and multiple cut-planes were attempted, until they revealed the bicuspid morphology. A complete raphe between the aortic "pseudo-cusps" was visualized. Even though no significant aortic regurgitation was noted, the dilation of the ascending aorta of more than 52 mm in the presence of bicuspid aortic valve prompted the indication for aortic surgery in this young patient (Fig 14.1).

Case 14.2

Fifty-four-year-old man presenting with ST-elevation acute anterior myocardial infarction, Killip I. Emergency coronary angiography is performed, with successful stenting of the left anterior descending coronary artery. Even though the

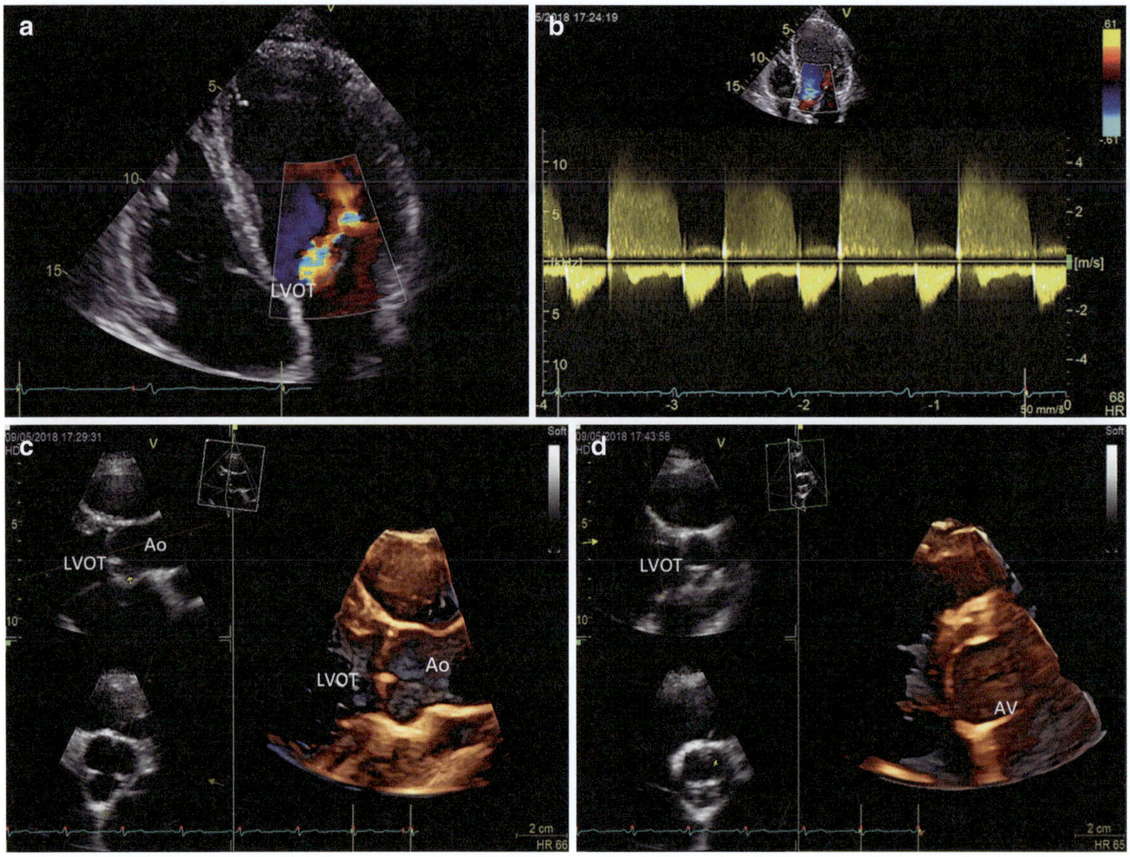

Fig. 14.6 Aortic regurgitation in a patient with aortic valve prolapse. (**a**) Shows an eccentric jet of aortic regurgitation. (**b**) Shows the Doppler curve of the aortic regurgitation. (**c**, **d**) Show the three-dimensional echocardiographic images of the aortic valve, with the evident prolapse revealed in the long axis view (**c**) and the regurgitant orifice in the short axis view (**d**). *Ao* aorta, *AV* aortic valve, *LVOT* left ventricular outflow tract

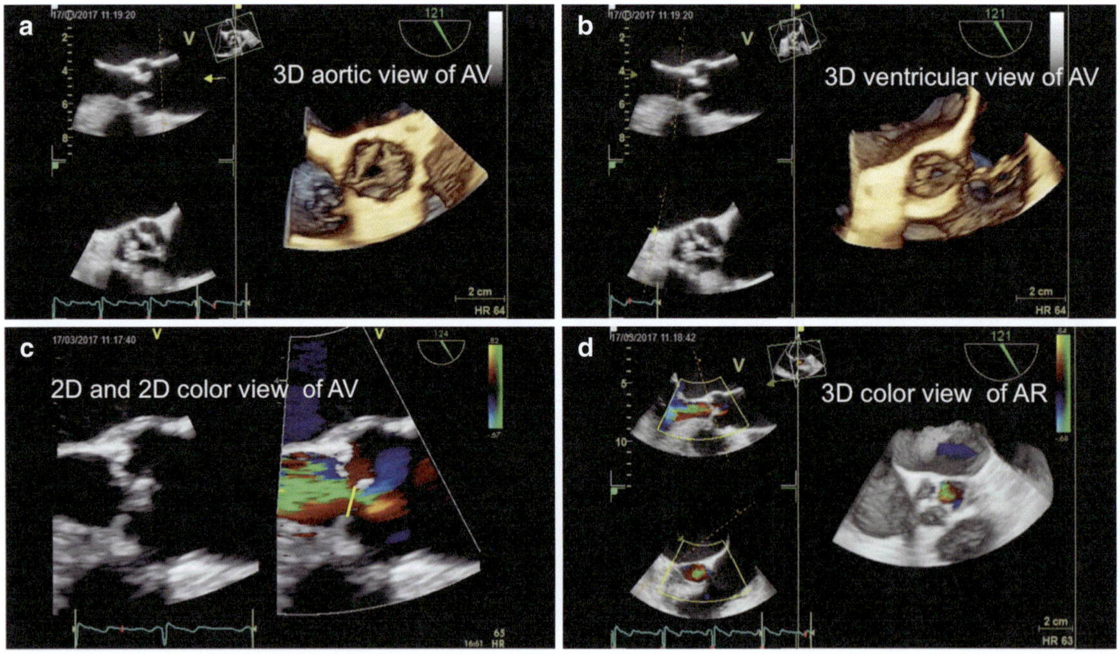

Fig. 14.7 Two- and three-dimensional echocardiography images of a rheumatic aortic valve in a patient with severe aortic regurgitation and moderate mitral regurgitation. (**a**) Shows the aortic side of the AV, with thickened and fused commissures; (**b**) shows the ventricular side of the AV, with the regurgitant orifice during proto-diastole; (**c**) shows the 2D color view of the aortic regurgitation jet from a parasternal long axis view; (**d**) shows the 3D color view of the aortic regurgitation jet, between the right and non-coronary cusps. *AV* aortic valve, *AR* aortic regurgitation

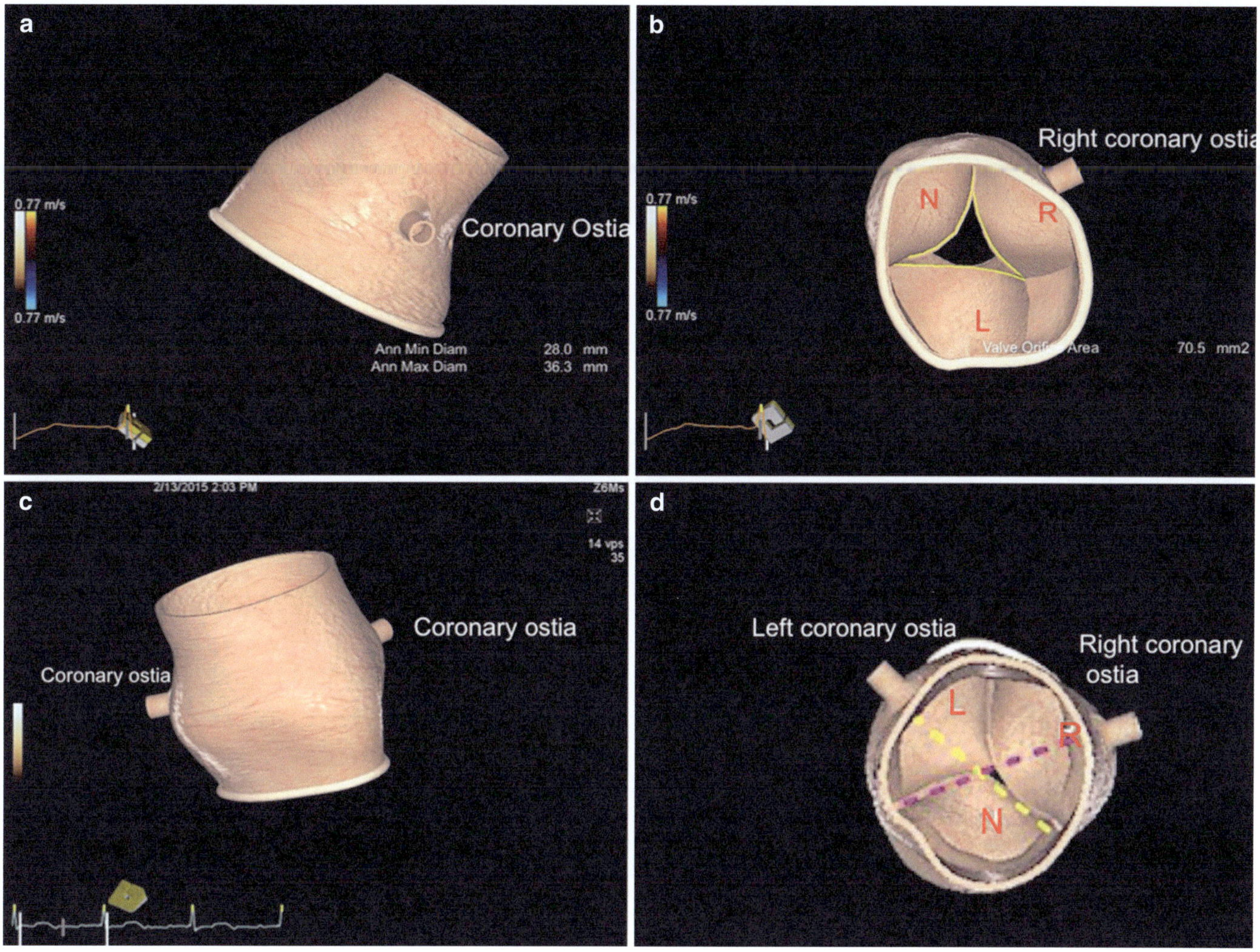

Fig. 14.8 Realistic model of the aortic valve complex obtained with three-dimensional echocardiography and dedicated software package. (**a**, **b**) Shows the reconstruction of a dilated aortic valve, with a regurgitant orifice due to dilation of the aortic annulus. Coronary ostia can be seen in (**a**, **c**), while right (R), left (L), and non-coronary (NC) aortic cusps are shown in (**b**). (**c**, **d**) Shows the reconstruction of a normal aortic valve and aortic root, with normal closure of the cusps

procedure was successful and the ECG changes were regressive, the patient developed progressive dyspnea. Echocardiography performed after the procedure revealed new onset of severe AR. However, the aortic valve did not show pathological features by two-dimensional echocardiography in both parasternal long and short axis views. A 3DE full volume, of the aortic valve was acquired from the parasternal short axis view and cropped below and above the aortic valve. The images showed a small "hole" in the left coronary cusp (Fig. 14.5). Complementary assessment using color 3DE showed that the orifice in the aortic cusp matched with the aortic regurgitant flow. Therefore, 3DE was pivotal to identify the true cause of the AR: a perforation of the aortic cusp during the procedure.

Case 14.3

Thirty-five-year-old man, with history of Ross procedure for bicuspid aortic valve 3 years prior, presenting with weight loss, anemia and exhertional dyspnea. Two-dimensional echocardiography revealed severe regurgitation of the bioprosthesis (Fig. 14.9) and a mobile mass attached to one of its cusps. 3DE revealed the true dimensions of the vegetation, its protrusion into the left ventricular outflow tract, and the flail of one of the valve cusps that causes severe regurgitation (Fig. 14.3). Moreover, 3DE showed a para-prosthetic abscess, which communicates with the left ventricular outflow tract and an inter-ventricular septal defect at the level of the membranous septum (Fig. 14.9).

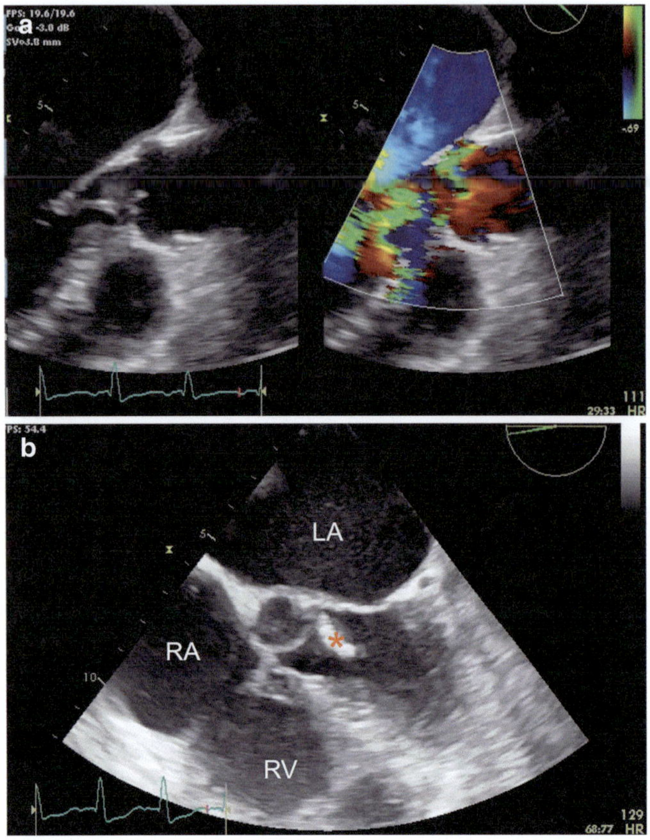

Fig. 14.9 Severe aortic regurgitation a patient with history of Ross procedure, due to endocarditis of the prosthesis. Two-dimensional echocardiography color Doppler of the aortic regurgitation (**a**), and the mobile mass seen into the left ventricular outflow tract (**b**). Three-dimensional images of the vegetation are shown in Fig. 14.3. *LA* left atrium, *RA* right atrium, *RV* right ventricle

References

1. Badano LP, Boccalini F, Muraru D, Bianco LD, Peluso D, Bellu R, et al. Current clinical applications of transthoracic three-dimensional echocardiography. J Cardiovasc Ultrasound. 2012;20(1):1–22.
2. Lang RM, Mor-Avi V, Sugeng L, Nieman PS, Sahn DJ. Three-dimensional echocardiography: the benefits of the additional dimension. J Am Coll Cardiol. 2006;48(10):2053–69.
3. Muraru D, Badano LP, Vannan M, Iliceto S. Assessment of aortic valve complex by three-dimensional echocardiography: a framework for its effective application in clinical practice. Eur Heart J Cardiovasc Imaging. 2012;13(7):541–55.
4. Mahmood F, Warraich HJ, Gorman JH 3rd, Gorman RC, Chen TH, Panzica P, et al. Changes in mitral annular geometry after aortic valve replacement: a three-dimensional transesophageal echocardiographic study. J Heart Valve Dis. 2012;21(6):696–701.
5. Veronesi F, Caiani EG, Sugeng L, Fusini L, Tamborini G, Alamanni F, et al. Effect of mitral valve repair on mitral-aortic coupling: a real-time three-dimensional transesophageal echocardiography study. J Am Soc Echocardiogr. 2012;25(5):524–31.
6. Joint Task Force on the Management of Valvular Heart Disease of the European Society of Cardiology, European Association for Cardio-Thoracic Surgery, Vahanian A, Alfieri O, Andreotti F, Antunes MJ, et al. Guidelines on the management of valvular heart disease (version 2012). Eur Heart J. 2012;33(19):2451–96.
7. Lang RM, Tsang W, Weinert L, Mor-Avi V, Chandra S. Valvular heart disease. The value of 3-dimensional echocardiography. J Am Coll Cardiol. 2011;58(19):1933–44.
8. Sadron Blaye-Felice MA, Seguela PE, Arnaudis B, Dulac Y, Lepage B, Acar P. Usefulness of three-dimensional transthoracic echocardiography for the classification of congenital bicuspid aortic valve in children. Eur Heart J Cardiovasc Imaging. 2012;13(12):1047–52.
9. Espinola-Zavaleta N, Munoz-Castellanos L, Attie F, Hernandez-Morales G, Zamora-Gonzalez C, Duenas-Carbajal R, et al. Anatomic three-dimensional echocardiographic correlation of bicuspid aortic valve. J Am Soc Echocardiogr. 2003;16(1):46–53.
10. Burri MV, Nanda NC, Singh A, Panwar SR. Live/real time three-dimensional transthoracic echocardiographic identification of quadricuspid aortic valve. Echocardiography. 2007;24(6):653–5.
11. Longobardo L, Coluccia V, Azzu A, Scarfo IS, Alfieri O, La Canna G. Three-dimensional echocardiography diagnosis of double perforation of bicuspid aortic valve. J Cardiovasc Med (Hagerstown). 2017;18(10):841–2.
12. Szymanski T, Maslow A, Mahmood F, Singh A. Three-dimensional echocardiographic assessment of coaptation after aortic valve repair. J Cardiothorac Vasc Anesth. 2017;31(3):993–1000.
13. Nemes A, Lagrand WK, McGhie JS, ten Cate FJ. Three-dimensional transesophageal echocardiography in the evaluation of aortic valve destruction by endocarditis. J Am Soc Echocardiogr. 2006;19(3):355 e13–4.
14. Veronesi F, Corsi C, Sugeng L, Mor-Avi V, Caiani EG, Weinert L, et al. A study of functional anatomy of aortic-mitral valve coupling using 3D matrix transesophageal echocardiography. Circ Cardiovasc Imaging. 2009;2(1):24–31.
15. Khosravi A, Sheykhloo H, Karbasi-Afshar R, Saburi A. Echocardiographic changes after aortic valve replacement: Does the failure rate of mitral valve change? ARYA Atheroscler. 2015;11(2):147–52.
16. Shiota T, Jones M, Delabays A, Li X, Yamada I, Ishii M, et al. Direct measurement of three-dimensionally reconstructed flow convergence surface area and regurgitant flow in aortic regurgitation: in vitro and chronic animal model studies. Circulation. 1997;96(10):3687–95.
17. Fang L, Hsiung MC, Miller AP, Nanda NC, Yin WH, Young MS, et al. Assessment of aortic regurgitation by live three-dimensional transthoracic echocardiographic measurements of vena contracta area: usefulness and validation. Echocardiography. 2005;22(9):775–81.
18. Mori Y, Shiota T, Jones M, Wanitkun S, Irvine T, Li X, et al. Three-dimensional reconstruction of the color Doppler-imaged vena contracta for quantifying aortic regurgitation: studies in a chronic animal model. Circulation. 1999;99(12):1611–7.
19. Li X, Jones M, Irvine T, Rusk RA, Mori Y, Hashimoto I, et al. Real-time 3-dimensional echocardiography for quantification of the difference in left ventricular versus right ventricular stroke volume in a chronic animal model study: improved results using C-scans for quantifying aortic regurgitation. J Am Soc Echocardiogr. 2004;17(8):870–5.
20. Chin CH, Chen CH, Lo HS. The correlation between three-dimensional vena contracta area and aortic regurgitation index in patients with aortic regurgitation. Echocardiography. 2010;27(2):161–6.
21. Grady L, Datta S, Kutter O, Duong C, Wein W, Little SH, et al. Regurgitation quantification using 3D PISA in volume echocardiography. Med Image Comput Comput Assist Interv. 2011;14(Pt 3):512–9.

15 Assessment After Surgery or Interventional Procedures on the Aortic Valve

Rebecca T. Hahn

Abstract

This chapter will cover the post-operative assessment of surgical and transcatheter aortic valves. Complications of surgical prostheses including paravalvular regurgitation and the use of three-dimensional imaging for guidance of prosthetic paravalvular regurgitation closure will also be discussed. Finally, the intra-procedural monitoring of transcatheter aortic valve replacement will be reviewed with case examples.

Keywords

Surgical aortic valve replacement · Bioprosthetic · Mechanical prosthesis · Transcatheter aortic valve replacement

Introduction

Three-dimensional echocardiography (3DE) has significantly changed the assessment of valvular pathology and has revolutionized not only patient selection for surgical repair but also for newer transcatheter procedures. This chapter will cover the post-operative assessment of surgical aortic valves, and the intra-procedural monitoring of transcatheter aortic valve replacements as well as of transcatheter treatment of aortic prosthetic paravalvular regurgitation.

Electronic Supplementary Material The online version of this chapter (https://doi.org/10.1007/978-3-030-14032-8_15) contains supplementary material, which is available to authorized users.

R. T. Hahn (✉)
Department of Cardiology/Structural Heart and Valve Center, Columbia University Medical Center, New York, NY, USA
e-mail: rth2@columbia.edu

Surgical Aortic Valve Replacement

The post-operative assessment of the aortic valve will depend on the primary valve lesion (i.e. stenosis versus regurgitation) and the surgical procedure performed (i.e. repair or replacement) as well as prosthetic valve type (mechanical or biologic). For surgical aortic valve replacement there has been a trend toward replacement with bioprosthetic valves, not only because randomized trials comparing biologic and mechanical valves in patients undergoing aortic valve replacement have shown no significant survival differences [1–3], but also with growing data showing the feasibility of transcatheter aortic valve implantation in failed bioprosthetic valves [4, 5]. If a biologic valve is appropriate, a number of options exist: stented and stentless valves, aortic homografts, and cadaveric recovered autografts.

The sutureless aortic bioprosthesis is another alternative to high risk surgical aortic valve replacement [4–7]. These valves use a self-expanding anchoring device into which the bioprosthetic valve is attached. There is no suture line, similar to the transcatheter aortic valve replacement (TAVR) devices. There are a number of advantages of this device over a TAVR: valve excision and annular decalcification and precise positioning. The advantages over traditional surgical aortic valve replacement include: reduced operative time and trauma, and the option for minimally invasive approaches [8]. Although some reports suggested a higher incidence of paravalvular regurgitation, a recent propensity matched comparison of the sutureless valve compared to transapical TAVR shows a lower incidence of paravalvular regurgitation but higher incidence of atrial fibrillation [6].

For aortic valve replacement in the setting of aortic stenosis, the pre-surgical evaluation should include a calculation of the ideal valve area for body surface area to avoid prosthesis-patient mismatch [9]. This requires a determination of annular area and determination of the maximum valve area with implantation of a specific size/type of prosthesis. If the esti-

L. P. Badano et al. (eds.), *Textbook of Three-Dimensional Echocardiography*, https://doi.org/10.1007/978-3-030-14032-8_15

mated effective orifice area indexed to body surface area is <0.85 cm^2/m^2, then aortic root enlargement or TAVR which yields typically larger valve areas for any given annular size, should be strongly considered. Although sizing for surgical aortic valve replacement has relied on surgical sizers, the TAVR literature clearly shows the accuracy of computed tomography and 3DE for measurement of the aortic annulus and sizing of the prosthesis [10, 11]. As new valve designs, in particularly the sutureless valves, are perfected, this complication of surgical aortic valve replacement may decrease.

Post-operative Assessment of Surgical Interventions

The immediate post-cardiopulmonary bypass assessment of the aortic valve includes an assessment of prosthesis seating and stability, prosthesis (or native if repaired) leaflet motion, impingement or trauma to adjacent structures (i.e. aorta), and an assessment of valve function. A comprehensive Doppler evaluation follows the same principles as for native valve stenosis and regurgitation assessment [12, 13]. Color Doppler, pulsed wave Doppler and continuous wave Doppler should be performed from multiple windows in order to minimize insonation angle, optimize imaging and accurately assess valve gradients and valve area, as well as the presence of aortic regurgitation. For calculations of effective orifice area or Doppler velocity index which require measurement of stroke volumes from different cardiac cycles and measurement of peak transvalvular velocity-time integral, matching the respective cycles lengths to within 10% is advised [14].

Increase velocities or gradients across the aortic valve may not always indicate prosthesis stenosis. Similarly, low gradients across the aortic valve, although comforting, may not always be normal. A flow-independent measure of valve area should always be performed to confirm that a low (or high) gradient is associated with normal function of the valve. In the setting of a high gradient, a standard algorithm should be followed to determine the etiology. First, the valve area should be calculated. If the effective orifice area is within the expected range for the valve type and size, then confirmation by a close evaluation of the prosthesis occluders (discs for a mechanical valve, and leaflets for a bioprosthetic valve) should confirm normal opening and closure. In addition, indexing the effective orifice area to body size may help determine if patient-prosthesis mismatch may be the cause of the high gradient. In the absence of patient-prosthesis mismatch, other etiologies of a high gradient but normal valve area should be sought, including a high output state, subvalvular obstruction or aortic regurgitation [15, 16].

Double envelope spectral Doppler profiles may often be seen in the setting of mechanical prostheses [17]. This is related to different flow characteristics of the mechanical orifices. In the setting of a single tilting disc, a large major and small minor orifice may create a dense and typically lower velocity jet arising from the major orifice, and a faint, higher velocity jet from the minor orifice. Similarly, the bileaflet disc mechanical valve generates a dense, lower velocity jet arising from the lateral orifices, with a faint, higher velocity jet from the central orifice. The faint, higher velocity profiles are created by pressure-recovery and do not represent flow from the main orifice(s); the dense, lower velocity jet should be used to assess function and calculate effective orifice area by continuity equation.

Long-term follow-up is required to determine the presence of prosthetic valve dysfunction. Prosthetic valve dysfunction may be categorized as structural or non-structural [18]. Structural valve dysfunction includes dysfunction or deterioration intrinsic to the valve, including calcification, leaflet tear or flail. This complication is more common in biologic valves, and may occur earlier in younger patients. Other patient comorbidities such as renal failure may increase the risk of calcification. Nonstructural valve dysfunction characteristically is seen early following implantation and is defined as any abnormality not intrinsic to the valve itself. These complications are usually related to technical issues and include suture dehiscence with associated paravalvular regurgitation, problems related to retained native mitral apparatus and prosthesis-patient mismatch. For the aortic prosthesis, motion discordant with the motion of the adjacent aortic root and native annulus usually indicates significant (40–90% of the annular circumference) dehiscence [19]. Other nonstructural problems such as pannus formation are late complications.

Significant complications that are not included in this simple classification system are thrombosis and endocarditis. Distinguishing pannus from thrombus may be difficult [14, 20]. Occurring almost exclusively on mechanical valves, thrombi are generally large, tissue-density masses which may interfere with occluder motion. The clinical history may give further clues since a short duration of symptoms (typically dyspnea or an embolic event) and inadequate anticoagulation or cause for increased coagulability are commonly associated [14, 21]. Lin et al. [22] formalized a grading scheme for predicting thrombus versus pannus. In this study of 53 patients with surgical confirmation, the transesophageal predictors of thrombus including: mobile mass [tissue-density], attachment to occluder, elevated gradient (peak aortic gradient ≥50 mmHg, mean mitral valve gradient ≥10 mmHg) and INR ≤2.5. The prevalence of thrombus was 14% with ≤1 predictor, 69% with 2 predictors, and 91% with ≥3 predictors. For the aortic position, pannus is more common than thrombus.

Echocardiography is an integral tool for the diagnosis and management of prosthetic valve endocarditis (Fig. 15.1, Video 15.1, Fig. 15.2, Videos 15.2a and 15.2b). Vegetations, valve dysfunction and periannular extension are the primary

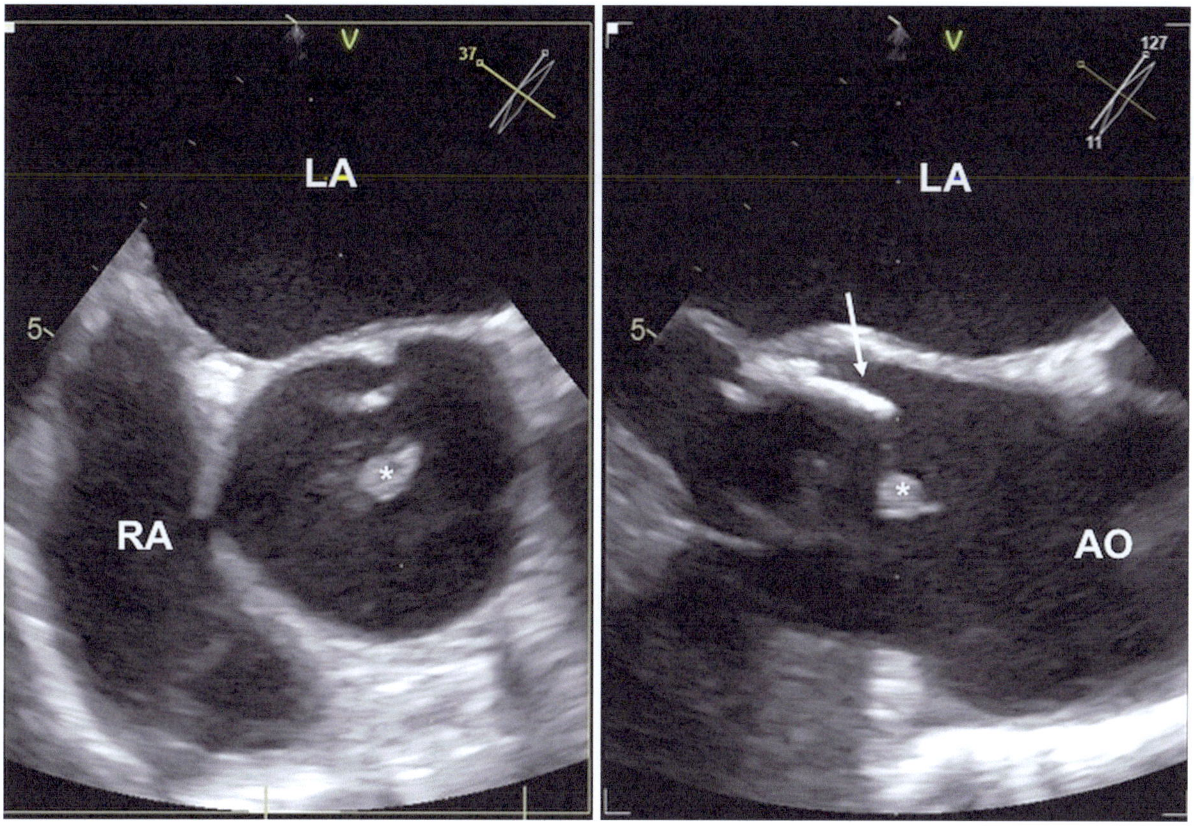

Fig. 15.1 Biplane display of aortic bioprosthesis endocarditis. *Left panel*, short axis view of a bioprosthetic valve in aortic position showing a mass (white asterisk) on the non-coronary sinus leaflet. By positioning the cursor on the mass, it is possible to see it in an orthogonal plane (*Right panel*) to increase our confidence in the diagnosis and better appreciate vegetation size and mobility (Video 15.1). *AO* aorta, *LA* left atrium, *RA* right atrium

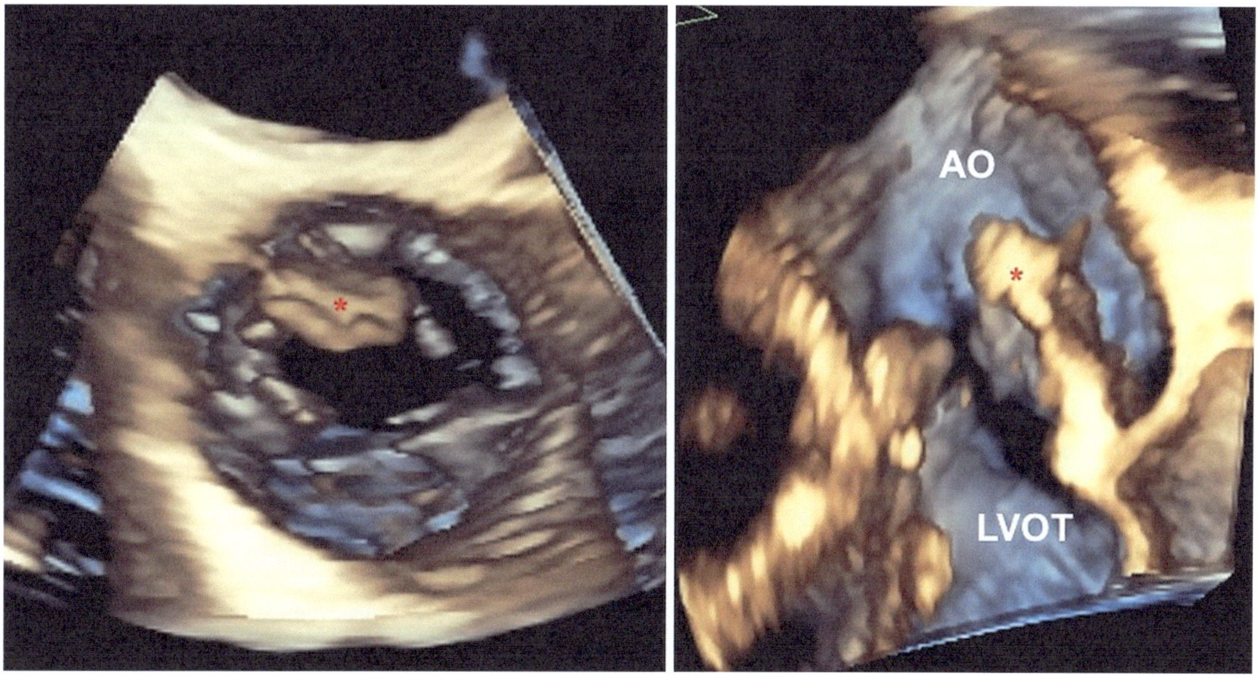

Fig. 15.2 Transesophageal volume rendering display of a vegetation (red asterisk) attached to the non-coronary sinus leaflet of the aortic bioprosthesis. *Left panel*, transversal cut-plane to visualize the prosthesis en face from the aortic perspective (Video 15.2a/left). *Right panel*, longitudinal cut-plane to appreciate vegetation's length and point of attachment. Three-dimensional echocardiography allows a better appreciation of the vegetation size (volume vs. linear dimensions) and mobility (no out-of-plane motion) (Video 15.2b/right). *AO* aorta, *LVOT* left ventricular outflow tract

findings. The diagnosis of a mitral-aortic intervalvular fibrosa pseudoaneurysm deserves special mention. Although most frequently a complication of aortic prosthetic valve endocarditis, it can be seen with mitral prosthetic valve endocarditis as well as in native valve endocarditis. The aortic root and mitral annulus are connected by a fibrous region called the "subaortic curtain" or "intervalvular fibrosa". This is not an uncommon site of infection following prosthetic valve implantation. The diagnosis of an abscess with fistula formation is made by visualization of an echo-free space in the mitral-aortic intervalvular fibrosa with systolic expansion and diastolic collapse with prominent pulsatility from a communication with the left ventricular outflow tract [23].

Further fistula formation between the pseudoaneurysm and the aorta or left atrium may reduce the pulsatility.

Monitoring Interventional Procedures: Paravalvular Closure and Transcatheter Aortic Valve Replacement

Prosthetic Paravalvular Regurgitation Closure

Peri-prosthetic paravalvular leak occurs in 2–10% of aortic prosthetic valves and 7–17% of mitral prosthetic valves [24]. Whereas most of these patients are asymptomatic, 1–3% of patients present clinically as heart failure if the regurgitant volume is large, hemolysis or both. Hemolysis with peri-prosthetic paravalvular leak has been ascribed to three basic mechanisms: fragmentation of erythrocites, collision and acceleration of the jet [25]. In symptomatic patients with severe paravalvular regurgitation the risk of adverse outcome with repeat surgery is up to 16% [2, 26] increasing with each reoperation [26]. Studies have shown that percutaneous closure of peri-prosthetic paravalvular leak is not only possible using a number of different devices [27–31], but successful in treating both heart failure and hemolysis with high procedural success rates [32–35]. Clinical success is determined by the procedural success and the presenting symptom. Improvement in heart failure symptoms is typically limited to patients with no or mild residual regurgitation following closure [34]. Patients with hemolytic anemia however, often fail to improve despite successful closure. Hein et al. [36] observed that 33% of patients requiring transfusions had worsening hemolysis after the procedure, and there was newly developed hemolysis in 10% of all patients. Persistent or worsening hemolysis may be due to the typical off-label use of devices used to close these leaks which are woven from a larger-caliber nitinol mesh which fail to conform to the irregular shapes of the paravalvular defects. More recently the Amplatzer vascular plug (AVP II and IV) devices have been used which have a smaller profile and conform to the shape of the defect allowing them to fit into the small, irregular paravalvular defects resulting in reduced para-device leak.

Transesophageal echocardiography and in particular 3DE, have been essential to procedural guidance of peri-prosthetic paravalvular leak closure, particularly for the mitral position [33, 37–39]. Intra-procedural transesophageal 3DE is used to: determine the exact number and location of the defect(s) in particular in relation to the prosthesis occluders, determine the exact size/dimensions of the defect, help determine the appropriate closure device and number, guide catheter positioning and device deployment, and determine the effectiveness of the procedure. For the aortic position, acoustic shadowing of much of the anterior sewing ring frequently limits the ability of echocardiographic guidance for peri-prosthetic paravalvular leak in this location, although off-axis (deep esophageal) or transgastric views can be also used. Alternatively intracardiac 3DE can be used, but the experience with this imaging modality during paravalvular leak closure is more limited.

Transcatheter Aortic Valve Replacement (TAVR)

Although many TAVR procedures are currently being performed under conscious sedation and fluoroscopic or transthoracic echocardiographic guidance only, the majority of patients in the randomized trials required transesophageal echocardiography guidance during valve implantation [40–43]. Transesophageal echocardiography has likely been instrumental in the reduction of complications such as paravalvular regurgitation [44], reduced use of contrast [45] and improved outcomes [46].

Prior to transcatheter valve deployment, a comprehensive transesophageal echocardiography study as recommended by the American Society of Echocardiography [47] should be performed to document baseline valvular and ventricular size and function. Pre-implant imaging is also used to confirm the annular and thus transcatheter valve size, as well as evaluate the "landing zone" of the transcatheter valve. The latter assessment will allow for anticipation and avoidance of complications such as paravalvular regurgitation (Fig. 15.3, Video 15.3, Fig. 15.4, Videos 15.4a and 15.4b), annular or aortic rupture (Fig. 15.5), or coronary occlusion. During the procedure, transesophageal echocardiography can be used to precisely position wires/catheters (i.e. pacing wires and left ventricular stiff wire) (Fig. 15.6, Videos 15.5a and 15.5b). Imaging during balloon aortic valvuloplasty may be enormously helpful in further procedural planning (Fig. 15.7, Video 15.6). Precise transcatheter valve positioning can be performed, also utilizing transesophageal echocardiography (Fig. 15.8, Video 15.7).

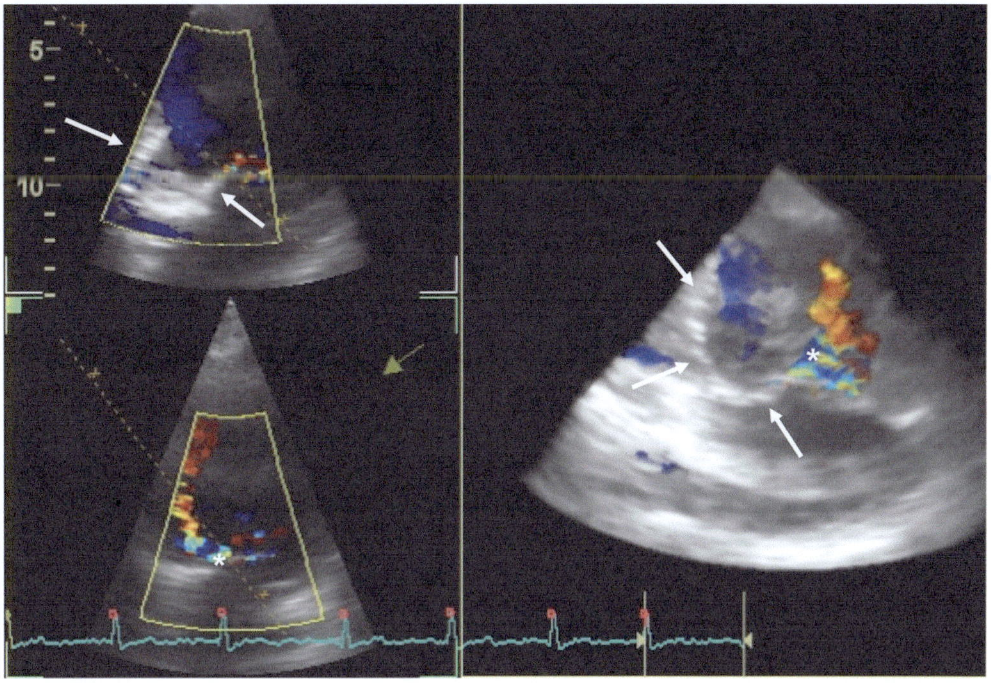

Fig. 15.3 Assessment of paravalvular regurgitation in a patient with poor parasternal acoustic window who received a TAVR (Video 15.3). The transthoracic 3DE color data set acquired from the apical approach can be sliced using a cut plane (broken yellow line) oriented perpendicular to the prosthesis stent (arrows) and passing through the distal part of it (*left panel*) in order to obtain an en face view of the valve from the ventricular perspective (*right panel*) which allows to assess the circumferential extension of the para-valvular leak (asterisk)

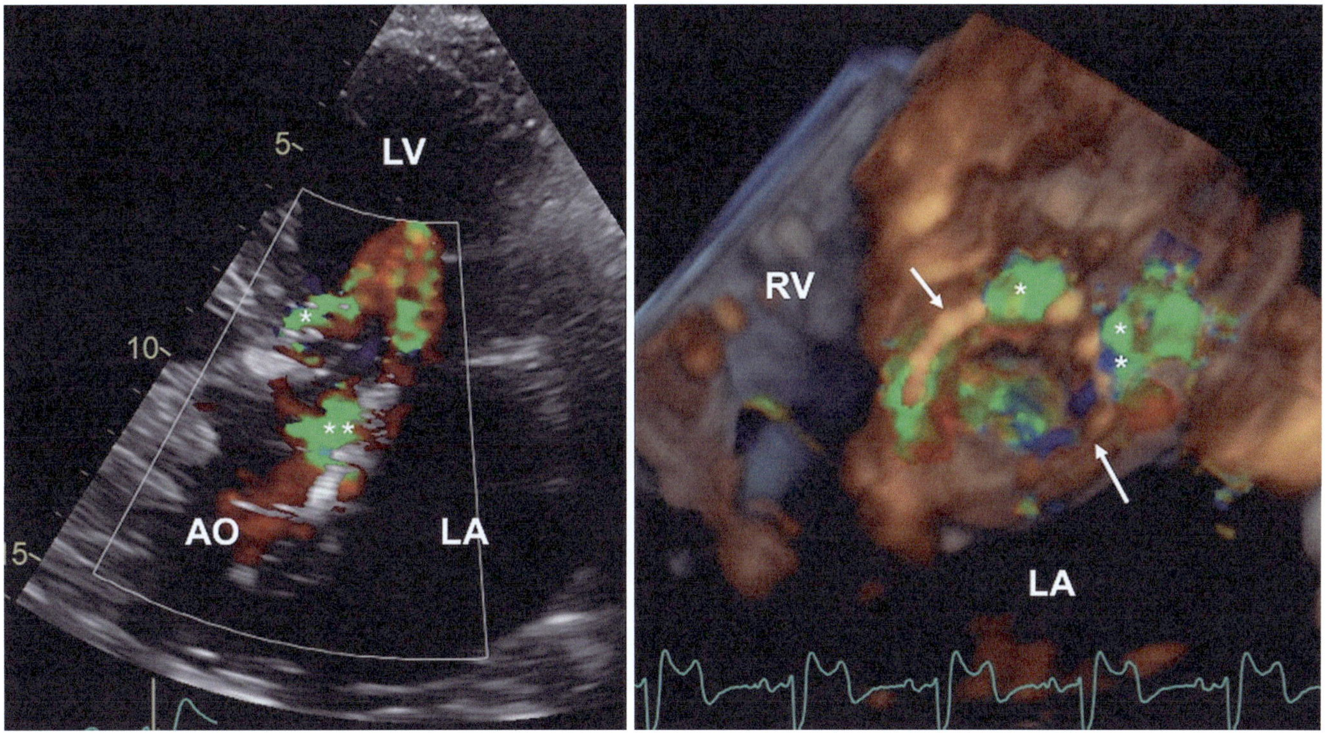

Fig. 15.4 Volume rendering of a severe para-valvular leak in a patients who received a TAVR. *Left panel*, five-chamber two-dimensional echocardiography with color Doppler showing multiple para-valvular leaks (asterisks) (Video 15.4a/left). *Right panel*, transthoracic volume rendered 3DE color acquisition showing the TAVR prosthesis en face from the ventricular perspective. There are two para-valvular leaks at 12 o'clock (asterisk) and from 1 to 3 o'clock (double asterisk). The prosthesis stent is indicated with arrows (Video 15.4b/Right). *AO* aorta, *LA* left atrium, *LV* left ventricle, *RV* right ventricle

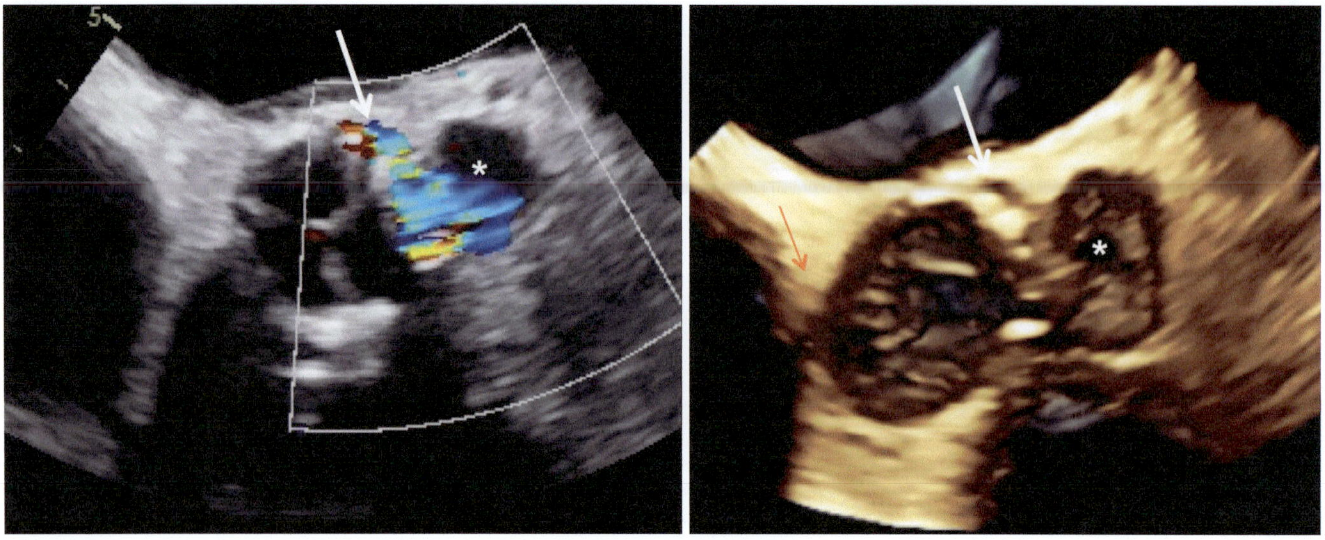

Fig. 15.5 Aortic annulus rupture after TAVR and pseudo aneurysm (asterisk) imaged by two-dimensional color echocardiography (*left panel*) and 3DE volume rendering of prosthesis and the pseudoaneurysm from the aortic perspective (*right panel*). The arrow shows the fistula between the aortic root and the pseudoaneurysm

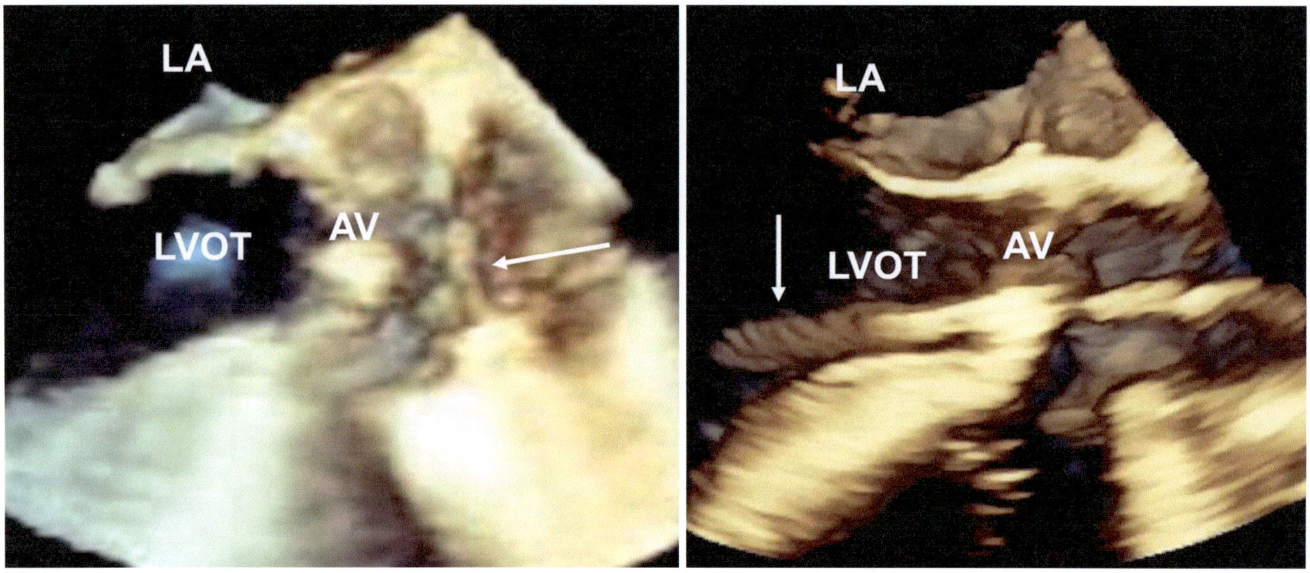

Fig. 15.6 Wire position check using real-time 3DE during TAVR procedure. *Left panel*, 3DE can help the interventional cardiologist to shorten the time needed to cross the stenotic aortic valve in difficult patients by imaging the wire (white arrow) and the valve orifice (Video 15.5a/Left). *Right panel*, after having crossed the valve, 3DE is also useful to check the wire (white arrow) position (Video 15.5b/Right) and the absence of wire related complications such as cardiac tamponade. *AV* aortic valve, *LA* left atrium, *LVOT* left ventricular outflow tract

Following valve deployment, transesophageal echocardiography provides rapid and accurate assessment of valve size/shape, position and function (Fig. 15.9, Video 15.8). But perhaps more importantly, transesophageal echocardiography can rapidly diagnose the etiology of acute hemodynamic compromise: acute valvular dysfunction (aortic or mitral regurgitation), tamponade physiology (chamber perforation or annular rupture), ventricular dysfunction (acute coronary obstruction or ischemic dysfunction) and aortic root catastrophe (aortic dissection or rupture).

Wire and Cannulation Position

The position of wires and catheters can easily be assessed by 3D TEE (Fig. 15.3, Video 15.3).

For transfemoral cases, the curve of the J-wire is ideally positioned in the apex of the ventricle and free of entanglement in the chordae, which on fluoroscopy may not be easily identified. The transapical TAVR approach requires additional imaging of the left ventricular apex (mid-esophageal view) to ensure optimal location of the apical puncture and

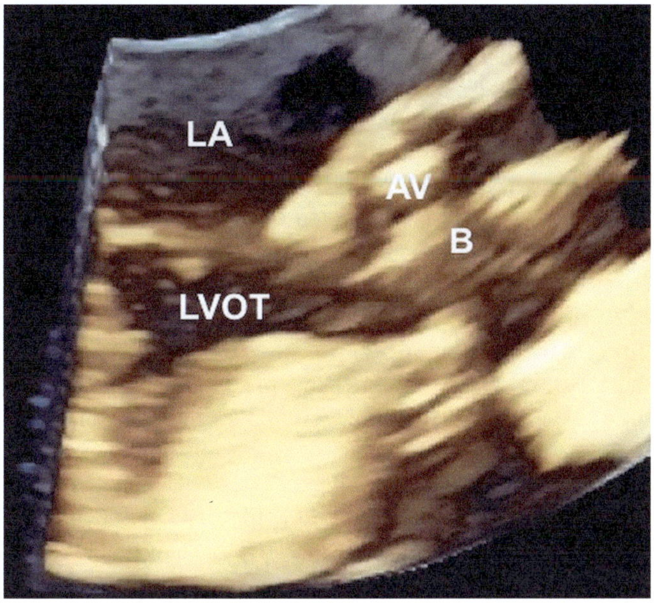

Fig. 15.7 Real-time volume rendering transesophageal 3DE of balloon valvuloplasty. In adjunct to fluoroscopy, echocardiography is useful to control the position of the balloon (B) before and during balloon inflation, and to check the effects of it on cusp mobility and calcium mobilization (Video 15.6). *AV* aortic valve, *LA* left atrium, *LVOT* left ventricular outflow tract

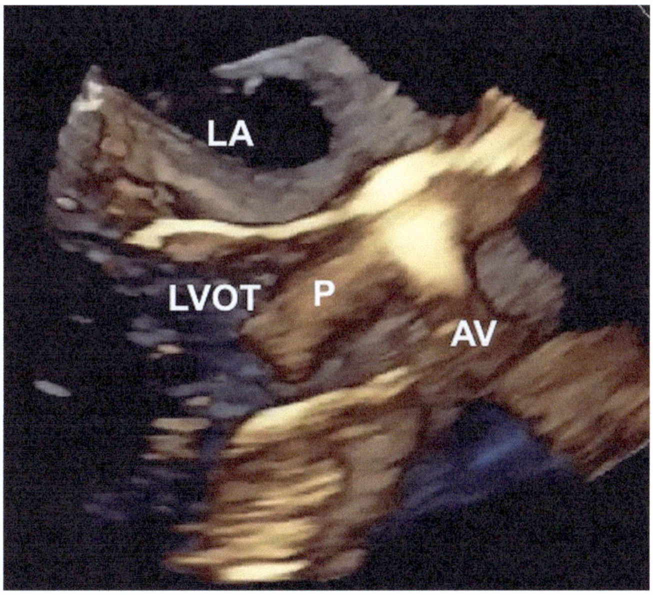

Fig. 15.8 Real-time volume rendering transesophageal 3DE to check prosthesis position before its release. In adjunct to fluoroscopy, echocardiography is useful to control the position of the prosthesis (P) before its release. In the case shown, the prosthesis (P) is too low in the LVOT and should be retracted at the level of the aortic valve (Video 15.7). *AV* aortic valve, *LA* left atrium, *LVOT* left ventricular outflow tract, *P* prosthesis

avoidance of the right ventricle, interventricular septum and papillary muscles.

3D imaging may help localize the cannulation site and guide the wire path within the ventricle.

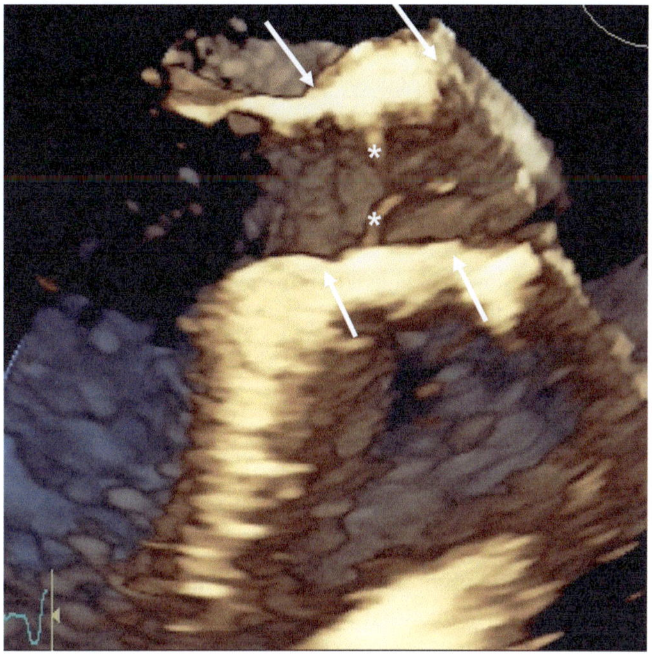

Fig. 15.9 Volume rendering transesophageal 3DE of a Sapien 3 prosthesis after it release. The arrows show the proximal and distal edges of the stent, the leaflets are indicated with the asterisks (Video 15.8)

Balloon Aortic Valvuloplasty

Imaging during balloon aortic valvuloplasty (Fig. 15.7, Video 15.6) is used not only to confirm annular sizing, but also to predict the displacement of calcium (i.e. near the annulus or left ventricular outflow tract) or calcified native structures (i.e. the left coronary cusp in relation to the left main coronary ostium) with valve deployment [48–50]. During balloon aortic valvuloplasty, the simultaneous multi-plane imaging mode is frequently utilized with imaging of the mid-esophageal long axis as the reference view, and short axis views view of the aortic valve or aortic root in the orthogonal lateral plane, depending on the specific high risk feature requiring imaging.

Adjustment of the imaging depth and sector size should be performed to ensure a frame rate of at least 10 Hz. It is important to remember that complications from balloon aortic valvuloplasty occur in up to 16% of patients [51] and echocardiographic imaging can help diagnose acute coronary occlusion, severe aortic regurgitation and tamponade. Finally, imaging following balloon aortic valvuloplasty should document an increase in leaflet opening after balloon aortic valvuloplasty, no significant change in mitral or aortic regurgitation, and no pericardial effusion.

Transcatheter Valve Positioning

Precise positioning the transcatheter heart valve is essential for procedural success and reduction in complications [52, 53]. Transesophageal echocardiography can play an important adjunctive role to fluoroscopy in this regard [54]. The crimped stent can typically be differentiated echocardiographically from the underlying balloon by both reducing overall gain, and angulating the transducer to identify an echodense, sharp-edged structure (as opposed to the heterogeneous appearance of the underlying deflated balloon) (Fig. 15.8, Video 15.7). When two-dimensional imaging is not sufficient, 3DE in the live, narrow-sector mode should be used since the additional depth of imaging may help differentiate the crimped valve and underlying balloon catheter.

The positioning of other valve designs may similarly be aided by the use of transesophageal 3DE however, the following discussion will be limited to the balloon-expandable SAPIEN 3 valve, and the self-expanding Evolut R valve.

Positioning of the SAPIEN 3 valve is different than prior iterations of the balloon-expandable valve. The cell design of this valve results in shortening of the valve only from the ventricular side with early anchoring of the outflow portion of the valve during balloon inflation. Thus positioning should focus on primarily the aortic or outflow end of the valve with the distal edge of the stent covering the native leaflets and below the sino-tubular junction.

Transesophageal 3DE may be useful in localizing calcium in the aortic root or left ventricular outflow tract which can then be avoided with fine-tuning. During valve deployment, transesophageal echocardiography offers the additional benefit of continuous, uninterrupted imaging of the pre-identified high risk features. When the aortic root or annulus appears stretched, balloon inflation can be slowed or even stopped, in order to avoid rupture of these structures.

Positioning of the self-expanding valve is primarily performed under fluoroscopic guidance however transesophageal echocardiography can be used as an adjunctive imaging modality which could reduce contrast use and reduce para-valvular regurgitation. Importantly, the optimal imaging plane of fluoroscopy is not the same as the sagittal (long-axis) transesophageal imaging plane. The posterior edge of the trans-catheter heart valve imaged on transesophageal echocardiography is typically the edge between the noncoronary and left coronary cusp, whereas the posterior edge of the trans-catheter heart valve on fluoroscopy is the edge adjacent to the left coronary cusp. Because of the curvature of the aorta, the transfemoral and often the transaortic approaches will typically result in the tip pointing posteriorly and to the left, such that when initial deployment begins, the posterior edge of the trans-catheter heart valve is "higher" (more aortic) than the anterior edge however as the valve is deployed, there is typically an operator-independent re-orientation of the valve to align more parallel to the long-axis of the aorta. A right subclavian approach however results in the tip pointing more medially and the "higher" edge of the valve is the medial aspect of the valve. The angle of deployment may influence the final non-coaxial position of the valve

Post-procedural Echocardiographic Imaging

Immediately following valve deployment, echocardiographic imaging provides rapid and accurate assessment of valve position, valve shape, leaflet motion (Fig. 15.9, Video 15.8) and gradients. Color Doppler imaging provides prompt and precise feedback to the interventionalists about the presence, location and qualitative severity of aortic regurgitation as well as coronary patency and mitral valve function (Fig. 15.10). In the setting of hemodynamic compromise, potential etiologies such as left and/or right ventricular dysfunction or aortic root catastrophe can be assessed within seconds.

Assessing para-valvular regurgitation is a major role of intra-procedural transesophageal echocardiography. There are a number of obvious differences between surgical and trans-catheter prosthetic valves which may result in significant differences in regurgitant jet anatomy and physiology.

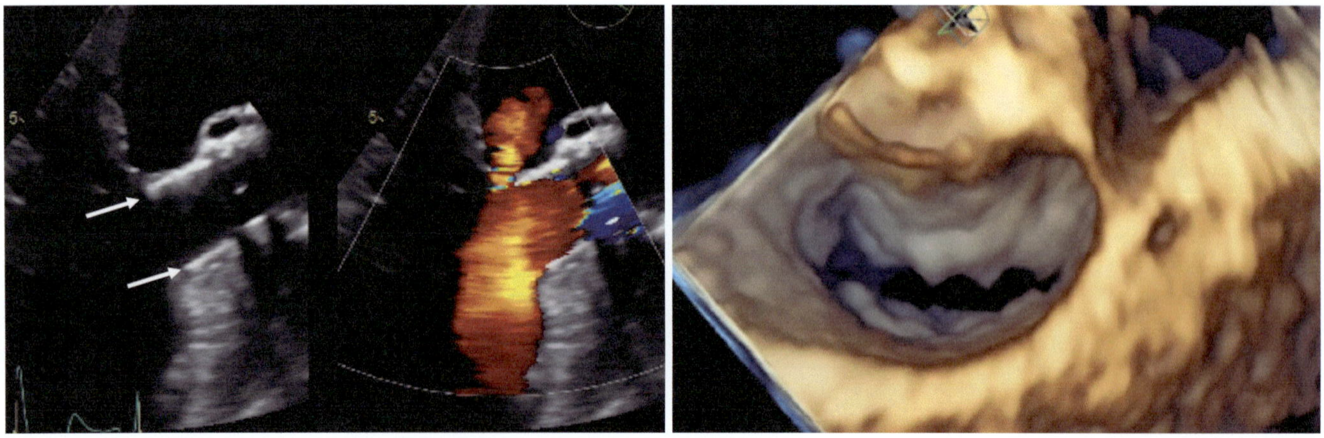

Fig. 15.10 Too low implant of a Sapien 3 valve which interferes with the motion of the anterior leaflet of the mitral valve. *Left panel*, the valve is too low in the left ventricular outflow tract (white arrows pointing at the distal edges of the stent), and interferes with the motion of the anterior leaflet causing mitral regurgitation. *Right panel*, volume rendering of the mitral valve seen en face from the atrial perspective. The stent position impacts on the morphology of the anterior mitral leaflet in the half open position

Transcatheter (and sutureless surgical) valves have no sewing ring and "dehiscence" by traditional definitions, will not occur although malposition or migration may. With transcatheter valves, the native aortic valve cusps and annulus are intact, reducing the space around the stent. Typically, there are multiple small paravalvular jets following TAVR, most commonly at the commissures of the native aortic valve leaflets [55]. In addition, the skirt at the proximal end of the transcatheter valve is specifically designed to reduce para-valvular regurgitation and only jets which extend beyond the skirt and into the left ventricle should be considered "real". Finally, para-valvular regurgitation jets frequently take an eccentric course with some jets directed perpendicular to the left ventricular outflow tract (instead of the typical parallel direction in the left ventricle). The goal of the imager must be to precisely document the origin, course and spatial extent of regurgitant jets and use multiparametric and multi-planar imaging.

Current echocardiographic guidelines [26] do not recommend using color Doppler jet length or vena contracta width to assess the severity of para-valvular regurgitation but in the acute setting post-TAVR, this is an even more important caveat. The aortic stenosis patient typically has a concentrically-hypertrophied ventricle with reduced ventricular compliance and/or diastolic dysfunction. In addition, with advanced age and high prevalence of hypertension, there is in addition significant reduction in aortic compliance. This complex physiology in addition to intra-operative hemodynamic changes, may significantly affect the color Doppler jet within the left ventricular outflow tract. Thus, 3DE may become the method of choice for directly measuring effective regurgitant orifice area and calculating aortic regurgitant volume (Fig. 15.11, Video 15.9). Validation of this technology for quantitating native aortic regurgitation is growing [56–58] and the utility of 3DE for the assessment of prosthetic regurgitation promising [59, 60]. Although a comprehensive, integrative approach must always be used when assessing regurgitation [14], 3D color Doppler can quickly be acquired from the mid-esophageal or deep transgastric views. With the use of off-line analysis packages, two orthogonal long-axis views of the jet, one with the narrowest and one with the broadest width of the jet, to identify plane of the vena contracta (Fig. 15.11, Video 15.9). The vena contracta is then directly planimetered from this short-axis view and a regurgitant volume can be calculated if a complete regurgitant spectral Doppler velocity-time-integral can be traced (Fig. 15.11, Video 15.9).

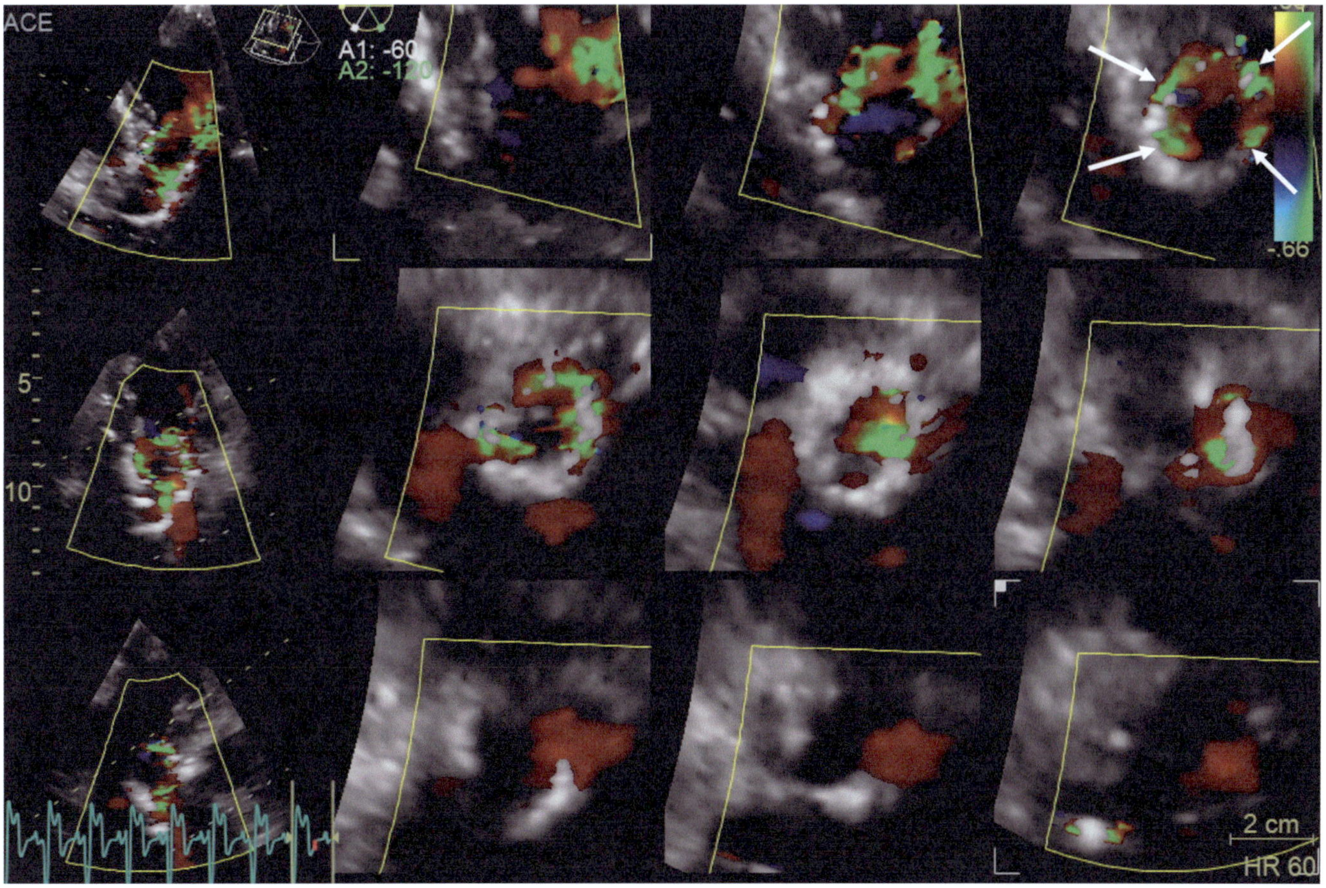

Fig. 15.11 Multislice display of a transthoracic 3DE color data set acquired from the apical approach to identify the origin and circumferential extension of multiple para-valvular leaks (arrows) (Video 15.9)

References

1. Oxenham H, Bloomfield P, Wheatley DJ, Lee RJ, Cunningham J, Prescott RJ, et al. Twenty year comparison of a Bjork-Shiley mechanical heart valve with porcine bioprostheses. Heart. 2003;89(7):715–21.
2. Hammermeister K, Sethi GK, Henderson WG, Grover FL, Oprian C, Rahimtoola SH. Outcomes 15 years after valve replacement with a mechanical versus a bioprosthetic valve: final report of the veterans affairs randomized trial. J Am Coll Cardiol. 2000;36(4):1152–8.
3. Stassano P, Di Tommaso L, Monaco M, Iorio F, Pepino P, Spampinato N, et al. Aortic valve replacement: a prospective randomized evaluation of mechanical versus biological valves in patients ages 55 to 70 years. J Am Coll Cardiol. 2009;54(20):1862–8.
4. D'Onofrio A, Messina A, Lorusso R, Alfieri OR, Fusari M, Rubino P, et al. Sutureless aortic valve replacement as an alternative treatment for patients belonging to the "gray zone" between transcatheter aortic valve implantation and conventional surgery: a propensity-matched, multicenter analysis. J Thorac Cardiovasc Surg. 2012;144(5):1010–6.
5. Flameng W, Herregods MC, Hermans H, Van der Mieren G, Vercalsteren M, Poortmans G, et al. Effect of sutureless implantation of the Perceval S aortic valve bioprosthesis on intraoperative and early postoperative outcomes. J Thorac Cardiovasc Surg. 2011;142(6):1453–7.
6. Martens S, Sadowski J, Eckstein FS, Bartus K, Kapelak B, Sievers HH, et al. Clinical experience with the ATS 3f enable(R) sutureless bioprosthesis. Eur J Thorac Cardiovasc Surg. 2011;40(3):749–55.
7. Phan K, Tsai YC, Niranjan N, Bouchard D, Carrel TP, Dapunt OE, et al. Sutureless aortic valve replacement: a systematic review and meta-analysis. Ann Cardiothorac Surg. 2015;4(2):100–11.
8. Gilmanov D, Farneti PA, Miceli A, Bevilacqua S, Glauber M. Perceval S sutureless aortic valve prosthesis implantation via a right anterior minithoracotomy. Multimed Man Cardiothorac Surg [Video-Audio Media]. 2013;2013:mmt012.
9. Pibarot P, Dumesnil JG. Hemodynamic and clinical impact of prosthesis-patient mismatch in the aortic valve position and its prevention. J Am Coll Cardiol. 2000;36(4):1131–41.
10. Achenbach S, Delgado V, Hausleiter J, Schoenhagen P, Min JK. Leipsic JA. SCCT expert consensus document on computed tomography imaging before transcatheter aortic valve implantation (TAVI)/transcatheter aortic valve replacement (TAVR). J Cardiovasc Comput Tomogr [Consensus Development Conference]. 2012;6(6):366–80.
11. Leipsic J, Gurvitch R, LaBounty TM, Min JK, Wood D, Johnson M, et al. Multidetector computed tomography in transcatheter aortic valve implantation. JACC Cardiovasc Imaging. 2011;4(4):416–29.
12. Zoghbi WA, Enriquez-Sarano M, Foster E, Grayburn PA, Kraft CD, Levine RA, et al. Recommendations for evaluation of the severity of native valvular regurgitation with two-dimensional and Doppler echocardiography. J Am Soc Echocardiogr. 2003;16(7):777–802.
13. Baumgartner H, Hung J, Bermejo J, Chambers JB, Evangelista A, Griffin BP, et al. Echocardiographic assessment of valve stenosis: EAE/ASE recommendations for clinical practice. J Am Soc Echocardiogr. 2009;22(1):1–23; quiz 101–2.
14. Zoghbi WA, Chambers JB, Dumesnil JG, Foster E, Gottdiener JS, Grayburn PA, et al. Recommendations for evaluation of prosthetic valves with echocardiography and doppler ultrasound: a report From the American Society of Echocardiography's Guidelines and Standards Committee and the Task Force on Prosthetic Valves, developed in conjunction with the American College of Cardiology Cardiovascular Imaging Committee, Cardiac Imaging Committee of the American Heart Association, the European Association of Echocardiography, a registered branch of the European Society of Cardiology, the Japanese Society of Echocardiography and the Canadian Society of Echocardiography, endorsed by the American College of Cardiology Foundation, American Heart Association, European Association of Echocardiography, a registered branch of the European Society of Cardiology, the Japanese Society of Echocardiography, and Canadian Society of Echocardiography. J Am Soc Echocardiogr. 2009;22(9):975–1014; quiz 82–4.
15. Pibarot P, Dumesnil JG. Prosthesis-patient mismatch: definition, clinical impact, and prevention. Heart. 2006;92(8):1022–9.
16. Pibarot P, Dumesnil JG. Prosthetic heart valves: selection of the optimal prosthesis and long-term management. Circulation. 2009;119(7):1034–48.
17. Gadhinglajkar S, Namboodiri N, Pillai V, Sreedhar R. Double-envelope continuous-wave Doppler flow profile across a tilting-disc mitral prosthesis: intraoperative significance. J Cardiothorac Vasc Anesth. 2011;25(3):491–4.
18. Akins CW, Miller DC, Turina MI, Kouchoukos NT, Blackstone EH, Grunkemeier GL, et al. Guidelines for reporting mortality and morbidity after cardiac valve interventions. J Thorac Cardiovasc Surg. 2008;135(4):732–8.
19. Effron MK, Popp RL. Two-dimensional echocardiographic assessment of bioprosthetic valve dysfunction and infective endocarditis. J Am Coll Cardiol. 1983;2(4):597–606.
20. Roudaut R, Serri K, Lafitte S. Thrombosis of prosthetic heart valves: diagnosis and therapeutic considerations. Heart. 2007;93(1):137–42.
21. Tong AT, Roudaut R, Ozkan M, Sagie A, Shahid MS, Pontes Junior SC, et al. Transesophageal echocardiography improves risk assessment of thrombolysis of prosthetic valve thrombosis: results of the international PRO-TEE registry. J Am Coll Cardiol. 2004;43(1):77–84.
22. Lin SS, Tiong IY, Asher CR, Murphy MT, Thomas JD, Griffin BP. Prediction of thrombus-related mechanical prosthetic valve dysfunction using transesophageal echocardiography. Am J Cardiol. 2000;86(10):1097–101.
23. Sudhakar S, Sewani A, Agrawal M, Uretsky BF. Pseudoaneurysm of the mitral-aortic intervalvular fibrosa (MAIVF): a comprehensive review. J Am Soc Echocardiogr. 2010;23(10):1009–18; quiz 112.
24. Taramasso M, Maisano F, Latib A, Denti P, Guidotti A, Sticchi A, et al. Conventional surgery and transcatheter closure via surgical transapical approach for paravalvular leak repair in high-risk patients: results from a single-centre experience. Eur Heart J Cardiovasc Imaging. 2014;15(10):1161–7.
25. Garcia MJ, Vandervoort P, Stewart WJ, Lytle BW, Cosgrove DM 3rd, Thomas JD, et al. Mechanisms of hemolysis with mitral prosthetic regurgitation. Study using transesophageal echocardiography and fluid dynamic simulation. J Am Coll Cardiol. 1996;27(2):399–406.
26. Echevarria JR, Bernal JM, Rabasa JM, Morales D, Revilla Y, Revuelta JM. Reoperation for bioprosthetic valve dysfunction. A decade of clinical experience. Eur J Cardiothorac Surg. 1991;5(10):523–6; discussion 7.
27. Hourihan M, Perry SB, Mandell VS, Keane JF, Rome JJ, Bittl JA, et al. Transcatheter umbrella closure of valvular and paravalvular leaks. J Am Coll Cardiol. 1992;20(6):1371–7.
28. Moore JD, Lashus AG, Prieto LR, Drummond-Webb J, Latson LA. Transcatheter coil occlusion of perivalvular mitral leaks associated with severe hemolysis. Catheter Cardiovasc Interv [Case Reports]. 2000;49(1):64–7.
29. Eisenhauer AC, Piemonte TC, Watson PS. Closure of prosthetic paravalvular mitral regurgitation with the Gianturco-Grifka vascular occlusion device. Catheter Cardiovasc Interv [Case Reports]. 2001;54(2):234–8.
30. Webb JG, Pate GE, Munt BI. Percutaneous closure of an aortic prosthetic paravalvular leak with an Amplatzer duct occluder. Catheter Cardiovasc Interv. 2005;65(1):69–72.

31. Nietlispach F, Johnson M, Moss RR, Wijesinghe N, Gurvitch R, Tay EL, et al. Transcatheter closure of paravalvular defects using a purpose-specific occluder. JACC Cardiovasc Interv. 2010;3(7):759–65.
32. Sorajja P, Cabalka AK, Hagler DJ, Rihal CS. Percutaneous repair of paravalvular prosthetic regurgitation: acute and 30-day outcomes in 115 patients. Circ Cardiovasc Interv. 2011;4(4):314–21.
33. Ruiz CE, Jelnin V, Kronzon I, Dudiy Y, Del Valle-Fernandez R, Einhorn BN, et al. Clinical outcomes in patients undergoing percutaneous closure of periprosthetic paravalvular leaks. J Am Coll Cardiol [Comparative Study]. 2011;58(21):2210–7.
34. Sorajja P, Cabalka AK, Hagler DJ, Rihal CS. Long-term follow-up of percutaneous repair of paravalvular prosthetic regurgitation. J Am Coll Cardiol. 2011;58(21):2218–24.
35. Moscucci M, Deeb GM, Bach D, Eagle KA, Williams DM. Coil embolization of a periprosthetic mitral valve leak associated with severe hemolytic anemia. Circulation [Case Reports]. 2001;104(16):E85–6.
36. Hein R, Wunderlich N, Robertson G, Wilson N, Sievert H. Catheter closure of paravalvular leak. EuroIntervention. 2006;2(3):318–25.
37. Rihal CS, Sorajja P, Booker JD, Hagler DJ, Cabalka AK. Principles of percutaneous paravalvular leak closure. JACC Cardiovasc Interv. 2012;5(2):121–30.
38. Bogunovic N, Faber L, Scholtz W, Mellwig KP, Horstkotte D, van Buuren F. Real-time three-dimensional transoesophageal echocardiography during percutaneous transcatheter occlusion of mitral periprosthetic paravalvular leak. Eur J Echocardiogr. 2011;12(3):E27.
39. Hoffmann R, Kaestner W, Altiok E. Closure of a paravalvular leak with real-time three-dimensional transesophageal echocardiography for accurate sizing and guiding. J Invasive Cardiol. 2013;25(11):E210–1.
40. Leon MB, Smith CR, Mack M, Miller DC, Moses JW, Svensson LG, et al. Transcatheter aortic-valve implantation for aortic stenosis in patients who cannot undergo surgery. N Engl J Med. 2010;363(17):1597–607.
41. Smith CR, Leon MB, Mack MJ, Miller DC, Moses JW, Svensson LG, et al. Transcatheter versus surgical aortic-valve replacement in high-risk patients. N Engl J Med. 2011;364(23):2187–98.
42. Popma JJ, Adams DH, Reardon MJ, Yakubov SJ, Kleiman NS, Heimansohn D, et al. Transcatheter aortic valve replacement using a self-expanding bioprosthesis in patients with severe aortic stenosis at extreme risk for surgery. J Am Coll Cardiol. 2014;63(19):1972–81.
43. Adams DH, Popma JJ, Reardon MJ. Transcatheter aortic-valve replacement with a self-expanding prosthesis. N Engl J Med. 2014;371(10):967–8.
44. Oguri A, Yamamoto M, Mouillet G, Gilard M, Laskar M, Eltchaninoff H, et al. Clinical outcomes and safety of transfemoral aortic valve implantation under general versus local anesthesia: subanalysis of the French Aortic National CoreValve and Edwards 2 registry. Circ Cardiovasc Interv. 2014;7(4):602–10.
45. Bagur R, Rodes-Cabau J, Doyle D, De Larochelliere R, Villeneuve J, Lemieux J, et al. Usefulness of TEE as the primary imaging technique to guide transcatheter transapical aortic valve implantation. JACC Cardiovasc Imaging. 2011;4(2):115–24.
46. de Brito FS Jr, Carvalho LA, Sarmento-Leite R, Mangione JA, Lemos P, Siciliano A, et al. Outcomes and predictors of mortality after transcatheter aortic valve implantation: Results of the Brazilian registry. Catheter Cardiovasc Interv. 2015;85(5):E153–62.
47. Hahn RT, Abraham T, Adams MS, Bruce CJ, Glas KE, Lang RM, et al. Guidelines for performing a comprehensive transesophageal echocardiographic examination: recommendations from the american society of echocardiography and the society of cardiovascular anesthesiologists. J Am Soc Echocardiogr. 2013;26(9):921–64.
48. Babaliaros VC, Liff D, Chen EP, Rogers JH, Brown RA, Thourani VH, et al. Can balloon aortic valvuloplasty help determine appropriate transcatheter aortic valve size? JACC Cardiovasc Interv. 2008;1(5):580–6.
49. Kasel AM, Cassese S, Bleiziffer S, Amaki M, Hahn RT, Kastrati A, et al. Standardized imaging for aortic annular sizing: implications for transcatheter valve selection. JACC Cardiovasc Imaging. 2013;6(2):249–62.
50. Patsalis PC, Al-Rashid F, Neumann T, Plicht B, Hildebrandt HA, Wendt D, et al. Preparatory balloon aortic valvuloplasty during transcatheter aortic valve implantation for improved valve sizing. JACC Cardiovasc Interv. 2013;6(9):965–71.
51. Ben-Dor I, Pichard AD, Satler LF, Goldstein SA, Syed AI, Gaglia MA Jr, et al. Complications and outcome of balloon aortic valvuloplasty in high-risk or inoperable patients. JACC Cardiovasc Interv. 2010;3(11):1150–6.
52. Dvir D, Lavi I, Eltchaninoff H, Himbert D, Almagor Y, Descoutures F, et al. Multicenter evaluation of Edwards SAPIEN positioning during transcatheter aortic valve implantation with correlates for device movement during final deployment. JACC Cardiovasc Interv. 2012;5(5):563–70.
53. Athappan G, Patvardhan E, Tuzcu EM, Svensson LG, Lemos PA, Fraccaro C, et al. Incidence, predictors, and outcomes of aortic regurgitation after transcatheter aortic valve replacement: meta-analysis and systematic review of literaturemeta-analysis and systematic review of literature. J Am Coll Cardiol. 2013;61(15):1585–95.
54. Hahn RT, Little SH, Monaghan MJ, Kodali SK, Williams M, Leon MB, et al. Recommendations for comprehensive intraprocedural echocardiographic imaging during TAVR. JACC Cardiovasc Imaging Dent Rev. 2015;8(3):261–87.
55. Pibarot P, Hahn RT, Weissman NJ, Monaghan MJ. Assessment of paravalvular regurgitation following TAVR: a proposal of Unifying Grading Scheme. JACC Cardiovasc Imaging Dent Rev. 2015;8(3):340–60.
56. Fang L, Hsiung MC, Miller AP, Nanda NC, Yin WH, Young MS, et al. Assessment of aortic regurgitation by live three-dimensional transthoracic echocardiographic measurements of vena contracta area: usefulness and validation. Echocardiography. 2005;22(9):775–81.
57. Pirat B, Little SH, Igo SR, McCulloch M, Nose Y, Hartley CJ, et al. Direct measurement of proximal isovelocity surface area by real-time three-dimensional color Doppler for quantitation of aortic regurgitant volume: an in vitro validation. J Am Soc Echocardiogr. 2009;22(3):306–13.
58. Poh KK, Levine RA, Solis J, Shen L, Flaherty M, Kang YJ, et al. Assessing aortic valve area in aortic stenosis by continuity equation: a novel approach using real-time three-dimensional echocardiography. Eur Heart J. 2008;29(20):2526–35.
59. Singh P, Manda J, Hsiung MC, Mehta A, Kesanolla SK, Nanda NC, et al. Live/real time three-dimensional transesophageal echocardiographic evaluation of mitral and aortic valve prosthetic paravalvular regurgitation. Echocardiography. 2009;26(8):980–7.
60. Singh P, Inamdar V, Hage FG, Kodali V, Karakus G, Suwanjutah T, et al. Usefulness of live/real time three-dimensional transthoracic echocardiography in evaluation of prosthetic valve function. Echocardiography. 2009;26(10):1236–49.

Left Atrium

16

Wendy Tsang, Kirk T. Spencer, and Roberto M. Lang

Abstract

The left atrium is a critical cardiac structure. Abnormalities in left atrial function affect not only left ventricular function but also predict poor cardiovascular outcomes. Depending on the population, increased rates of atrial fibrillation, stroke and hospitalization have been associated with increased left atrial size. The left atrium is best assessed with transthoracic echocardiography using dedicated two-dimensional imaging views. While three-dimensional echocardiography-derived volumes are more accurate, current use is limited by lack of normal values and automated analysis packages that allow rapid measurement in clinical practice. Available left atrial cut-offs are based on maximum volumes indexed for body-surface area and do not differ between genders. While much of the available data is on maximum left atrial volume, other measurements may provide more important information on pathological processes and better prognosticate outcomes. These measurements include: changes in left atrial volumes during the cardiac cycle; left atrial contractile function measured through strain; and left atrial shape. Finally, monitoring of left atrial changes and recognition of reverse remodelling may lead to the use of left atrium as therapeutic target in clinical practice and trials.

Keywords

Left atrium · Function · Volume · Normal · Strain · Two-dimensional echocardiography · Three-dimensional echocardiography · Measurement

Introduction

The left atrium plays an important role in normal left ventricular function. It not only acts as a contractile pump that delivers 15–30% of the entire left ventricular filling volume but also acts as a reservoir that collects pulmonary venous return during ventricular systole allowing passage of the atrial stored blood into the left ventricle during early ventricular diastole (Fig. 16.1) [1, 2]. Given its important role, changes to normal left atrial size or function have been associated with adverse cardiovascular outcomes [3–8]. For example, enlargement of the left atrium is associated with a higher incidence of atrial fibrillation and stroke [1, 9–11]. As well, patients with enlarged left atriums have a higher risk of hospitalization, major cardiac events or mortality if they experience either a myocardial infarction, dilated cardiomyopathy or diabetes mellitus [12–16]. These adverse outcomes develop because, in the absence of mitral valve disease, an increase in left atrial size most commonly reflects increased wall tension as a result of chronic augmentation of left atrial pressure [17–19]. This increase in left atrial size also results in impaired left atrial function due to atrial myopathy [20]. Thus, left atrial enlargement is both a marker of severity and chronicity of diastolic dysfunction and magnitude of left atrial pressure elevation [7, 17–19, 21].

Electronic Supplementary Material The online version of this chapter (https://doi.org/10.1007/978-3-030-14032-8_16) contains supplementary material, which is available to authorized users.

W. Tsang (✉)
Cardiology, Toronto General Hospital, University Health Network, University of Toronto, Toronto, ON, Canada
e-mail: wendy.tsang@uhn.ca

K. T. Spencer
Department of Medicine/Section of Cardiology, University of Chicago Medical Center, Chicago, IL, USA
e-mail: kspencer@uchicago.edu

R. M. Lang
Noninvasive Cardiac Imaging Laboratories, Department of Medicine/Section of Cardiology, University of Chicago Medical Center, Chicago, IL, USA
e-mail: rlang@medicine.bsd.uchicago.edu, rlang@bsd.uchicago.edu

L. P. Badano et al. (eds.), *Textbook of Three-Dimensional Echocardiography*, https://doi.org/10.1007/978-3-030-14032-8_16

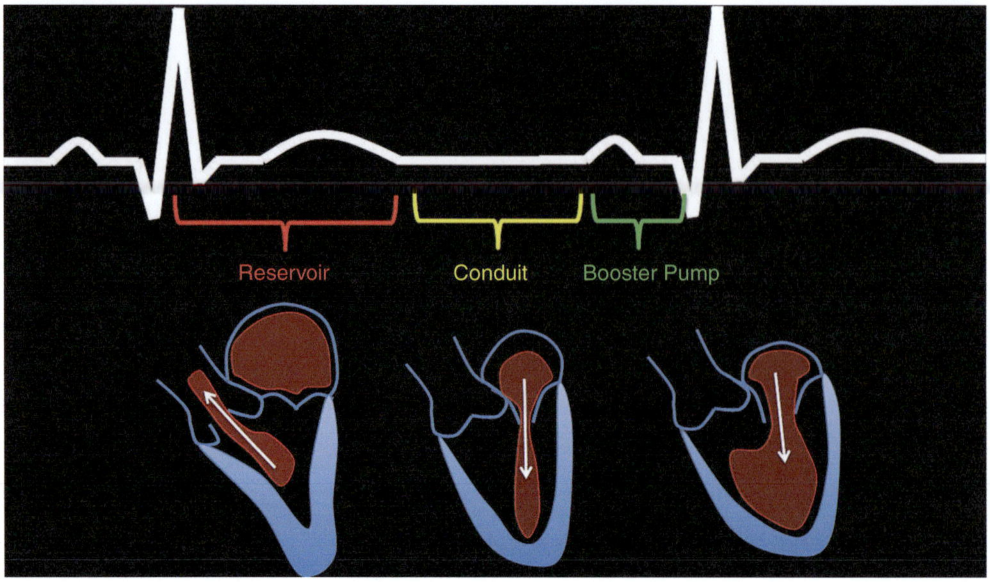

Fig. 16.1 Function of the left atrium through the cardiac cycle

Imaging of the Left Atrium

Left atrial size assessment is best accomplished with transthoracic echocardiography, which allows complete visualization of the left atrium. With transesophageal echocardiography, the entire left atrium frequently cannot be fit in the image sector thereby precluding the ability to measure left atrial size (Fig. 16.2). Care should be taken to avoid foreshortening the left atrium when acquiring images to measure left atrial size and volume. As the longitudinal axis of the left atrium often lies in a different plane from the left ventricle, dedicated acquisitions of the left atrium from the apical transducer position should be obtained for accurate left atrial measurements (Fig. 16.3) [22–24]. In the correct plane and time of the cardiac cycle, the base of the left atrium should be at its largest size, indicating that the imaging plane passes through the maximal short-axis area. The left atrial length should also be maximized to ensure alignment along the true long axis of the left atrium.

Measurements should be taken at the end of left ventricular systole, as this is when the left atrial chamber is at its greatest dimension (Fig. 16.4). When using the biplane disc summation method to calculate left atrial volumes, the length of the long-axes measured in the 2- and 4-chamber views should be similar. When tracing the borders of the left atrium, the confluences of the pulmonary veins, and left atrial appendage should be excluded. The atrio-ventricular interface should be represented by the mitral annulus plane and not by the tip of the mitral leaflets.

Left Atrial Measurement

There are three measurements of left atrial size that are frequently reported: left atrial antero-posterior dimension, left atrial area and left atrial volume. Of these, the recommended parameter by current guidelines is left atrial volume [25]. However, for years, the most reported parameter has been the linear antero-posterior left atrial measurement obtained from the parasternal long-axis view using M-mode or two-dimensional transthoracic echocardiography [1, 9, 14, 26–28]. This was due to the fact that the antero-posterior dimension is highly reproducible. However, caution must be advised when interpreting antero-posterior dimensions as they may not represent an accurate metric of left atrial size [29, 30]. This is because the antero-posterior diameter assumes that, when the left atrium enlarges, all of its dimensions change similarly, which is often not the case during left atrial remodelling, especially when the enlargement is eccentric [31, 32]. Therefore, antero-posterior linear dimension should not be used as the sole measurement of left atrial size.

Left atrial area measurements can be obtained by planimetry in the apical 4- and 2-chamber views. Measurements should be obtained by contouring orthogonally around the long-axis of the left atrium from good quality images that avoid left atrial foreshortening [25]. These tracings should exclude the pulmonary veins and left atrial appendage. Once the left atrial areas have been traced in these views, all software packages will automatically compute left atrial volume, by either the method of disks or by the area-length technique. Thus, given the ease with which left atrial volumes can be

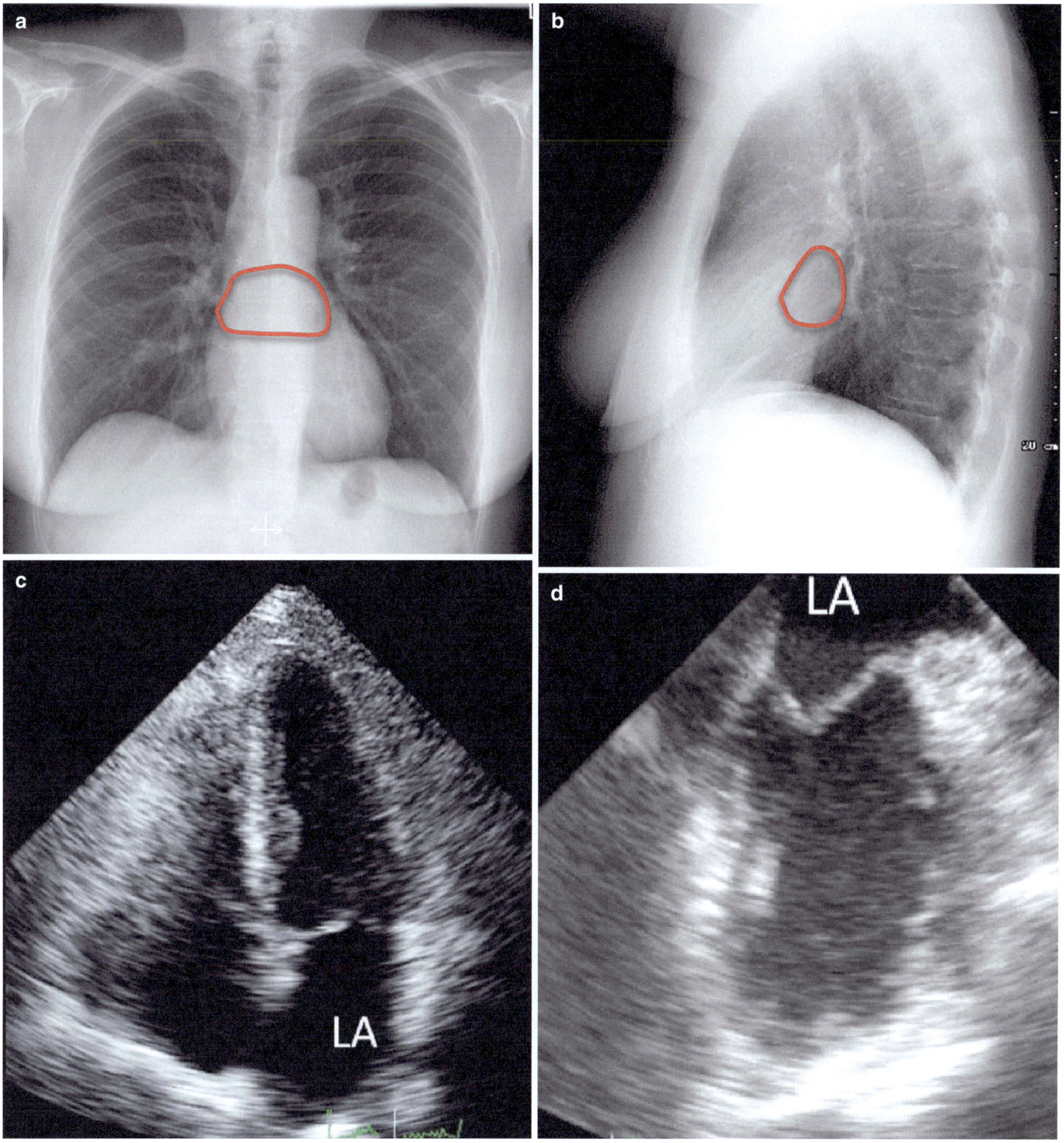

Fig. 16.2 The left atrium (LA) is best assessed through imaging tests due to its location in the chest as seen on chest X-ray (**a**, **b**). With echocardiography, measurement is best performed on transthoracic imaging (**c**), as the entire left atrium is not seen with transesophageal echocardiography (**d**)

obtained in clinical practice, it has been recommended that left atrial volumes be reported over left atrial area.

The preference for reporting left atrial volume over area or dimension is because left atrial volumes accounts for alterations in left atrial chamber size in all directions and consequently has been shown to be a more powerful prognostic variable in a variety of cardiac disease states when compared with antero-posterior diameter or area. Overall, left atrial volume measurements better reflect the burden and chronicity of elevated left ventricular filling pressures and are stronger predictors of outcomes [12, 13, 15, 33–38].

Four different methods can be used to measure left atrial volumes: (1) prolate ellipse method, (2) biplane area-length method, (3) biplane Simpson method, and (4) three-dimensional echocardiography (3DE). With two-dimensional

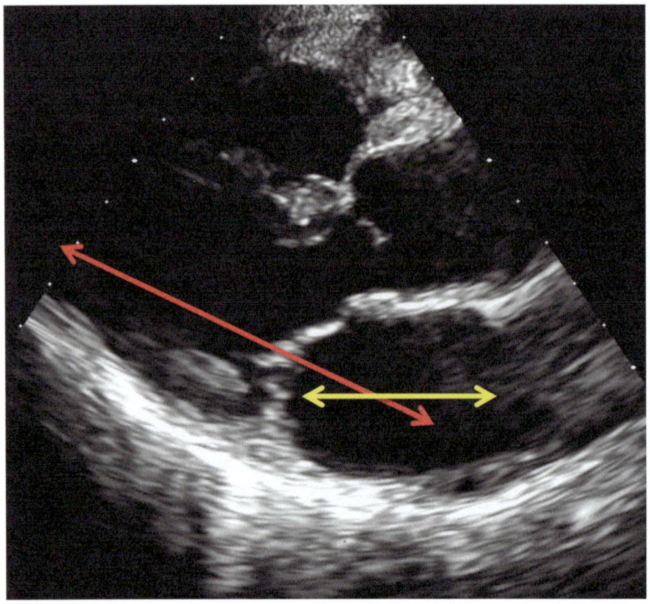

Fig. 16.3 The long-axis of the left atrium is not in the same plane as the long-axis of the left ventricle. This is best seen in the parasternal long-axis view. Here the long-axis of the left ventricle (red arrow) is in a different plane from the long-axis of the left atrium (yellow arrow). Thus, dedicated apical views of the left atrium focused to obtain the longest axes are required to measure the left atrium accurately

echocardiographic images, left atrial volume should be measured using the Simpson method. The left atrial endocardial border is traced and volume computed by adding the volume of a stack of 20 cylinders of length (L) and area calculated by orthogonal minor and major transverse axes (a_l and b_l) assuming an oval shape (Fig. 16.4):

$$\text{LA volume} = \left(\frac{\pi}{4}\right) \times \underset{i=1}{20} a_i \times b_i \times \frac{L}{20}$$

The left atrial endocardial borders should be traced in both the apical 4- and 2-chamber views. A single plane approach based on the geometric assumption that the left atrium is circular in the short axis cut plane has also been used. While this assumption may not be always accurate, this approach could be used in cases when performing planimetry in both views is difficult [39].

Alternatively, a biplane calculation could also be performed using the LA areas and length measured from both the apical 4- (A1) and 2-chamber (B1) views. LA volume is calculated as:

$$\text{LA volume} = \frac{\left(\frac{8}{3\pi}\right) \times A1 \times B1}{L} = \frac{0.85 \times A1 \times B1}{L}$$

L is the shortest distance between the mid-line of the plane of mitral annulus to the opposite superior side (roof) of the left atrium measured in either the 4- or 2-chamber views. As well, it is assumed that the difference between L measured in the 2- and 4-chambers views is less than 1 cm. While the area–length method still assumes an ellipsoidal left atrial shape, it has the advantage of reducing linear dimensions to a single measurement [7, 40]. It must be noted that measurements obtained using the area-length method are not inter-

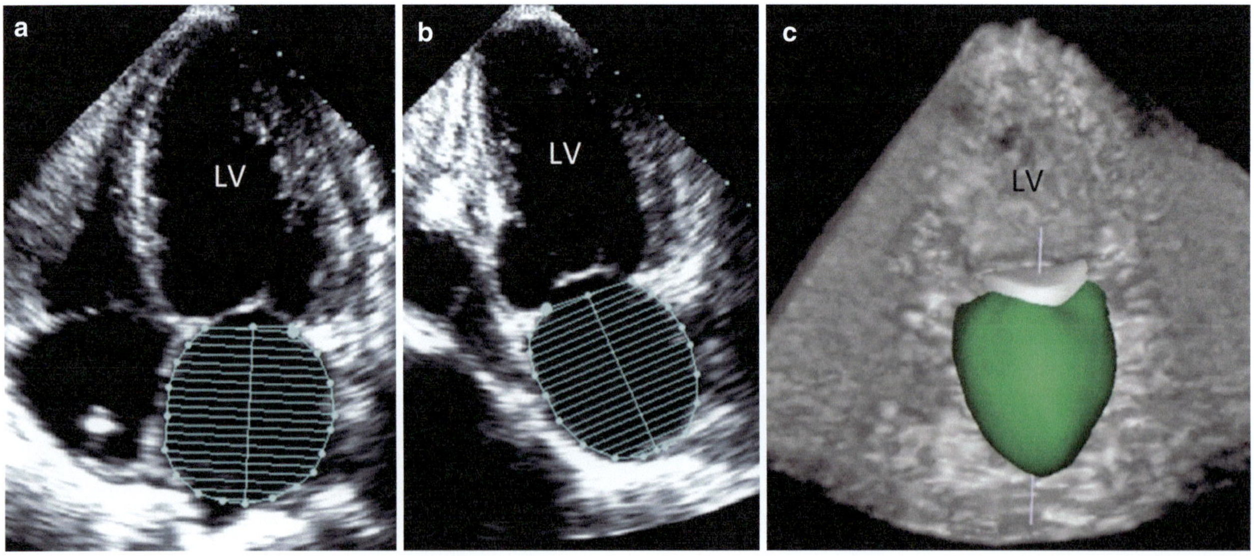

Fig. 16.4 Left atrial volume should be measured using the Simpson's method on dedicated left atrial 4- and 2-chamber views (**a**, **b**). 3D echocardiography allows more accurate measurements of left atrial volume (**c**) but normal values have not been established. *LV* left ventricle

changeable with the Simpson's method and different normal values exist for each method [41]. However, the prognostic power of left atrial volumes calculated with both two-dimensional algorithms is similar [42].

The prolate ellipse method requires measurement of left atrial dimensions from the parasternal long-axis view (D_1) and the long-and short-axis (D_2, D_3) from the apical 4-chamber view. Left atrial volume is calculated as $D_1 \times D_2 \times D_3 \times 0.523$. Overall, this method is not recommended due to the relative inaccuracy of the linear measurements required for its calculation.

If 3DE is possible, left atrial volumes are more accurate when measured using 3DE dataset than calculated from conventional two-dimensional echocardiography views [22, 24, 43]. This avoids errors in measuring left atrial volumes (i.e. geometrical assumptions about left atrial shape and/or foreshortening of the two-dimensional views) that come from using two-dimensional echocardiographic images. This is because the shape of the left atrium in cross-section perpendicular to the left atrial long-axis is not circular but ellipsoid and that the two-dimensional views used for calculations may not cut through the correct major and minor axis of the left atrium. However, measurement by 3DE requires dedicated quantitative software packages (Fig. 16.5) and was time-consuming [44–46]. Recently, new, fully automated algorithms have been developed to provide quick and reproducible measurement of maximal left atrial volume [47]. Clinically, 3DE measurements of left atrial volume have been demonstrated to have a stronger and additive prognostic value [48–50]. Therefore, with the development of automated 3DE chamber quantification software packages [47], the integration of 3DE left atrial volume measurements into practice will be more practical and add clinical value.

Finally, it must be noted though that two-dimensional echocardiography derived left atrial volumes are typically smaller than those reported from computed tomography, cardiac magnetic resonance imaging or 3DE [22, 31, 32].

Normal Values

Left atrial size is dependent on gender. However, the gender differences in left atrial size are generally accounted for when adjusting for body size. Several indexing methods have been proposed [38, 53], but indexing to body-surface area has yielded the most available data. Thus, only the indexed value should be reported [2, 38]. A normal indexed left atrial volume, calculated with two-dimensional echocardiography, is 25 ± 4 mL with an upper normal volume based on two standard deviations of 33 mL. This is supported by studies documenting increased morbidity in patients with left atrial volumes >32–34 mL and with American Society of Echocardiography/European Association Cardiovascular Imaging guideline document on evaluation of diastolic function, which recommends the use of an indexed left atrial volume >34 mL/m^2 as abnormal [16, 36, 37, 54]. Although not recommended by current guidelines [25], there is growing evidence to support the use of 3DE to measure left atrial volume based on its superior accuracy. If 3DE is used to measure left atrial volumes, the upper limit of normal is larger than the one used for two dimensional echocardiography (Table 16.1).

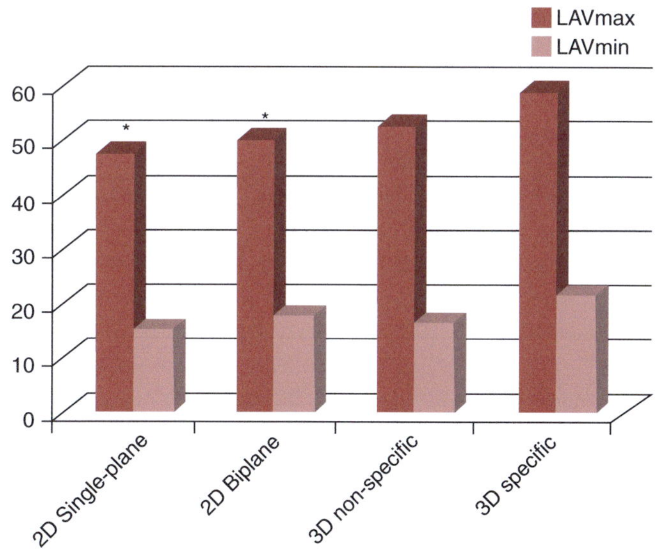

Fig. 16.5 Comparison of left atrial volumes calculated with two-dimensional echocardiography algorithms (either single- and bi-plane), non-dedicated 3DE software package (adaptation of tools developed for the measurement of left ventricular volumes) and dedicated 3DE software package. Left atrial volumes are smaller when calculated using two-dimensional echocardiography than 3DE. 3DE software packages dedicated to the left atrium provide larger volumes than measurement performed using non dedicated software packages

Table 16.1 Comparison of normal values and upper limits of normality of left atrial volumes measured with three-dimensional echocardiography and calculated with two-dimensional echocardiography [22, 44–46, 50]

Reference	Study characteristics	Left atrial volume	3DE (mL/m^2)	2DE (mL/m^2)	Upper limit of normality 3DE (mL/m^2)	Upper limit of normality 2DE (mL/m^2)
Aune et al. [44]	Prospective. 166 healthy subjects. Non dedicated software package (Q-Lab®, Philips Medical Systems)	Maximum			41	
		Minimum			22	
Badano et al. [22]	Prospective. 244 healthy volunteers. Dedicated software package (4D LA function, TomTec Imaging Systems, Unterschleissen, D)	Maximum	32 ± 7	24 ± 6	46	34
		Minimum	11 ± 3	8 ± 3	17	14
		Pre-A	18 ± 5	15 ± 5	28	25
Azar et al. [45]	Prospective. 63 healthy volunteers. Non dedicated software package (Q-Lab®, Philips Medical Systems)	Maximum	24 ± 6			
		Minimum	10 ± 4			
Russo et al. [50]	Prospective. 142 elderly (66 ± 9 years) healthy volunteers. Non dedicated software package (Q-Lab®, Philips Medical Systems)	Maximum			34	36
		Minimum			21	
Sugimoto et al. [46]	Prospective. 371 healthy subjects. Non-dedicated software package (4D Cardio View, TomTec Imaging Systems, Unterschleissen, D)	Maximum	41 ± 1			

Left Atrial Function and Volume

As mentioned earlier, the left atrium has three major functions during the cardiac cycle: a "reservoir", a "conduit" and a "booster pump". During these phases, left atrial volume will vary to reflect the mechanical function of the left atrium [55]. While maximal left atrial volume is routinely measured in clinical practice, changes in left atrial volumes more accurately describe left atrial phasic function (Fig. 16.6). Reservoir volume is estimated by measuring the total left atrial emptying volume. This is calculated from the difference between the maximum left atrial volume just before mitral valve opening and minimal left atrial volume when the mitral valve closes. Total left atrial emptying fraction is determined by dividing the total left atrial emptying volume by left atrial maximal volume. Conduit volume is estimated by measuring the left atrial passive emptying volume, which is the difference between the maximal left atrial volume and the left atrial volume preceding atrial contraction. Left atrial passive ejection fraction is calculated by dividing left atrial passive emptying volume by the maximum left atrial volume. The contractile or booster function volume is measured through the left atrial active emptying volume, which is the difference between the left atrial volume measured pre-atrial contraction and the minimum left atrial volume. The difference between left ventricular stroke volume and the total left atrial emptying volume is left atrial passive conduit volume. Finally, a novel measure that incorporates left atrial emptying fraction, left ventricular outflow tract velocity time integral and maximal left atrial volume indexed to body surface area is left atrial functional index [56]. This parameter has been demonstrated to predict heart failure hospitalization in patients with coronary artery disease and preserved left ventricular ejection fraction.

It must be noted that left ventricular diastolic properties affect the contribution of left atrial phasic function to left ventricular function. As age affects diastolic function, age also affects the relationship between left atrial and left ventricular function. When diastolic function is normal, the relative contribution of left atrial reservoir, conduit and contractile functions to left ventricular filling is 40%, 35% and 25%, respectively [55]. With abnormal LV relaxation, the contribution of the left atrial reservoir and contractile function increases and conduit function decreases. However, with advanced LV diastolic dysfunction, the left atrium functions predominantly as a conduit.

Assessment of Left Atrial Function

Left atrial function can also be assessed using pulsed-wave Doppler interrogation of the transmitral and pulmonary venous blood flow velocities (Table 16.2). Normally, the pulmonary venous flow pattern from the pulmonary veins to the left atrium consists of an early ventricular systolic wave followed by a late ventricular systolic/isovolumic relaxation wave and then an early ventricular diastolic wave and finally reversal of flow from the left atrium to the pulmonary veins during atrial systole. Note that the early ventricular systolic

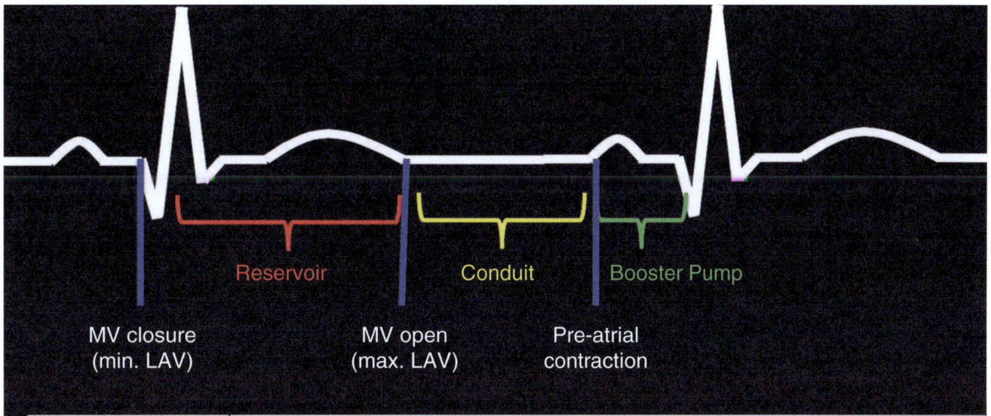

Function	Calculation
Global Function	LA EF = (Max. LAV – Min. LAV)/Max. LAV
Reservoir	Total LA Emptying Volume = (Max. LAV – Min. LAV)
Conduit	LA Passive Emptying Volume = (Max. LAV – LAV pre-atrial contraction)
Contractile/ Booster Pump	LA Active Emptying Volume = (LAV pre-atrial contraction – Min. LAV)

Fig. 16.6 Determination of left atrial function through volume assessment. *EF* emptying fraction, *LA* left atrial, *LAV* left atrial volume, *Max* maximal, *Min* minimum, *MV* mitral valve

Table 16.2 Spectral and tissue Doppler indices of left atrial function

LA function	Transmitral flow	Pulmonary venous flow	Composite indices	Tissue velocity	Strain	Strain rate
Global function			• LA functional index = (LA EF × $LVOT_{VTI}$)/(LAV/BSA)			
Reservoir		• S wave vel • S wave VTI		• S′	• Systolic strain • Total strain	• Ventricular systolic strain rate
Conduit	• E wave vel • E wave VTI • E/A	• D wave vel • D wave VTI		• E′	• Early diastolic strain • Positive strain	• Early ventricular diastolic strain rate
Booster pump	• A wave vel • A wave VTI • E/A • Atrial filling fraction • LA appendage velocity	• Pulmonary venous reversal velocity	• Ejection force • Left atrial kinetic energy	• A′	• Late diastolic strain • Negative strain	• Late ventricular diastolic strain rate

BSA body surface area, *EF* emptying fraction, *LA* left atrial, *LAV* left atrial volume, *LVOT* left ventricular outflow tract, *VTI* velocity-time integral

wave is only distinctly seen in 30% of transthoracic studies [55]. Overall pulmonary vein systolic waves are indicators of left atrial reservoir function and diastolic waves are an indicator of left atrial conduit function.

Factors that affect phasic left atrial pressure affect pulmonary vein waves. For instance, left ventricular systolic function and left atrial relaxation affects the magnitude and velocity-time integral of the early pulmonary vein systolic wave. Whereas, left atrial compliance affects both pulmonary vein systolic waves. Late systolic pulmonary wave reflects propagation of the right ventricular pressure pulse through the pulmonary circulation and so right ventricular stroke volume affects it. Pulmonary vein diastolic wave is an indicator of conduit function and so factors affecting left atrial afterload (left ventricular relaxation, mechanical mitral valve obstruction) affect it.

Left atrial booster pump function can be assessed by examining flows caused by left atrial contraction into the left ventricle. Transmitral flow waves such as the A-wave velocity, A-wave velocity time integral and the atrial-filling fraction) all provide information of left atrial booster pump function.

Other methods that can provide assessments of global and regional atrial contractile function include two-dimensional pulsed wave and color tissue Doppler echocardiographic imaging as well as speckle tracking strain. It must be noted that the choice of zero baseline for reporting left atrial strain may cause some confusion. If the ventricular cycle is used, ventricular end-diastole is the zero reference and the peak positive longitudinal strain corresponds to atrial reservoir function and the strain during early and late diastole correspond to conduit and atrial booster function (Fig. 16.7). In contrast, if the atrial cycle is used where the atrial end-diastole at the onset of the p-wave is the zero reference, the first negative peak strain represents the atrial booster pump function. Peak positive strain represents the conduit function and the sum is reservoir function.

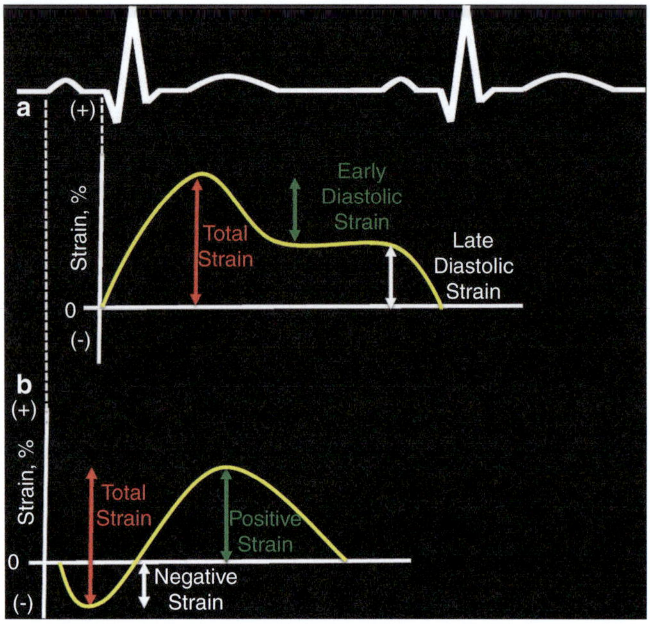

Fig. 16.7 The zero reference point determines strain nomenclature. The QRS complex (**a**) or the electrocardiographic p-wave (**b**) can be used as the zero reference point

Left atrial strain from two-dimensional echocardiography is subjected to the limitations of tomographic imaging. It is unable to capture the true 3D motion of the left atrial myocardium. Three-dimensional speckle tracking echocardiography may address issues such as through-plane motion that occurs with two dimensional imaging. In addition to allowing measurement of longitudinal and circumferential strain, three-dimensional strain will allow evaluation of left atrial endocardial area strain. However, similar to two-dimensional left atrial strain, the clinical utility of these measurements is unclear at this time.

3DE has been used to measure left atrial phasic function (Fig. 16.8, Video 16.1) and normative values have been reported [22, 46].

Left Atrial Remodeling

Left atrial remodeling occurs in response to two conditions: pressure and volume overload. Left atrial enlargement from volume overload occurs in those with valvular regurgitation or high output states such as anemia or athlete's heart. Generally, myocyte relaxation is normal under these conditions.

Pressure overload typically results in left atrial enlargement due to increased left atrial afterload such as in mitral valve disease or left ventricular dysfunction and often results in abnormal myocyte relaxation. Overall, there is strong cor-

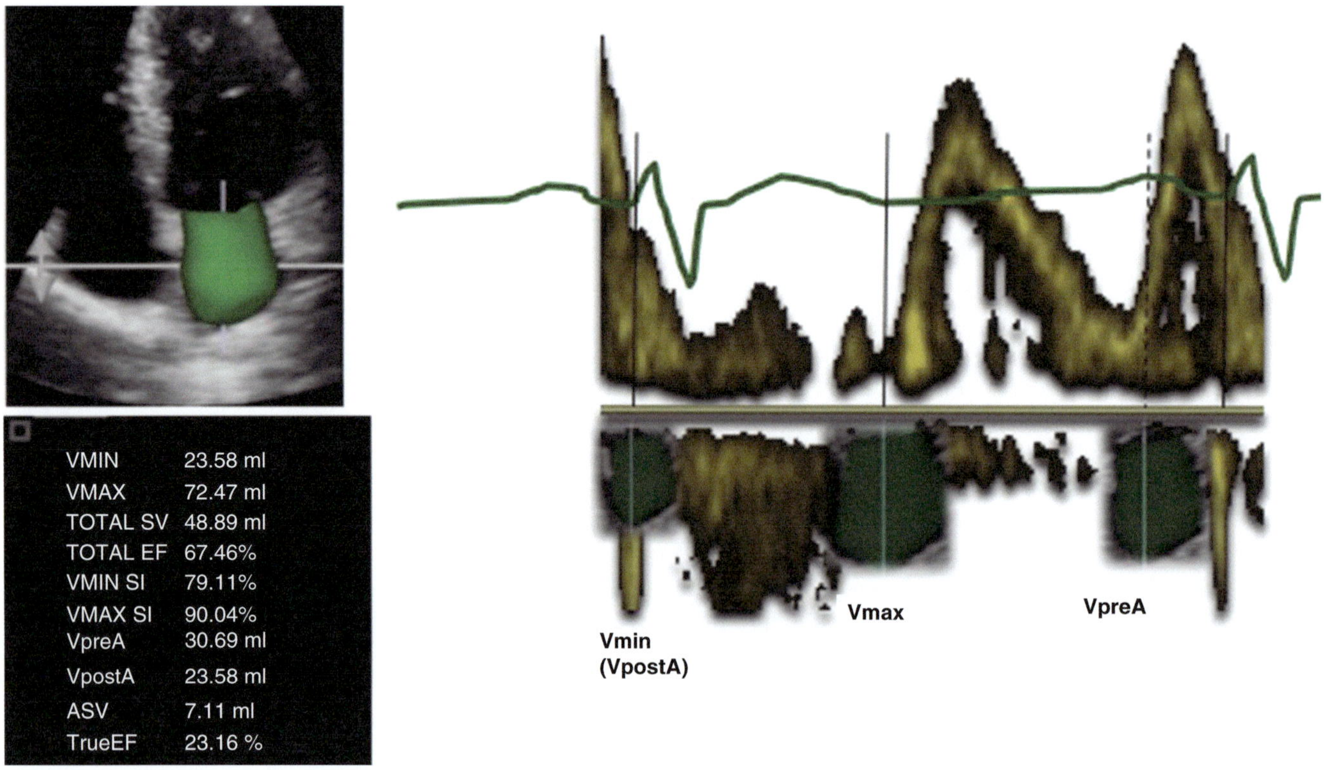

Fig. 16.8 Measurement of phasic left atrial volumes (minimum, maximum and pre-A) using 3DE. Electrocardiographic tracing and mitral valve inflow Doppler tracing are shown as time references. The table shows the volumes at different timing and calculated function indexes (Video 16.1). *EF* emptying fraction, *SV* stroke volume, *Vmax* Left atrial maximal volume, *Vmin* left atrial minimal volume, *VpreA* left atrial volume pre-atrial contraction

relation between the severity of left ventricular diastolic dysfunction and left atrial volume in the absence of mitral valve disease, atrial fibrillation and conditions with higher cardiac output. During ventricular diastole, the left atrium is exposed to left ventricular pressure. In the case of left ventricular diastolic dysfunction, with increased left ventricular stiffness, left atrial pressures increases to maintain adequate left ventricular filling. The increase in left atrial pressure leads to chamber dilatation and stretching of the atrial myocardium. Thus, left atrial volume increases both with severity of diastolic dysfunction and chronicity of the dysfunction and therefore can serve as a marker of long-term control of diastolic filling pressures. One exception to the relationship between left atrial size and diastolic function exists when atrial fibrillation is present.

In addition to conditions where left atrial afterload is increased, there is a clinical scenario called "stiff left atrium syndrome" where pressure overload from left atrial fibrosis and/or calcification results in left atrial enlargement [57]. This is due to decreased left atrial compliance resulting in an increase in left atrial and pulmonary pressures and right heart failure.

Left atrial enlargement is often found in patients with atrial fibrillation. However, it has been difficult to establish a relationship between atrial fibrillation and left atrial enlargement [58]. Studies have demonstrated that sustained atrial tachyarrhythmias can result in atrial structural, contractile and electrical remodeling but this may also be the result of high ventricular rates and high ventricular filling pressures [59, 60].

Reverse Remodeling

Reverse remodeling occurs when the left atrial size and function improves and reverses to a more normal form. This has been demonstrated to be feasible with the use of medical therapy independent of changes to blood pressure [61, 62]. While the clinical implication of these changes is unclear, it suggests the possibility of using left atrial size as a therapeutic target.

Assessment of Left Atrial Shape

Left atrial dilatation does not occur in a uniform manner. Thus, left atrial shape may be a better measure of left atrial remodeling. With 3DE, left atrial shape can be assessed. This has provided insight into the mechanism that determines blood stasis, which predisposes to embolic events in patients with mitral stenosis. It has been reported that patients in whom the left atrium remodels from an ellipsoidal to a more spherical shape are at greater risk of embolic events independent on the cardiac rhythm [63]. Spherical remodeling is felt to result in an increase in atrial wall tension that: (1) predisposes patients to atrial fibrillation; and (2) is less effective for atrial contraction. While this information is physiologically important, at this time the clinical utility of left atrial shape is still unclear.

Prognostic Value of Left Atrial Size

Left ventricular size is a strong predictor and prognosticator of outcomes in many clinical disease processes. Increased maximal and minimal left atrial size have been demonstrated to be associated with the development of adverse cardiovascular outcomes such as death, heart failure, and stroke in patients without a history of atrial fibrillation or significant valvular disease [55]. For those with dilated cardiomyopathy, minimal left atrial volume predicts mortality and the need for cardiac transplantation [55]. Increased left atrial size also predicts outcomes associated with atrial fibrillation. It predicts the development of a first or recurrent episode of atrial fibrillation, the likelihood of maintaining sinus rhythm post-cardioversion/ablation/heart failure [64]. When compared, left atrial volume is a stronger predictor of these adverse outcomes compared to left atrial area or diameter measurements [65]. Generally, left atrial volumes $\geq$32 mL/m^2 are associated with increased risk of first stroke or heart failure independent of age and other risk factors [33, 36]. It must be noted though that left atrial volume is a continuous variable and the larger the size the greater the risk [66].

Summary

Left atrial size assessment is important in routine clinical practice as it has important clinical and prognostic significance. Left atrial volumes should be measured using dedicated optimized views and reported indexed to body-surface area. While two dimensional echocardiographic methods for measuring left atrial volumes are recommended, 3DE methods are likely more accurate. However, the use of three-dimensional echocardiography to obtain left atrial volume values is limited by the time required to analyze the dataset to obtain this measurement and the lack of large population based normal values. These issues will be addressed by the development of automated chamber quantification programs for 3DE data and large 3D echocardiographic studies on left atrial size in normal and abnormal patients. Finally, further study is needed into understanding the clinical value of measurements left atrial contractile function.

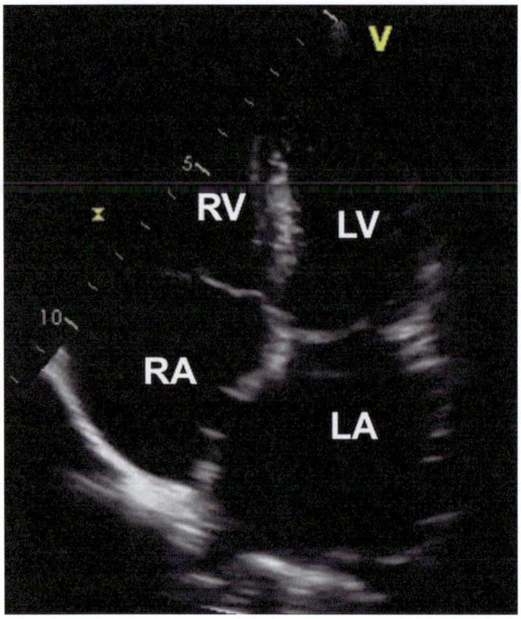

Fig. 16.9 Apical 4-chamber view optimized for left atrial size measurement. The left atrium appears large. *LA* left atrium, *LV* left ventricle, *RA* right atrium, *RV* right ventricle

Clinical Case 16.1

Fifty-four-year-old woman with no history of cardiovascular disease and no cardiovascular risk factor. Echocardiographic study indicated as part of her pre-operative work-up before undergoing abdominal surgery.

The conventional two-dimensional echocardiographic study was normal except a moderately enlarged left atrium (64 mL, 43 mL/m^2) when volume was computed using the biplane discs' summation algorithm (Fig. 16.9). However, when a 3DE data set of the left atrium was acquired and the left atrial volume was measured, it was found to be normal (52 mL, 34 mL/m^2). Figure 16.10 shows the asymmetric shape of the left atrium of this lady that is not accounted by the two-dimensional algorithm.

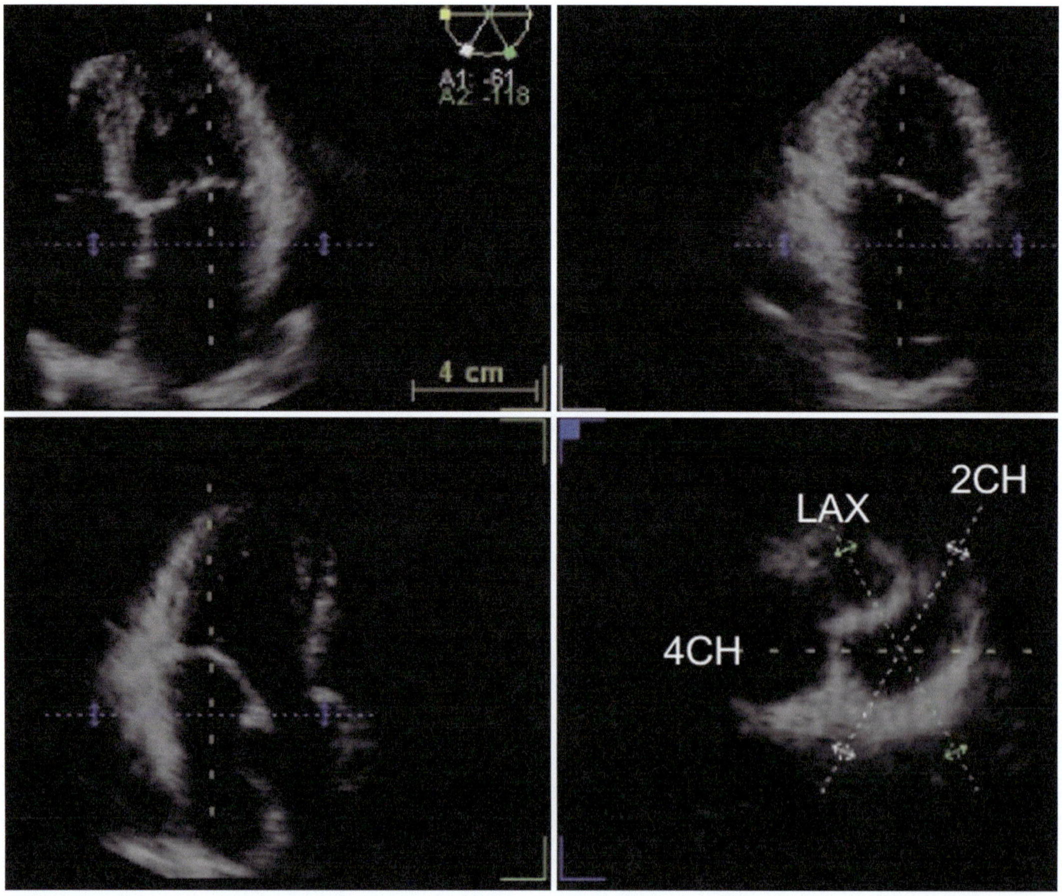

Fig. 16.10 Multislice (triplane) display of a 3DE data set including the left atrium. The right lower panel shows the positions of the three longitudinal cut planes (4-, 2-chamber and long axis views) on a transversal cut plane of the left atrium to appreciate the asymmetric shape of it, the non-orthogonal position of the 4- and 2-chamber views and the fact that the narrow long-axis view (flattened left atrium) has not been taken into account by the two-dimensional algorithm. *2CH* two-chamber view (right upper panel), *4CH* four-chamber view (left upper panel), *LAX* longitudinal axis (left lower panel)

References

1. Rosca M, Lancellotti P, Popescu BA, Pierard LA. Left atrial function: pathophysiology, echocardiographic assessment, and clinical applications. Heart. 2011;97:1982–9.
2. Spencer KT, Mor-Avi V, Gorcsan J, et al. Effects of aging on left atrial reservoir, conduit, and booster pump function: a multi-institution acoustic quantification study. Heart. 2001;85:272–7.
3. Bouzas-Mosquera A, Broullon FJ, Alvarez-Garcia N, et al. Left atrial size and risk for all-cause mortality and ischemic stroke. CMAJ. 2011;183:E657–64.
4. Kizer JR, Bella JN, Palmieri V, et al. Left atrial diameter as an independent predictor of first clinical cardiovascular events in middle-aged and elderly adults: The Strong Heart Study (SHS). Am Heart J. 2006;151(2):412–8.
5. Lancellotti P, Donal E, Magne J, et al. Risk stratification in asymptomatic moderate to severe aortic stenosis: the importance of the valvular, arterial and ventricular interplay. Heart. 2010;96:1364–71.
6. Le Tourneau T, Messika-Zeitoun D, Russo A, et al. Impact of left atrial volume on clinical outcome in organic mitral regurgitation. J Am Coll Cardiol. 2010;56:570–8.
7. Tsang TSM, Barnes ME, Gersh BJ, Bailey KR, Seward JB. Left atrial volume as a morphophysiologic expression of left ventricular diastolic dysfunction and relation to cardiovascular risk burden. Am J Cardiol. 2002;90:1284–9.
8. Tsang TSM, Barnes ME, Gersh BJ, et al. Prediction of risk for first age-related cardiovascular events in an elderly population: the incremental value of echocardiography. J Am Coll Cardiol. 2003;42:1199–205.
9. Benjamin EJ, Dagostino RB, Belanger AJ, Wolf PA, Levy D. Left atrial size and the risk of stroke and death—the Framingham Heart-Study. Circulation. 1995;92:835–41.
10. Tsang TS, Gersh BJ, Appleton CP, et al. Left ventricular diastolic dysfunction as a predictor of the first diagnosed nonvalvular atrial fibrillation in 840 elderly men and women. J Am Coll Cardiol. 2002;40:1636–44.
11. Tsang TSM, Barnes ME, Gersh BJ, Bailey KR, Seward JB. Risks for atrial fibrillation and congestive heart failure in patients >= 65 years of age with abnormal left ventricular diastolic relaxation. Am J Cardiol. 2004;93:54–8.
12. Beinart R, Boyko V, Schwammenthal E, et al. Long-term prognostic significance of left atrial volume in acute myocardial infarction. J Am Coll Cardiol. 2004;44:327–34.
13. Moller JE, Hillis GS, Oh JK, et al. Left atrial volume—a powerful predictor of survival after acute myocardial infarction. Circulation. 2003;107:2207–12.
14. Dini FL, Cortigiani L, Baldini U, et al. Prognostic value of left atrial enlargement in patients with idiopathic dilated cardiomyopathy and ischemic cardiomyopathy. Am J Cardiol. 2002;89:518–23.
15. Sabharwal N, Cemin R, Rajan K, Hickman M, Lahiri A, Senior R. Usefulness of left atrial volume as a predictor of mortality in patients with ischemic cardiomyopathy. Am J Cardiol. 2004;94:760–3.
16. Poulsen MK, Dahl JS, Henriksen JE, et al. Left atrial volume index: relation to long-term clinical outcome in type 2 diabetes. J Am Coll Cardiol. 2013;62(25):2416–21.
17. Appleton CP, Galloway JM, Gonzalez MS, Gaballa M, Basnight MA. Estimation of left ventricular filling pressures using two-dimensional and Doppler echocardiography in adult patients with cardiac disease. Additional value of analyzing left atrial size, left atrial ejection fraction and the difference in duration of pulmonary venous and mitral flow velocity at atrial contraction. J Am Coll Cardiol. 1993;22:1972–82.
18. Geske JB, Sorajja P, Nishimura RA, Ommen SR. The relationship of left atrial volume and left atrial pressure in patients with hypertrophic cardiomyopathy: an echocardiographic and cardiac catheterization study. J Am Soc Echocardiogr. 2009;22:961–6.
19. Guron CW, Hartford M, Rosengren A, Thelle D, Wallentin I, Caidahl K. Usefulness of atrial size inequality as an indicator of abnormal left ventricular filling. Am J Cardiol. 2005;95:1448–52.
20. Ersboll M, Andersen MJ, Valeur N, Mogensen UM, Waziri H, Moller JE, et al. The prognostic value of left atrial peak reservoir strain in acute myocardial infarction is dependent on left ventricular longitudinal function and left atrial size. Circ Cardiovasc Imaging. 2013;6:26–33.
21. Simek CL, Feldman MD, Haber HL, Wu CC, Jayaweera AR, Kaul S. Relationship between left ventricular wall thickness and left atrial size: comparison with other measures of diastolic function. J Am Soc Echocardiogr. 1995;8:37–47.
22. Badano LP, Miglioranza MH, Mihaila S, et al. Left atrial volumes and function by three-dimensional echocardiography: reference values, accuracy, reproducibility, and comparison with two-dimensional echocardiographic measurements. Circ Cardiovasc Imaging. 2016;9:e004229.
23. Kebed K, Kruse E, Addetia K, et al. Atrial-focused views improve the accuracy of two-dimensional echocardiographic measurements of the left and right atrial volumes: a contribution to the increase in normal values in the guidelines update. Int J Cardiovasc Imaging. 2017;33:209–18.
24. Iwataki M, Takeuchi M, Otani K, et al. Measurement of left atrial volume from transthoracic three-dimensional echocardiographic datasets using the biplane Simpson's technique. J Am Soc Echocardiogr. 2012;25:1319–26.
25. Lang RM, Badano LP, Mor-Avi V, et al. Recommendations for cardiac chamber quantification by echocardiography in adults: an update from the American Society of Echocardiography and the European Association of Cardiovascular Imaging. Eur Heart J Cardiovasc Imaging. 2015;16:233–70.
26. Di Tullio MR, Sacco RL, Sciacca RR, Homma S. Left atrial size and the risk of ischemic stroke in an ethnically mixed population. Stroke. 1999;30:2019–24.
27. Olshansky B, Heller EN, Mitchell LB, et al. Are transthoracic echocardlographic parameters associated with atrial fibrillation recurrence or stroke? Results from the atrial fibrillation follow-up investigation of rhythm management (AFFIRM) study. J Am Coll Cardiol. 2005;45:2026–33.
28. Rusinaru D, Tribouilloy C, Grigioni F, et al. Left atrial size is a potent predictor of mortality in mitral regurgitation due to flail leaflets results from a large international multicenter study. Circ Cardiovasc Imaging. 2011;4:473–U43.
29. Schabelman S, Schiller NB, Silverman NH, Ports TA. Left atrial volume estimation by two-dimensional echocardiography. Catheter Cardio Diag. 1981;7:165–78.
30. Wade MR, Chandraratna PAN, Reid CL, Lin SL, Rahimtoola SH. Accuracy of nondirected and directed M-mode echocardiography as an estimate of left atrial size. Am J Cardiol. 1987;60:1208–11.
31. Vyas H, Jackson K, Chenzbraun A. Switching to volumetric left atrial measurements: impact on routine echocardiographic practice. Eur J Echocardiogr. 2011;12(2):107–11.
32. Badano LP, Pezzutto N, Marinigh R, et al. How many patients would be misclassified using M-mode and two-dimensional estimates of left atrial size instead of left atrial volume? A three-dimensional echocardiographic study. J Cardiovasc Med (Hagerstown). 2008;9:476–84.
33. Barnes ME, Miyasaka Y, Seward JB, et al. Left atrial volume in the prediction of first ischemic stroke in an elderly cohort without atrial fibrillation. Mayo Clin Proc. 2004;79:1008–14.
34. Gottdiener JS, Kitzman DW, Aurigemma GP, Arnold AM, Manolio TA. Left atrial volume, geometry, and function in systolic and diastolic heart failure of persons >= 65 years of age (The Cardiovascular Health Study). Am J Cardiol. 2006;97:83–9.

35. Rossi A, Cicoira M, Zanolla L, et al. Determinants and prognostic value of left atrial volume in patients with dilated cardiomyopathy. J Am Coll Cardiol. 2002;40:1425–30.
36. Takemoto Y, Barnes ME, Seward JB, et al. Usefulness of left atrial volume in predicting first congestive heart failure in patients >= 65 years of age with well-preserved left ventricular systolic function. Am J Cardiol. 2005;96:832–6.
37. Tsang TSM, Abhayaratna WP, Barnes ME, et al. Prediction of cardiovascular outcomes with left atrial size—is volume superior to area or diameter? J Am Coll Cardiol. 2006;47:1018–23.
38. Pritchett AM, Jacobsen SJ, Mahoney DW, Rodeheffer RJ, Bailey KR, Redfield MM. Left atrial volume as an index of left atrial size: a population-based study. J Am Coll Cardiol. 2003;41:1036–43.
39. Russo C, Hahn RT, Jin ZZ, Homma S, Sacco RL, Di Tullio MR. Comparison of echocardiographic single-plane versus biplane method in the assessment of left atrial volume and validation by real time three-dimensional echocardiography. J Am Soc Echocardiogr. 2010;23:954–60.
40. Nistri S, Galderisi M, Ballo P, et al. Determinants of echocardiographic left atrial volume: implications for normalcy. Eur J Echocardiogr. 2011;12:826–33.
41. Kou S, Caballero L, Dulgheru R, et al. Echocardiographic reference ranges for normal cardiac chamber size: results from the NORRE Study. Eur Heart J Cardiovasc Imaging. 2014;15(6):680–90.
42. Surkova E, Badano LP, Genovese D, et al. Clinical and prognostic implications of methods and partition values used to assess left atrial volume by two-dimensional echocardiography. J Am Soc Echocardiogr. 2017;30:1119–29.
43. Mor-Avi V, Yodwut C, Jenkins C, et al. Real-time 3D echocardiographic quantification of left atrial volume: multicenter study for validation with CMR. JACC Cardiovasc Imaging. 2012;5: 769–77.
44. Aune E, Baekkevar M, Roislien J, Rodevand O, Otterstad JE. Normal reference ranges for left and right atrial volume indexes and ejection fractions obtained with real-time three-dimensional echocardiography. Eur J Echocardiogr. 2009;10:738–44.
45. Azar F, Perez de Isla L, Moreno M, et al. Three-dimensional echocardiographic assessment of left atrial size and function and the normal range of asynchrony in healthy individuals. Rev Esp Cardiol. 2009;62:816–9.
46. Sugimoto T, Robinet S, Dulgheru R, et al. Echocardiographic reference ranges for normal left atrial function parameters: results from the EACVI NORRE study. Eur Heart J Cardiovasc Imaging. 2018;19:630–8.
47. Tsang W, Salgo IS, Medvedofsky D, et al. Transthoracic 3D echocardiographic left heart chamber quantification using an automated adaptive analytics algorithm. JACC Cardiovasc Imaging. 2016;9:769–82.
48. Wu VC, Takeuchi M, Kuwaki H, et al. Prognostic value of LA volumes assessed by transthoracic 3D echocardiography: comparison with 2D echocardiography. JACC Cardiovasc Imaging. 2013;6:1025–35.
49. Suh IW, Song JM, Lee EY, et al. Left atrial volume measured by real-time 3-dimensional echocardiography predicts clinical outcomes in patients with severe left ventricular dysfunction and in sinus rhythm. J Am Soc Echocardiogr. 2008;21:439–45.
50. Russo C, Jin Z, Homma S, et al. LA phasic volumes and reservoir function in the elderly by real-time 3D echocardiography: normal values, prognostic significance, and clinical correlates. JACC Cardiovasc Imaging. 2017;10:976–85.
51. Rodevand O, Bjornerheim R, Ljosland M, Maehle J, Smith HJ, Ihlen H. Left atrial volumes assessed by three- and two-dimensional echocardiography compared to MRI estimates. Int J Cardiac Imag. 1999;15:397–410.
52. Stojanovska J, Cronin P, Patel S, et al. Reference normal absolute and indexed values from ecg-gated MDCT: left atrial volume, function, and diameter. Am J Roentgenol. 2011;197:631–7.
53. Vasan RS, Levy D, Larson MG, Benjamin EJ. Interpretation of echocardiographic measurements: a call for standardization. Am Heart J. 2000;139:412–22.
54. Nagueh SF, Appleton CP, Gillebert TC, et al. Recommendations for the evaluation of left ventricular diastolic function by echocardiography. J Am Soc Echocardiogr. 2009;22:107–33.
55. Abhayaratna WP, Seward JB, Appleton CP, et al. Left atrial size: physiologic determinants and clinical applications. J Am Coll Cardiol. 2006;47:2357–63.
56. Welles CC, Ku IA, Kwan DM, Whooley MA, Schiller NB, Turakhia MP. Left atrial function predicts heart failure hospitalization in subjects with preserved ejection fraction and coronary heart disease: longitudinal data from the Heart and Soul Study. J Am Coll Cardiol. 2012;59:673–80.
57. Mehta S, Charbonneau F, Fitchett DH, Marpole DG, Patton R, Sniderman AD. The clinical consequences of a stiff left atrium. Am Heart J. 1991;122:1184–91.
58. Thamilarasan M, Klein AL. Factors relating to left atrial enlargement in atrial fibrillation: "chicken or the egg" hypothesis. Am Heart J. 1999;137:381–3.
59. Allessie M, Ausma J, Schotten U. Electrical, contractile and structural remodeling during atrial fibrillation. Cardiovasc Res. 2002;54:230–46.
60. Schoonderwoerd BA, Ausma J, Crijns HJ, Van Veldhuisen DJ, Blaauw EH, Van Gelder IC. Atrial ultrastructural changes during experimental atrial tachycardia depend on high ventricular rate. J Cardiovasc Electrophysiol. 2004;15:1167–74.
61. Tsang TS, Barnes ME, Abhayaratna WP, et al. Effects of quinapril on left atrial structural remodeling and arterial stiffness. Am J Cardiol. 2006;97:916–20.
62. Gerdts E, Wachtell K, Omvik P, et al. Left atrial size and risk of major cardiovascular events during antihypertensive treatment: losartan intervention for endpoint reduction in hypertension trial. Hypertension. 2007;49:311–6.
63. Nunes MC, Handschumacher MD, Levine RA, et al. Role of LA shape in predicting embolic cerebrovascular events in mitral stenosis: mechanistic insights from 3D echocardiography. JACC Cardiovasc Imaging. 2014;7:453–61.
64. Vaziri SM, Larson MG, Benjamin EJ, Levy D. Echocardiographic predictors of nonrheumatic atrial fibrillation. The Framingham Heart Study. Circulation. 1994;89:724–30.
65. Tsang TS, Abhayaratna WP, Barnes ME, Miyasaka Y, Gersh BJ, Bailey KR, et al. Prediction of cardiovascular outcomes with left atrial size: is volume superior to area or diameter? J Am Coll Cardiol. 2006;47:1018–23.
66. Thomas L, Marwick TH, Popescu BA, Donal E, Badano LP. Left Atrial Structure and Function, and Left Ventricular Diastolic Dysfunction. J Am Coll Cardiol. 2019;73 (15):1961–77.

Assessment of the Right Ventricle

17

Denisa Muraru, Monica Luiza de Alcantara, Elena Surkova, and Basma Elnagar

Abstract

Right ventricular (RV) size and function have been found to be important predictors of cardiovascular morbidity and mortality in patients with various clinical conditions. However, assessment of the RV using conventional two-dimensional echocardiography is a challenging task due to the complex anatomy and the location of the RV in the chest. Although cardiac magnetic resonance is considered a "gold standard" for RV assessment, the development of three-dimensional echocardiography (3DE) opened new exciting opportunities in RV imaging. 3DE has proven accurate in measuring RV volumes and ejection fraction when compared with cardiac magnetic resonance. During the last decade, the added prognostic value of using 3DE to assess RV geometry and function over conventional two-dimensional and Doppler echocardiography has been increasingly reported.

Keywords

Right ventricular volume · Right ventricular ejection fraction · Right ventricular shape · Three-dimensional echocardiography · Reference values · Normal values

Electronic Supplementary Material The online version of this chapter (https://doi.org/10.1007/978-3-030-14032-8_17) contains supplementary material, which is available to authorized users.

Right ventricular (RV) volumes and ejection fraction (EF) are independent determinants of patient clinical status and adverse outcome [1–4]. Specifically, RV dysfunction has been associated with increased morbidity and mortality in patients with congenital heart disease, valvular disease, coronary artery disease, pulmonary hypertension, and heart failure. The assessment of RV size and function is pivotal for the diagnostic and therapeutic strategy in many clinical situations, such as arrhythmogenic cardiomyopathy, right-sided valvular heart disease, congenital heart disease, candidates for cardiac surgery, heart transplantation or left ventricular assist device therapy.

Transthoracic echocardiography is the primary imaging modality for the assessment of RV size and systolic function. As a result of the complex shape of the RV, the use of simple geometric modeling for the calculation of RV volumes and EF from two-dimensional echocardiographic images remains challenging. Conventional assessment of RV chamber function is commonly based on regional analyses applied only on a single slice of the RV (i.e. the apical 4-chamber view of the RV inflow), which may not always reflect the true global RV systolic performance. Three-dimensional echocardiography (3DE) enables accurate and reproducible measurements of RV volumes and EF [5]. The 3DE-derived RVEF is the only true global measure of RV pump function that can be measured by echocardiography. Albeit affected by inherent limitations (i.e. load dependency), EF is an established standard measure of chamber function, easy to use and interpret by clinicians, as it is routinely employed in practice for reporting left ventricular

D. Muraru (✉)
University of Milano-Bicocca, and Istituto Auxologico Italiano, IRCCS, San Luca Hospital, Milano, Italy
e-mail: denisa.muraru@unimib.it

M. L. de Alcantara
Department of Echocardiography, Ecocardiografia Americas Medical City, Hospital Samaritano and Cardiologia Proecho, Rio de Janeiro, Brazil

E. Surkova
Department of Echocardiography, Cardiac Division, Royal Brompton Hospital, Royal Brompton and Harefield NHS Foundation Trust, London, UK
e-mail: e.surkova@rbht.nhs.uk

B. Elnagar
Tanta Faculty of Medicine, Tanta University, Tanta, Egypt

Department of Cardiology, Tanta University Hospital, Tanta, Egypt

L. P. Badano et al. (eds.), *Textbook of Three-Dimensional Echocardiography*, https://doi.org/10.1007/978-3-030-14032-8_17

systolic function using two-dimensional echocardiography, as well as both left and RV systolic function using different imaging modalities. 3DE quantitation of RV size and function is not affected by plane position error or unverified geometric assumptions, and therefore it is more accurate and reproducible than two-dimensional echocardiography indices when image quality is adequate [6]. Moreover, 3DE-derived RV systolic function has shown prognostic value [7, 8], and age-and gender-specific normative values of RV volumes and EF have been identified [9]. Accordingly, the current ASE/EACVI guidelines on cardiac chamber quantification recommend that any echocardiography laboratory with proper 3DE equipment and expertise should consider using 3DE to assess RV size and function [5].

In this chapter, we will review the basics of 3DE acquisition and analysis, the clinical applications, with a special emphasis on the added value and limitations of current 3DE technology.

Acquisition and Display of RV Data Sets

In general, the 3DE assessment of the RV is performed at the end of a standard echocardiographic examination. The matrix-array probe is usually placed in the apical position or on the left anterior axillary line, and oriented towards the right heart in order to obtain the "RV-focused" view (with the RV in the center of the image sector and the apex-forming left ventricle on the right) (Fig. 17.1). For RV acquisition from "RV-focused view" approach, the use of a scanning bed with an apical cut is extremely useful, since it allows to position the patient in the left lateral position (almost forming 90° angle with the bed) and to accommodate more easily the probe in the correct position (more lateral than the usual position used to acquire the left ventricle) in order to obtain higher quality images. When the apical window is unsatisfactory, a low parasternal or subcostal window can be used,

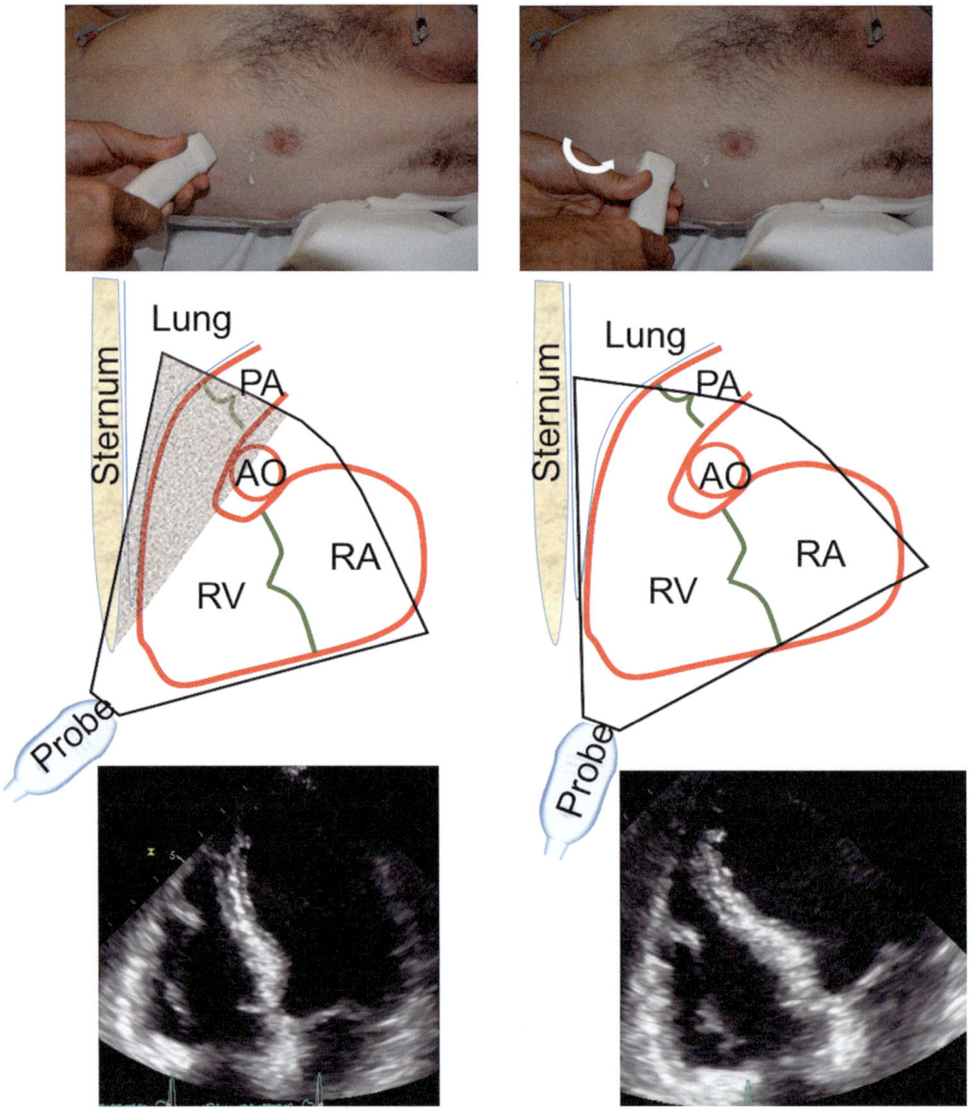

Fig. 17.1 Correct probe orientation (*right upper panel*) to obtain of the right ventricular focused apical 4-chamber views (*right lower panel*) compared to the conventional probe position (*left upper panel*) to obtain the classic apical 4-chamber view (*left lower panel*). Note that, using the conventional 4-chamber view, the right ventricular anterior wall and the right ventricular outflow tract cannot be acquired in the 3DE data set because of the interference of the sternum and lungs (*see charts in mid panels*). To obtain complete 3DE data sets of the right ventricle the patient should be in a forced left lateral decubitus (laying at almost 90° with the bed) and the probe should be placed more laterally and more anteriorly oriented than it is usually positioned when acquiring the left ventricle. *AO* aorta, *PA* pulmonary artery, *RA* right atrium, *RV* right ventricle

provided that the entire RV can be included in the pyramidal data set with good endocardial definition.

In order to maximize the temporal resolution, the volume depth and the volume size (in both lateral and elevation directions) should be minimized to include only the RV and the tricuspid valve throughout the cardiac cycle, and to exclude the basal part of the right atrium. For instance, a normal-sized RV can be usually imaged adequately using a 60° × 60° volume size; conversely, dilated RVs and/or with rounded apex require a larger volume size (up to 90° × 90°, at the expense of a lower temporal resolution). In any case, it is recommended that the left ventricle should be at least partially included in the RV dataset, since the available software analysis tools require the identification of left ventricular apex and mitral valve landmarks for spatial orientation purposes.

Routinely, the RV is imaged using a multi-beat full-volume 3D acquisition from 4 to 6 consecutive cardiac cycles. In specific situations when multi-beat RV acquisition is not feasible (irregular heart rhythm, dyspnea, lack of cooperation for breathhold, etc.), single-beat RV data sets can be also used, particularly if the 3D ultrasound system is equipped with high volume-rate real-time scanning capabilities [10]. However, it should be kept in mind that an accurate assessment of RV EF relies on a sufficient temporal resolution (at least 20–25 vps), which on most systems can be achieved using only a multi-beat acquisition mode.

The acquisition of an optimal RV 3D data set is more challenging than of the LV, and requires skill, coordination and patience. The key is to optimize the image quality and to stabilize it just before initiating the multi-beat acquisition. With few exceptions, this requires the application of respiratory maneuvers, changes of the probe position, orientation and pressure, or a steeper lateral position of the patient, until the entire RV walls are adequately visualized within the data set. While performing these maneuvers, we prefer to check their effect on the image quality by visualizing the RV in multiple slices (preferably short-axes), displayed side-by-side in real-time (Fig. 17.2, Video 17.1). If the 3DE system

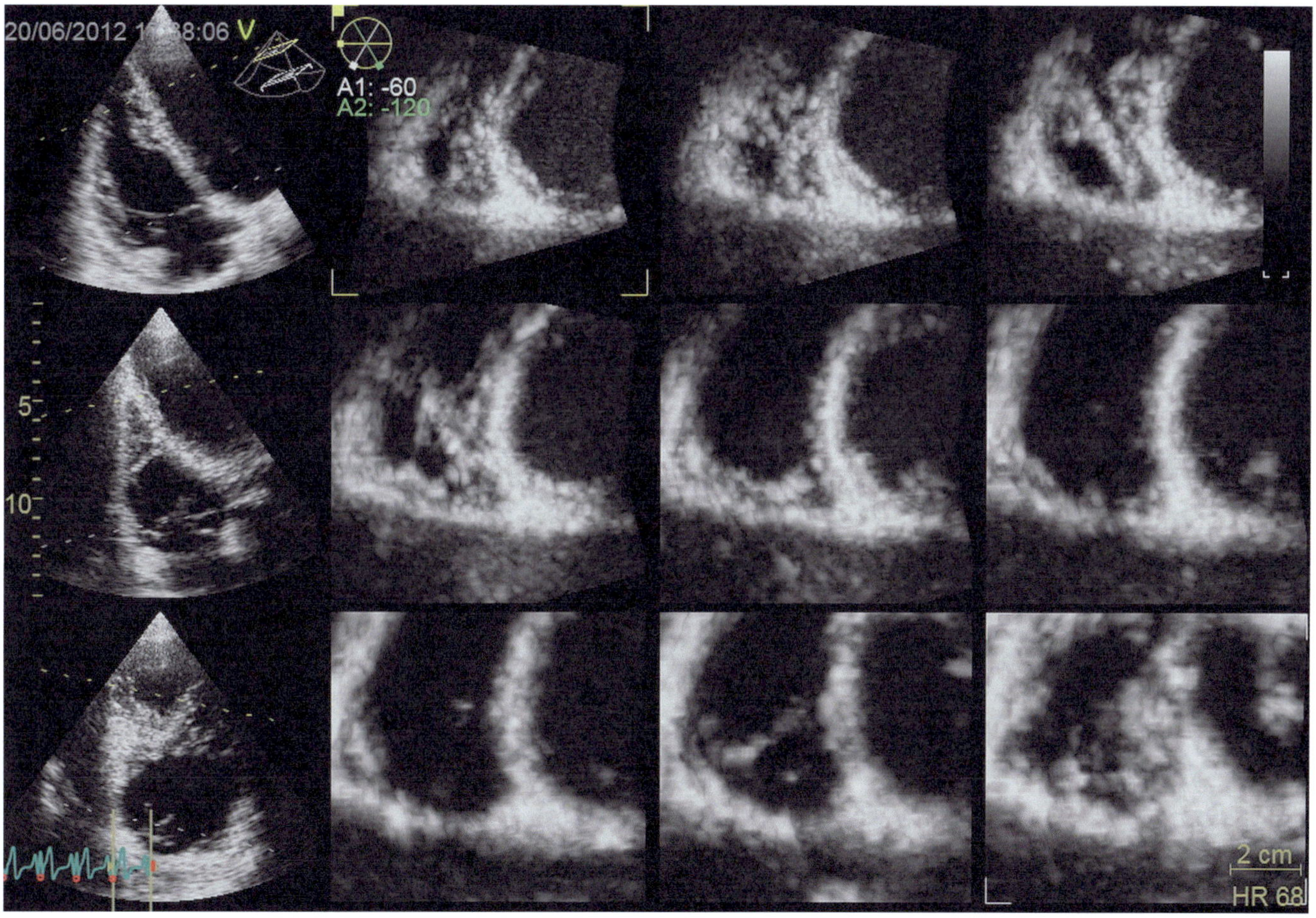

Fig. 17.2 Multislice (12-slice) display of 3DE data set of the right ventricle. The right ventricle has been acquired from the apical approach using the right ventricular focused view as reference (*left upper panel*). To check that the whole right ventricle is included in the data set, the data set has been sliced in three longitudinal views (the reference one and the views at 60° and 120° from the reference one) and nine transversal slices. The position and the orientation of the apical and the basal transversal slices can be controlled by adjusting the dashed lines on the longitudinal slices, the other seven are automatically sliced at equidistant space (Video 17.1)

does not allow for multi-slice display in real time, the RV image quality can be verified also after the acquisition and, if unsatisfactory, the acquisition sequence should be repeated.

Some ultrasound systems provide the possibility of obtaining three equidistant apical views of the RV (triplane imaging), which can be also steered manually around the central long-axis of the RV for a more complete evaluation of RV regional and global function than possible by conventional two-dimensional echocardiography (Fig. 17.3, Video 17.2). This is a viable alternative to the full volume multi-beat acquisition of the RV, whenever the latter cannot be performed (irregular atrial fibrillation, dyspnea, lack of cooperation, etc.). Of note, the presence of atrial fibrillation itself is not a contraindication to attempt the multi-beat acquisition (particularly on 3DE scanners performing a continuous multi-beat acquisition), as a set of relatively regular four consecutive beats can be stitched together sometimes without visible stitching artifacts.

3DE imaging of the RV should not be performed in patients with poor acoustic windows or large amounts of dropout. While the use of contrast is recommended for enhancing the endocardial definition of RV in two-dimensional echocardiography, for 3DE imaging of RV it is only rarely used at present due to unsatisfactory results due to partial volume effect. These patients should be addressed to other imaging modalities for RV quantification (Cardiac magnetic resonance, Computed Tomography, etc.).

RV Anatomy

Knowledge of the RV anatomy and of its spatial relationships with the other cardiac structures is pivotal for an accurate orientation and interpretation of the 3D images. For a detailed description of RV anatomy and physiology, the reader may consult some excellent reviews dedicated to this topic [11, 12].

Briefly, the normal RV is more triangular in shape when viewed from the front (Fig. 17.4a, Video 17.3a), and crescent-shaped when viewed in cross-section (Fig. 17.4b, Video 17.3b). Under normal loading conditions, the septum is concave towards the LV in both systole and diastole (Fig. 17.4). In adults, the RV volume is larger than the left ventricular volume, while the stroke volume of RV and the left ventricle are similar.

The RV outflow tract presents a "cross-over" relationship with the left ventricular outflow tract when the RV and left ventricular outflow tracts lack this characteristic "cross-over", this can be a sign of congenital heart disease, such as complete transposition.

The RV chamber has three component parts: inlet, apical trabecular and outlet. Because of the complex shape of the RV, commonly the three components cannot be seen simultaneously in a single cross-sectional view with two-dimensional echocardiography (Fig. 17.5a, b, Video 17.3b). The recognition of apical trabecular part, together with several other anatomical characteristics is of particular significance in congenital patients, for the distinction of morphologically RV versus morphologically left ventricle:

1. The septal insertion of the tricuspid valve is located more apically than the mitral valve.
2. Apical trabecular component of the RV has coarser trabeculations than the left ventricular apex.
3. The ventriculo-infundibular fold separates the tricuspid from the pulmonary valve, while in the left ventricle, there is the mitral-aortic fibrous continuity.
4. The moderator band, which continues the septomarginal band, is characteristic for RV, being absent in the left ventricle.

Regional Function

The assessment of RV regional function by echocardiography is important for diagnosis and therapy, particularly in ischemic heart disease, pulmonary embolism, cardiomyopathies, and athletes. Localized RV dyskinesia or aneurysm is an important diagnostic criterion for arrythmogenic RV cardiomyopathy [13]. Hypokinesia of the RV free wall combined with the normal contraction of the RV apex (McConnell sign) in presence of RV pressure overload is a typical echocardiographic sign of acute pulmonary embolism [14]. RV wall motion abnormalities could be also seen in patients with RV myocardial infarction, chronic pulmonary hypertension, sarcoidosis and congenital heart disease. Although clinically important, imaging the RV wall motion remains challenging because of its myocardial fiber orientation, complex anatomy that prevents the visualization of the same segments from orthogonal views, thin myocardial wall and peculiar myocardial mechanics. RV wall motion and shape sometimes is interpreted in a way similar to LV counterpart, which may be misleading: while the LV is symmetric and ellipsoidal, the geometry of the RV is complex; tethering of the free-wall by the moderator band and a nonlinear shape of the RV significantly contribute to a lack of understanding of the normal and pathological RV wall motion patterns [15].

Due to the thinness and limited visualization of RV walls, standard two-dimensional echocardiography has a rather limited sensitivity in comparison with cardiac magnetic resonance for detecting local abnormalities, such as hypokinetic segments, small aneurysms or bulging. Often these abnormalities are not

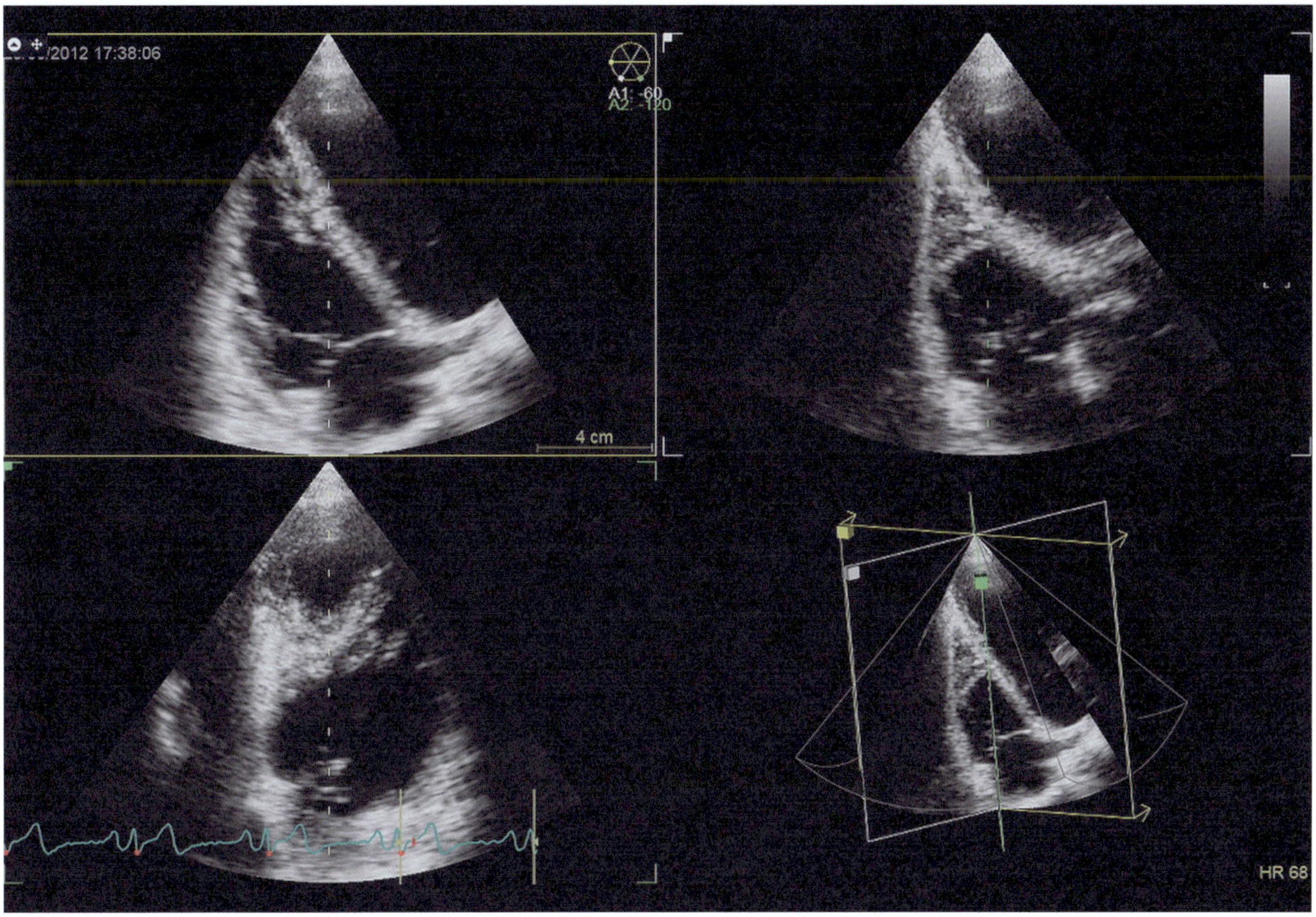

Fig. 17.3 Triplane display of the right ventricle (Video 17.2). The reference plane is shown in the left upper panel (*yellow plane*). The secondary planes are set by default at 60° (white plane, *right upper panel*) and 120° (green plane, *left lower panel*). The position and the orientation of the cut planes is shown in the right lower panel. Orientation of secondary planes can be adjusted only during acquisition (see also Chap. 2)

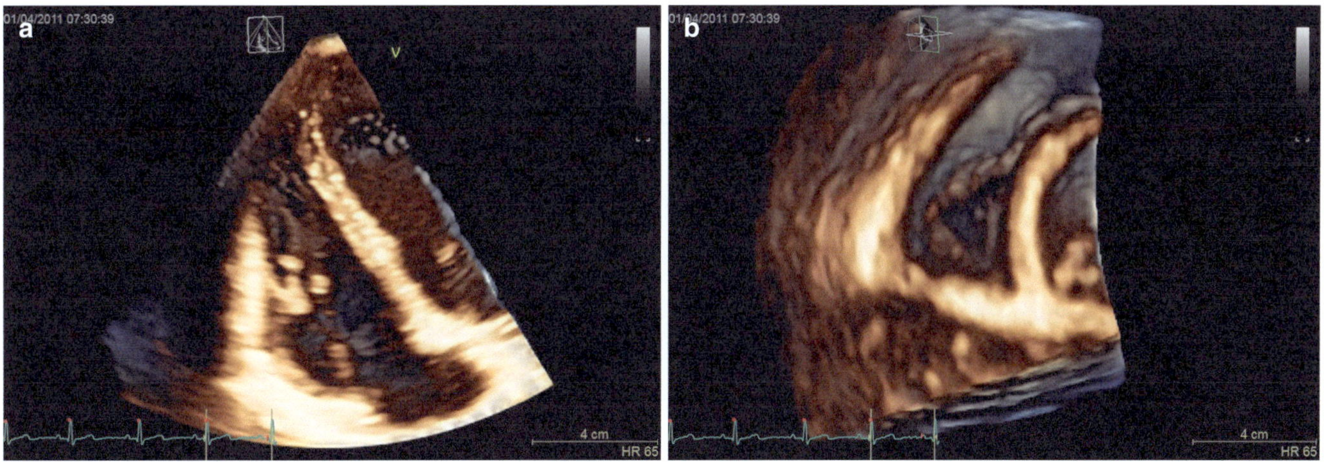

Fig. 17.4 Volume rendering of the right ventricular data set showing a frontal (**a**, Video 17.3a) and a trasversal (**b**, Video 17.3b) views of the cavity to appreciate its complex geometry

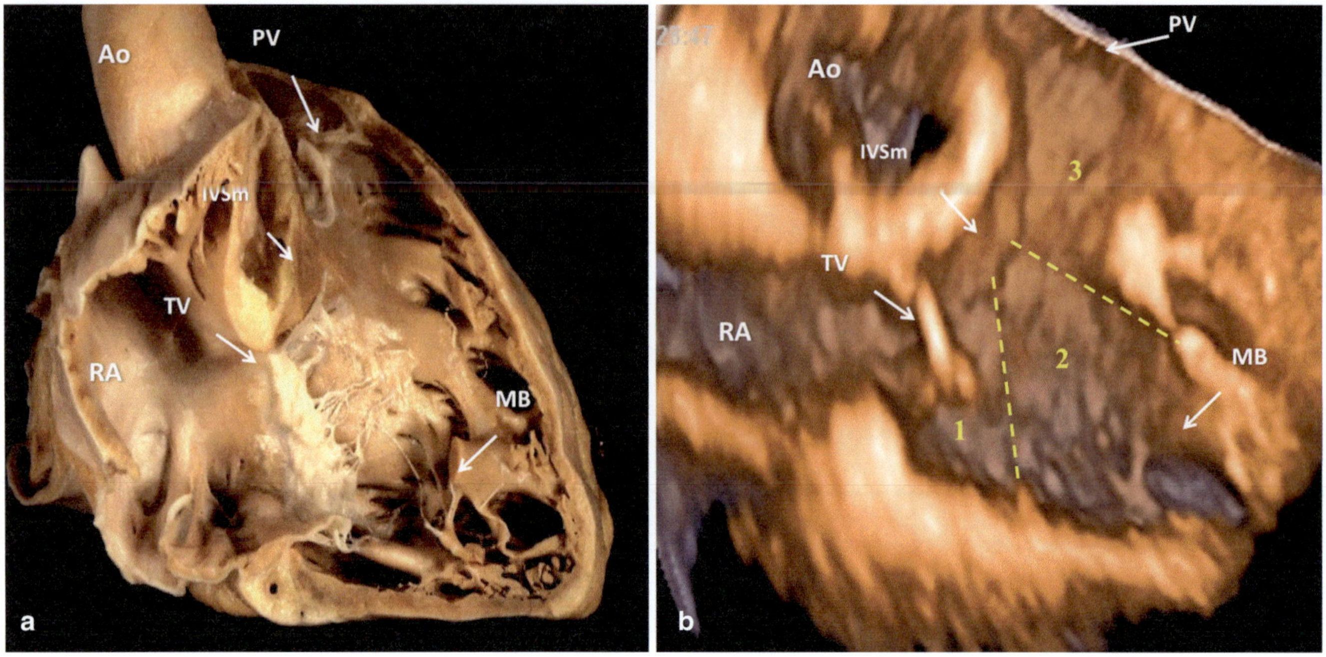

Fig. 17.5 Careful cropping of the 3DE right ventricular data set allows to assess the detailed anatomy of the right ventricular cavity and its three components: (1) Inlet; (2) apical trabecular; and (3) Outlet (**b**, Video 17.3b). On the left (**a**), anatomical specimen reproducing the same cut plane of the 3DE data set (Courtesy of prof Cristina Basso, Cardiovascular Pathology, University of Padua, Padova, Italy)

confined to standard two-dimensional echocardiography views of the RV, requiring skill and experience to perform multiple scans from off-axis views of RV. By its ability to acquire the entire RV walls within a single data set, that can be sliced in unlimited number of longitudinal or transversal slices (Fig. 17.3), 3DE is likely to improve the sensitivity of echocardiography to detect regional RV abnormalities.

Quantitative Analysis of RV Geometry and Function

Because of its complex shape, there is no geometrical model that can allow a reliable calculation of RV volumes and EF by standard two-dimensional echocardiography. For this reason, surrogate parameters of RV size (diameters and areas derived from standard two-dimensional views) and systolic function (TAPSE, tricuspid annulus plane systolic excursion; FAC, fractional area change; TDI S wave, systolic anterior wall myocardial velocity measure by tissue Doppler imaging; RIMP, Right ventricular Index of Myocardial Performance etc.) are routinely used. However, these parameters are affected by significant limitations, mainly related to their regional nature and view- and/or angle-dependency [16].

With the advent of 3DE, the accurate and reproducible quantification of RV volumes and EF by echocardiography has finally become possible, as it is routinely done for the LV. While all 3DE systems are equipped with their own specific algorithms for LV quantitation, the RV analysis from 3DE data sets has been traditionally performed with a single software package able to post-process 3DE data sets in DICOM format from all 3DE companies (i.e. 4D-RV Function 1.1/1.2 by TomTec Imaging Systems, Unterschlessheim, Germany) [17] (Fig. 17.6, Video 17.4). Recently GE Vingmed (Horten, N) has developed its own software package to measure RV volumes, EF and several two-dimensional echocardiography parameters (diameters, TAPSE, RV fractional area change) using data sets acquired with GE ultrasound systems (Fig. 17.7).

Feasibility

Feasibility depends on both acquisition and analysis issues. In general, the reported feasibility of multi-beat 3DE for the RV is around 85% (ranging from 52 to 93%, depending on how strict is the patient selection based on two-dimensional image quality) [9, 18] and lower than for the LV. As one may expect, single-beat real-time acquisition is more feasible (96–97%) than multi-beat [10, 19]. Feasibility of RV 3DE analysis is limited by the quality of the 2DE acoustic window ("bad 2D images lead to worse 3DE images…"), artifacts and dropouts affecting the RV anterior wall and the RV outflow tract. The overall image quality of RV data sets increases with the experience in 3DE and appears better in patients than in healthy subjects [19].

Image quality interpretation is inherently subjective; however if the ultrasound drop-out is present in more than one-half of the RV free wall in the coronal or short-axis views [20, 21], then the data set should be considered of poor quality and not feasible for quantitation.

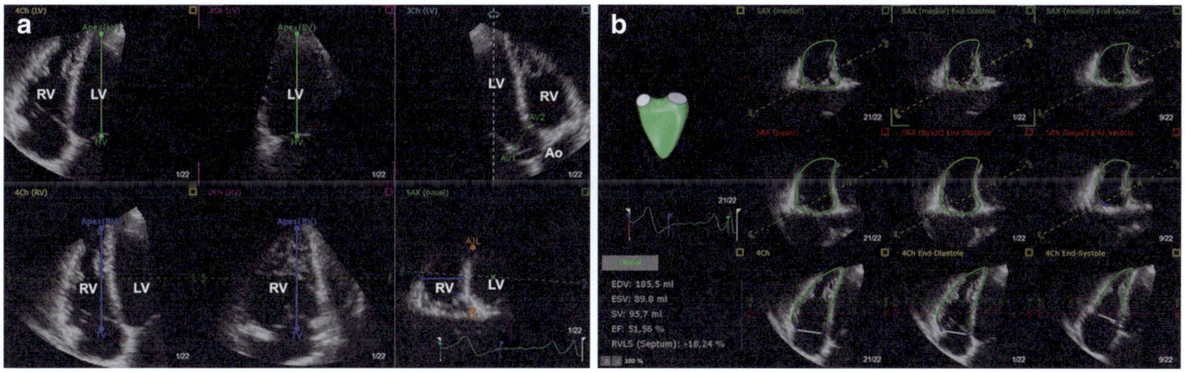

Fig. 17.6 Measurement of right ventricular volumes and ejection fraction by 4D RV function 2.0 (TomTec Imaging Systems, Unterschleisse, D). (**a**) Initialization of the three-dimensional echocardiography data set of the right ventricle for the measurement of right ventricular volumes. See text for details. (**b**) After the initialization of the data set a semiautomated endocardial border detection by the algorithm provides a first estimate of the beutel of the right ventricle on the left. The position of endocardial border traced by the algorithm is displayed on mid-cavity (SAX (medial)) and basal (SAX (basal) transversal cut planes, and 4-chamber equivalent (4Ch) longitudinal cut plane, both at end-diastole and end-systole, for manual editing. *2Ch* 2-chamber view-equivalent cut plane, *3CH* apical long-axis view-equivalent cut plane, *4Ch* 4-chamber view-equivalent cut plane, *AJL* anterior junction of the right ventricular free wall with the interventricular septum, *Ao* aorta, *AV* aortic valve, *EDV* end-diastolic volume, *EF* ejection fraction, *ESV* end-systolic volume, *LV* left ventricle, *PJL* posterior junction of the right ventricular free wall with the interventricular septum, *RV* right ventricle, *RVLS* right ventricular longitudinal strain, *SAX* short axis view

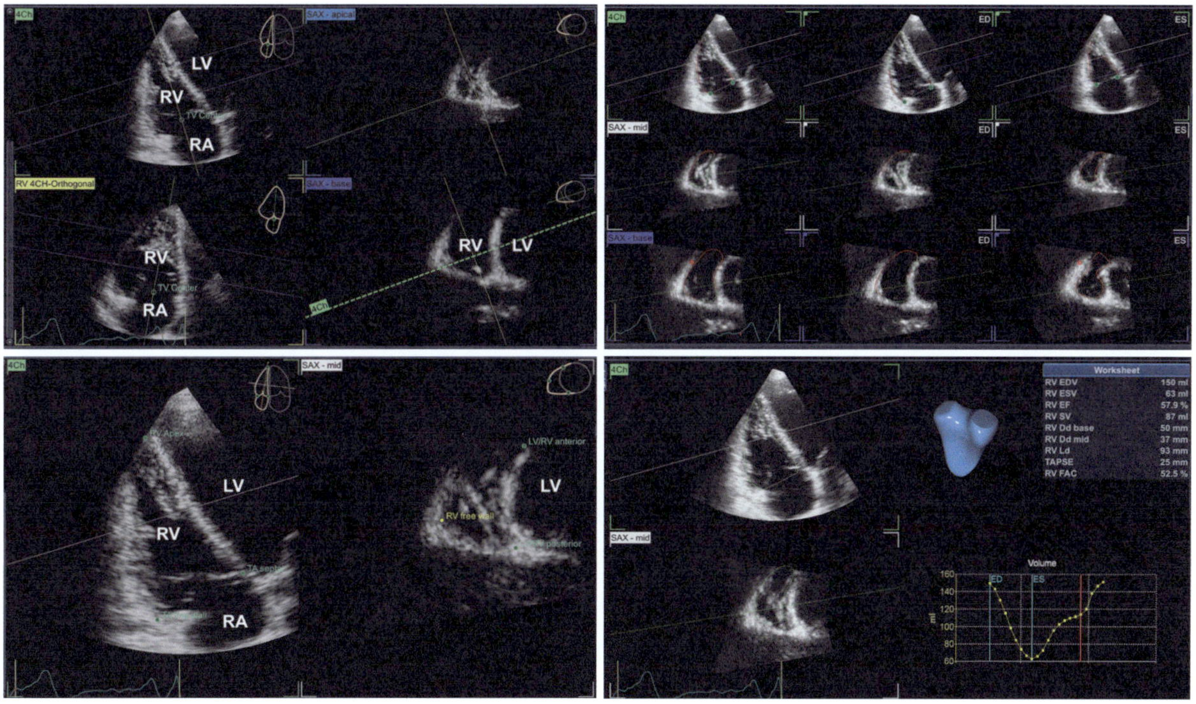

Fig. 17.7 Measurement of right ventricular volumes and ejection fraction by 4D AutoRVQ (GE Vingmed, Horten, N). *Left upper panel*, initialization of the software package by positioning the yellow vertical line passing through the right ventricular apex and the center of the tricuspid valve in the apical RV focused view (upper left quadrant) and its orthogonal view (lower left quadrant). The center of the tricuspid valve is also identified. The green line is positioned across the largest part of the cescentic transversal apical and basal views on the right. *Left lower panel*, Tricuspid annulus points at the insertion of septal and anterior tricuspid valve leaflets are localized as well as the right ventricular apex (left quadrant), and the anterior and posterior insertion points of right ventricular free wall on interventricular septum, and right ventricular free-wall endocardium (right quadrant. *Right upper panel*, the semiautomatically detected endocardial border can be edited by the operator by clicking on the part of the border needing editing (highlighted in red) and dragging the line to the desired position by moving the mouse. The position of the two transversal cut planes: Sax-base and SAX-mid is shown by the corresponding blue and white lines on the 4 chamber view, respectively. They can be adjusted by the operator. *Right lower panel*, the final endocardial border detection is shown dynamically in both longitudinal and transversal cut-planes (left quadrants) and the surface rendering of the dynamic right ventricular cavity is shown in blue. Results are displayed as numerical values and also as a Volume-time curve (right lower quadrant). *4Ch* 4-chamber view, *Dd* diastolic diameter, *EDV* end-diastolic volume, *EF* ejection fraction, *ESV* end-systolic volume, *FAC* fractional area contraction, *Ld* diastolic length, *LV* left ventricle, *RA* right atrium, *RV* right ventricle, *SAX-base* transversal cut plane taken at the base of the right ventricle, *SAX-mid* transversal cut plane taken at mid right ventricular length, *SV* stroke volume, *TAPSE* tricuspid annulus plane systolic excursion

Accuracy

In general, the 3DE provides accurate data on RV volumes and EF. On average, there is a small negative bias with respect to end-diastolic volumes measure with cardiac magnetic resonance (15 mL), while the agreement on RVEF is excellent, with negligible negative bias in the range of 1–4% [17, 21]. Larger bias between cardiac magnetic resonance and 3DE volumes were reported in congenital heart diseases [22]. In older subjects, 3DE overestimated RV volumes and underestimated RVEF. The accuracy of RV 3DE volumes is limited by the difficulty to include the RV outflow tract in the data set in case of very dilated RVs (end-diastolic volume >200 mL), and blurring of RV endocardial contour [17].

Reproducibility

Intraobserver reproducibility of 3DE volumes and EF by 3DE is excellent, and comparable with that reported for cardiac magnetic resonance [21]. Intercenter, interobserver and test-retest reproducibility are good and acceptable for clinical use, albeit they are generally lower than those reported for cardiac magnetic resonance [9, 19, 23, 24]. Poor image quality of 3DE data set and lower levels of experience in 3DE may adversely affect reproducibility. This is due to the fact that current semi-automated software packages for RV 3DE quantification still require a significant amount of manual input from the operator for endocardial border corrections, which may increase the measurement variability even when performed on the same images by different operators with different training or levels of experience [21].

Reference Values

In healthy subjects, RV volumes increase with body size. Men have lower EF and larger RV volumes than women of similar age, even after indexing for body surface area. Older age is associated with smaller volumes and higher EF. These relationships were consistently demonstrated in large normative studies using both 3DE [9] and cardiac magnetic resonance [25, 26] for RV analysis. The availability of normative tables and equations specifically developed for 3DE [5, 9] could allow for a more accurate and earlier detection of RV impairment, avoiding the confounding effects of age, sex and body size on RV 3DE measurements (Table 17.1). Both 3DE and cardiac magnetic resonance agree about the lower limit of normality for RV EF that is 45% [5, 9, 23].

Recently, reference values for RV volumes and EF have been derived from a population of 360 healthy children (136 children <7 years of age), group II (106 girls and 118 boys 7–18 years of age) [27].

Clinical Significance of 3DE Volumes and EF

The superiority of 3DE for assessing the RV size and function in comparison with standard echocardiographic indices translates into a greater accuracy of detecting RV

Table 17.1 Normative values for 3D echocardiographic right ventricular volumes and ejection fraction by gender and age decade [9]

		RV end-diastolic volume (mL)			RV end-systolic volume (mL)		
Age (years)	n (women, men)	All	Women	Men	All	Women	Men
<30	114 (46,68)	105 (69,183)	88 (66,136)	122 (80,189)	46 (18,88)	35 (14,71)	51 (30,94)
30–39	98 (50,48)	92 (64,147)	85 (63,117)	114 (72,153)	36 (18,67)	31 (17,52)	45 (25,66)
40–49	98 (53,45)	90 (63,132)	82 (64,106)	101 (75,137)	35 (16,54)	30 (15,44)	40 (23,62)
50–59	91 (49,42)	90 (62,138)	79 (62,117)	101 (72,138)	33 (18,62)	29 (18,46)	37 (22,63)
60–69	69 (39,30)	85 (47,139)	79 (43,100)	98 (76,149)	32 (14,61)	30 (13,40)	37 (20,68)
≥70	37 (23,14)	77 (50, 125)	70 (51,86)	98 (64,129)	23 (11,53)	20 (12,32)	34 (18,54)
All	507 (260,247)	91 (61,150)	81 (58,120)	107 (74,163)	35 (16,72)	30 (15,52)	44 (22,80)

		RV stroke volume (mL)			RV ejection fraction (%)		
Age (years)	n (women, men)	All	Women	Men	All	Women	Men
<30	114 (46,68)	63 (41,95)	56 (42,77)	69 (41,101)	58 (42,75)	60 (45,80)	56 (42,68)
30–39	98 (50,48)	60 (36, 93)	56 (38,72)	68(37,97)	61 (48,76)	63 (52,77)	60 (48,72)
40–49	98 (53,45)	56 (37,82)	51 (39,71)	63 (39,86)	63 (51,79)	65 (50,79)	61 (51,75)
50–59	91 (49,42)	56 (35,78)	50 (35,68)	63 (44,84)	62 (46,75)	62 (47,76)	62 (45,73)
60–69	69 (39,30)	52 (28,85)	49 (25,61)	64 (48,88)	61 (50,79)	61 (53,75)	63 (50,78)
≥70	37 (23,14)	54 (31,77)	49 (31,64)	61 (45,79)	68 (56,81)	71 (60,81)	65 (56,75)
All	507 (260,247)	57 (36,87)	52 (35,72)	66 (40,91)	62 (47,77)	63 (49,79)	60 (45,75)

Modified from Maffessanti F, Muraru D, Esposito R, et al. Age-, body size-, and sex-specific reference values for right ventricular volumes and ejection fraction by three-dimensional echocardiography: a multicenter echocardiographic study in 507 healthy volunteers. Circulation: Cardiovascular Imaging. 2013;6(5):700-10

Data expressed median (5th, 95th percentile)

RV right ventricular

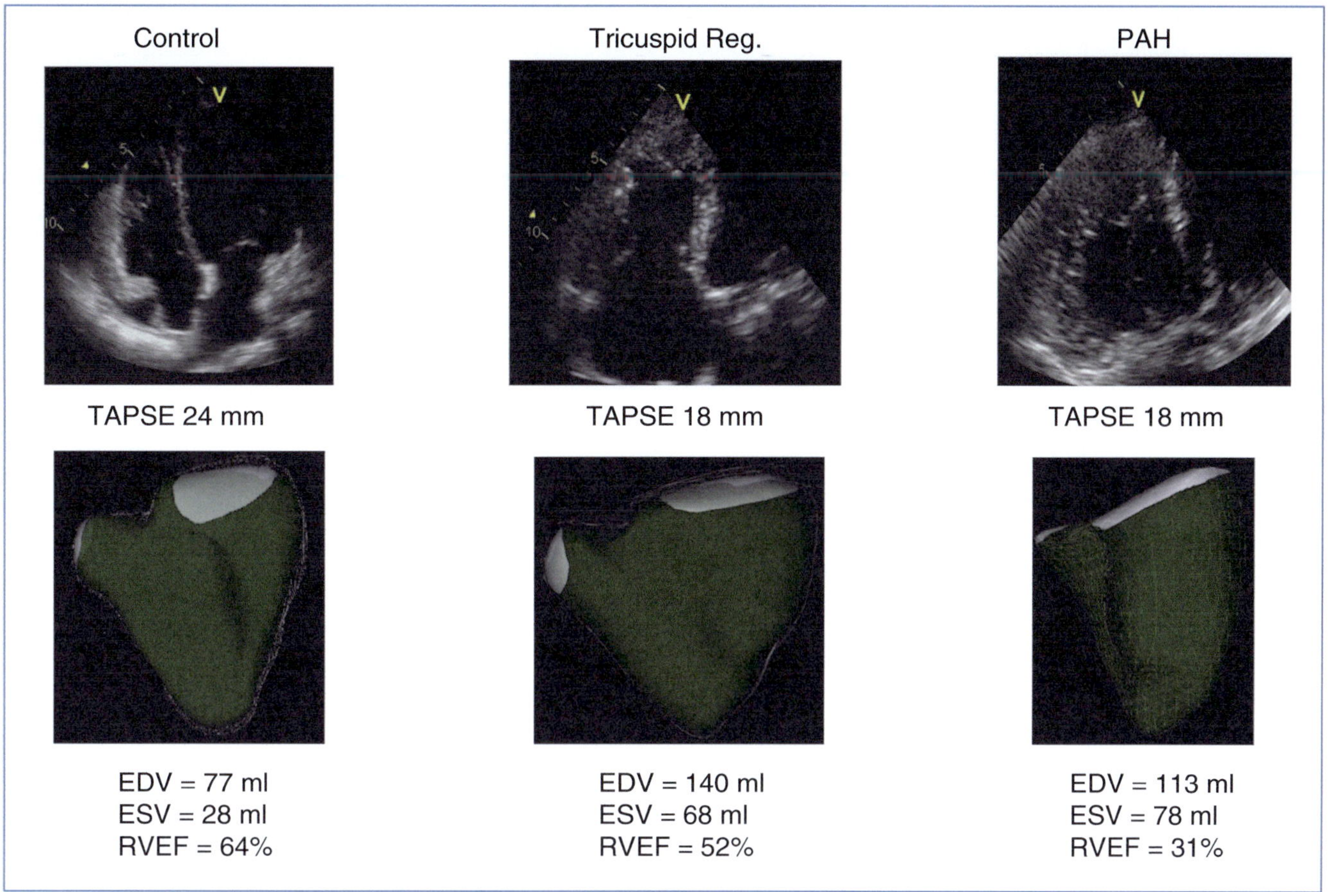

Fig. 17.8 Comparison of TAPSE and 3DE data among a normal subject (on the left), a patients with right ventricular volume overload (in the center) and a patient with right ventricular pressure overload (on the right). Despite the fact that the TAPSE is reduced in both patients compared to the normal subjects, TAPSE values in patients are still within normal ranges and do not tell much about the pathophysiologic condition. Conversely, 3DE measurements allow to understand the pathophysiologic condition. In the normal subject, both right ventricular volumes and ejection fraction are normal. In the patient with right ventricular volume overload, volumes are enlarged but ejection fraction is normal. In the patient with right ventricular pressure overload, volumes are normal but ejection fraction is reduced

dysfunction (Fig. 17.8). Comparative studies have shown that TAPSE is the worst predictor of RV dysfunction (i.e. TAPSE <19 mm had 56% sensitivity to detect RVEF <50% by cardiac magnetic resonance), while RV fractional area change having intermediate value and 3DE RVEF had the best ability (94% sensitivity) to identify RV dysfunction [19]. TAPSE is influenced by overall heart motion (rocking) and translation, being insensitive to reductions in RV radial function that typically occur in RV pressure overload. RV fractional area change is the only two-dimensional echocardiography parameter accounting for both longitudinal and radial function of the RV, however it is applied to RV inflow only. In patients after cardiac surgery, pulmonary thrombendarterectomy or heart transplant recipients, commonly TAPSE has low values and can no longer be used as a correlate of overall RV performance [28, 29]. In patients with thoracic deformities (pectus excavatum), the interpretation of RV morphology and function based on a single two-dimensional echocardiography 4-chamber slice can be misleading, as the RV free wall is often impressed by the deformed sternum [30]. In these settings, 3DE may have an important incremental role in assessing RV function by ultrasound.

Recently Nagata et al. [31] reported the independent prognostic value of RV EF in predicting cardiac mortality and MACEs (including cardiac death, nonfatal myocardial infarction, ventricular fibrillation, and heart failure exacerbation requiring hospitalization) in unselected consecutive patients undergoing echocardiography. Preliminary data from our laboratory confirmed the results of Nagata and coworkers [31] showing that, among 412 consecutive, unselected patients followed for 3.7 years, those with reduced RV EF (i.e. RV EF < 45%) had significantly reduced survival (Fig. 17.9 data on file). Moreover, we were able to stratify RV function according to prognosis and provide cut-off values of RV EF able to identify group of patients with significantly different and increasing risk of mortality and MACE (Fig. 17.10). Finally, in the same patients we showed that RV EF had an incremental prognostic value over left ventricular ejection fraction (Fig. 17.11).

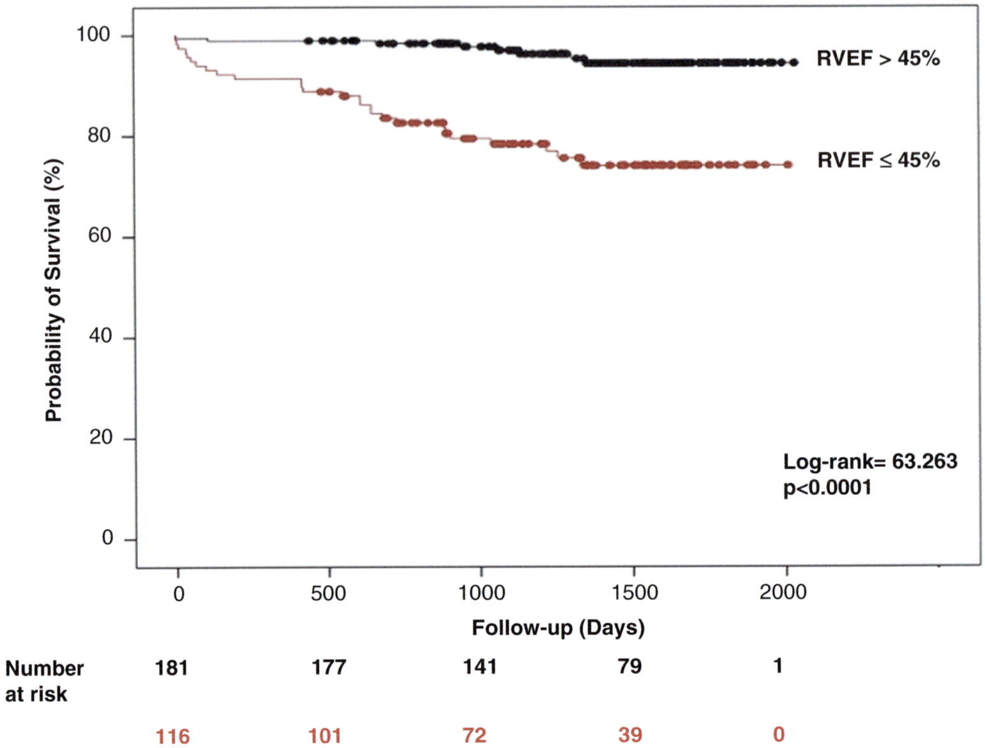

Fig. 17.9 Kaplan-Meier estimates of survival to cardiac death according to right ventricular ejection fraction in 412 consecutive, unselected patients undergoing echocardiography for clinical indications (data on file)

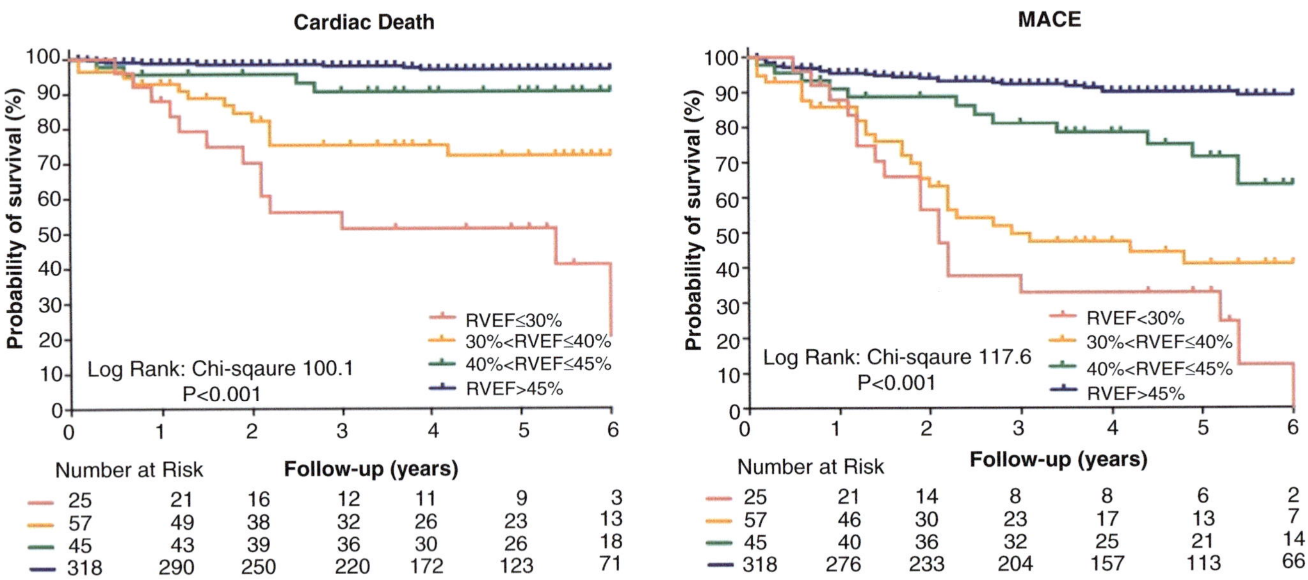

Fig. 17.10 Kalan-Meier estimates of survival to cardiac death (*right panel*) and freedom from MACE (*left panel*) in 409 unselected patients using the new partition values to grade the severity of right ventricular dysfunction

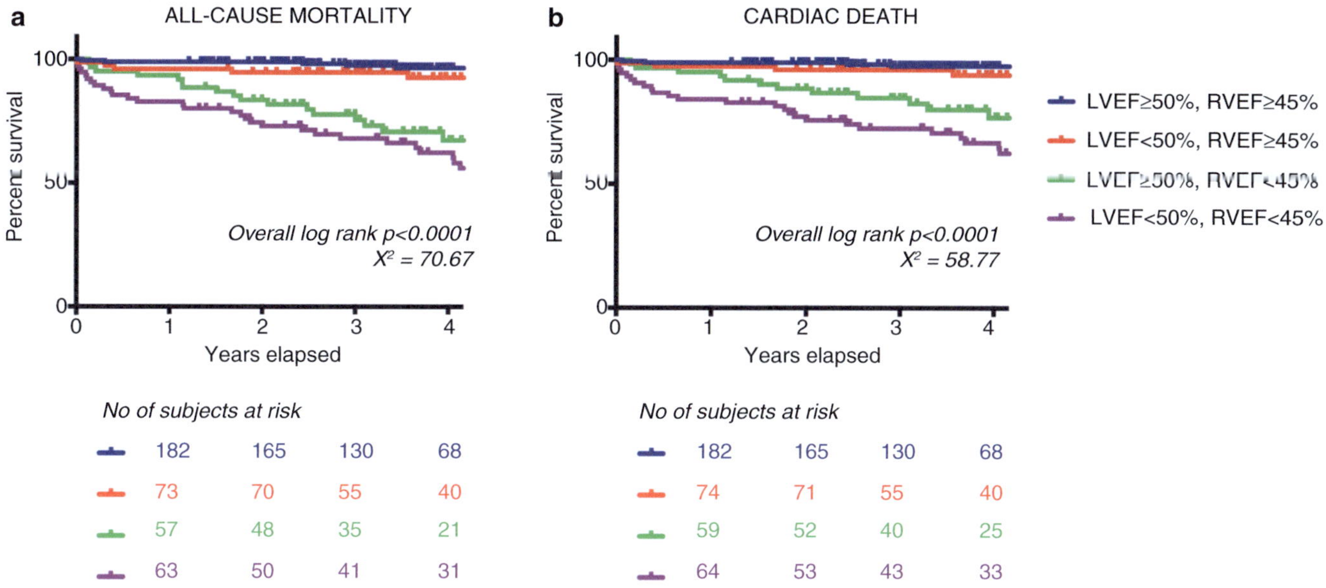

Fig. 17.11 Kaplan-Meier survival analysis for all-cause mortality (**a**) and cardiac death (**b**) associated with the different combinations of 3DE-derived left and right ventricular ejection fraction. Color of numbers of subjects at risk correspond to the relevant groups. *LVEF* left ventricular ejection fraction, *RVEF* right ventricular ejection fraction

Advanced RV Analysis from 3DE

Longitudinal Versus Radial Shortening

Both longitudinal and radial (or transverse) displacements contribute to RV pump function, and their reciprocal interplay varies in different pathological conditions.

In heart transplant recipients and after cardiac surgery, it has been demonstrated that longitudinal function parameters (TAPSE, S wave velocity at tissue Doppler echocardiography) are reduced and may no longer be representative of overall RV systolic function [28, 32, 33]. It is not yet clear if impaired RV longitudinal systolic function as measured by TAPSE after heart transplant or cardiac surgery is reflective of true RV dysfunction or just a consequence of abnormal RV geometry and increased translation after pericardiectomy. This is a critically important issue, as RV failure is a common and much feared complication after heart transplant, being the single most important cause of death in the early post period.

In pulmonary hypertension patients, RV ejection fraction is better reflected by transverse rather than longitudinal wall motion (TAPSE) [34]. This abnormal RV wall motion in pulmonary hypertension could be explained by impaired RV myocardial contractility due to altered fiber orientation, which become more transversally oriented as the chamber dilates.

Traditional echocardiographic parameters (TAPSE, fractional area change, RV longitudinal strain, etc.) are not adequate to study these insights, since they lack a dedicated measure of RV radial shortening, and evaluate only the RV inflow. Thus, they underestimate the contribution of inward motion of entire RV free wall surface to the overall RV pump function.

Recently, a software package was developed and applied to the 3D beutel of the RV, allowing to discriminate between the relative contribution of the longitudinal and radial displacement to the global RV pump function [35] (Fig. 17.12). Recent preliminary results showed that the impairment of RV pump function in pulmonary hypertension patients is mainly driven by the progressive reduction of RV radial function. Similarly, in HT patients, 3DE confirmed a shift in relative contribution of longitudinal and radial motion to global RV function in comparison with healthy RV (data on file) (Fig. 17.13a, b).

Separate quantification of the longitudinal versus radial component of RV shortening by 3DE may advance our understanding of RV adaptation to different pathological conditions and is likely to detect earlier the RV function impairment.

RV Shape

RV remodeling involves not only changes in size and function, but also in shape. In pulmonary hypertension patients, septal curvature assessed by two-dimensional echocardiography and cardiac magnetic resonance images has been correlated with the severity of pulmonary hypertension and two-dimensional echocardiography-derived eccentricity indices have been shown to differentiate pressure from volume

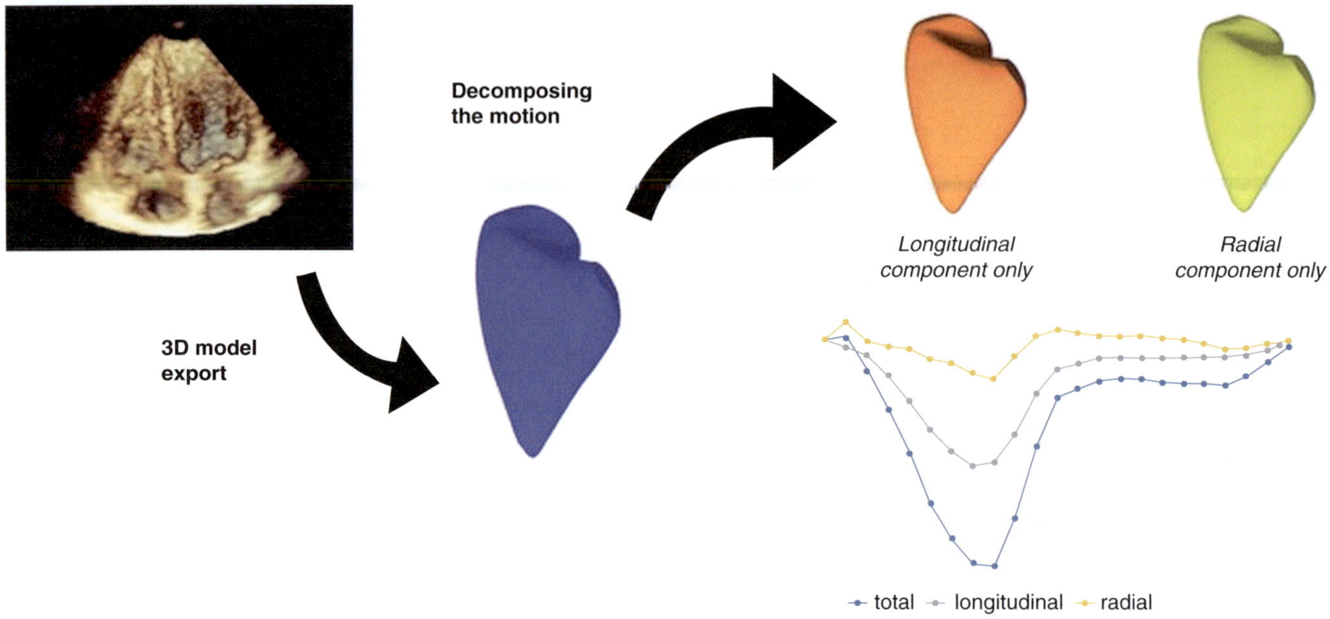

Fig. 17.12 Assessment of the relative contribution of longitudinal and radial displacement to right ventricular ejection fraction by three-dimensional echocardiography. A 3DE data set of the right ventricle is post-processed to generate a right ventricular beutel (blue beutel) to quantitate global right ventricular ejection fraction. Then the longitudinal and radial vectors of the knot points of the surface rendering can be measured to split the longitudinal (orange beutel) and radial (yellow beutel) components

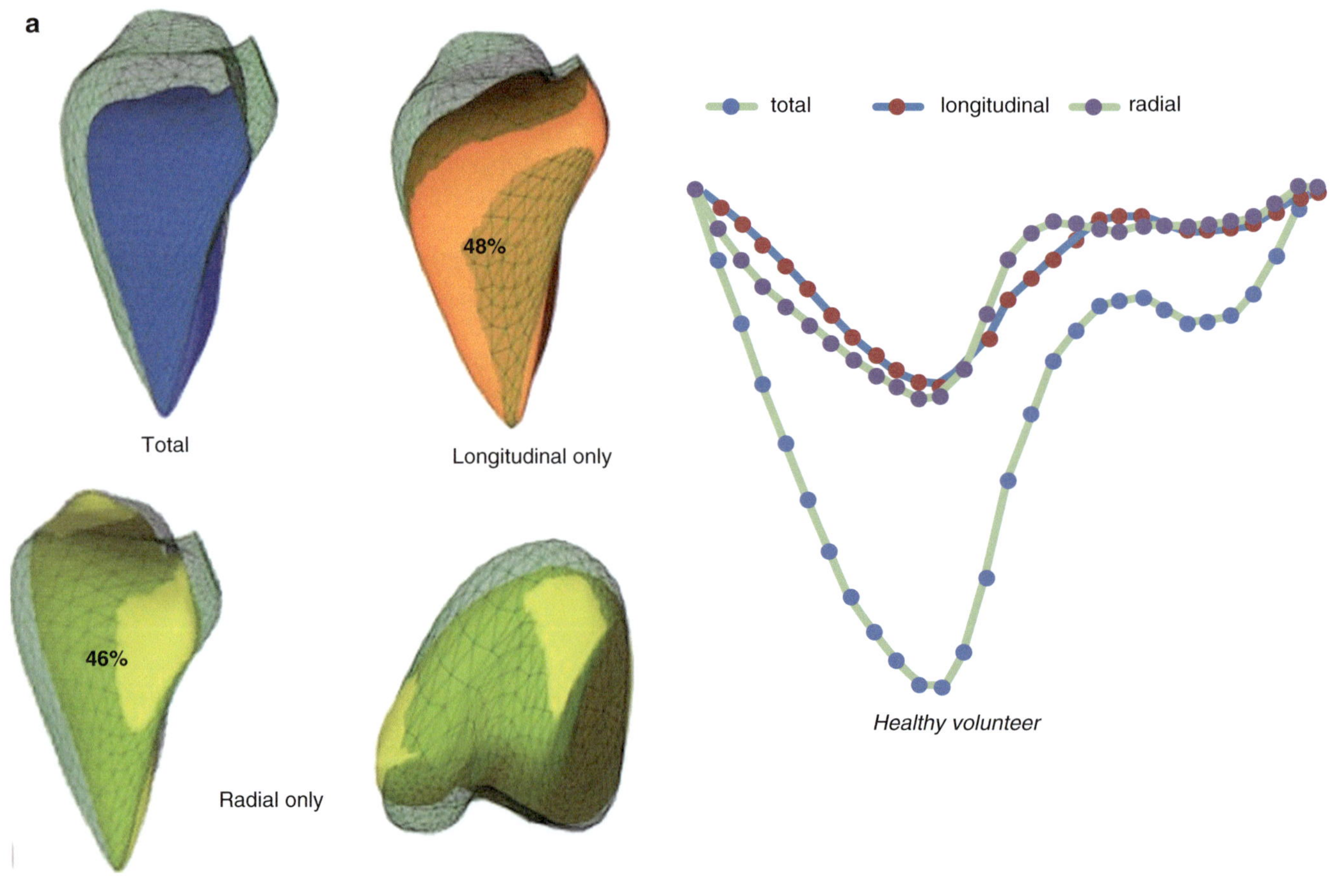

Fig. 17.13 (**a**) In normal subjects the contribution of the longitudinal (orange dotted line) and the radial (purple dotted line) components to global right ventricular pump function is very similar. (**b**) In patients with pressure overload, the radial component is diminished whereas the longitudinal one is increased to maintain ejection fraction

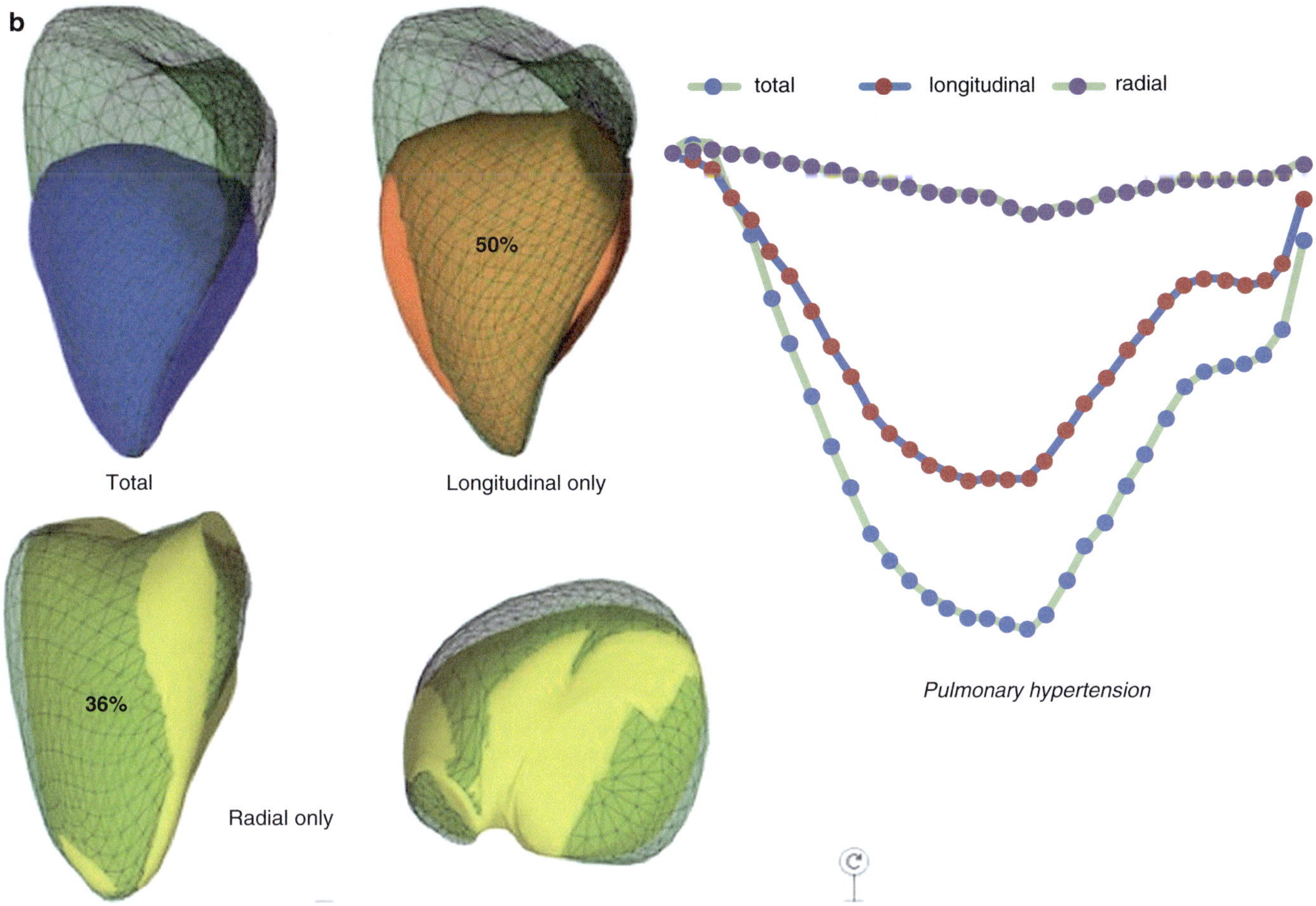

Fig. 17.13 (continued)

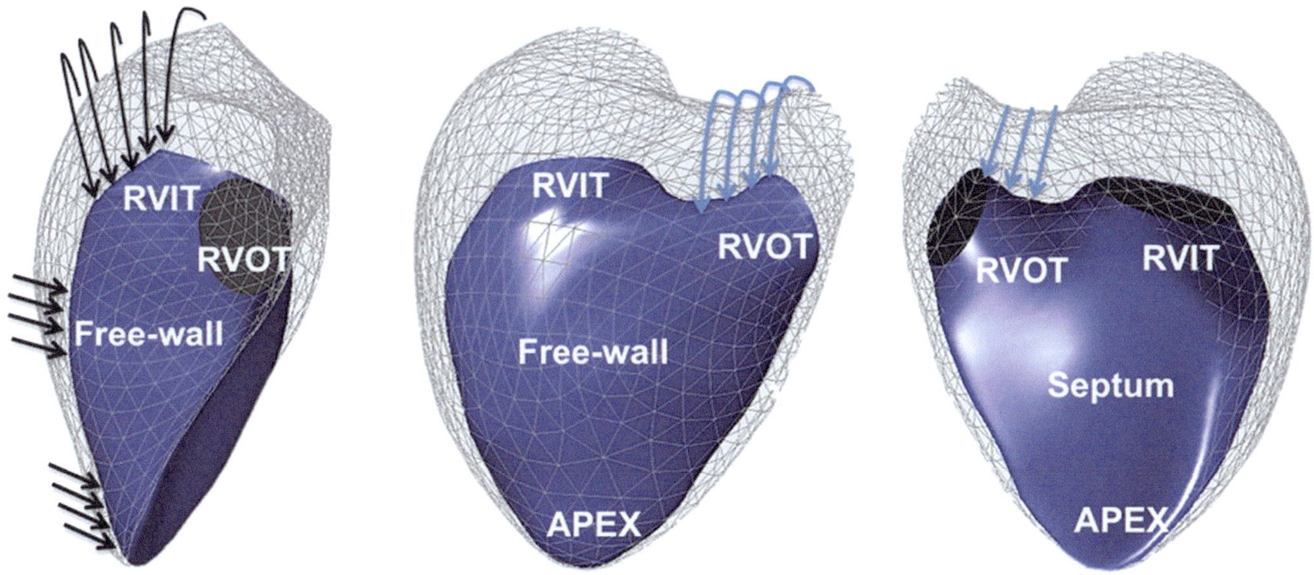

Fig. 17.14 Charts showing the changes of right ventricular curvature from end-diastole to end-systole. The *gray mesh* shows the right ventricle in end-diastole and the *blue solid frame* the right ventricle in end-systole in a healthy subject. The apical free wall becomes more pointed (*black arrows* at apex), whereas the body free wall flattens, as do the right ventricular outflow (RVOT) and inflow (RVIT) tracts (see *arrows* at respective positions). Conversely, septal curvature does not change from end-diastole to end-systole [36]. Reprinted from Journal of the American Society of Echocardiography, Vol. 31, Issue 5, Morphologic Analysis of the Normal Right Ventricle Using Three-Dimensional Echocardiography-Derived Curvature Indices, Addetia K, Muraru D, singh A, Surkova E, Mor-Avi V, Badano LP, Lang RM, pages 614-623, © 2018, with permission from Elsevier/The American Society of Echocardiography

overload states. 3DE offers the unique opportunity to quantify the true 3D RV shape from the same data set on which volumes and EF are measured [36] (Fig. 17.14). RV shape might provide outcome information that is independent of that predicted by size and function parameters [37]. Preliminary data showed that RV inflow curvature was a more robust predictor of death than RV ejection fraction, RV volumes, or other regional curvature indices, suggesting that patients who die have more flat RV inflow regions. This is likely due to the presence of significant functional tricuspid regurgitation in these patients, which can cause annular dilatation, as well as dilatation and flatt of RV inflow [37].

Future studies in various clinical conditions leading to RV failure will allow to explore the clinical value of RV regional shape parameters derived from 3DE.

RV Strain

3DE allows to derive several indices of RV systolic myocardial deformation based on 3D speckle-tracking technology, such as 3D longitudinal, circumferential, radial and area strain [38]. Confirming previous observations in pulmonary hypertension patients, circumferential and area strain were more closely correlated with RV ejection fraction than longitudinal strain [8]. Moreover, 3D strain parameters were able to predict survival in pulmonary hypertension patients. Present limitations relate to the scarce evidence on the added clinical value of 3D strain for RV function analysis and to the lack of an analysis tool dedicated for RV myocardial strain.

Conclusions

Right ventricular function and mechanics have proven to be important parameters of overall cardiac function and strong predictors of cardiovascular morbidity and mortality. However, accurate evaluation of the RV geometry and performance with conventional two-dimensional and Doppler echocardiography remains challenging due to existing limitations of this imaging modality. Recent developments of 3DE allows more accurate, anatomically sound, and reproducible assessment of the RV geometry and functions and enables advanced assessment of RV function in this technically challenging cardiac chamber.

References

1. Knauth AL, Gauvreau K, Powell AJ, et al. Ventricular size and function assessed by cardiac MRI predict major adverse clinical outcomes late after tetralogy of Fallot repair. Heart. 2008;94:211–6.
2. van Wolferen SA, Marcus JT, Boonstra A, et al. Prognostic value of right ventricular mass, volume, and function in idiopathic pulmonary arterial hypertension. Eur Heart J. 2007;28:1250–7.
3. Meyer P, Filippatos GS, Ahmed MI, et al. Effects of right ventricular ejection fraction on outcomes in chronic systolic heart failure. Circulation. 2010;121:252–8.
4. Bourantas CV, Loh HP, Bragadeesh T, et al. Relationship between right ventricular volumes measured by cardiac magnetic resonance imaging and prognosis in patients with chronic heart failure. Eur J Heart Fail. 2011;13:52–60.
5. Lang RM, Badano LP, Mor-Avi V, et al. Recommendations for cardiac chamber quantification by echocardiography in adults: an update from the American Society of Echocardiography and the European Association of Cardiovascular Imaging. J Am Soc Echocardiogr. 2015;28:1–39.e14.
6. Lang RM, Badano LP, Tsang W, et al. EAE/ASE recommendations for image acquisition and display using three-dimensional echocardiography. Eur Heart J Cardiovasc Imaging. 2012;13:1–46.
7. Vitarelli A, Barilla F, Capotosto L, et al. Right ventricular function in acute pulmonary embolism: a combined assessment by three-dimensional and speckle-tracking echocardiography. J Am Soc Echocardiogr. 2014;27:329–38.
8. Smith BC, Dobson G, Dawson D, Charalampopoulos A, Grapsa J, Nihoyannopoulos P. Three-dimensional speckle tracking of the right ventricle: toward optimal quantification of right ventricular dysfunction in pulmonary hypertension. J Am Coll Cardiol. 2014;64:41–51.
9. Maffessanti F, Muraru D, Esposito R, et al. Age-, body size-, and sex-specific reference values for right ventricular volumes and ejection fraction by three-dimensional echocardiography: a multicenter echocardiographic study in 507 healthy volunteers. Circ Cardiovasc Imaging. 2013;6:700–10.
10. Zhang QB, Sun JP, Gao RF, et al. Feasibility of single-beat full-volume capture real-time three-dimensional echocardiography for quantification of right ventricular volume: validation by cardiac magnetic resonance imaging. Int J Cardiol. 2013;168:3991–5.
11. Haddad F, Hunt SA, Rosenthal DN, Murphy DJ. Right ventricular function in cardiovascular disease, part I: anatomy, physiology, aging, and functional assessment of the right ventricle. Circulation. 2008;117:1436–48.
12. Ho SY, Nihoyannopoulos P. Anatomy, echocardiography, and normal right ventricular dimensions. Heart. 2006;92(Suppl 1):i2–13.
13. Haugaa KH, Basso C, Badano LP, et al. Comprehensive multimodality imaging approach in arrhythmogenic cardiomyopathy-an expert consensus document of the European Association of Cardiovascular Imaging. Eur Heart J Cardiovasc Imaging. 2017;18:237–53.
14. Konstantinides SV, Torbicki A, Agnelli G, et al. 2014 ESC guidelines on the diagnosis and management of acute pulmonary embolism. Eur Heart J. 2014;35:3033–69, 3069a–k.
15. Quick S, Speiser U, Kury K, Schoen S, Ibrahim K, Strasser R. Evaluation and classification of right ventricular wall motion abnormalities in healthy subjects by 3-tesla cardiovascular magnetic resonance imaging. Neth Heart J. 2015;23:64–9.
16. Badano LP, Ginghina C, Easaw J, et al. Right ventricle in pulmonary arterial hypertension: haemodynamics, structural changes, imaging, and proposal of a study protocol aimed to assess remodelling and treatment effects. Eur J Echocardiogr. 2010;11:27–37.
17. Shimada YJ, Shiota M, Siegel RJ, Shiota T. Accuracy of right ventricular volumes and function determined by three-dimensional echocardiography in comparison with magnetic resonance imaging: a meta-analysis study. J Am Soc Echocardiogr. 2010;23:943–53.
18. Khoo NS, Young A, Occleshaw C, Cowan B, Zeng IS, Gentles TL. Assessments of right ventricular volume and function using three-dimensional echocardiography in older children and adults with congenital heart disease: comparison with cardiac magnetic resonance imaging. J Am Soc Echocardiogr. 2009;22:1279–88.
19. Knight DS, Grasso AE, Quail MA, et al. Accuracy and reproducibility of right ventricular quantification in patients with pressure and volume overload using single-beat three-dimensional echocardiography. J Am Soc Echocardiogr. 2015;28(3):363–74.

20. Sugeng L, Mor-Avi V, Weinert L, et al. Multimodality comparison of quantitative volumetric analysis of the right ventricle. JACC Cardiovasc Imaging. 2010;3:10–8.
21. Muraru D, Spadotto V, Cecchetto A, et al. New speckle-tracking algorithm for right ventricular volume analysis from three-dimensional echocardiographic data sets: validation with cardiac magnetic resonance and comparison with the previous analysis tool. Eur Heart J Cardiovasc Imaging. 2016;17(11):1279–89.
22. van der Zwaan HB, Helbing WA, McGhie JS, et al. Clinical value of real-time three-dimensional echocardiography for right ventricular quantification in congenital heart disease: validation with cardiac magnetic resonance imaging. J Am Soc Echocardiogr. 2010;23:134–40.
23. Addetia K, Bhave NM, Tabit CE, et al. Sample size and cost analysis for pulmonary arterial hypertension drug trials using various imaging modalities to assess right ventricular size and function end points. Circ Cardiovasc Imaging. 2014;7:115–24.
24. van der Zwaan HB, Geleijnse ML, Soliman OI, et al. Test-retest variability of volumetric right ventricular measurements using real-time three-dimensional echocardiography. J Am Soc Echocardiogr. 2011;24:671–9.
25. Foppa M, Arora G, Gona P, et al. Right ventricular volumes and systolic function by cardiac magnetic resonance and the impact of sex, age, and obesity in a longitudinally followed cohort free of pulmonary and cardiovascular disease: the Framingham Heart Study. Circ Cardiovasc Imaging. 2016;9:e003810.
26. Kawut SM, Lima JA, Barr RG, et al. Sex and race differences in right ventricular structure and function: the multi-ethnic study of atherosclerosis-right ventricle study. Circulation. 2011;123:2542–51.
27. Laser KT, Karabiyik A, Korperich H, et al. Validation and reference values for three-dimensional echocardiographic right ventricular volumetry in children: a multicenter study. J Am Soc Echocardiogr. 2018. pii: S0894-7317(18)30150-0. https://doi.org/10.1016/j.echo.2018.03.010. [Epub ahead of print].
28. Maffessanti F, Gripari P, Tamborini G, et al. Evaluation of right ventricular systolic function after mitral valve repair: a two-dimensional Doppler, speckle-tracking, and three-dimensional echocardiographic study. J Am Soc Echocardiogr. 2012;25:701–8.
29. Giusca S, Dambrauskaite V, Scheurwegs C, et al. Deformation imaging describes right ventricular function better than longitudinal displacement of the tricuspid ring. Heart. 2010;96:281–8.
30. Mocchegiani R, Badano L, Lestuzzi C, Nicolosi GL, Zanuttini D. Relation of right ventricular morphology and function in pectus excavatum to the severity of the chest wall deformity. Am J Cardiol. 1995;76:941–6.
31. Nagata Y, Wu VC, Kado Y, et al. Prognostic value of right ventricular ejection fraction assessed by transthoracic 3D echocardiography. Circ Cardiovasc Imaging. 2017;10(2). pii: e005384.
32. Tamborini G, Muratori M, Brusoni D, et al. Is right ventricular systolic function reduced after cardiac surgery? A two- and three-dimensional echocardiographic study. Eur J Echocardiogr. 2009;10:630–4.
33. Badano LP, Miglioranza MH, Edvardsen T, et al. European Association of Cardiovascular Imaging/Cardiovascular Imaging Department of the Brazilian Society of Cardiology recommendations for the use of cardiac imaging to assess and follow patients after heart transplantation. Eur Heart J Cardiovasc Imaging. 2015;16:919–48.
34. Kind T, Mauritz GJ, Marcus JT, van de Veerdonk M, Westerhof N, Vonk-Noordegraaf A. Right ventricular ejection fraction is better reflected by transverse rather than longitudinal wall motion in pulmonary hypertension. J Cardiovasc Magn Reson. 2010;12:35.
35. Lakatos B, Toser Z, Tokodi M, et al. Quantification of the relative contribution of the different right ventricular wall motion components to right ventricular ejection fraction: the ReVISION method. Cardiovasc Ultrasound. 2017;15:8.
36. Addetia K, Maffessanti F, Muraru D, et al. Morphologic analysis of the normal right ventricle using three-dimensional echocardiography-derived curvature indices. J Am Soc Echocardiogr. 2018;31(5):614–23.
37. Addetia K, Maffessanti F, Yamat M, et al. Three-dimensional echocardiography-based analysis of right ventricular shape in pulmonary arterial hypertension. Eur Heart J Cardiovasc Imaging. 2016;17(5):564–75.
38. Ishizu T, Seo Y, Atsumi A, et al. Global and regional right ventricular function assessed by novel three-dimensional speckle-tracking echocardiography. J Am Soc Echocardiogr. 2017;30:1203–13.

The Normal Tricuspid Valve

18

Karima Addetia, Denisa Muraru, Andrada-Camelia Guta, Luigi P. Badano, and Roberto M. Lang

Abstract

The interest of both cardiologists (echocardiographers and interventional cardiologists) and cardiac surgeons about the tricuspid valve has been fueled by the association of better understanding of the role of tricuspid regurgitation as an independent determinant of patients' morbidity and mortality, and the advent of novel transcatheter devices to treat severe tricuspid regurgitation in high surgical risk patients. However, conventional two-dimensional echocardiography is unsuitable to study the anatomy and the pathophysiological mechanisms of the regurgitant tricuspid valve because of the complex three-dimensional geometry of the valve and its anterior position in the mediastinum (just behind the sternum). Three-dimensional echocardiography has emerged as a very cost-effective imaging modality to: (1) Assess the anatomy of the tricuspid valve; (2) Measure the size/geometry of the tricuspid annulus; (3) Identify the mechanism of tricuspid regurgitation; (4) analyze the anatomic relationships between the tricuspid valve apparatus and the surrounding cardiac structures; (5) Measure the volumes and function of the right atrium and right ventricle.

This chapter will describe the normal anatomy of the tricuspid valve apparatus and how to use three-dimensional echocardiography to acquire, display and perform quantitative analyses of the tricuspid valve using both transthoracic and transesophageal approaches.

Keywords

Tricuspid valve · Tricuspid leaflets · Tricuspid annulus · Transthoracic three-dimensional echocardiography · Transesophageal three-dimensional echocardiography

Introduction

Echocardiography is the first-line imaging modality for the assessment of the tricuspid valve (TV) anatomy and function. With respect to other imaging modalities, its low cost, immediate access, safety and portability, and excellent temporal resolution represent significant advantages, enabling to assess the TV wherever necessary (e.g. in the echocardiography laboratory, catheterization laboratory, operating room or at bedside). However, the use of two-dimensional echocardiography to assess the TV is rather challenging because of the complex non-planar geometry of the annulus, the highly variable anatomy of the valve and its position in the anterior mediastinum, just behind the sternum [1]. Moreover, with two-dimensional echocardiography, it is difficult to visualize all three leaflets simultaneously in a single tomographic view (Fig. 18.1, Videos 18.1a and 18.1b) and there are uncertainties about which leaflet can be visualized in any single two-dimensional

Electronic Supplementary Material The online version of this chapter (https://doi.org/10.1007/978-3-030-14032-8_18) contains supplementary material, which is available to authorized users.

K. Addetia (✉) · R. M. Lang
Noninvasive Cardiac Imaging Laboratories, Department of Medicine/Section of Cardiology, University of Chicago Medical Center, Chicago, IL, USA
e-mail: kaddetia@medicine.bsd.uchicago.edu; rlang@medicine.bsd.uchicago.edu

D. Muraru · L. P. Badano
University of Milano-Bicocca, and Istituto Auxologico Italiano, IRCCS, San Luca Hospital, Milano, Italy
e-mail: denisa.muraru@unimib.it; luigi.badano@unimib.it

A.-C. Guta
Department of Cardiac, Thoracic and Vascular Sciences, University of Padua School of Medicine, Padua, Italy

Department of Cardiology, "Prof. Dr. C.C. Iliescu" Institute of Cardiovascular Diseases, Bucharest, Romania

L. P. Badano et al. (eds.), *Textbook of Three-Dimensional Echocardiography*, https://doi.org/10.1007/978-3-030-14032-8_18

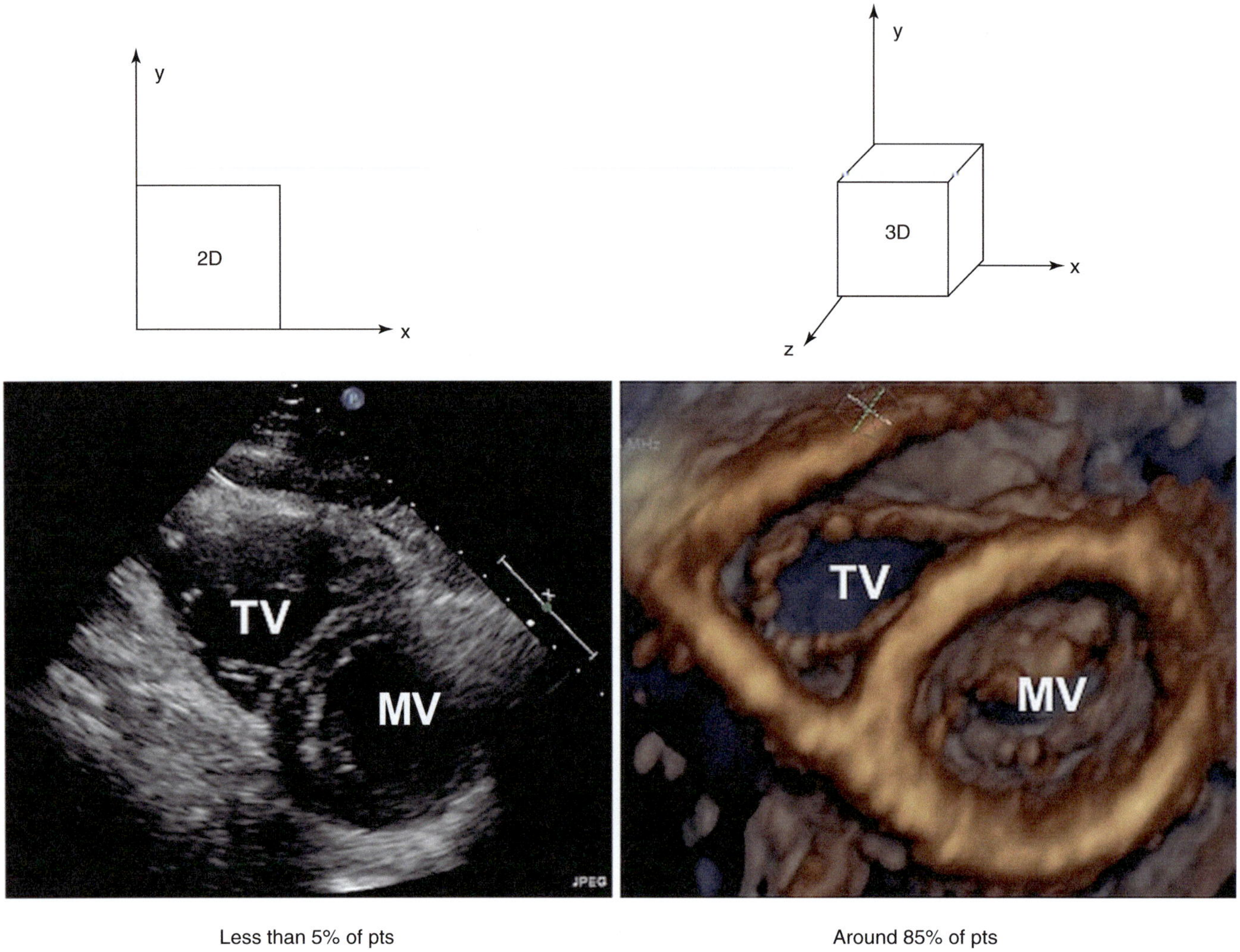

Fig. 18.1 Echocardiographic imaging of the tricuspid valve using transthoracic two-dimensional (left panel, Video 18.1a Left) and transthoracic three-dimensional (central panel, Video 18.1b Right) techniques with the corresponding estimated rates of successful visualization in routine patients. *2D TTE* two-dimensional transthoracic echocardiography, *3D TTE* three-dimensional transthoracic echocardiography, *MV* mitral valve, *TV* tricuspid valve

echocardiographic view [2–4]. Nowadays, three-dimensional echocardiography (3DE) allows to fully appreciate the TV complexity in the beating heart and has become the preferred imaging modality to assess the anatomy and function of the TV [5–7].

In this chapter, we will review the anatomy of the TV complex, strategies for 3DE acquisition and display, as well as describe the contemporary methods to perform a quantitative assessment of the TV.

Functional Anatomy of the Tricuspid Valve and Comparison with the Mitral Valve

The TV is larger and more caudally located than the mitral valve. Moreover, TV is quite complex and variable in morphology (Fig. 18.2, Video 18.2). Compared to the two-leaflet mitral valve, the TV classically consists of three unequal leaflets named (according to their anatomical orientation) as the anterior (the largest, with quadrangular shape), the septal (the smallest, semicircular in shape) and the posterior (also named mural or inferior, intermediate in size, with triangular shape and scalloped indentations). However, the classic "tricuspid" morphology of the valve does not apply to all patients since autopsy studies have reported quite a large variability in the number of TV leaflets (from 2 to 6, Fig. 18.3, Videos 18.3a and 18.3b) in up to 38% of patients [8]. Due to the lower atrio-ventricular pressure gradient, normal TV leaflets are thinner than mitral valve leaflets. The septal leaflet is attached to a part of the annulus which is relatively fixed, due to its position between the fibrous trigons, and its insertion is more apical than the insertion of the anterior leaflet of the mitral valve. Differently from the mitral valve, TV has a unique connection with the interventricular septum (multiple chordae from the septal leaflet are inserted directly on the septal myocardium) and no continuity with the semilunar valve (i.e. the pulmonary valve) due to the interposition of the crista supraventricularis.

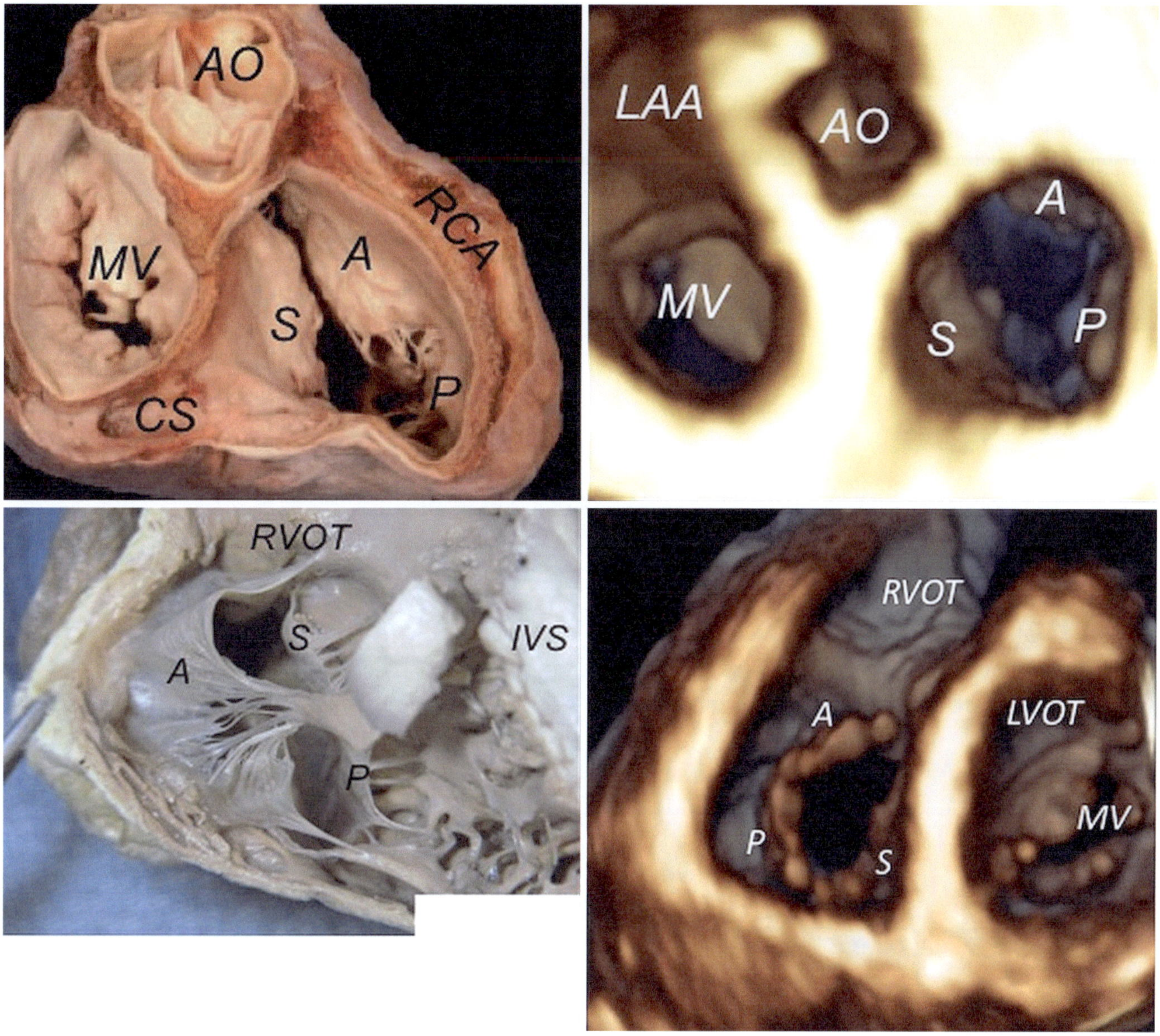

Fig. 18.2 Volume rendered display of the tricuspid valve acquired using transthoracic three-dimensional echocardiography side by side with anatomical specimens. Upper panels, tricuspid vale seen from the atrial perspective (Video 18.2). Lower panels, tricuspid valve seen from the ventricular perspective (Video 18.1b Right). *A* anterior tricuspid leaflet, *Ao* aortic valve, *CS* coronary sinus, *LAA* left atrial appendage, *LVOT* left ventricular outflow tract, *MV* mitral valve, *P* posterior tricuspid leaflet, *RCA* right coronary artery, *RVOT* right ventricular outflow tract, *S* septal tricuspid leaflet. Bottom left image—Courtesy of Dr. Stephen P. Sanders, Professor of Pediatrics, Harvard Medical School, Departments of Cardiology, Pathology and Cardiac Surgery. Boston Children's Hospital, Boston

Competency of the TV depends on the structural integrity and functional coordination of the various components of the TV apparatus: annulus, papillary muscles, *chordae tendineae* and ventricular myocardium. The normal tricuspid annulus has a complex elliptical non-planar shape, with the antero-septal portion being the highest, close to the right ventricular outflow tract and the aortic valve, and the postero-lateral being the lowest (towards the right ventricle) (Fig. 18.4). The tricuspid annulus is about 20% larger and less symmetric than the "saddled-shaped" mitral annulus. Normal tricuspid annulus diameter depends on many factors including age, gender, right atrial and right ventricular size and loading conditions [9, 10]. Moreover, the shape and the size of the tricuspid annulus varies continuously throughout the cardiac cycle with a complex and constant changing segmental movement evoking that of waves [11]. The diastolic opening of the leaflets along with the corresponding expansion of the tricuspid annulus determines a tricuspid orifice area of 7–9 cm^2. Differences in the anatomic structures surrounding the tricuspid and the mitral annulus may explain the wide dynamicity of the former (approximately, its circumference and area change by 19% and 30%, respectively, during cardiac cycle). The mitral annulus has two major fibrous structures, the right and left fibrous trigones, whereas

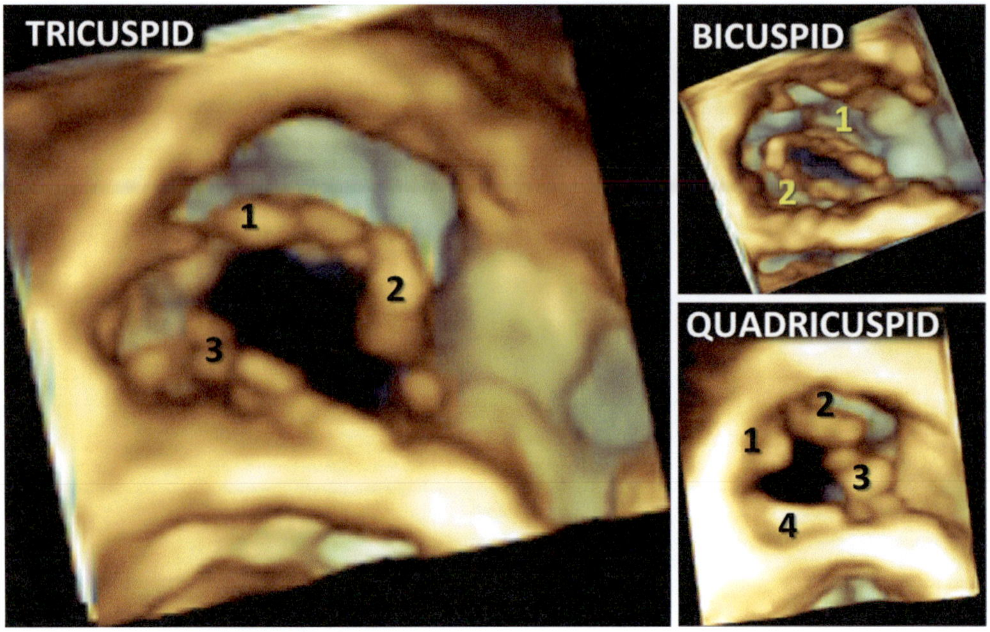

Fig. 18.3 Anatomical variants of the tricuspid valve displayed in volume rendering from the ventricular perspective: tricuspid valve (Video 18.1b Right); bicuspid valve (Video 18.3a Upper); quadricuspid valve (Video 18.3b Lower)

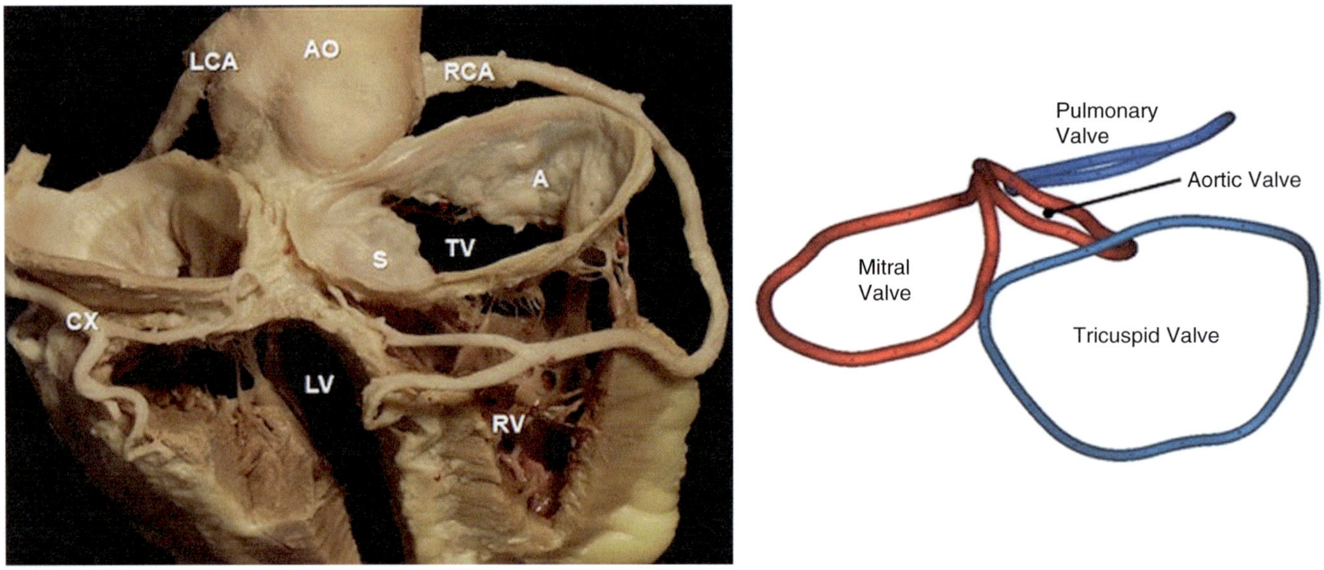

Fig. 18.4 Non-planar geometry of tricuspid annulus. *Left panel*, Anatomical specimen showing the complex three-dimensional shape of the tricuspid annulus and its spatial relationships with the surrounding anatomical structures. Courtesy of Drs. Edgardo Bonacina and Horia Muresian, Clinical Pathology Unit, ASST Grande ospedale metropolitano Niguarda, Milan, Italy. *Right panel*, computer reconstruction of the stereoscopic geometry of the annuli of the four cardiac valves. *A* anterior tricuspid leaflet, *Ao* aorta, *Cx* circumflex branch of the left coronary artery, *LCA* left coronary artery, *LV* left ventricle, *RCA* right coronary artery, *RV* right ventricle, *S* septal tricuspid leaflet, *TV* tricuspid valve

the tricuspid annulus has only a single right fibrous trigone. The mitral annulus is not in contact with the myocardium along the base of the anterior mitral leaflet which is positioned between the fibrous trigones. Conversely, most of the circumference of the tricuspid annulus is directly in contact with the myocardium (Fig. 18.4), whose contractility affects tricuspid annulus size changes. Tricuspid annulus dilation is, together with leaflet tethering, one of the mechanisms leading to functional tricuspid regurgitation. Since the septal leaflet is fixed and the posterior leaflet id attached to the inferior wall of the right ventricle (whose displacement is limited by the diaphragm), the tricuspid annulus can only dilate along the anterior leaflet attachment as the right ventricular free wall expands outward.

Differently form the mitral valve which is usually supported by two papillary muscles, each of them providing chordae to both mitral leaflets, the papillary muscles supporting the TV are smaller, often multiple, widely separated, and carrying chordae only to the homolateral leaftet(s). In addition, there may be accessory chordal attachments to the right ventricuar free wall and to the moderator band (Fig. 18.5). This different arrangement of the subvalvular apparatus may explain the higher propensity to regurgitate of the TV compared to mitral valve. Whereas the separation of mitral leaflet caused by annular enlargement is limited by the crossing of the chordae tendineae (as each papillary muscle provides chordae to both leaflets), the connection of TV leaflets to homolateral papillary muscles only allows wide separation of the leaflets with TA and cavity enlargement.

However, due to the complexity of TV embryologic development, the anatomic arrangement of leaflets, *chordae tendineae*, and papillary muscles is highly variable and may be "as unique to each individual as one's finger print" [12]. Accordingly, there is a need of a detailed study of the anatomy of the regurgitant TV that cannot be obtained with a tomographic imaging technique like two-dimensional echocardiography [3, 4] and requires a three-dimensional imaging [1, 13, 14].

Last, but particularly important for devices targeting the tricuspid annulus, are the relationships of the TV with the surrounding structures. The right coronary artery runs in the atrio-ventricular groove separated only by 5–6 mm from the septal and posterior portion of the tricuspid annulus and 7 mm by its anterior portion. However, the course of the right coronary artery in the atrio-ventricular groove is highly variable and, with the emerging role of percutaneous approaches to functional tricuspid regurgitation repair, computed tomography plays a pivotal role in visualizing the spatial relationships between the right coronary artery and tricuspid annulus. Other relevant adjacent structures include the atrioventricular node, the ostium of the coronary sinus, and the tendon of Todaro which form the triangle of Koch.

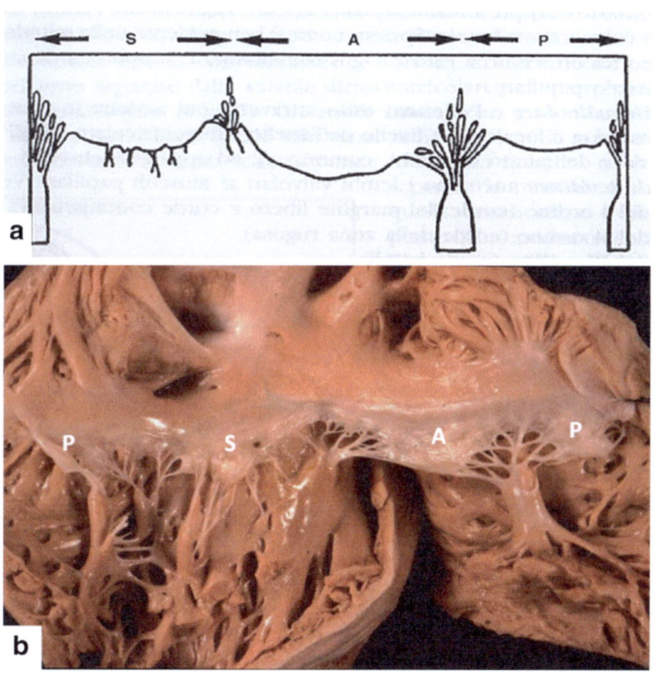

Fig. 18.5 Anatomic specimens showing the tricuspid valve and its subvalvular apparatus. (**a**) Schematic drawing showing the topographic position of the tricuspid leaflets. (**b**) Tricuspid valve subvalvular apparatus is characterized by multiple, widely separated papillary muscles (yellow arrow) which carry chordae to a single tricuspid valve leaflet. Accessory chordal attachments to the right ventricular free wall can also be noted

Impact of Knowledge Derived From 3D

As previously mentioned, the most valuable contribution of 3D echocardiography for assessment of the tricuspid valve is the ability to simultaneously visualize all three TV leaflets (Fig. 18.1). This is extremely important for the correct anatomic localization of leaflet pathology [5, 13].

Without the use of 3DE it is not possible to be sure which combination TV leaflets is being imaged in the standard two-dimensional TV views i.e. the right ventricular inflow, parasternal short axis and apical four-chamber views [1, 3, 4, 15]. Multiple textbooks describe with certainty the specific leaflets that are seen in the standard two-dimensional echocardiography views. With some variations, it has been generally stated that the posterior and anterior TV leaflets are visualized in the right ventricular inflow view, the septal and anterior leaflets in the parasternal short-axis view, and the anterior and septal leaflets in the apical four-chamber view [16–18]. With careful studies using 3D and 2D acquisitions from the identical transducer position it had been shown that it is impossible to describe with certainty which leaflets are being imaged in each of the standard views [3, 4]. However, when taking into account adjacent structures, it is possible to reliably predict specific leaflet combinations. For instance, in the apical transducer position, the septal leaflet is always adjacent to the septum. When the aortic valve is seen, as in the five-chamber view, the anterior and septal leaflets are being imaged. When the coronary sinus is visualized, the posterior and septal leaflets are the ones being imaged. In the RV inflow view, when the septum is seen the anterior and septal TV leaflets are being imaged (Fig. 18.6). Also if a single leaflet is seen in the parasternal short axis view this leaflet is almost always the anterior TV leaflet. This form of targeted imaging allows localization of pathology on 2D echocardiography with subsequent confirmation using 3D [17, 18].

3D Acquisition and Display of the Tricuspid Valve

Transthoracic 3DE acquisitions of data sets including the TV can be performed from any of the conventional acoustic windows (parasternal, apical and subcostal). There is no *a priori* preferred acoustic window from which to acquire a transthoracic 3DE data set of TV. The acoustic window from which the TV is best visualized by conventional two-dimensional echocardiography is usually used to acquire a 3DE data set of the TV. However, due to the close proximity of the TV and the right ventricle to the chest wall, and the spatial orientation of the leaflets perpendicular to the direction of ultrasound beams, an optimal transthoracic 3DE acquisition of the TV is often best achieved from the apical approach, using a right ventricu-

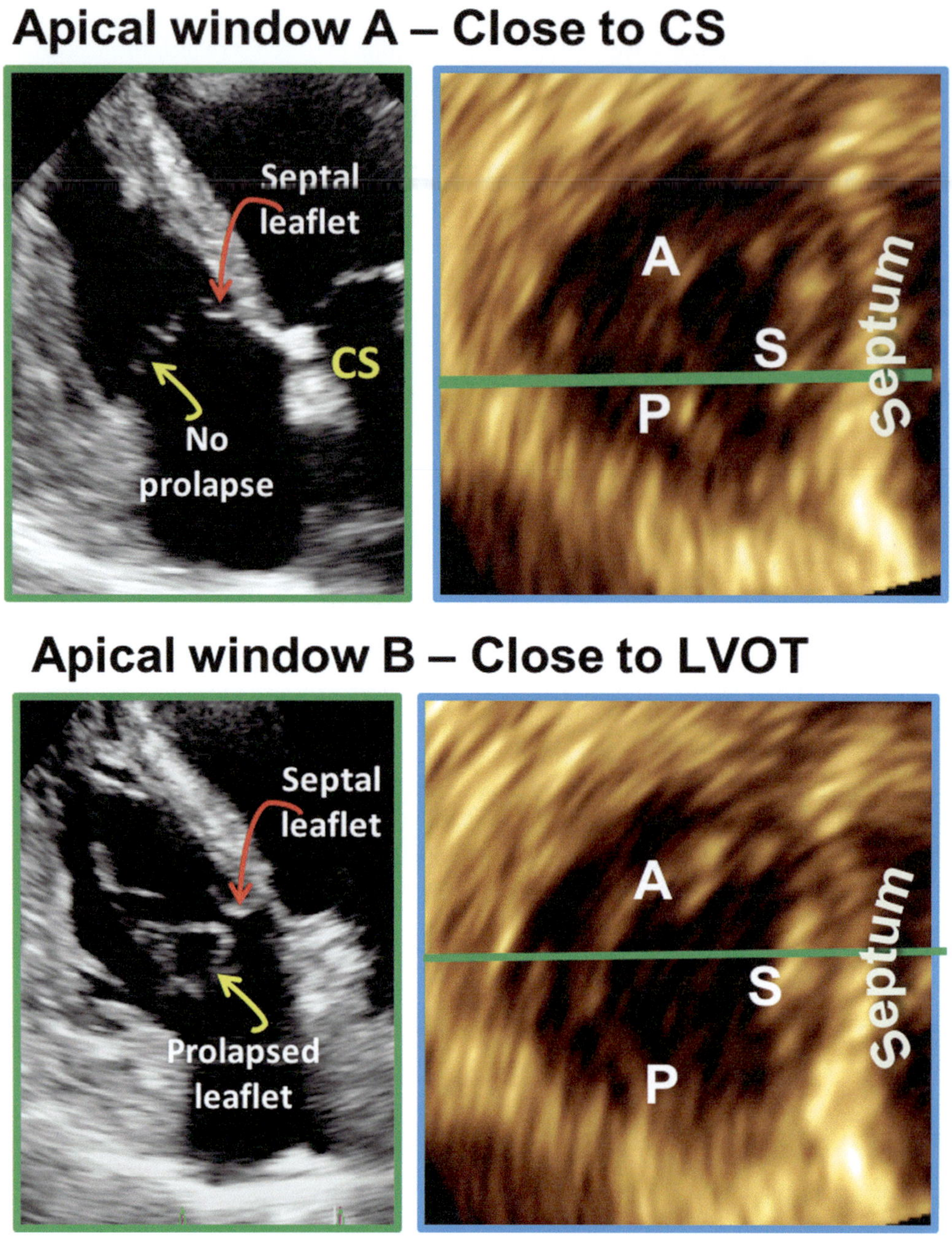

Fig. 18.6 Two-dimensional views obtained from the same 3D data set to illustrate the effect of small changes of the position of the cut plane (i.e. two-dimensional view), shown by the green horizontal line on the 3DE images on the left, on two-dimensional visualization of the tricuspid leaflets. In the apical view with coronary sinus (CS) present (left, upper quadrant), the posterior (P) and the septal (S) tricuspid valve leaflets are shown in the two-dimensional vie. In the apical view with left ventricular outflow tract present (left, lower quadrant), the anterior (A) and the septal (S) tricuspid leaflets are visualized in the two-dimensional view

lar focused or a foreshortened 4-chamber view, which allows to include the entire TV in the data set. Often, a modified high parasternal view with the transducer angulated towards the right hip, or the parasternal short axis window can be also used to obtain good quality 3DE data sets of TV. With the parasternal approaches, the TV is situated in the near field and the resulting 3DE images may have a better spatial resolution than images acquired from the apical approach. However, since the quality of apical window is usually better than parasternal window in many adult patients, both approaches are valid as long as all three TV leaflets are completely visualized.

To achieve the best spatial resolution, it is pivotal that the TV is located in the center of the pyramidal volume acquisition (see also Chap. 2). The acquisition volume size and shape will be adjusted in order to encompass the entire TV complex in the data set, including the leaflets, their attachment to the septum and to the anterior wall, and the annulus. The initial step for a good 3DE acquisition is to optimize the two-dimensional image of the TV to ensure clear delineation of the valve structures with high tissue-blood contrast and absent/minimal noise. Next is to ensure that the TV complex is encompassed within the smallest possible acquisition volume during the entire cardiac cycle. Because of the complex anatomy of the valve, it is recommended that the acquisition volume encompasses also surrounding anatomical structures to help to interpret TV anatomy: the right ventricular outflow tract/aorta to identify the anterior leaflet, the interatrial septum/mitral valve to identify the septal leaflet, and the coronary sinus to identify

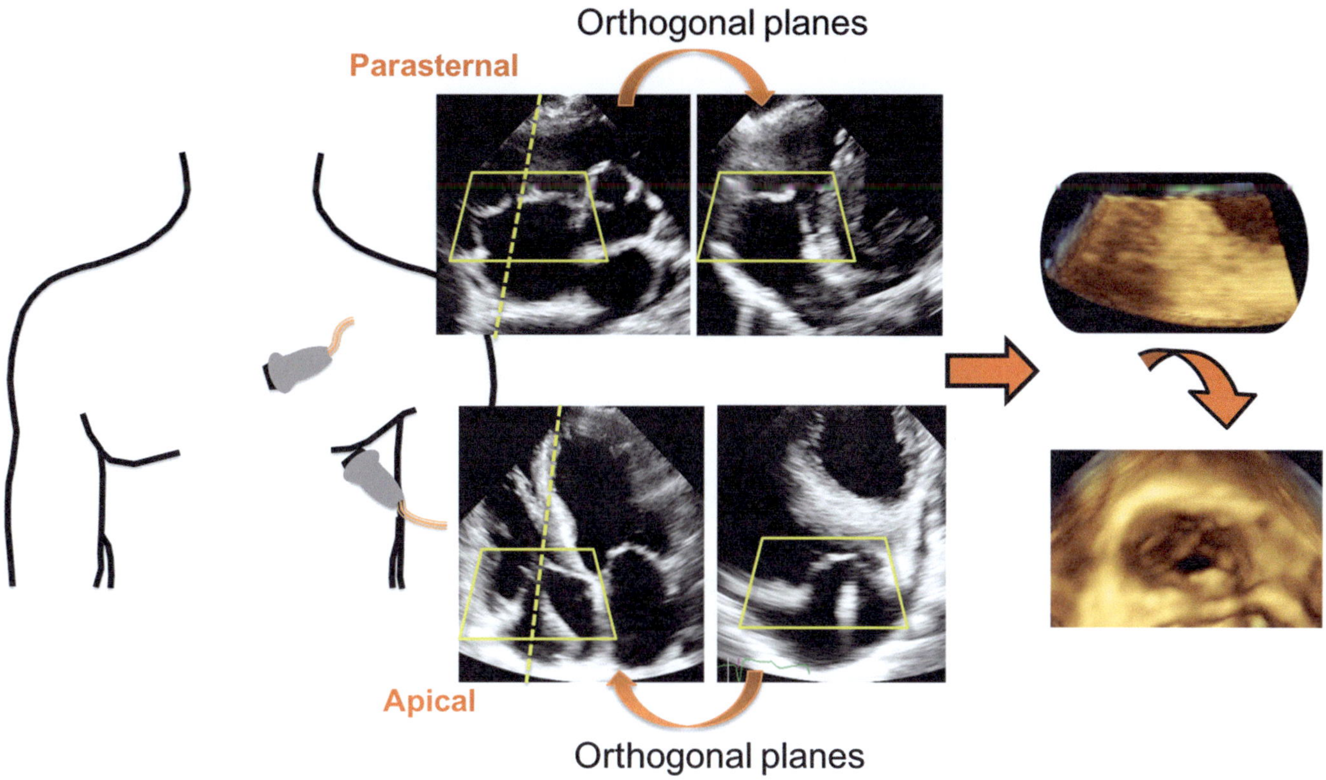

Fig. 18.7 Three-dimensional data sets of the tricuspid valve can be acquired using the transthoracic approach from the apical four-chamber view, parasternal long-axis right ventricular inflow views and parasternal basal short-axis view. In this figure, the transducer positions for both the parasternal short axis and the apical four-chamber acquisitions are appreciated (left panel). Biplane positioning of the scan box prior to data acquisition is illustrated in in the middle panel. At this stage it is important to ensure that the entire valve is included in the pyramidal dataset throughout the cardiac cycle. The final 3DE image is positioned for assessment so that the septal leaflet is in the 6 o'clock position (right panel)

the commissure between the septal and the posterior leaflet. Accordingly, the region of interest is usually sized and positioned using two orthogonal cut planes (Fig. 18.7).

Important limitations of the use of 3DE in imaging the cardiac valves are the difficulties to appreciate tissue characteristics (i.e. presence of calcifications, fibrosis or vegetations, etc.) and to evaluate leaflet thickness. In 3DE, color maps are used to code the position (depth) of the voxels and not tissue texture abnormality. Moreover, 3DE usually shows leaflets thicker than they actually are [19]. This phenomenon is due to blurring or amplification artifacts. The different resolution in axial, lateral, and elevation direction of the 3D volumetric data set (with the axial resolution being higher than lateral, and lateral higher than elevation) actually produces 3D "non-isotropic voxels." In the assembly process, if the system uses in one specific perspective prevalently the elevation resolution (i.e. *en face* view of the valves obtained from 3D data sets acquired using transthoracic approach and apical position), thin and long structures, such as tricuspid leaflets, may appear with increased thickness.

The right heart and the TV are located in the anterior mediastinum, quite far from the standard mid-esophageal position of the probe with the left heart structures interposed between the probe and the TV. Since images in the far field may be subject to beam widening and attenuation, often transesophageal 3DE data sets from this position are of lower quality than transthoracic 3DE data sets obtained in patients with good transthoracic acoustic window. Because the right heart structures in part rest on the diaphragm, the distance between the transducer and TV can be reduced by advancing the probe to the distal esophagus, proximal to the gastroesophageal junction to obtain unobstructed views of the TV and acquire an optimal transesophageal 3DE data set. From this position, there is no left atrium in the near field and only the right heart structures are visualized (Fig. 18.8). However, this acquisition may provide good 3DE images of the valve leaflets only when they are in the closed position (during systole), when leaflets are perpendicular to the insonation beam, whereas the leaflets may be poorly visualized in the open position (during diastole) when they are parallel to the insonation beam. Conversely, acquisitions from the transgastric approach frequently allow good visualization of the TV leaflets in diastole, since they will be perpendicular to the insonation beam, but not in systole (Fig. 18.9). Accordingly, it is often necessary to obtain multiple transesophageal 3DE data sets from different probe positions in order to fully assess the TV and the tricuspid annulus.

There are a number of limitations of transesophageal 3DE imaging of the TV. First, the position of the esophagus in relation to the plane of the tricuspid annulus typically places the annular plane 0–45° to the insonation beam from every imaging plane. Differences in resolution in axial, lateral, and elevation direction of the 3DE volumetric data set (with the

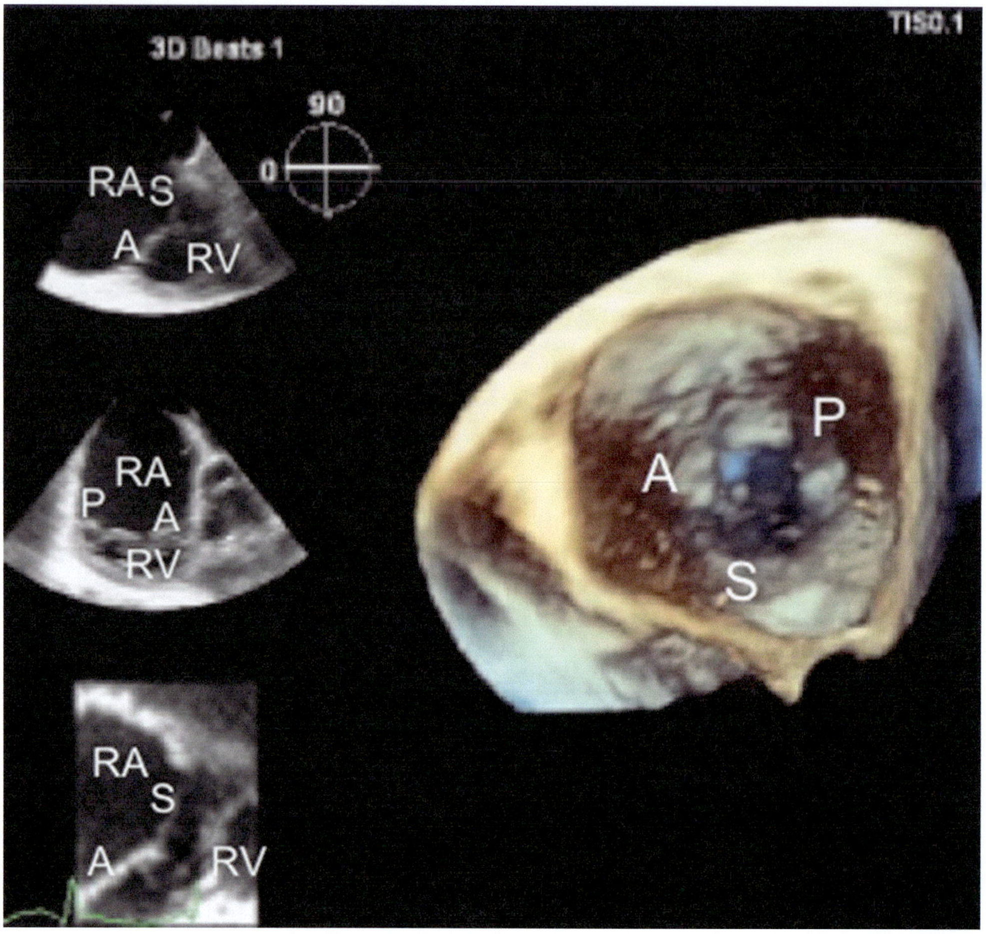

Fig. 18.8 Simultaneous biplane image from the low-esophageal position with only the right heart structures seen (Left panels). The septal (S) and anterior (A) leaflets of the tricuspid valve can be seen in the left upper quadrant. In the central left quadrant, which is the orthogonal view of the upper, the anterior and posterior (P) tricuspid valve leaflets are seen. From this position of the transesophageal probe, the three-dimensional data set of the tricuspid valve can be acquired (right quadrant), in this instance, shown from the atrial perspective and rotated into the "surgical" *en face* view with the septal leaflet at 6 o'clock. Image courtesy of Dr. Rebecca T. Hahn. *RA* right atrium, *RV* right ventricle

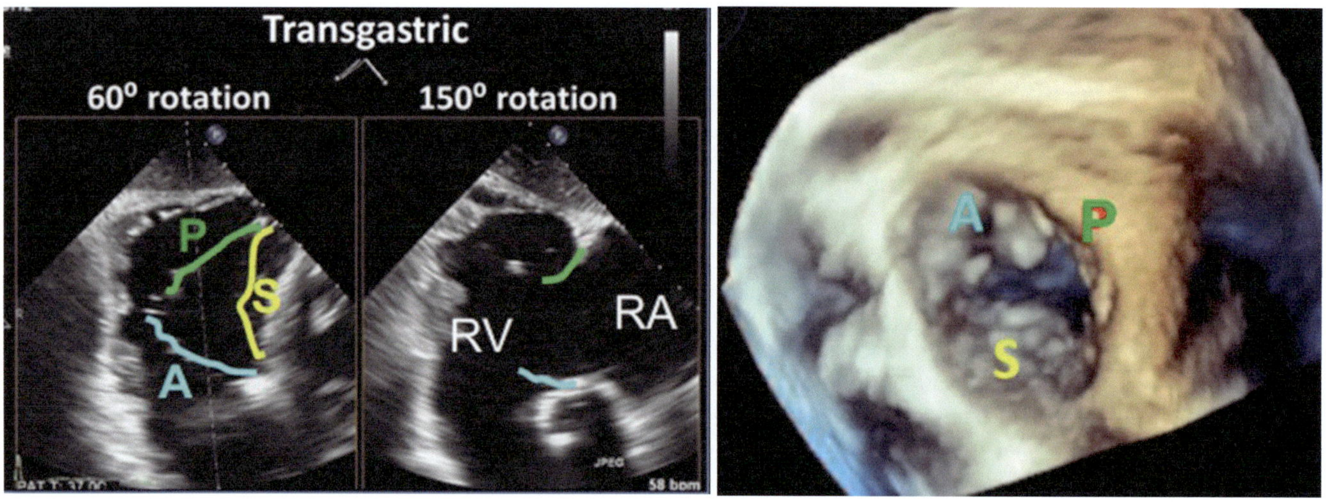

Fig. 18.9 Simultaneous biplane image from the transgastric position (left panel). The short-axis view of the tricuspid valve (left quadrant, left panel) images all three leaflet tips; the septal (S), anterior (A), and posterior (P) leaflets whereas the long-axis orthogonal view (right quadrant of the left panel) images the anterior and posterior leaflets (see colors as reference). From this position of the transesophageal probe, the three-dimensional data set of the tricuspid valve can be acquired (right panel), shown from the atrial perspective and rotated into the "surgical" *en face* view with the septal leaflet at 6 o'clock. Image courtesy of Dr. Rebecca T. Hahn. *RA* right atrium, *RV* right ventricle

axial resolution being higher than lateral, and lateral higher than elevation) actually produces 3D "non-isotropic voxels". When the leaflets are more parallel to the insonation beam (i.e. at 0°), lateral and elevational gain resolution will limit structural definition. Patients with an annular plane perpendicular to the insonation beam (i.e. at 90°) may have better imaging of the tricuspid leaflets in systole, whereas the reverse is true for imaging leaflets in diastole. Second, the tricuspid leaflets are much thinner than the mitral leaflets, resulting in poor echo definition of the body of the leaflets and significant echo-dropout. The thin leaflets and their oblique orientation respect to the ultrasound beam produce weaker and scattered than strong and specular echoes. The assembly algorithms therefore are unable to reconstruct valve leaflet surfaces without dropout artifacts [19].

However, if the system optimizes the elevational plane, then thin and long structures, such as tricuspid leaflets, may appear with indistinct edges and increased thickness. Third, the fibrous body of the heart as well as any prosthetic material in the left heart (i.e. prosthetic valves) may cause acoustic shadowing or reverberations in the far field of imaging, commonly masking the TV. Although this can frequently be overcome by inserting the probe further into the esophagus (thus removing the near field left heart structure causing the artifact), this also changes the angle of insonation with the problems already mentioned. All of these issues become even more problematic for 3DE color Doppler imaging.

The two most commonly used 3DE acquisition modes are real-time and multi-beat full-volume [6]. The trade-offs between the two modes should be taken into consideration as per patient and according to the objectives of the 3DE acquisition.

Real-Time 3DE Acquisition of TV

Real-time 3DE refers to a volume of information acquired over a single or multiple heart-beats. Real-time, single-beat 3DE acquisition is not limited by motion artifacts (i.e. breathing or patient movement) or R-R cycle variability (i.e. arrhythmias). Since the TV in the parasternal views is in the near field, the scan sector can be increased with less reduction of volume rate due to the minimal depth required for the acquisition, and it is sometimes possible to visualize the complete TV with a single beat real-time transthoracic 3DE acquisition. Real-time single beat transesophageal 3DE, with and without color Doppler, may be most useful when assessing respiratory variations of the regurgitant orifice size and for intra-procedural guidance of interventional procedures on the TV.

Multibeat 3DE Acquisition of TV

Multibeat, full-volume data sets are composed of several sub-volumes that are stitched together to create a single, larger volumetric data set with higher temporal and spatial resolution compared to the same volume acquired using single beat acquisitions. Multi-beat 3DE data sets may be acquired with or without color Doppler. The 3DE color Doppler acquisition is usually performed to obtain an assessment of the severity of tricuspid regurgitation independent of the geometric assumptions about the shape of the regurgitant orifice affecting the measurements of the diameter of the vena contracta or the calculation of the effective regurgitant orifice area by proximal isovelocity surface area (PISA) [5]. However, multi-beat acquisitions could be limited by stitching artifacts due to respiration, arrhythmias or patient's movements. Stitching artifacts could be an issue that precludes accurate interpretation of the 3DE data set and can be avoided by acquiring the data set during relatively stable R-R intervals on the ECG, breath-holding, with the patient immobile and without moving the probe [6]. The number of cardiac cycles to acquire depends on patient's characteristics (cardiac rhythm, ability to cooperate etc.), the size of the TV complex and the acquisition depth. However, for quantitative analyses, a data set should have a minimum temporal resolution of 20 volumes per second, with higher frame rates needed for assessing normal annular dynamics or in presence of tachycardia. In order to capture the volume with minimal stitching artifacts, imaging the elevational plane (either by two- or 3DE *en face* view) can be used (See Chap. 2).

3DE Display and Quantitative Analysis of the TV

To assess the anatomy of the TV, 3DE data sets are typically displayed in volume rendering mode, visualizing the valve *en face* from both the ventricular and the atrial perspectives (Fig. 18.2). Usually, the atrial perspective (also called "surgical view" since it resembles the view of the surgeon when he/she opens the right atrium) is used to assess patients with primary TR (degenerative, traumatic, etc.). The ventricular perspective is mainly used to evaluate the commissures and the regurgitant or stenotic orifice in patients with functional TR or stenotic tricuspid valves. Additional longitudinal cut planes can be used to evaluate the motion of single leaflets, the chordae tendineae and the papillary muscle position (Fig. 18.10, Video 18.4).

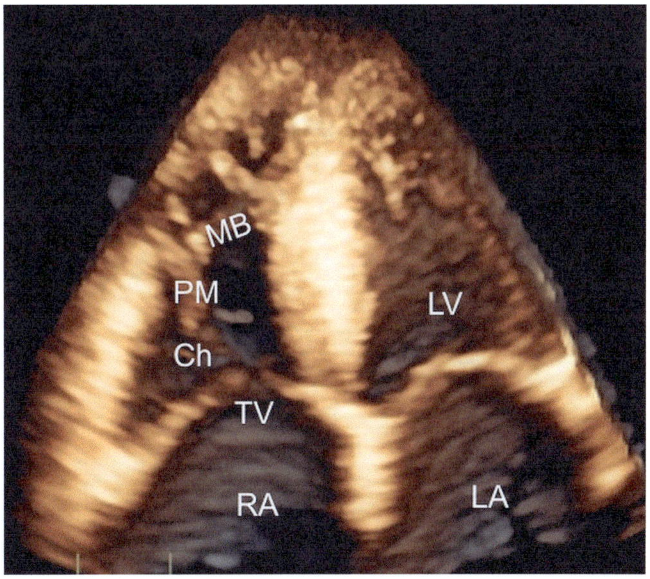

Fig. 18.10 Transthoracic three-dimensional echocardiography. Volume rendering of the tricuspid valve complex (Video 18.4). Longitudinal cut planes of the data set allow the assessment of leaflet motion and of the anatomy of subvalvular apparatus. *APM* anterior papillary muscle, *LA* left atrium, *LV* left ventricle, *Ch* chordae tendineae, *MB* moderator band, *RA* right atrium, *RV* right ventricle, *TV* tricuspid valve

Despite the fact that current recommendations (6) advocate orienting the 3D *en face* view with the TV septal leaflet placed inferiorly (at 6 o'clock position), regardless of the atrial or ventricular perspective, these recommendations were written at the end of the last decade, when interventional procedures on the TV were not available, and the proposed orientation of the TV was aimed to replicate the surgical view. Today, when 3DE is mainly used to guide interventional procedures in the catheterization laboratory, we propose a more anatomically oriented display of the TV (Fig. 18.2). Alternatively, Hausleiter et al. [20] recently proposed orienting the *en face* volumes in a way similar to the orientation of a 2D transgastric image; septal leaflet between 12–5 o'clock and the aorta at 5 o'clock. This orientation eliminates the third step (rotation of the image) that is always required by current guidelines since the anterior leaflet (not the septal leaflet) is in the far field of imaging from all imaging planes.

Since there is no commercially available, dedicated software package to perform an echocardiographic quantitative analysis of either TV leaflets size and position, or annulus geometry, measurements are obtained from dedicated cut-planes obtained by slicing the 3DE data set. A transversal cut plane positioned at the level of the tricuspid annulus and oriented in order to cross the junction with TV leaflets in two orthogonal planes, will allow the planimetry of tricuspid annulus area and perimeter, and to obtain anatomically sound measurements of its major and minor axis (Fig. 18.11). These measurements are likely to be relatively

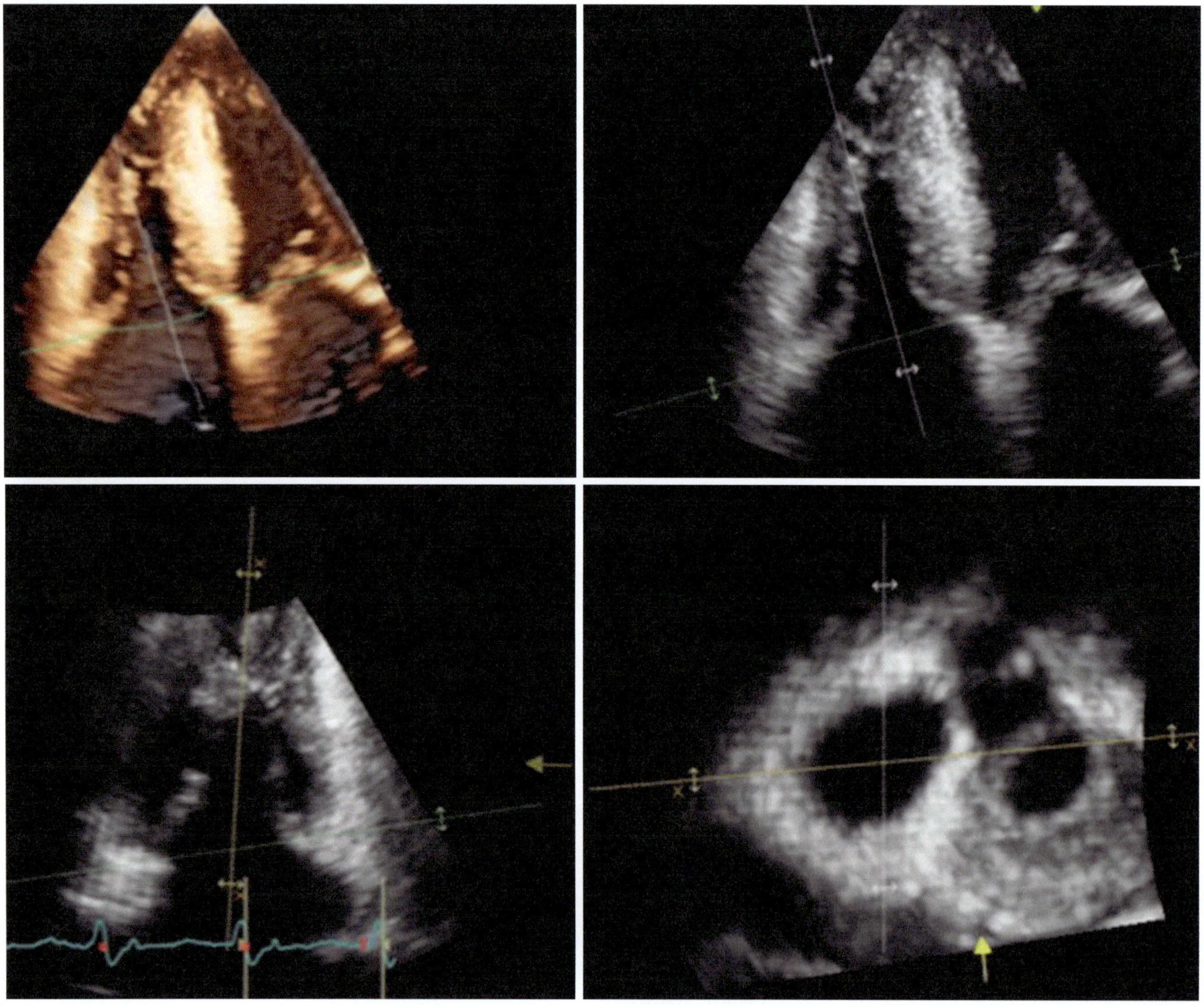

Fig. 18.11 Quantitative assessment of the geometry of the tricuspid annulus by slicing the transthoracic three-dimensional data set of the tricuspid valve. The 3DE data set (left upper panel) is sliced in two orthogonal cut planes: the four chamber (yellow right upper quadrant) and its orthogonal view (white lower left quadrant) crossing at the center of the tricuspid annulus (white and yellow vertical lines). Then, the green plane (horizontal dashed line) is positioned at the level of the tricuspid annulus in both views to obtain a transversal cut plane at the level of the annulus (green right lower quadrant) on which the diameters, the perimeter and the projected 2D area of the tricuspid annulus can be measured. *LA* left atrium, *LV* left ventricle, *RA* right atrium, *RV* right ventricle

accurate in patients with severe functional TR in whom the tricuspid annulus is flattened [21]. Conversely, in normal subjects and in patients in whom the 3D geometry of the tricuspid annulus is preserved, measurements obtained by 3D reconstruction of the annulus are significantly different from those obtained by direct planimetry of tomographic cut planes [10]. A dedicated software package for a 3D reconstruction of the tricuspid annulus will allow initialization of the annulus in a series of rotated planes around it in order to factor the non-planar nature of the TV into the tricuspid annulus measurements (Fig. 18.12, Videos 18.5a, 18.5b, and 18.5c). This feature is not possible with the commercially available slicing method of TA assessment, which provides only planar tomographic views [22]. When performing annular measurements using the slicing method, the position of the annular plane is chosen by the operator. However, the choice of the position of this plane is quite difficult because of the non-planarity of the annulus. If the chosen annular plane is located at the hinge points of the annulus in one longitudinal view, it may not be possible to ensure that it is at the hinge points in the orthogonal plane. As a compromise, the plane is often placed above the annulus, towards the right atrium. As a result: *i.* the operator measures a projected or planar area instead of the actual annular area; *ii.* part of the right atrial wall will be incorrectly identified as tricuspid annular boundary, results in smaller end-diastolic measurements, because at this time the right atrium is the smallest. These findings explain why there is a need for dedicated software packages that account for the non-planarity of the TV annulus to provide a more reliable and semi-automated quantification of tricuspid annulus size and dynamics [10, 23].

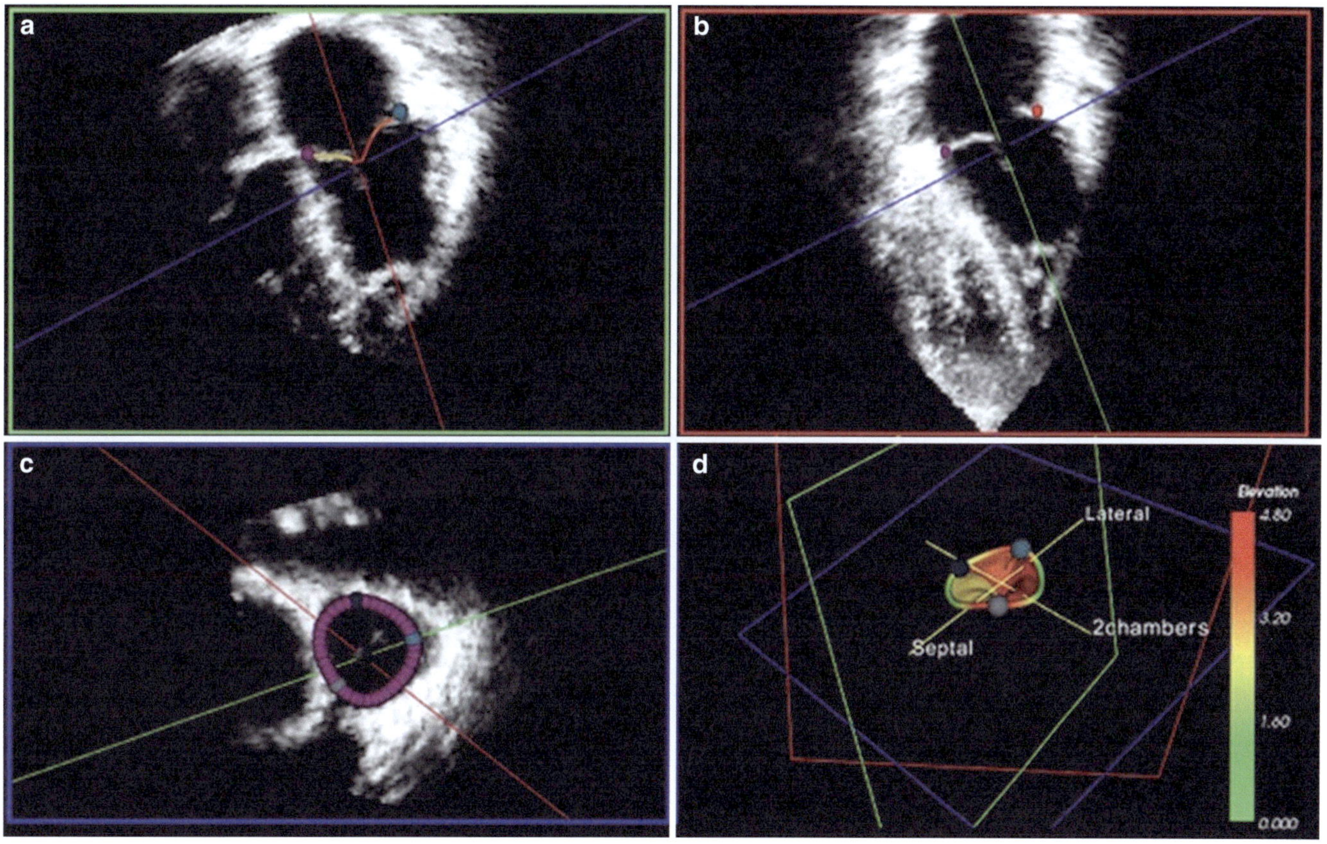

Fig. 18.12 Custom-made software package for anatomically sound quantitation of tricuspid annulus and leaflet geometry using 3DE data sets. Initialization starts with multi-planar reconstruction to allow the operator to identify the correct 4-chamber view (**a**) in combination with the orthogonal longitudinal view (**b**). Then, initialization of the tricuspid annulus will be manually performed in the mid-systolic frame by marking valve leaflet hinge points at both end-diastole and end-systole (Video 18.5a). This initialization will be performed in eight rotated planes around the tricuspid valve center point. Further editing will be allowed on any user-identified rotational plane (Video 18.5b). Input from the user will be interactively resampled to 80 points along the annulus using smooth spline interpolation (**c**). These 80 points will then be automatically tracked throughout the cardiac cycle to obtain the following TA measurements: area (computed as the sum of the triangles composing the 3D mesh connecting all the annulus points), instantaneous area change, perimeter (computed as the sum of the distances between consecutive annulus points), long- and short-axis dimensions and circularity (ratio of short- to long-axis dimensions) (Video 18.5c). The three commissural points will then be manually identified on the 3D looping image with the superimposed annulus. Then, an automatic algorithm will identify the surface defining the three TV leaflets using edge detection techniques. Finally, a surface rendering of the valve can be displayed and eventually printed (**d**)

In addition, dedicated longitudinal cut planes positioned in the center of each leaflet will allow the measurements of the length of the leaflets (Fig. 18.13), the leaflet-to-annular plane tethering angle of each leaflet, and of the coaptation depth of TV leaflets (Fig. 18.14). Tenting volume of TV leaflets by 3DE—accounting for both annulus dilation and leaflet tethering—is a predictor of residual TR following surgical tricuspid annuloplasty [24].

Finally, the 3De data set of the TV can be printed [25] to appreciate valve morphology and perform qualitative and quantitative analysis useful for pre-procedural (surgical or interventional) planning and teaching (See Fig. 2.15, Chap. 2).

Future Directions

Despite the growing need for better characterization of the tricuspid valve in patients considered for left valve surgery, there is no commercially available software package dedicated to tricuspid valve geometry quantitation. With the advent of more studies showing the benefits of 3D imaging specifically as it relates to surgical outcomes and to guide interventional procedures perhaps there will be a greater push towards developing specific tools to be incorporated into daily routine.

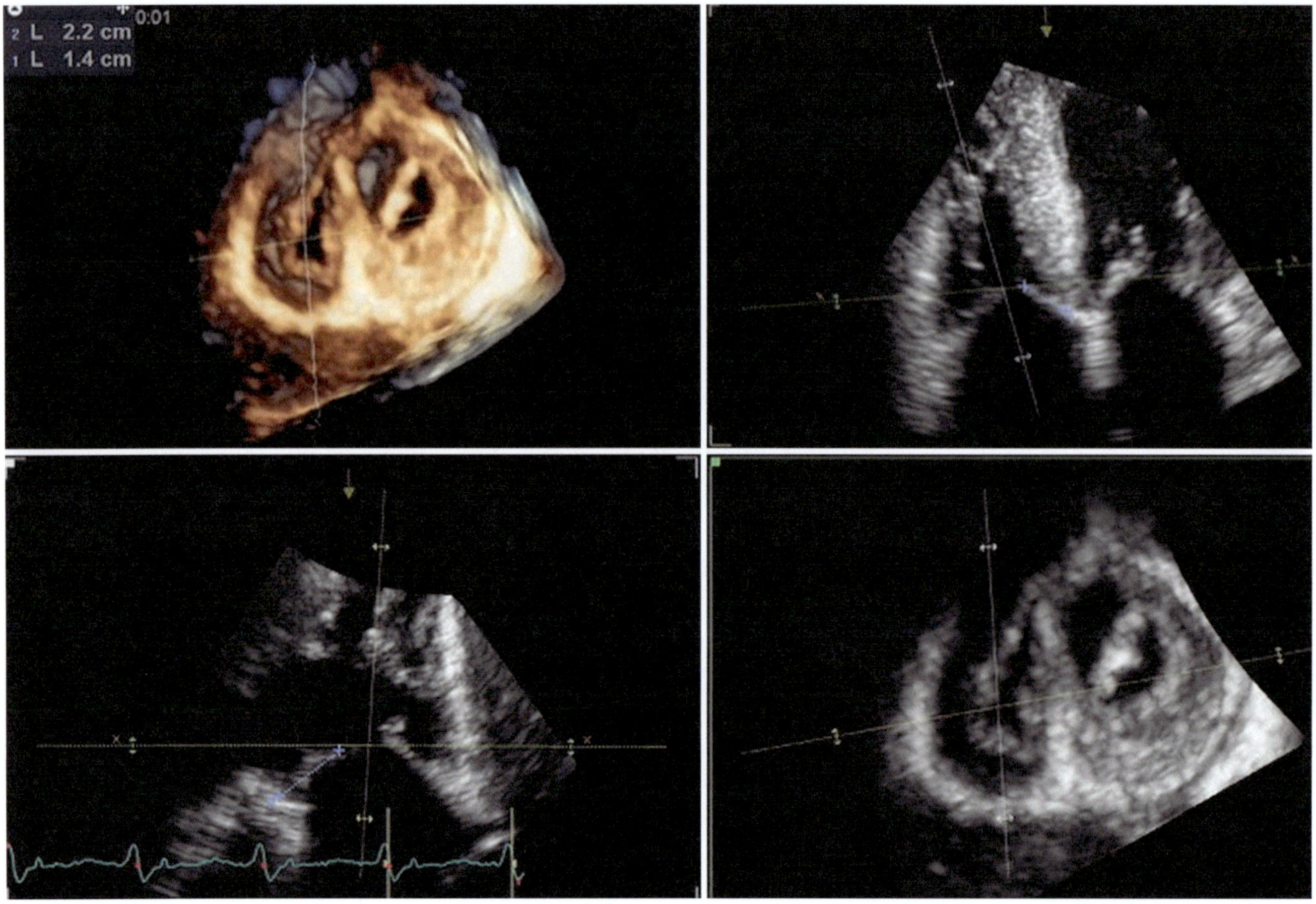

Fig. 18.13 Slicing of the three-dimensional echocardiography data set of the tricuspid valve to obtain cut planes in the center of each tricuspid valve leaflet to measure their diastolic length. In the example, the cut planes have been oriented to pass through the center of the septal (yellow line and right upper quadrant) and the posterior (white line and left lower quadrant) leaflets as they are seen in the volume rendered image (left, upper quadrant)

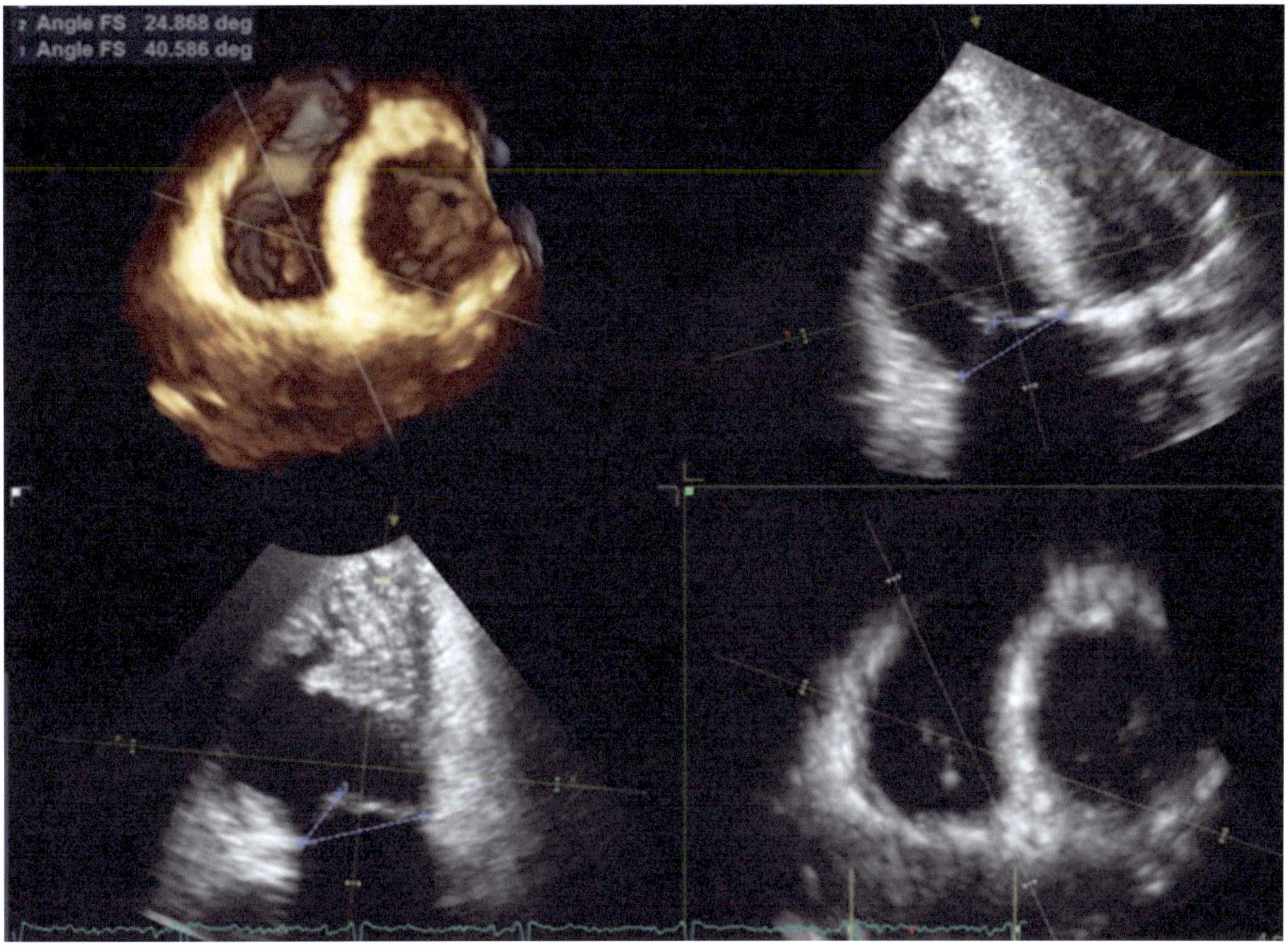

Fig. 18.14 Slicing of the three-dimensional echocardiography data set of the tricuspid valve to obtain cut planes in the center of each tricuspid valve leaflet to measure their tethering angle (right panel) in systole. In the example, the cut planes have been oriented to pass through the center of the septal (yellow line and right upper quadrant) and the anterior (white line and left lower quadrant) leaflets as they are seen in the volume rendered image (left, upper quadrant)

Acknowledgements We would like to acknowledge Dr. Stephen P. Sanders, Professor of Pediatrics (Cardiology), Harvard Medical School, Departments of Cardiology, Pathology, and Cardiac Surgery, Boston Children's Hospital for providing Fig. 18.2 for this chapter. We would also acknowledge Dr Rebecca T Hahn, Director of Interventional Echocardiography NewYork-Presbyterian/ Columbia University Medical Center and professor of medicine at Columbia University Medical Center for providing Figs. 18.8 and 18.9.

References

1. Badano LP, Agricola E, Perez de Isla L, Gianfagna P, Zamorano JL. Evaluation of the tricuspid valve morphology and function by transthoracic real-time three-dimensional echocardiography. Eur J Echocardiogr. 2009;10(4):477–84.
2. Anwar AM, Geleijnse ML, Soliman OI, McGhie JS, Frowijn R, Nemes A, et al. Assessment of normal tricuspid valve anatomy in adults by real-time three-dimensional echocardiography. Int J Cardiovasc Imaging. 2007;23(6):717–24.
3. Stankovic I, Daraban AM, Jasaityte R, Neskovic AN, Claus P, Voigt JU. Incremental value of the en face view of the tricuspid valve by two-dimensional and three-dimensional echocardiography for accurate identification of tricuspid valve leaflets. J Am Soc Echocardiogr. 2014;27(4):376–84.
4. Addetia K, Yamat M, Mediratta A, Medvedofsky D, Patel M, Ferrara P, et al. Comprehensive two-dimensional interrogation of the tricuspid valve using knowledge derived from three-dimensional echocardiography. J Am Soc Echocardiogr. 2016;29(1):74–82.
5. Hahn RT. State-of-the-art review of echocardiographic imaging in the evaluation and treatment of functional tricuspid regurgitation. Circ Cardiovasc Imaging. 2016;9(12). pii: e005332.

6. Lang RM, Badano LP, Tsang W, Adams DH, Agricola E, Buck T, et al. EAE/ASE recommendations for image acquisition and display using three-dimensional echocardiography. Eur Heart J Cardiovasc Imaging. 2012;13(1):1–46.
7. Muraru D, Hahn RT, Soliman OI, Faletra FF, Basso C, Badano LP. 3-Dimensional Echocardiography in Imaging the Tricuspid Valve. JACC Cardiovasc Imaging. 2019;12(3):500–15.
8. Sutton JP, Ho SY, Vogel M, Anderson RH. Is the morphologically right atrio-ventricular valve tricuspid? J Heart Valve Dis. 1995;4:571–5.
9. Miglioranza MH, Mihaila S, Muraru D, Cucchini U, Iliceto S, Badano LP. Variability of tricuspid annulus diameter measurement in healthy volunteers. JACC Cardiovasc Imaging. 2015;8(7):864–6.
10. Addetia K, Muraru D, Veronesi F, Jenei C, Cavalli G, Besser SA, et al. 3-Dimensional echocardiographic analysis of the tricuspid annulus provides new insights into tricuspid valve geometry and dynamics. JACC Cardiovasc Imaging. 2019;12(3):401–12.
11. Acar C, Perier P, Fontaliran F, Deloche A, Carpentier A. Anatomical study of the tricuspid valve and its variations. Surg Radiol Anat. 1990;12(3):229–30.
12. Victor S, Nayak VM. The tricuspid valve is bicuspid. J Heart Valve Dis. 1994;3(1):27–36.
13. Muraru D, Badano LP, Sarais C, Solda E, Iliceto S. Evaluation of tricuspid valve morphology and function by transthoracic three-dimensional echocardiography. Curr Cardiol Rep. 2011;13(3):242–9.
14. David TE. Functional tricuspid regurgitation: a perplexing problem. J Am Soc Echocardiogr. 2009;22(8):904–6.
15. Anwar AM, Geleijnse ML, Ten Cate FJ, Meijboom FJ. Assessment of tricuspid valve annulus size, shape and function using real-time three-dimensional echocardiography. Interact Cardiovasc Thorac Surg. 2006;5(6):683–7.
16. Otto CM. Textbook of clinical echocardiography. 4th ed. Philadelphia: W.B. Saudenrs; 2004.
17. Armstrong WF, Ryan T. Feigenbaum's echocardiography. 7th ed. Philadelphia: Lippincott Williams & Wilkins; 2010.
18. Lancellotti P, Moura L, Pierard LA, Agricola E, Popescu BA, Tribouilloy C, et al. European Association of Echocardiography recommendations for the assessment of valvular regurgitation. Part 2: mitral and tricuspid regurgitation (native valve disease). Eur J Echocardiogr. 2010;11(4):307–32.
19. Faletra F, Ramamuthi A, De Quarti MC, Leo LA, Moccetti T, Pandian N. Artfacts in three-dimensional echocardiography. J Am Soc Echocardiogr. 2014;27:453–62.
20. Hausleiter J, Braun D, Orban M, Latib A, Lurz P, Boekstegers P, et al. Patient selection, echocardiographic screening and treatment strategies for interventional tricuspid repair using the edge-to-edge repair technique. EuroIntervention 2018. pii: EIJ-D-17-01136. https://doi.org/10.4244/EIJ-D-17-01136. [Epub ahead of print].
21. Fukuda S, Gillinov AM, McCarthy PM, Matsumura Y, Thomas JD, Shiota T. Echocardiographic follow-up of tricuspid annuloplasty with a new three-dimensional ring in patients with functional tricuspid regurgitation. J Am Soc Echocardiogr. 2007;20:1236–12242.
22. Prihadi EA, Delgado V, Hahn RT, Leipsic J, Min JK, Bax JJ. Imaging needs in novel transcatheter tricuspid valve interventions. JACC Cardiovasc Imaging. 2018;11(5):736–54.
23. Miglioranza MH, Mihaila S, Muraru D, Cucchini U, Iliceto S, Badano LP. Dynamic changes in tricuspid annular diameter measurement in relation to the echocardiographic view and timing during the cardiac cycle. J Am Soc Echocardiogr. 2015;28(2):226–35.
24. Min SY, Song JM, Kim JH, Jang MK, Kim YJ, Song H, et al. Geometric changes after tricuspid annuloplasty and predictors of residual tricuspid regurgitation: a real-time three-dimensional echocardiography study. Eur Heart J. 2010;31(23):2871–80.
25. Muraru D, Veronesi F, Maddalozzo A, Dequal D, Frajhof L, Rabischoffsky A, et al. 3D printing of normal and pathologic tricuspid valves from transthoracic 3D echocardiography data sets. Eur Heart J Cardiovasc Imaging. 2017;18(1):802–8.

Tricuspid Valve: Congenital Abnormalities and Stenosis

19

Pei-Ni Jone and Shelby Kutty

Abstract

Three-dimensional echocardiography (3DE) has incremental diagnostic value over two-dimensional echocardiography in the evaluation of the tricuspid valve. 3DE provides en face view of all leaflets of the tricuspid valve. The understanding of tricuspid valve leaflet morphology and mechanisms of valvular regurgitation from 3DE provides valuable insights into tricuspid valve function, and assists in the planning for surgical interventions. Congenital abnormalities of the tricuspid valve and illustrative clinical cases are presented in this chapter.

Keywords

Three-dimensional echocardiography · Tricuspid valve · Tricuspid valve dysplasia · Ebstein anomaly · Tricuspid valve prolapse · Functional abnormalities of the tricuspid valve · Tricuspid valve in corrected transposition · Tricuspid valve stenosis · Tricuspid regurgitation.

Congenital Abnormalities of the Tricuspid Valve

The tricuspid valve is the largest of the four valves in the heart and has three leaflets [1–3]. The anterior leaflet is the largest of the three leaflets and is supported by a large papillary muscle that attaches to the moderator band and a small papillary muscle of the conus. The septal leaflet of the tricuspid valve has chordae that insert directly into the septum with no papillary muscles. The posterior leaflet is probably the smallest leaflet and it is supported by the smaller, more posteriorly situated papillary muscle. The annulus of the tricuspid valve is elliptical in shape.

Congenital anomalies of the tricuspid valve includes tricuspid valve dysplasia, Ebstein anomalies, tricuspid valve prolapse, functional abnormalities of the tricuspid valve, tricuspid valve in corrected transposition, and tricuspid stenosis from congenital tricuspid stenosis and from rheumatic heart disease. Evaluation of the tricuspid valve is limited from two-dimensional echocardiography, as the three leaflets cannot be displayed simultaneously. With three-dimensional echocardiography (3DE), evaluation of the leaflets is precise and accurate [4]. An en face view of the tricuspid valve from the right atrium allows accurate identification of the anterior, septal, and posterior leaflets (Fig. 19.1 and Video 19.1). Transthoracic 3DE has an equivalent diagnostic yield as transesophageal 3DE for the tricuspid valve in most subjects, especially the young. 3DE allows for several enface views of the tricuspid valve from the transthoracic approach including parasternal short axis view, apical four chamber view, and subcostal views. 3DE can readily define the morphologic features of the valve and the associated mechanism(s) for regurgitation, which are key pieces of information to the surgeon for pre-operative planning of valve repair. Each of the congenital tricuspid anomalies will be described in the clinical cases below with its findings on 3DE.

Clinical Cases

Tricuspid Valve Dysplasia

In tricuspid valve dysplasia, there is no downward displacement of the septal leaflet. This in an anomaly often observed in the neonate. The leaflets are usually thickened, deficient, and

Electronic Supplementary Material The online version of this chapter (https://doi.org/10.1007/978-3-030-14032-8_19) contains supplementary material, which is available to authorized users.

P.-N. Jone (✉)
Department of Pediatric Cardiology, Children's Hospital Colorado, University of Colorado School of Medicine, Aurora, CO, USA
e-mail: pei-ni.jone@childrenscolorado.org

S. Kutty
Taussig Heart Center, The Johns Hopkins Hospital and School of Medicine, Baltimore, MD, USA

L. P. Badano et al. (eds.), *Textbook of Three-Dimensional Echocardiography*, https://doi.org/10.1007/978-3-030-14032-8_19

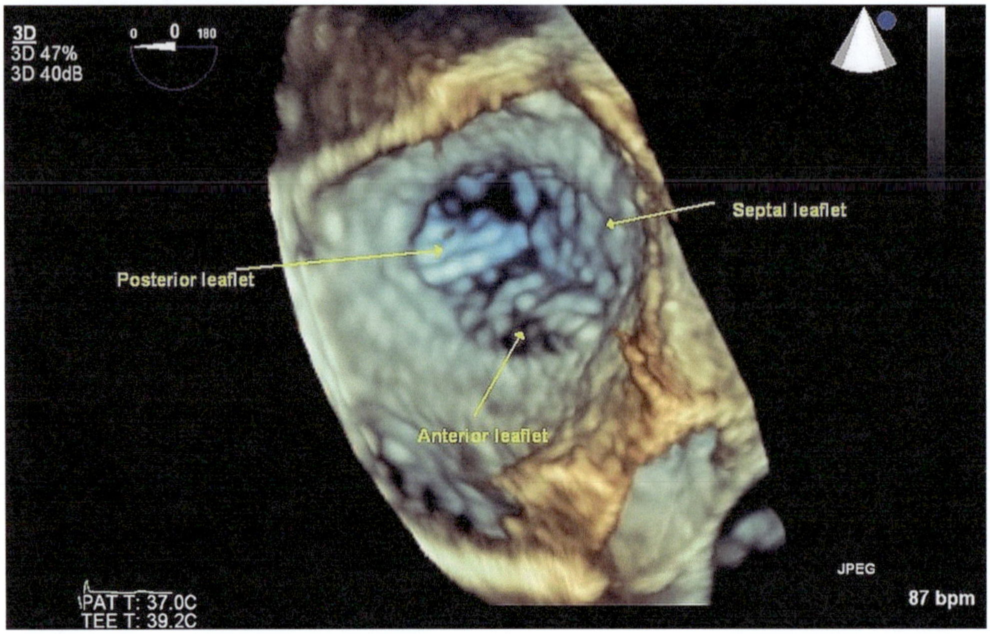

Fig. 19.1 3DE transesophageal image of the normal tricuspid valve looking down from the right atrium. (Video 19.1)

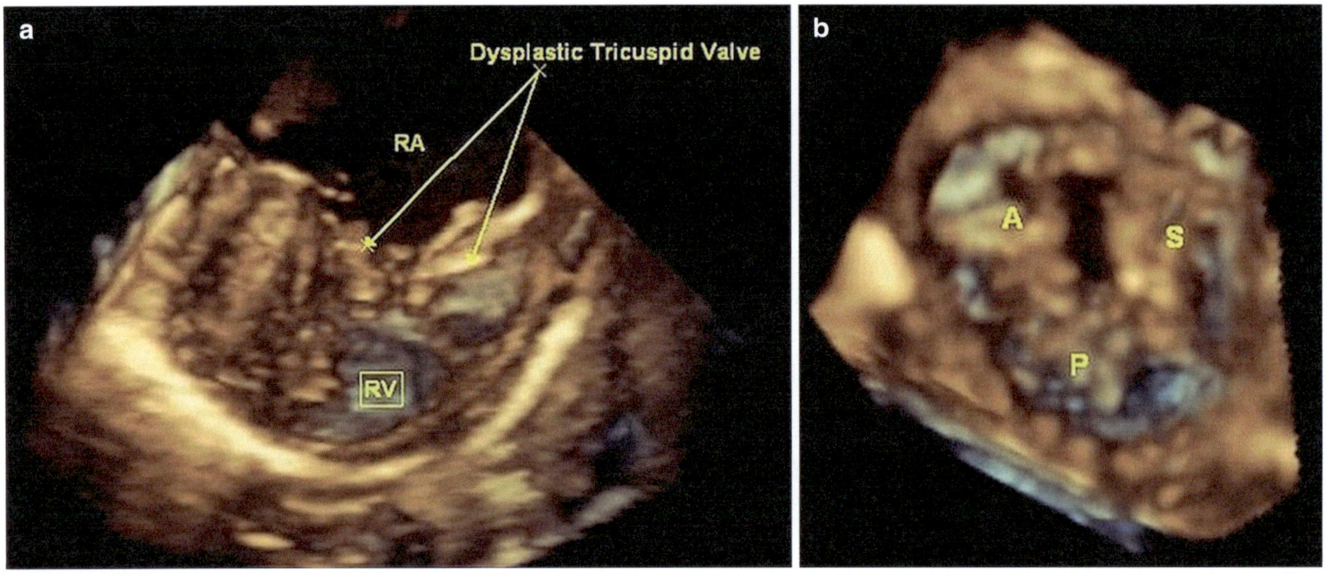

Fig. 19.2 (**a**) Transthoracic three-dimensional echocardiography demonstrates tricuspid valve dysplasia with septal leaflet tethered to the septum and thickened tricuspid valve leaflets in the left panel. (**b**) There is noncoaptation of the dysplastic tricuspid valve leaflets looking from the ventricle up. *A* anterior leaflet, *P* posterior leaflet, *RA* right atrium, *RV* right ventricle, *S* septal leaflet (Videos 19.2a and 19.2b)

have short chordae that tether the valve so that the leaflets do not have the ability to coapt. The anterior and posterior leaflets are tethered by the shortened chordae, and cannot abut against the septal leaflet, resulting in tricuspid valve regurgitation. A hypoplastic papillary muscle may be seen in conjunction with this lesion [5]. Tricuspid valve dysplasia can occur in isolation or can be associated with other congenital heart disease, such as pulmonary atresia with intact ventricular septum.

A 3-day-old neonate presented with cyanosis and a dysplastic tricuspid valve. The leaflets are thickened and dysplastic that resulted in inability of the septal leaflet to coapt with the anterior or posterior leaflets, causing moderate to severe tricuspid valve regurgitation (Fig. 19.2, Videos 19.2a and 19.2b).

Ebstein Anomaly

Ebstein anomaly of the tricuspid valve, first described in 1866, comprises <1% of all congenital heart disease and occurs in 1 per 200,000 live births [6]. It involves the apical (downward) displacement of insertion of the septal leaflet of the tricuspid valve (≥8 mm/m^2), redundant elongated anterior tricuspid valve leaflet, adherence of the septal and posterior leaflets to the underlying myocardium (failure of delamination), dilation of the atrioventricular junction, and right ventricular thinning, enlargement, and dysfunction [5, 7–9]. The anterior leaflet may have distal linear attachments to the anterior wall of the right ventricle and in some cases can result in right ventricular outflow tract obstruction. There can be significant tricuspid valve regurgitation with right atrial and right ventricular volume overload. Altered electrical synchrony and Wolff-Parkinson-White syndrome are associated with the disease [6, 10]. Progressive right heart failure can affect these patients early in life and many of these patients need surgery to correct this anomaly. With 3DE, the anterior leaflet of the Ebstein valve can be seen attaching to the anterior wall of the right ventricle and right ventricular outflow tract.

A 7-year-old female with Ebstein anomaly of tricuspid valve is shown. Note that the anterior leaflet is displaced anteriorly (Fig. 19.3, Videos 19.3a and 19.3b) into the right ventricular outflow tract with moderate to severe valvular regurgitation (Fig. 19.4 and Video 19.4). In an 11-year-old male with Ebstein anomaly, the non-coapting tricuspid valve is viewed from the ventricular side (Fig. 19.5 and Video 19.5).

Tricuspid Valve Prolapse

Congenital tricuspid valve prolapse is seen in patients with elastin abnormalities, whereas acquired tricuspid valve prolapse occurs in the setting of anterior chest wall trauma, secondary to closure of ventricular septal defect, subendocardial ischemia, or papillary muscle dysfunction. Rarely, it presents as cleft of the anterior leaflet of the tricuspid valve with prolapse, resulting in severe tricuspid regurgitation. Isolated congenital cleft of the anterior tricuspid valve leaflet is very rare with a reported incidence of 0.018% [11].

A 15-year-old female, diagnosed at 3 years of age with severe tricuspid valve regurgitation, presented to cardiology clinic with fatigue and palpitations. There was no prior history of infection or trauma to the chest. The two-dimensional echocardiogram showed severe prolapse of the tricuspid valve and severe regurgitation in addition to severe dilation of the right heart. There was mildly to moderately decreased systolic function. 3DE demonstrated a congenital cleft of the tricuspid anterior leaflet with severe prolapse and thickening (Fig. 19.6, Videos 19.6a and 19.6b). There were two septal papillary muscles; one attaching to the septal leaflet and the other attaching to the posterior leaflet. The chordal attachment to the anterior leaflet was disrupted, with severe tricuspid regurgitation (Fig. 19.7 and Video 19.7). Intra-operative findings confirmed the diagnosis of cleft anterior tricuspid valve leaflet with significant prolapse and thickening.

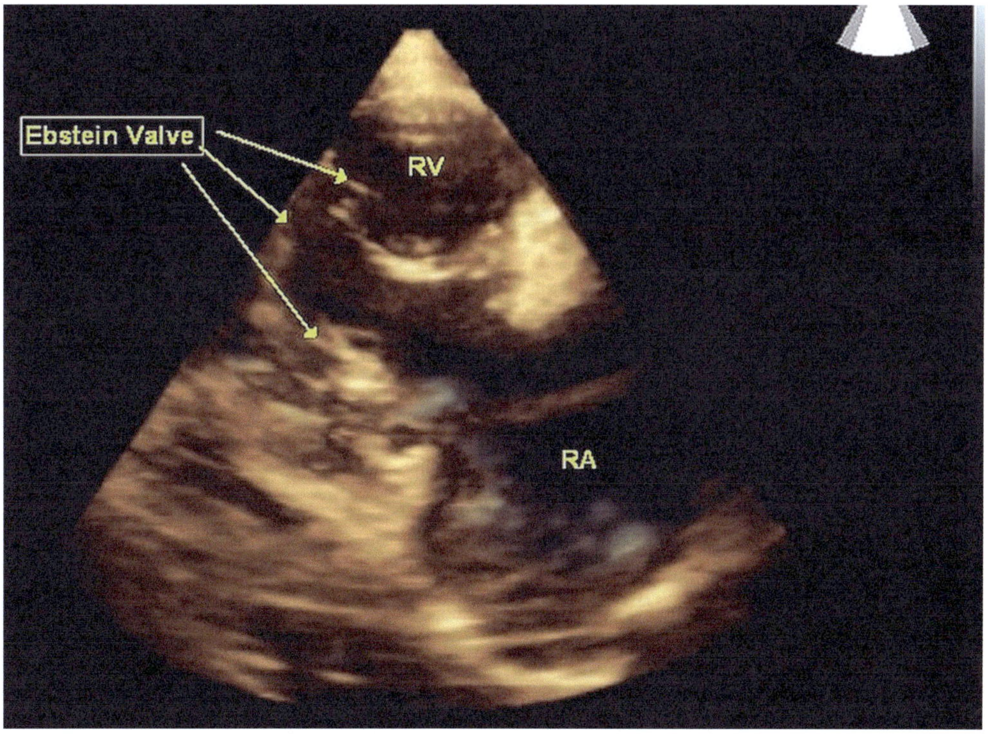

Fig. 19.3 Transthoracic parasternal long axis view of the tricuspid valve in Ebstein anomaly. Note the septal leaflet displaced down to the right ventricle. *RA* right atrium and *RV* right ventricle (Videos 19.3a and 19.3b)

Functional Abnormalities of the Tricuspid Valve

Functional abnormalities of the tricuspid valve are encountered when there is secondary dilation of the tricuspid valve annulus from diverse etiology, including pulmonary valve regurgitation, pulmonary hypertension, orthotopic heart transplant, left-sided valvular heart disease, all forms of cardiomyopathy, or surgical damage to the valve at the time of the ventricular septal defect repair [12–17]. The underlying mechanism for functional tricuspid regurgitation is likely annular dilatation and septal leaflet tethering [15]. In patients with pulmonary hypertension (idiopathic or secondary to left heart disease or cardiomyopathy), the mechanism of tricuspid regurgitation is possibly leaflet tethering combined with alteration to a more circular annulus secondary to right ventricular pressure load [17]. In patients with low-pressure volume-loaded right ventricle, annular dilation is usually the mechanism of tricuspid regurgitation, resulting in poor coaptation of the valve leaflets. In hearts where ventricular septal defect has been repaired, the mechanism of tricuspid regurgitation is the result of damage to the anteroseptal commissure or tethering of the septal leaflet. In patients with right heart endomyocardial biopsy after heart transplantation, bioptome induced injury and avulsion of the papillary muscle of the conus results in tricuspid valve prolapse and regurgitation, typically arising from the anteroseptal commissure. Finally, in patients with hypoplastic left heart syndrome (HLHS), the mechanism(s) of tricuspid regurgitation include annular dilation, increased tricuspid valve tethering volume, increased prolapse volume, and flatter bending angle [18–21].

TR FROM EBSTEIN ATRIAL VIEW

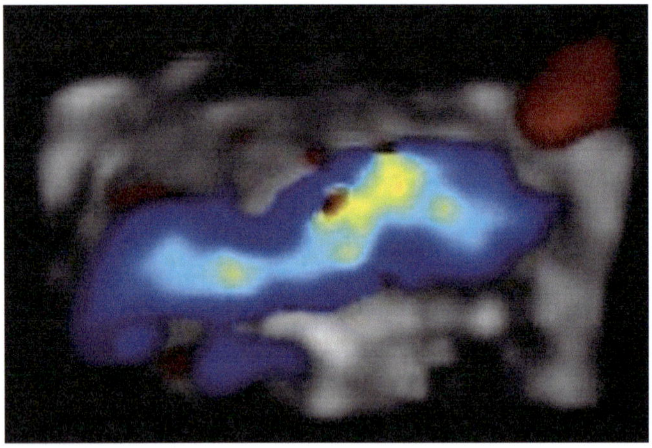

Fig. 19.4 Three-dimensional echocardiography color Doppler demonstrating severe regurgitation of the tricuspid valve in Ebstein anomaly (right atrial view) (Video 19.4)

Tricuspid regurgitation is an important risk factor associated with morbidity and mortality in HLHS. Using 3DE, Takahashi et al. elucidated that those patients with tethering of the tricuspid valve have flattened tricuspid valve annulus and a more laterally displaced papillary muscle, whereas patients with prolapse have dilated annulus and smaller septal leaflet [18]. Kutty et al. demonstrated that tricuspid valve prolapse evolves in patients with HLHS as leaflet growth is an important factor in maintaining normal leaflet coaptation [19]. Tricuspid valve failure in HLHS may represent an inability of the valve to adapt to the increase demand of tethering, and rapid annular dilation that accompanies the volume and pressure loading stressors after stage one palliation

Fig. 19.5 Tricuspid valve non-coaptation in Ebstein anomaly shown from the ventricular side (Video 19.5)

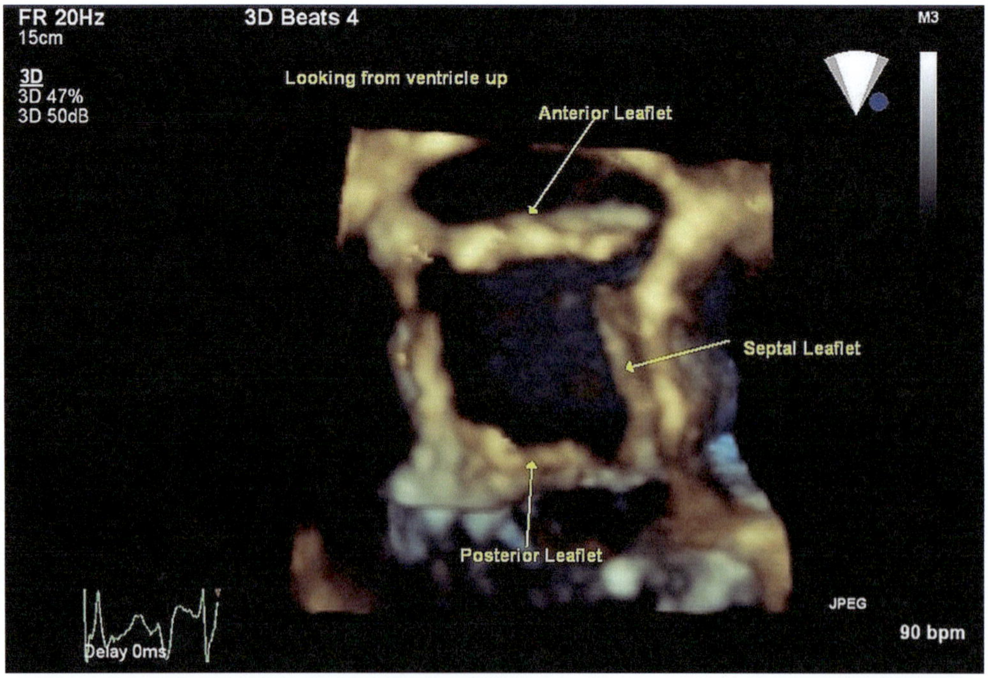

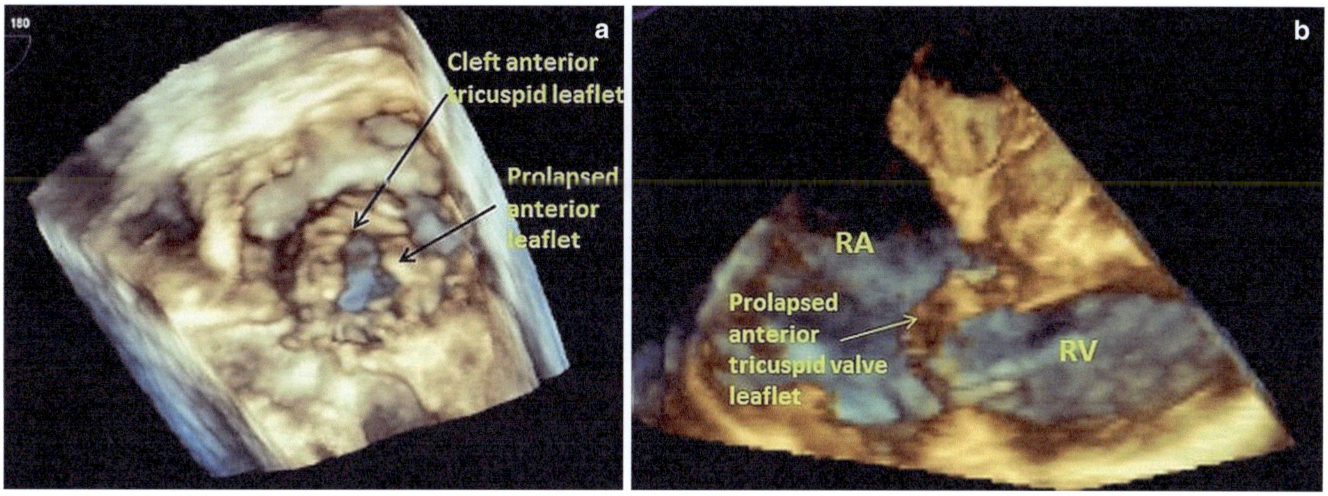

Fig. 19.6 (**a**) Cleft anterior tricuspid valve leaflet is demonstrated in en face view. There is also prolapse of the anterior leaflet above the tricuspid valve annulus. (**b**) Four-chamber view shows dilated right atrium (RA) and right ventricle (RV) with anterior leaflet prolapse. Image courtesy of Dr. Gerald Marx at Boston's Children's Hospital (Videos 19.6a and 19.6b)

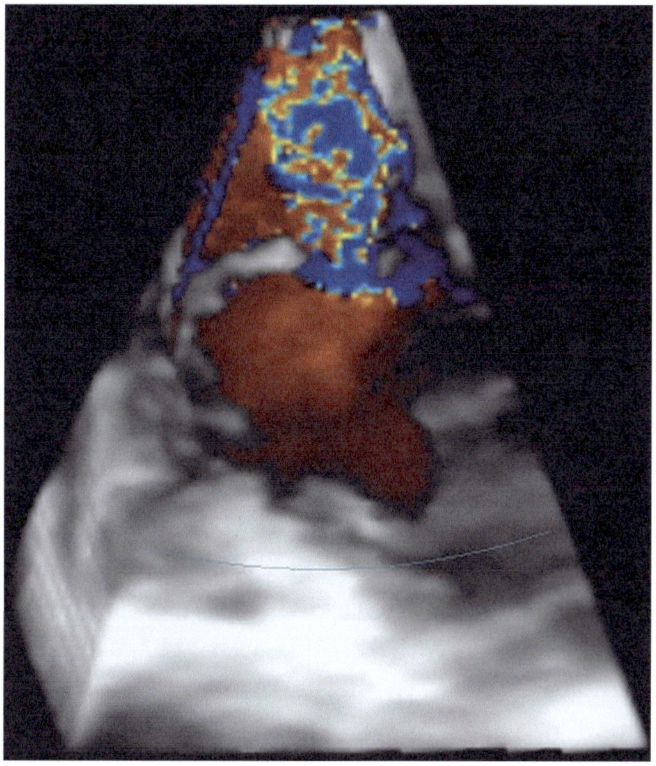

Fig. 19.7 Color Doppler demonstration of severe tricuspid regurgitation (Video 19.7)

of this disease [19]. Regurgitation begets more regurgitation as demonstrated in the patient below. With increasing regurgitation, there is more annular dilation as the tricuspid valve becomes more circular, which compromises the normal function of the elliptical tricuspid valve.

A 20-month-old male with hypoplastic left heart syndrome, status-post bidirectional cavopulmonary shunt operation had progressive tricuspid valve regurgitation (Fig. 19.8).

Tricuspid Valve in Corrected Transposition of the Great Arteries

The tricuspid valve in corrected transposition of the great arteries is dysplastic consisting of thickened leaflets and associated short chordae, which results in leaflet tethering. Occasionally one of the leaflets can be displaced, the posterior leaflet being the frequently displaced leaflet. Moreover, the valve is under systemic pressure and has a more circular annulus. All these features, in combination with valve dysplasia and chordal abnormalities lead to progressive tricuspid regurgitation. Regurgitation causes more ventricular dilation which results in more annular dilation. This in turn causes inability of the leaflets to coapt, worsening regurgitation and perpetuating a vicious cycle. Prolapse or straddling of the valve can also occur in some patients with correct transposition of the great arteries.

A 12-year-old male with corrected transposition has prolapse of the tricuspid valve. This patient underwent a cardiac catheterization procedure for hemodynamic evaluation (Video 19.8a). A 5-day-old female with straddling tricuspid valve in corrected transposition (Fig. 19.9 and Video 19.8b).

Tricuspid Stenosis

In congenital tricuspid stenosis, the valve annulus appears relatively large with leaflets that are thickened with commissural fusion and shortened chordae [22, 23]. This lesion is usually associated with other anomalies such as right ventricular outflow tract obstruction or atresia secondary to hypoplasia of the right ventricle. Isolated congenital tricuspid valve stenosis is extremely rare. In adults, tricuspid stenosis occurs as sequelae of rheumatic heart disease.

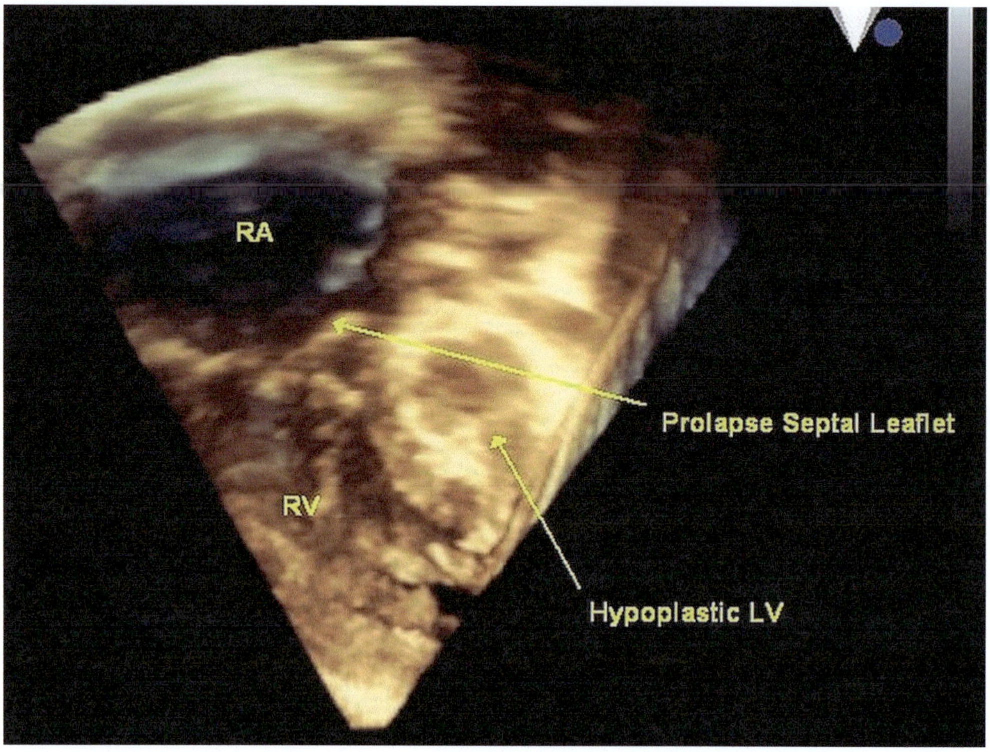

Fig. 19.8 Transthoracic apical four-chamber three-dimensional echocardiography image demonstrating tricuspid valve prolapse in a patient with hypoplastic left heart syndrome

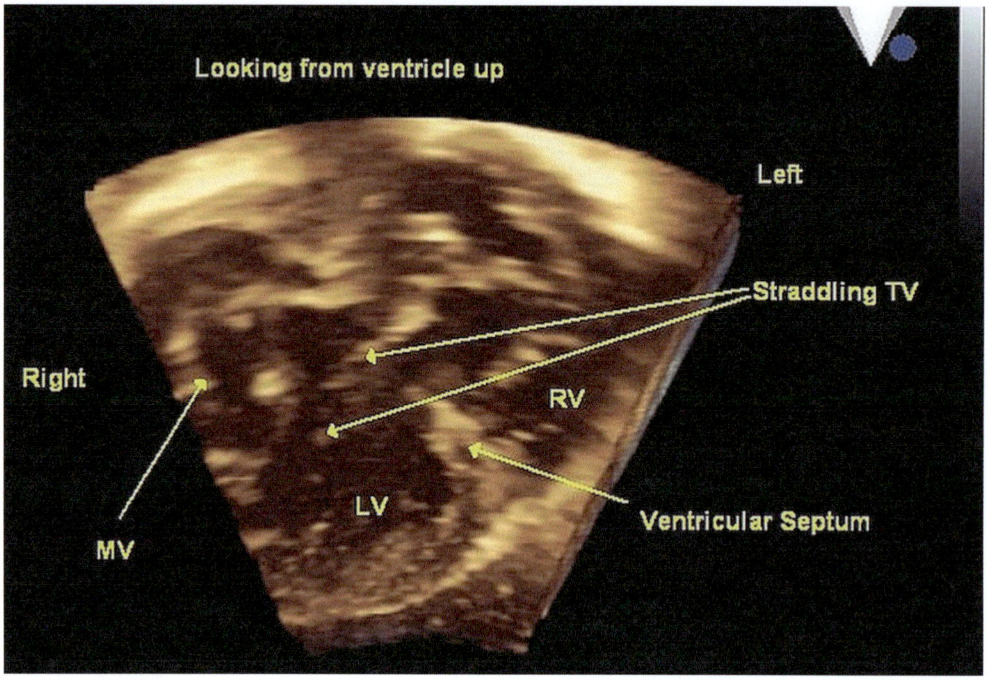

Fig. 19.9 Three-dimensional transthoracic subxiphoid image in a patient with corrected transposition of the great arteries. The straddling tricuspid valve is on the 'left side' of the heart. *LV* left ventricle, *MV* mitral valve, *RV* right ventricle, *TV* tricuspid valve (Videos 19.8a and 19.8b)

Patients who have had porcine bioprosthetic valves in the tricuspid position for treatment of Ebstein anomaly may develop tricuspid stenosis over time [24].

Clinical Case of Tricuspid Stenosis

An 8-year-old male with bioprosthetic valve in the tricuspid position, which became stenotic (Fig. 19.10 and Video 19.9) requiring catheter mediated placement of Melody valve prosthesis (Fig. 19.11 and Video 19.10). Evaluation of the bioprosthetic tricuspid valve has been established in the adult literature but not in the pediatric population [25]. Doppler parameters of prosthetic tricuspid valve function in adults that would meet criteria for stenosis include peak instantaneous velocity of >1.7 m/s, mean gradient ≥6 mmHg, and pressure half-time ≥230 ms [25–28]. There are currently no established indices for effective

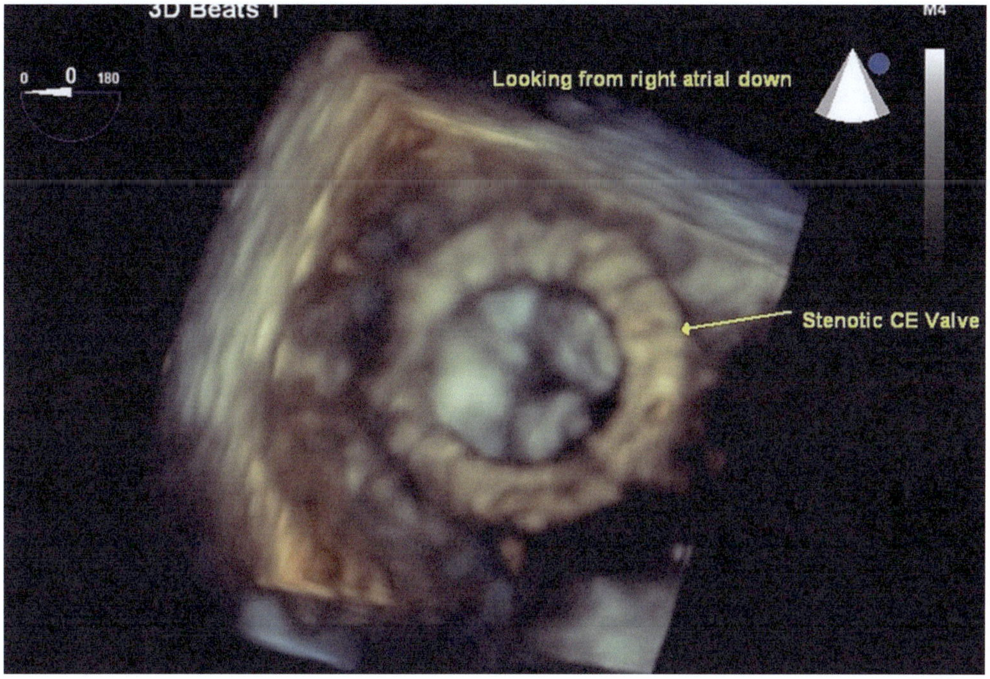

Fig. 19.10 Transesophageal three-dimensional image of the stenotic Carpentier-Edwards valve imaged from the right atria down. *CE* Carpentier-Edwards (Video 19.9)

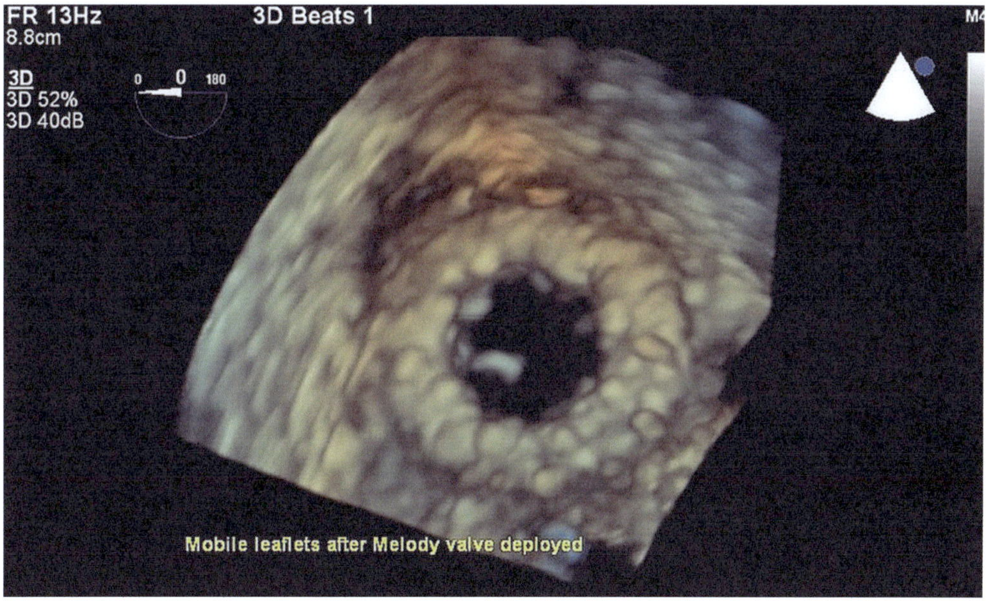

Fig. 19.11 Three-dimensional echocardiographic image status-post deployment of a Melody valve within the Carpentier-Edwards valve. Note the thin and mobile leaflets of the Melody prosthesis (Video 19.10)

orifice area quantification of the prosthetic tricuspid valve in children or adults. Further research in this area is needed.

References

1. Silver MD, Lam JH, Ranganathan N, Wigle ED. Morphology of the human tricuspid valve. Circulation. 1971;43(3):333–48.
2. Lamers WH, Viragh S, Wessels A, Moorman AF, Anderson RH. Formation of the tricuspid valve in the human heart. Circulation. 1995;91(1):111–21.
3. Addetia K, Yamat M, Mediratta A, Medvedofsky D, Patel M, Ferrara P, et al. Comprehensive two-dimensional interrogation of the tricuspid valve using knowledge derived from three-dimensional echocardiography. J Am Soc Echocardiogr. 2016;29(1):74–82.
4. Stankovic I, Daraban AM, Jasaityte R, Neskovic AN, Claus P, Voigt JU. Incremental value of the en face view of the tricuspid valve by two-dimensional and three-dimensional echocardiography for accurate identification of tricuspid valve leaflets. J Am Soc Echocardiogr. 2014;27(4):376–84.
5. Ammash NM, Warnes CA, Connolly HM, Danielson GK, Seward JB. Mimics of Ebstein's anomaly. Am Heart J. 1997;134(3):508–13.
6. Attenhofer Jost CH, Connolly HM, Dearani JA, Edwards WD, Danielson GK. Ebstein's anomaly. Circulation. 2007;115(2):277–85.
7. Lev M, Liberthson RR, Joseph RH, Seten CE, Eckner FA, Kunske RD, et al. The pathologic anatomy of Ebstein's disease. Arch Pathol. 1970;90(4):334–43.

8. Ho SY, Goltz D, McCarthy K, Cook AC, Connell MG, Smith A, et al. The atrioventricular junctions in Ebstein malformation. Heart. 2000;83(4):444–9.
9. Anderson KR, Zuberbuhler JR, Anderson RH, Becker AE, Lie JT. Morphologic spectrum of Ebstein's anomaly of the heart: a review. Mayo Clin Proc. 1979;54(3):174–80.
10. Celermajer DS, Bull C, Till JA, Cullen S, Vassillikos VP, Sullivan ID, et al. Ebstein's anomaly: presentation and outcome from fetus to adult. J Am Coll Cardiol. 1994;23(1):170–6.
11. Eichhorn P, Ritter M, Suetsch G, von Segesser LK, Turina M, Jenni R. Congenital cleft of the anterior tricuspid leaflet with severe tricuspid regurgitation in adults. J Am Coll Cardiol. 1992;20(5):1175–9.
12. Song JM, Fukuda S, Lever HM, Daimon M, Agler DA, Smedira NG, et al. Asymmetry of systolic anterior motion of the mitral valve in patients with hypertrophic obstructive cardiomyopathy: a real-time three-dimensional echocardiographic study. J Am Soc Echocardiogr. 2006;19(9):1129–35.
13. Sukmawan R, Watanabe N, Ogasawara Y, Yamaura Y, Yamamoto K, Wada N, et al. Geometric changes of tricuspid valve tenting in tricuspid regurgitation secondary to pulmonary hypertension quantified by novel system with transthoracic real-time 3-dimensional echocardiography. J Am Soc Echocardiogr. 2007;20(5):470–6.
14. Ton-Nu TT, Levine RA, Handschumacher MD, Dorer DJ, Yosefy C, Fan D, et al. Geometric determinants of functional tricuspid regurgitation: insights from 3-dimensional echocardiography. Circulation. 2006;114(2):143–9.
15. Park YH, Song JM, Lee EY, Kim YJ, Kang DH, Song JK. Geometric and hemodynamic determinants of functional tricuspid regurgitation: a real-time three-dimensional echocardiography study. Int J Cardiol. 2008;124(2):160–5.
16. Ring L, Rana BS, Kydd A, Boyd J, Parker K, Rusk RA. Dynamics of the tricuspid valve annulus in normal and dilated right hearts: a three-dimensional transoesophageal echocardiography study. Eur Heart J Cardiovasc Imaging. 2012;13(9):756–62.
17. Spinner EM, Buice D, Yap CH, Yoganathan AP. The effects of a three-dimensional, saddle-shaped annulus on anterior and posterior leaflet stretch and regurgitation of the tricuspid valve. Ann Biomed Eng. 2012;40(5):996–1005.
18. Takahashi K, Inage A, Rebeyka IM, Ross DB, Thompson RB, Mackie AS, et al. Real-time 3-dimensional echocardiography provides new insight into mechanisms of tricuspid valve regurgitation in patients with hypoplastic left heart syndrome. Circulation. 2009;120(12):1091–8.
19. Kutty S, Colen T, Thompson RB, Tham E, Li L, Vijarnsorn C, et al. Tricuspid regurgitation in hypoplastic left heart syndrome: mechanistic insights from 3-dimensional echocardiography and relationship with outcomes. Circ Cardiovasc Imaging. 2014;7(5):765–72.
20. Kutty S, Graney BA, Khoo NS, Li L, Polak A, Gribben P, et al. Serial assessment of right ventricular volume and function in surgically palliated hypoplastic left heart syndrome using real-time transthoracic three-dimensional echocardiography. J Am Soc Echocardiogr. 2012;25(6):682–9.
21. Khoo NS, Smallhorn JF. Mechanism of valvular regurgitation. Curr Opin Pediatr. 2011;23(5):512–7.
22. Svane S. Congenital tricuspid stenosis. A report on six autopsied cases. Scand J Thorac Cardiovasc Surg. 1971;5(3):232–8.
23. Lewis T. Congenital tricuspid stenosis. Clin Sci. 1945;5(3–4):261–73.
24. Williams DB, Danielson GK, McGoon DC, Puga FJ, Mair DD, Edwards WD. Porcine heterograft valve replacement in children. J Thorac Cardiovasc Surg. 1982;84(3):446–50.
25. Zoghbi WA, Chambers JB, Dumesnil JG, Foster E, Gottdiener JS, Grayburn PA, et al. Recommendations for evaluation of prosthetic valves with echocardiography and doppler ultrasound: a report From the American Society of Echocardiography's Guidelines and Standards Committee and the Task Force on Prosthetic Valves, developed in conjunction with the American College of Cardiology Cardiovascular Imaging Committee, Cardiac Imaging Committee of the American Heart Association, the European Association of Echocardiography, a registered branch of the European Society of Cardiology, the Japanese Society of Echocardiography and the Canadian Society of Echocardiography, endorsed by the American College of Cardiology Foundation, American Heart Association, European Association of Echocardiography, a registered branch of the European Society of Cardiology, the Japanese Society of Echocardiography, and Canadian Society of Echocardiography. J Am Soc Echocardiogr. 2009;22(9):975–1014, quiz 1082–4
26. Connolly HM, Miller FA Jr, Taylor CL, Naessens JM, Seward JB, Tajik AJ. Doppler hemodynamic profiles of 82 clinically and echocardiographically normal tricuspid valve prostheses. Circulation. 1993;88(6):2722–7.
27. Kobayashi Y, Nagata S, Ohmori F, Eishi K, Nakano K, Miyatake K. Serial doppler echocardiographic evaluation of bioprosthetic valves in the tricuspid position. J Am Coll Cardiol. 1996;27(7):1693–7.
28. Aoyagi S, Nishi Y, Kawara T, Oryoji A, Kosuga K, Ohishi K. Doppler echocardiographic evaluation of St. Jude Medical valves in the tricuspid position. J Heart Valve Dis. 1993;2(3):279–86.

Organic Tricuspid Regurgitation

20

Denisa Muraru, Karima Addetia, Fabiana Jarjour, Roberto M. Lang, and Luigi P. Badano

Abstract

It is usually reported that only 10–15% of patients with tricuspid regurgitation have an organic (primary) etiology of the valve disease. However, it is likely that the actual prevalence of organic etiology of tricuspid regurgitation has been underestimated because of the technical limitations of conventional two-dimensional echocardiography to visualize the anatomy and assess the function of the tricuspid valve. However, the correct diagnosis of tricuspid regurgitation etiology and the assessment of valve anatomy are pivotal either to plan surgery or to select the most appropriate device and approach in interventional cardiology in patients who need tricuspid valve repair.

In this chapter we will review the added value of three-dimensional echocardiography to assess the anatomy and the severity of the various forms of organic (primary) tricuspid regurgitations.

Keywords

Three-dimensional echocardiography · Tricuspid valve · Tricuspid valve disease · Tricuspid regurgitation · Tricuspid valve repair · Rheumatic tricuspid stenosis · Carcinoid disease · Pacemaker interference · Infective endocarditis · Traumatic tricuspid regurgitation · Degenerative tricuspid regurgitation

Electronic Supplementary Material The online version of this chapter (https://doi.org/10.1007/978-3-030-14032-8_20) contains supplementary material, which is available to authorized users.

D. Muraru (✉) · L. P. Badano
University of Milano-Bicocca, and Istituto Auxologico Italiano, IRCCS, San Luca Hospital, Milan, Italy
e-mail: denisa.muraru@unimib.it, denisa.muraru@unipd.it; luigi.badano@unimib.it

K. Addetia · R. M. Lang
Noninvasive Cardiac Imaging Laboratories, Department of Medicine/Section of Cardiology, University of Chicago Medical Center, Chicago, IL, USA
e-mail: kaddetia@medicine.bsd.uchicago.edu; rlang@medicine.bsd.uchicago.edu, rlang@bsd.uchicago.edu

F. Jarjour
Department of Cardiac, Thoracic and Vascular Sciences, University of Padua School of Medicine, Padua, Italy

Despite the fact that, in the majority of patients, tricuspid regurgitation (TR) is secondary to diseases affecting the left side of the heart, pulmonary hypertension, atrial fibrillation or pulmonary diseases (functional TR, see also Chap. 21), there is a consistent number of patients with primary (organic) TR [1]. Prevalence of primary TR has been underestimated mainly due to the limited capability of conventional two-dimensional and Doppler echocardiography in visualizing tricuspid valve (TV) anatomy and diagnosing its defects [2–5] (see also Chap. 18). The advent of three-dimensional echocardiography (3DE), the relatively high feasibility of the acquisition of 3DE data sets of the TV from the transthoracic approach [1, 6], and the availability of transcatheter procedures to correct severe TR has completely changed our approach to patients with TR (Table 20.1).

Accurate anatomic characterization of the TV and of the underlying mechanism of dysfunction is the first step in the evaluation of patients with TR. The accurate identification of TV leaflets, orientation of the commissures, their spatial relationship with adjacent structures, correct anatomic and functional relationships with the other components of the TV complex, recognition of the anatomical right ventricle (RV) from the systemic ventricle and of the true congenital abnormalities of the TV from normal anatomic variants are key to diagnose primary TR and plan proper treatment. In this regard the possibility to visualize the whole TV from any perspective offered by 3DE has greatly enhanced our diagnostic accuracy

In this chapter we will review the added value of 3DE to diagnose and assess the severity of the main conditions determining primary TR.

L. P. Badano et al. (eds.), *Textbook of Three-Dimensional Echocardiography*, https://doi.org/10.1007/978-3-030-14032-8_20

Table 20.1 Additive diagnostic value of three-dimensional echocardiography over current two-dimensional technique in various tricuspid valve diseases

Tricuspid valve disease	Added diagnostic value of 3DE
Functional tricuspid regurgitation	– Exclusion of organic etiology of tricuspid regurgitation – Measurement of size and shape of tricuspid annulus – Right ventricular volumes and ejection fraction – Right atrial volume – Measurement of tricuspid valve tenting volume – Estimation of regurgitation severity independent on geometric assumptions about regurgitant orifice geometry
Tricuspid valve prolapse	– Precise identification of the prolapsing leaflet/s – Extent of the prolapse/flail – Estimation of regurgitation severity independent on geometric assumptions about regurgitant orifice geometry – Right ventricular volumes and ejection fraction – Right atrial volume
Traumatic tricuspid regurgitation	Visualization of papillary muscle and/or chordal rupture
Ebstein anomaly	– Precise morphology of tricuspid leaflets, extent of development of their formation, level of their attachment, and degree of coaptation – Visualization of the mechanism of regurgitation or stenosis – Visualization of subvalvular apparatus – Volume of the functional right ventricle
Interference from cardiac implantable electronic devices	– Precise identification of regurgitation mechanism: Valve injury during lead placement or manipulation (e.g. leaflet perforation or laceration) Mechanical interference of leads with normal leaflet excursion/coaptation Leaflet entrapment Subvalvular apparatus structure entanglement (e.g. transection of papillary muscles or chordae tendineae) Endocarditis
Infective endocarditis	– Comprehensive assessment of TV anatomy – Location of vegetation point of attachment – Vegetation characteristics and sizing (volume) – Regurgitation mechanism
Rheumatic heart disease	– Detailed leaflet anatomy – Extent of commissural fusion – Leaflet shortening and thickening – Involvement of subvalvular apparatus – Direct planimetry of residual orifice area – Right atrial volume
Carcinoid disease	– Comprehensive assessment of TV anatomy – Identification of the regions of ineffective leaflet coaptation and the lack of commissural fusion – Better assessment of regurgitation severity – Direct planimetry of residual orifice area

TV tricuspid valve

Ebstein's Anomaly

Among the congenital abnormalities of the TV, Ebstein's anomaly is the most frequent (see also Chap. 19). Ebstein's anomaly is a congenital defect of the TV in which the origins of the septal or posterior leaflets, or both, are displaced downward into the right ventricle by more than 8 mm/m^2, resulting in the atrialization of the right ventricular inflow (Fig. 20.1, Videos 20.1a and 20.1b). The leaflets are usually deformed and the commissure between the posterior and the anterior leaflet may be absent. A redundant, sail-like anterior leaflet with several fenestrations is generally present. There is a wide spectrum of the severity of TV malformation and the outcome of patients with Ebstein's anomaly is mainly dependent on its severity (Fig. 20.2, Videos 20.2a, 20.2b, and 20.2c). Although two-dimensional echocardiography can visualize the characteristic displacement of the septal leaflet attachment and the redundant and elongated anterior leaflet, the complex anatomy of the disease and the mechanisms of valve regurgitation are very difficult to assess using conventional tomographic views [7]. 3DE can provide a comprehensive morphological and quantitative assessment of anatomical abnormalities occurring in Ebstein's anomaly in most of the patients [8–10].

In adult patients with Ebstein's anomaly, 3DE is particularly useful in delineating the chordal attachment of the three leaflets of the TV. Multiple systematic cropping and sectioning of the 3DE data sets of the TV will enable the visualization of the characteristic "bubble-like" appearance of the leaflets, resulting from the bulging of the nontethered leaflet areas. In addition, an en face view of the TV is easily obtainable with 3DE, to measure the leaflet surface areas and to visualize the regions of ineffective leaflet coaptation (Fig. 20.3, Videos 20.3a and 20.3b). The ability to measure the surface and the free leaflet margin length by 3DE are particularly noteworthy in view of the current repair techniques that involve the reconstruction of a monocuspid TV using the tissue of the large anterior leaflet. Moreover, 3DE can be useful in evaluating the size of the functional right ventricle, and in estimating the severity of TR by measuring the vena contracta area on cross-sectional planes placed at the narrowest region of the 3D color Doppler jet.

Carcinoid Heart Disease

The TV is the most frequently affected valve in carcinoid heart disease [11, 12]. The valvular involvement consists of leaflet thickening with excessive fibrosis and markedly restricted motion. The fibrotic leaflets move in a stiff "board-like" fashion rather than the normal undulating motion and their restricted opening leads to the RV inflow obstruction. The TV

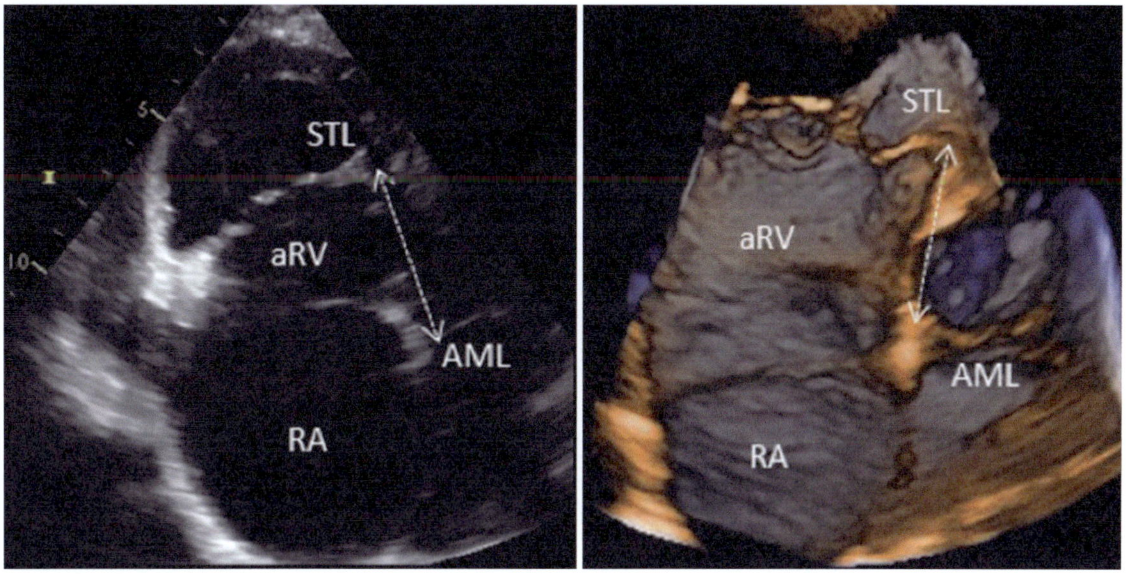

Fig. 20.1 Ebstein's anomaly. Left, two-dimensional echocardiography (Video 20.1a left). Right, three-dimensional echocardiography (Video 20.1b right). Downward displacement of the septal leaflet of the tricuspid valve (double arrow dashed line). The position of the tricuspid annulus is also visible making possible to measure the extent of the atrialized portion of the right ventricle. *AML* anterior mitral leaflet, *aRV* atrialized right ventricle, *RA* right atrium, *STL* septal tricuspid leaflet

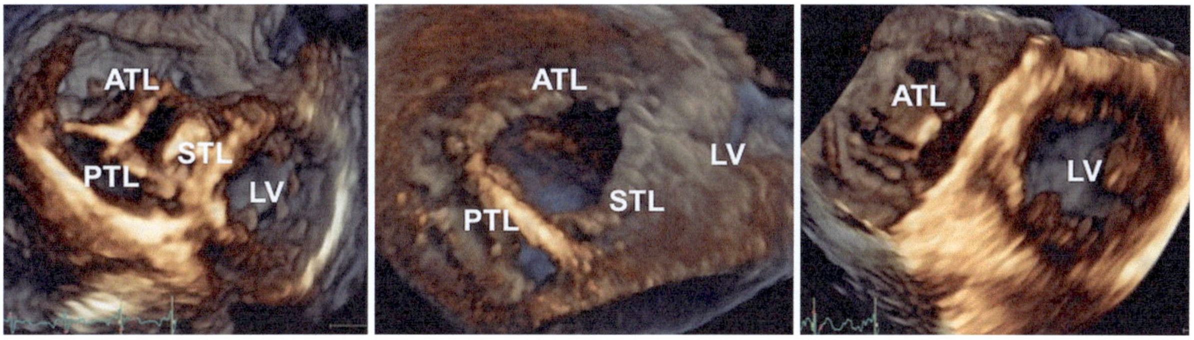

Fig. 20.2 Volume rendered *en face* view of the tricuspid valve from the ventricular perspective in three patients with Ebstein's anomaly and various degrees of valve leaflet malformation from the left (the three leaflets are well visualized with a large coaptation gap, Video 20.2a left), to the center (three leaflets with malformation of the posterior one and very large coaptation gap, Video 20.2b center) to the right (large and grossly malformed anterior leaflet with large fenestrations, Video 20.2c right). *ATL* anterior tricuspid leaflet, *LV* left ventricle, *PTL* posterior tricuspid leaflet, *STL* septal tricuspid leaflet

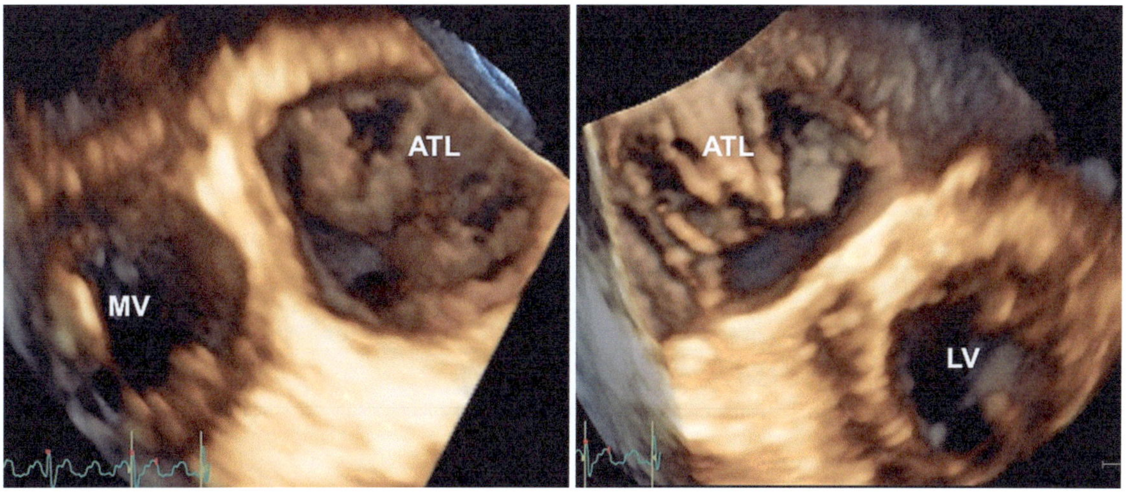

Fig. 20.3 Volume rendering of a grossly deformed tricuspid valve in a patient with Ebstein's anomaly. *En face* view of the valve from the atrial (*left,* Video 20.3a Left) and ventricular (*right,* Video 20.3b right) perspectives. *ATL* anteriori tricuspid leaflet, *LV* left ventricle, *MV* mitral valve

leaflets are usually retracted and held partially open during both systole and diastole, thus resulting in a combined tricuspid stenosis and regurgitation, the latter being predominant [1, 13] (Fig. 20.4a–d, Videos 20.4a, 20.4b, 20.4c, and 20.4d).

3DE allows an en face view of the valve from either atrial or ventricular side, as well as a detailed assessment of subvalvular apparatus (Fig. 20.5a–d, Videos 20.5a, 20.5b, 20.5c, and 20.5d). Because individual leaflet involvement can be highly variable and associated with various extents of subvalvular apparatus thickening and fibrosis, 3DE is particularly valuable in assessing patients with carcinoid disease, due to its ability to visualize simultaneously all three TV

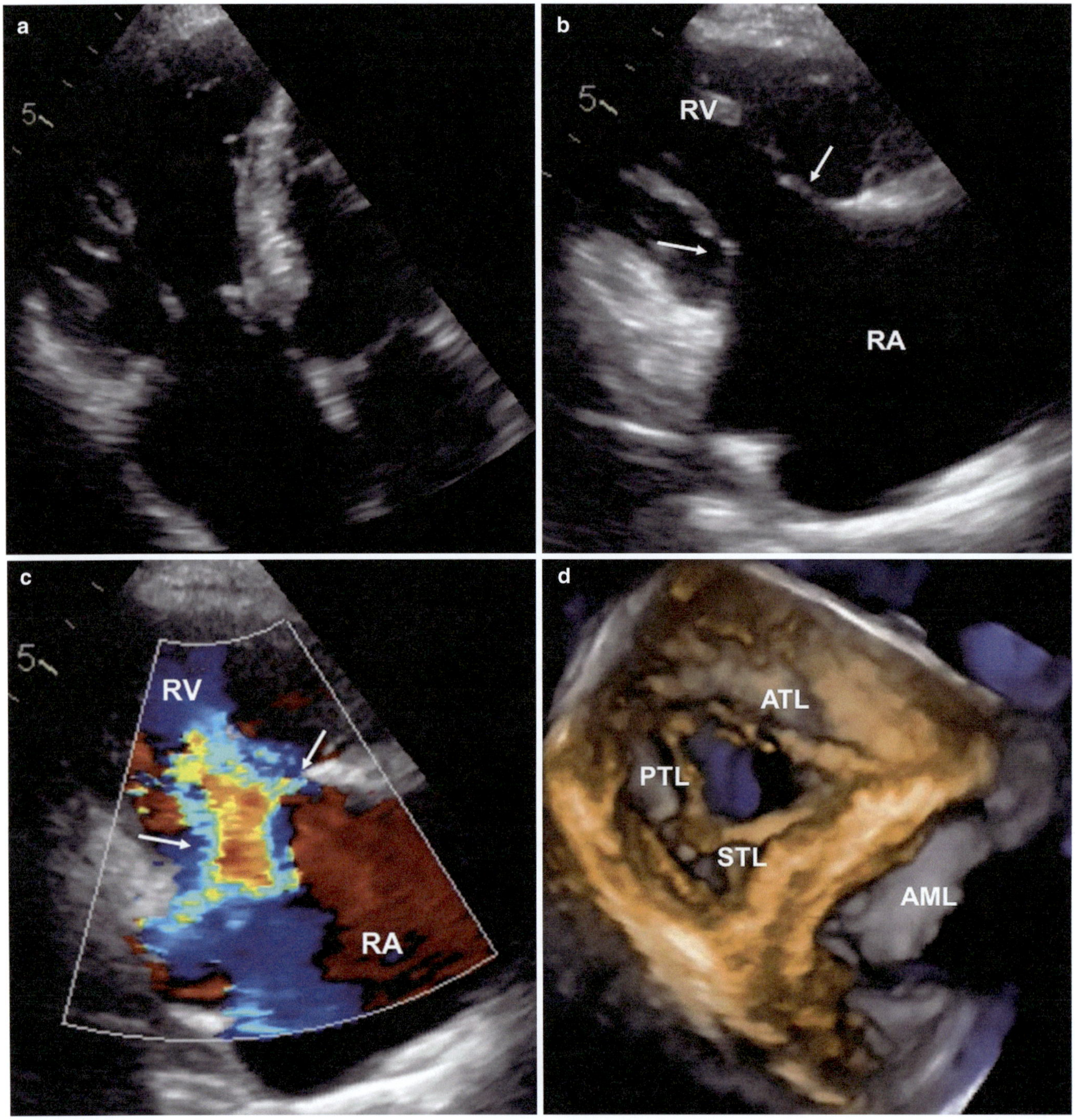

Fig. 20.4 Tricuspid valve involvement in carcinoid disease. ***Left*/(a) *and right*/(*b*) *upper panels***, two-dimensional 4-chamber and parasternal long axis views showing the thickened and retracted leaflets of the tricuspid valve (white arrows), fixed in open position in systole and in diastole (Videos 20.4a and 20.4b). ***Left lower panel*/(*c*)** Two-dimensional color Doppler in parasternal long-axis view showing the cohesistence of both stenosis and massive tricuspid regurgitation (Video 20.4c). ***Right lower panel*/(*d*)** 3D volume rendering of the tricuspid valve seen *en face* from the ventricular perspective, depicting the thickened and retracted tricuspid leaflets with a large central orifice which shows little variation in size from systole to diastole (Video 20.4d). *AML* anterior mitral leaflet, *ATL* anterior tricuspid leaflet, *PTL* posterior tricuspid leaflet, *RA* right atrium, *RV* right ventricle, *STL* septal tricuspid leaflet

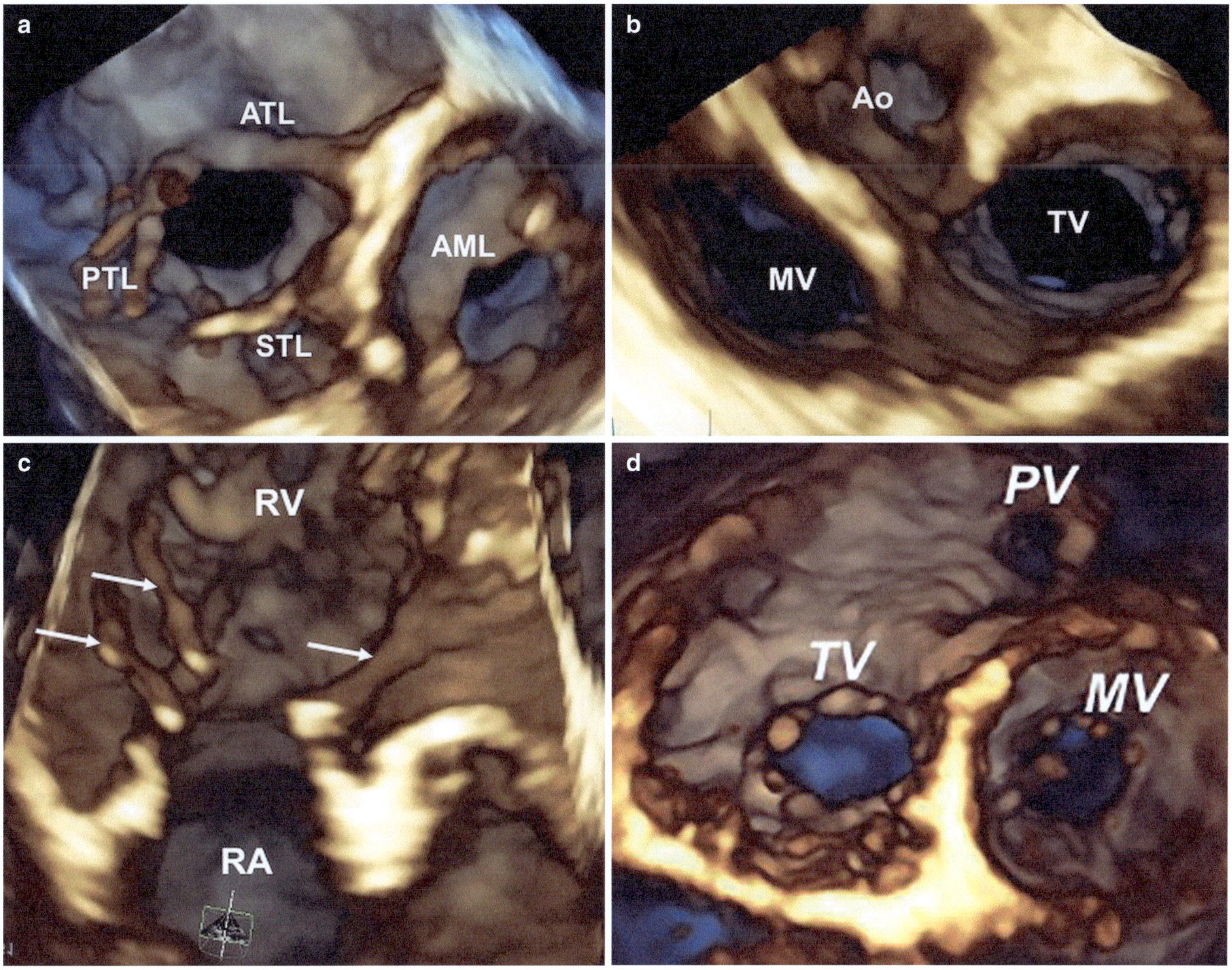

Fig. 20.5 Three-dimensional echocardiography in a patient with carcinoid disease and cardiac involvement. Volume rendering of the tricuspid valve seen from the ventricular (**a**)/***left upper panel,*** Video 20.5a) and atrial (**b**)/***right upper panel,*** Video 20.5b) perspectives. The leaflets are thickened, retracted and hypomobile. The mitral valve is thickened and hypomobile due to extension of the carcinoid to the left side through a patent foramen ovale. Longitudinal cut of the data set to assess the subvalvular apparatus (**c**)/***left lower panel,*** Video 20.5c) showing thickening and retraction of the chordae (white arrows) with fibrous plaques. Transversal cut plane showing the involvement of the pulmonary valve which shows the same anatomo-pathological features of the tricuspid valve leading to steno-insufficiency. (**d**)/***right lower panel,*** Video 20.5d) (Courtesy of Alex Felix, Rio de Janeiro, Brazil). *Ao* aortic valve, *AML* anterior mitral leaflet, *ATL* anterior tricuspid leaflet, *PTL* posterior tricuspid leaflet, *MV* mitral valve, *PV* pulmonary valve, *RA* right atrium, *RV* right ventricle, *STL* septal tricuspid leaflet, *TV* tricuspid valve

leaflets and their chordal attachments from unique perspectives. Occasionally, the pulmonary valve is involved in carcinoid disease as well (Fig. 20.5d, Lower right panel).

Cardiac Implantable Electronic Devices and Tricuspid Regurgitation

It is now well established that: (1) a sizable number of patients with permanent pacemaker, cardiac resynhronization therapy device or implantable cardioverter-defibrillator may present significant TR; (2) the leads of such devices may be the primary cause of symptomatic TR; and (3) moderate or severe TR caused by cardiac implantable electronic devices is associated to increased mortality and heart failure hospitalization rates [14]. Structural damages to the TV during implantation of cardiac electronic devices may occur by damaging the valve during lead placement or manipulation (e.g. leaflet perforation or laceration), mechanical interference of leads with normal leaflet excursion/coaptation, leaflet entrapment, subvalvular apparatus structure entanglement (e.g. transection of papillary muscles or chordae tendineae), and endocarditis.

The diagnosis of lead-induced TR may be challenging using conventional two-dimensional echocardiography, because of the difficulties in identifying the anatomical relationship between the lead and the TV complex structures. Sensitivity of transthoracic two-dimensional echocardiography for diagnosing a lead-related TR ranges between 12% and 17% [15, 16] and, till the advent of 3DE the diagnosis of lead-related TR was made, with few (intraoperative) exceptions, during post-mortem examinations.

The possibility offered by 3DE to obtain an *en face* view of all three TV leaflets in a single cut plane allows one to precisely identify the route of the lead across the right heart cavities, its position at the TV level, and its spatial relationships with the individual leaflets (Fig. 20.6a–d, Videos 20.6a, 20.6b, 20.6c, and 20.6d). Seo et al. [16] reported that in almost all patients with mild to moderate tricuspid regurgitation, the pacemaker lead position was in between the tricuspid leaflets, particularly between the posterior and the anterior or the septal leaflet. This may explain the poor performance of 2DE for an accurate diagnosis in this clinical scenario, because the TV commissures cannot be visualized by 2DE, and the posterior leaflet can be usually seen in the parasternal RV inflow view only (especially challenging in the not so rare case of a poor parasternal acoustic window). The main mechanism of severe pacemaker lead-induced

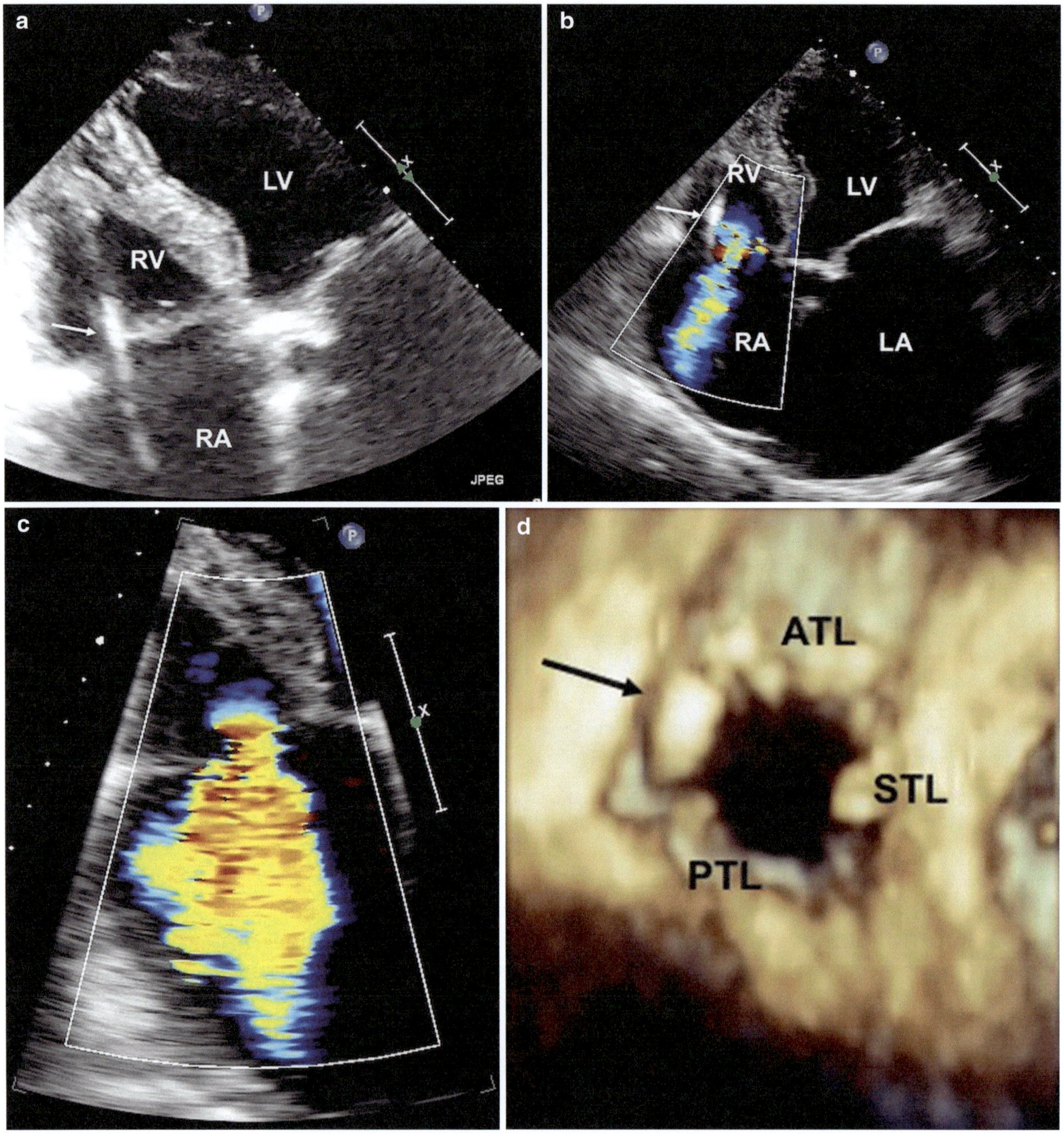

Fig. 20.6 Pacemaker lead interference with anterior leaflet mobility creating severe tricuspid regurgitation. (**a**)/***Upper left panel***, two-dimensional right ventricular focused view. Tricuspid annulus was mildly dilated (22 mm/m^2) and there was no apparent abnormality of the tricuspid valve leaflets. The pacemaker lead (white arrow) is clearly visible, but presence/absence of interference with anterior leaflet motion was difficult to assess (Video 20.6a). (**b**)/***Upper right panel***, color Doppler shows significant tricuspid regurgitation in a patient with dilated atria (Video 20.6b). (**c**)/***Lower left panel***, Vena contracta and PISA radius (at 30 cm/s) were 8 and 9 mm, respectively (Video 20.6c). (**d**)/***Lower right panel***, Volume rendering of the tricuspid valve seen *en face* from the ventricular perspective showing the position of the pacemaker lead (black arrow) which restricts the motion of the anterior tricuspid leaflet (Video 20.6d). *ATL* anterior tricuspid leaflet, *LA* left atrium, *LV* left ventricle, *PTL* posterior tricuspid leaflet, *RA* right atrium, *RV* right ventricle, *STL* septal tricuspid leaflet

tricuspid regurgitation was the interference with the effective TV leaflet coaptation (7/12 patients), the posterior leaflet being obstructed in four patients, and the septal leaflet in three. Importantly, this study confirmed the findings of Schnabel et al. [17], who reported an easier visualization of the TV leaflets by transthoracic 3DE in patients with RV dysfunction than in healthy subjects.

Mediratta et al. [18] used transthoracic 3DE to examine 121 patients with implanted cardiac devices and found that lead position was clearly identifiable in 90% of the patients. They showed that leads positioned against TV leaflets impinge upon or restrict leaflet motion and cause TR (Fig. 20.6). Conversely, leads positioned in one of the commissures (Fig. 20.7a, b, Videos 20.7a and 20.7b) or those which remain mobile in the center of the TV orifice, do not interfere with leaflet mobility. Addetia et al. [19] used transthoracic 3DE to study 100 patients before and after implantation of cardiac electronic devices. They found that device leads interfered with TV leaflet mobility in 45%, being the septal tricuspid leaflet the most frequently affected (in almost 50% of the cases). On multivariable analysis, only pre-implantation vena contracta width of the TR flow and the presence of an interfering device lead were independently associated to post-device TR. Furthermore, the presence of an interfering device lead was the only factor associate to post-implant TR worsening.

Traumatic Tricuspid Regurgitation

Traumatic TR is a rare cardiovascular complication that may occur as a consequence of blunt chest trauma, with disruption of chordal structures, or from internal (usually iatrogenic) trauma from a pacemaker lead, a stiff guidewire, a bioptome during RV endomyocardial biopsy, or during radiofrequency ablation for treatment of arrhythmias when devices can perforate TV leaflets or damage subvalvular chordal apparatus.

Injures of heart valves during blunt chest trauma are relatively rare. However, the TV is relatively often involved because the RV is situated just behind the sternum and has a predisposition to anteroposterior compression injuries. A sudden increase in RV pressure during the end-diastolic phase may cause a serious traction on both the valvular and subvalvular apparatus that may result in papillary muscle/chordal rupture or leaflet damage. Usually, the anterior papillary muscle is the most frequently involved

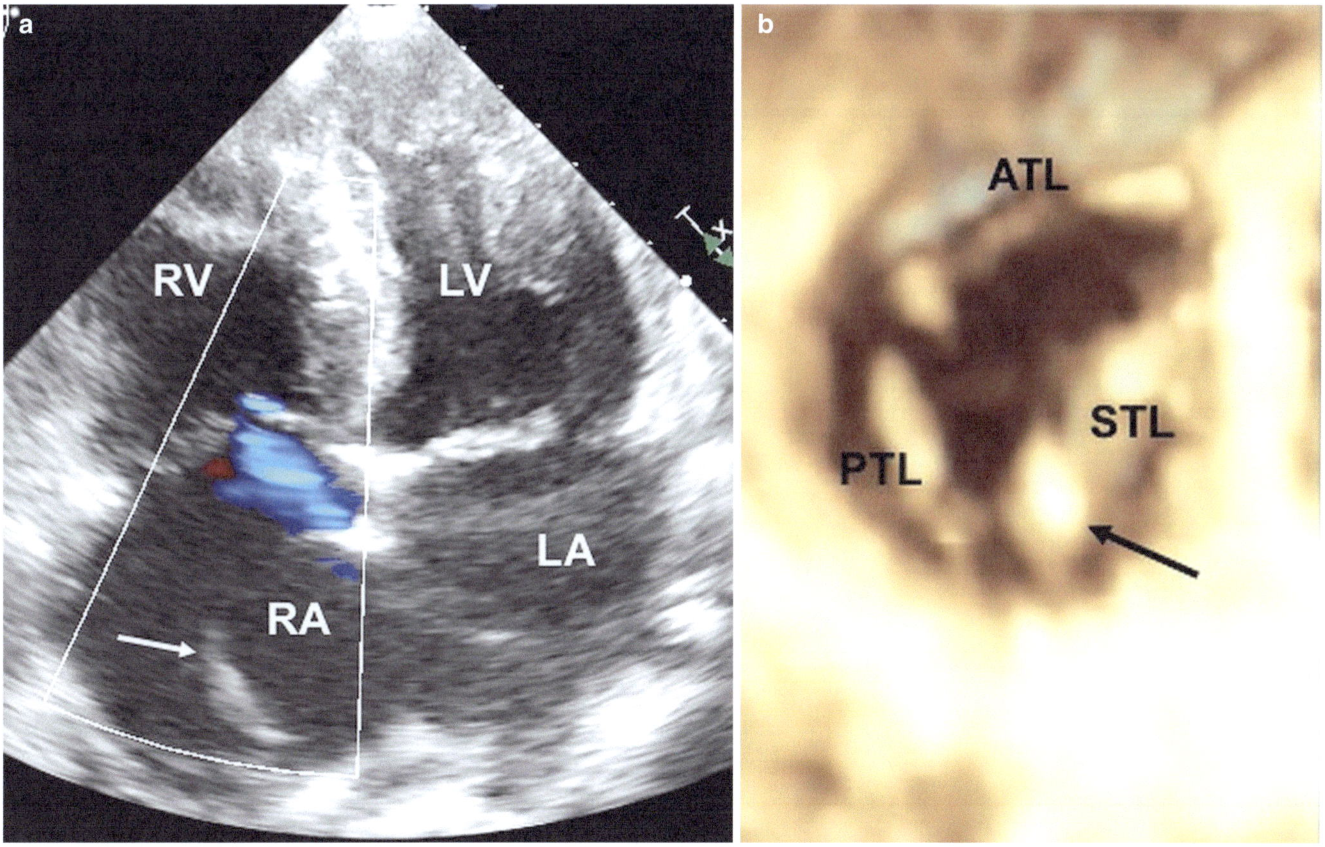

Fig. 20.7 Normal pace-maker lead position in a patient with mild tricuspid regurgitation. (**a**)/***Left***, Two-dimensional apical 4-chamber view with color Doppler showing a mild tricuspid regurgitation after pacemaker implantation (Video 20.7a Left). (**b**)/***Right***, Volume rendering of the tricuspid valve seen *en face* from the ventricular perspective the black arrow shows the pace-maker lead positioned in the commissure between the posterior and the septal tricuspid leaflets with no interference with valve leaflet motion (Video 20.7b Right). *ATL* anterior tricuspid leaflet, *LA* left atrium, *LV* left ventricle, *PTL* posterior tricuspid leaflet, *RA* right atrium, *RV* right ventricle, *STL* septal tricuspid leaflet

TV structure, but any of the components of the TV apparatus may be damaged. This complication may remain asymptomatic for years and traumatic TR remains undetected for years in many patients until they undergo occasional physical examination or echocardiography for other indications, or RV failure occurs. When echocardiography is performed many years after the trauma (often the patients do not remember it anymore) the etiology of the severe TR is difficult to identify with conventional two-dimensional echocardiography. 3DE can accurately delineate the anatomy of the TV and identify the flail leaflet(s) and the involvement of the subvalvular apparatus (ruptured chordae and/or papillary muscle), and may help in the decision making and in planning the surgical correction [20] (Fig. 20.8a–d, Videos 20.8a, 20.8b, 20.8c, and 20.8d, Fig. 20.9, Videos 20.9a and 20.9b).

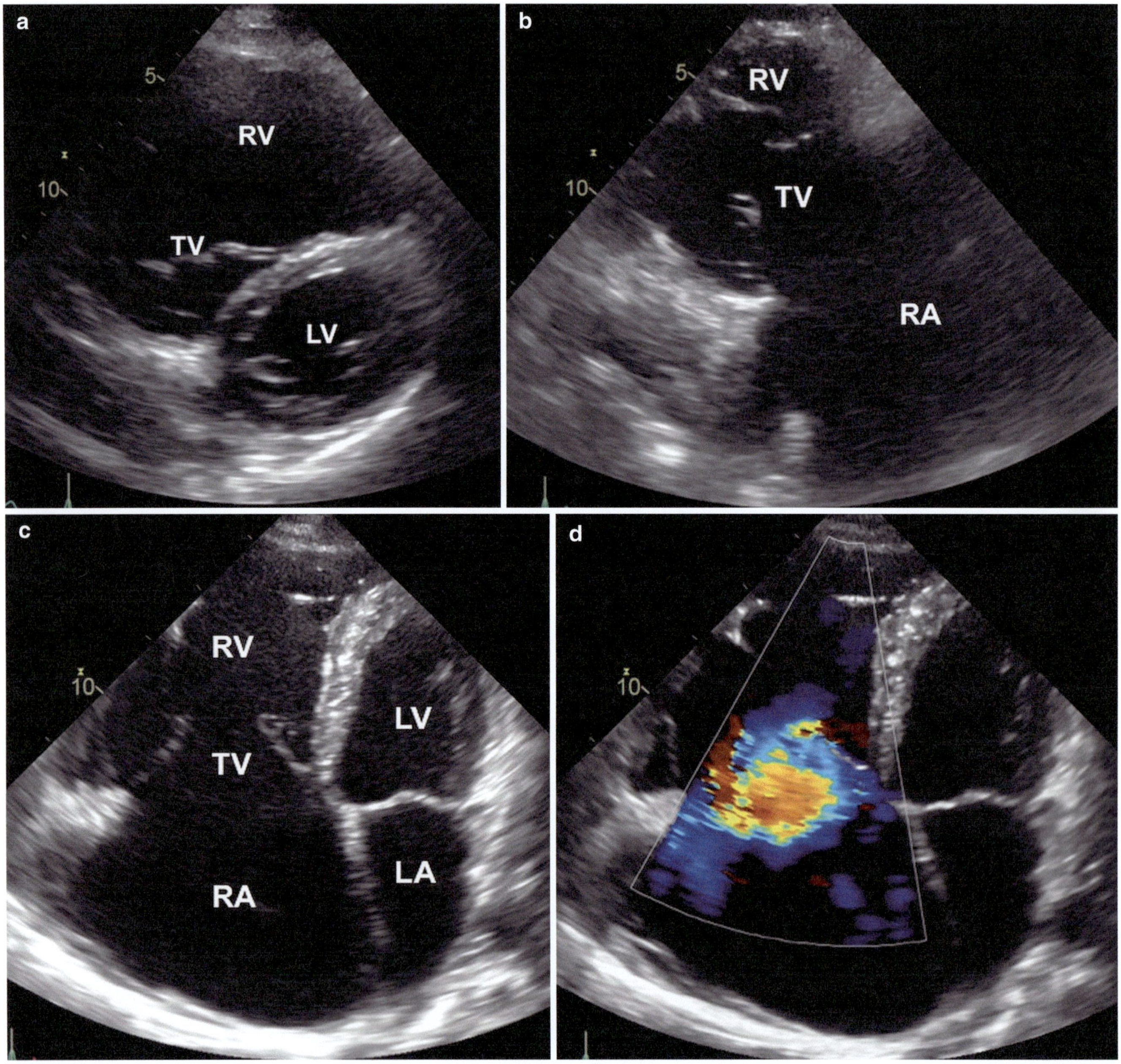

Fig. 20.8 Conventional two-dimensional and color Doppler echocardiography in a patient with blunt chest trauma occurred 25 years before the echocardiographic study. (**a**)/***Upper left panel***, parasternal short-axis view of the tricuspid valve (Video 20.8a). (**b**)/***Upper right panel***, parasternal long-axis view of right ventricular inflow showing two tethered tricuspid leaflets and a large coaptation gap (Video 20.8b). (**c**)/***Lower left panel***, apical 4-chamber view (Video 20.8c). (**d**)/***Lower right panel***, same apical 4-chamber view as in the left panel with color Doppler showing severe tricuspid regurgitation (Video 20.8d). *LA* left atrium, *LV* left ventricle, *RA* right atrium, *RV* right ventricle, *TV* tricuspid valve

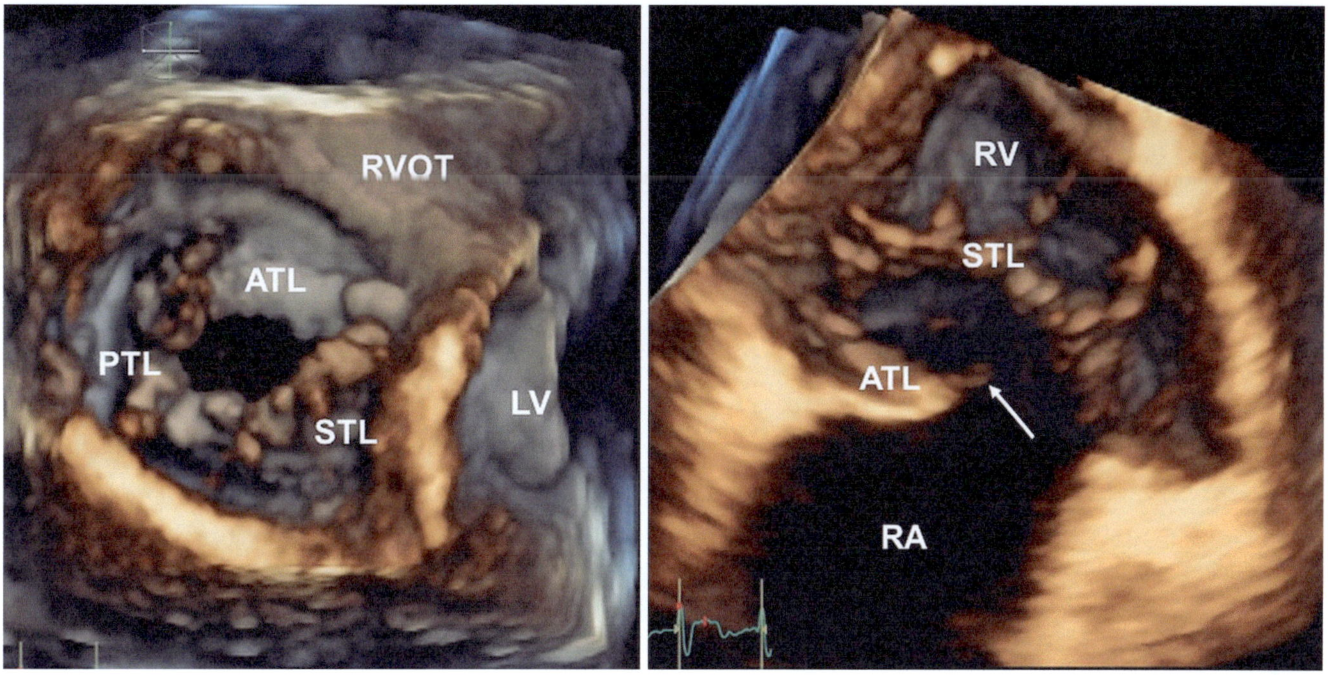

Fig. 20.9 Transthoracic three-dimensional echocardiography with volume rendering of the same tricuspid valve illustrated in Fig. 20.8. *Left panel*, en-face view from the ventricular perspective showing that only the septal and posterior tricuspid leaflets are tethered, whereas the anterior leaflet is flailing (Video 20.9a left). *Right panel*, Longitudinal cut at the level of the anterior leaflet showing its flail and the ruptured chorda (white arrow, Video 20.9b Right). *ATL* anterior tricuspid leaflet, *PTL* posterior tricuspid leaflet, *RA* right atrium, *RV* right ventricle, *RVOT* right ventricular outflow tract, *STL* septal tricuspid leaflet

Tricuspid Valve Diseases With Restricted Leaflet Mobility

Although the mitral and the aortic valve are the two most involved valves in rheumatic heart disease, the TV is frequently involved too. A recent echocardiographic study performed in Bangladesh reported that out of 173 patients with chronic rheumatic disease, 36 (21%) had evidence of TV involvement (15 patients with prevalent tricuspid stenosis and 21 with prevalent regurgitation) [21]. In addition to carcinoid heart disease (see above), valvulopathies associated with Fen-Phen and methysergide are also characterized by thickened fibrotic and hypomobile tricuspid leaflets, with various degrees of valve stenosis and regurgitation.

Conventional two-dimensional images show thickening and shortening of the TV leaflets, which may exhibit some doming in diastole. Doppler recordings of transtricuspid flow velocity allow the calculation of mean gradient and of the valve area by pressure half-time method, as described for the mitral valve. However, unlike what is routinely done for assessing mitral stenosis severity, neither transthoracic nor transesophageal two-dimensional echocardiography can provide en face views of the stenotic orifice and the fused commissures of the TV (Fig. 20.10a–d, Videos 20.10a, 20.10b, 20.10c, and 20.10d). Using 3DE, the stenotic orifice of the TV can be clearly visualized from the ventricular side and planimetered [1, 22] (Fig. 20.11).

Degenerative Tricuspid Valve Regurgitation

The same myxomatous changes that occur in mitral valve disease may also affect TV leaflets and chordae tendineae resulting in TV prolapse and regurgitation (Fig. 20.12, Video 20.11). Prolapse of the mitral valve is usually present in these patients as well. Prolapse of the TV has been reported in about 20% of patients with mitral valve prolapse (Fig. 20.13, Video 20.12). TV prolapse may also be associated with atrial septal defect.

Infective Endocarditis of the Tricuspid Valve

Vegetations or masses of the TV apparatus can be nicely characterized as location, shape and size more readily and accurate with 3DE (Fig. 20.14, Videos 20.13a and 20.13b, Fig. 20.15, Video 20.14). 3DE can also depict leaflet perforations/prolapse and color Doppler supports the diagnosis with information on the mechanism and the severity of TR. 3DE is particularly useful in patients with prosthetic devices (e.g., pacemaker or intracardiac defibrillator leads, or TV prostheses) to assess the precise location of the vegetations and their relationship with the prosthetic structures [23] (Fig. 20.16, Video 20.15).

It is a fact that two-dimensional echocardiography has a good sensitivity to detect pathologic masses and to assess

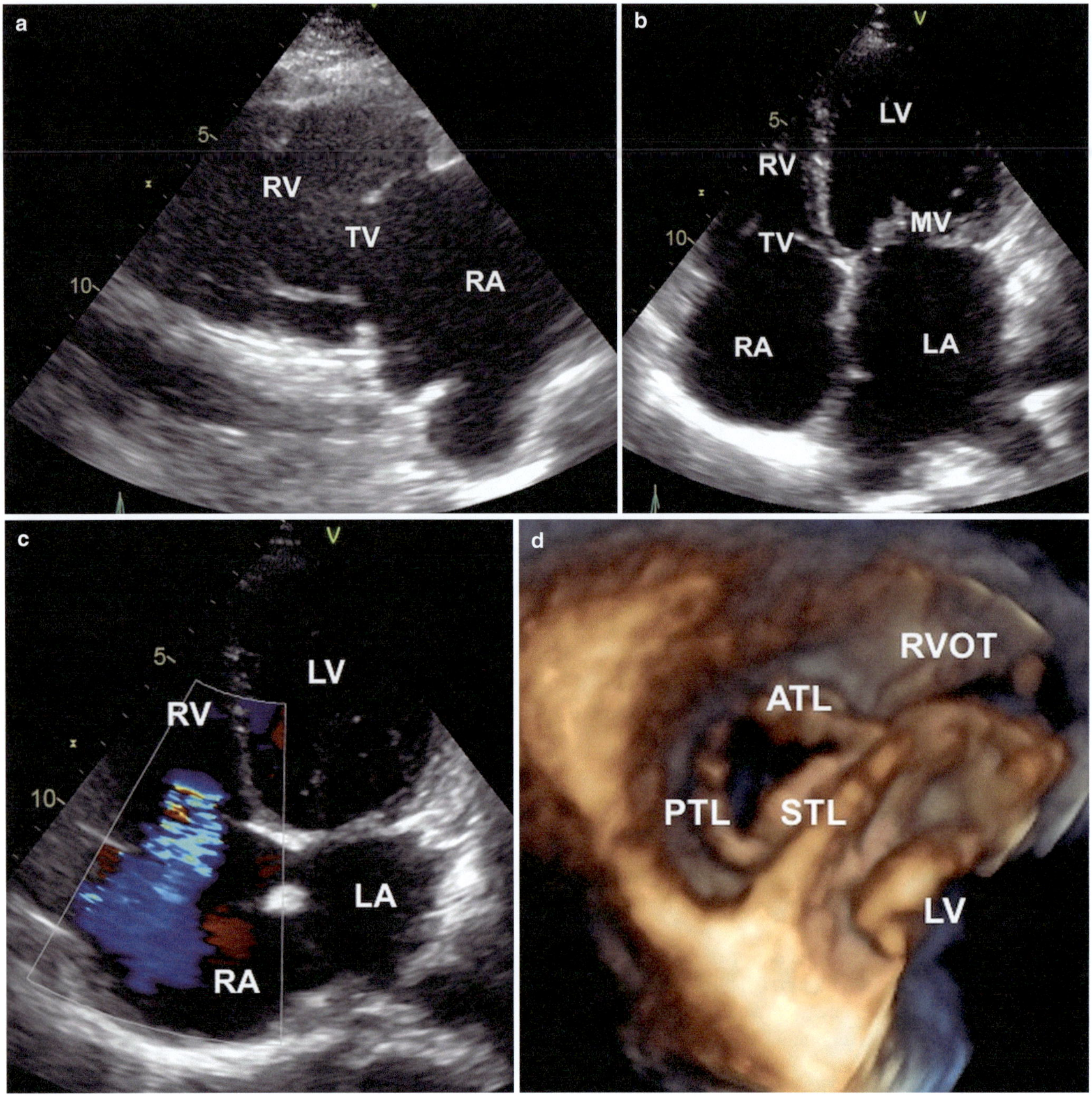

Fig. 20.10 Rheumatic tricuspid valve diseases with prevalent regurgitation. (**a**)/***Upper left panel,*** parastenal long axis view of right ventricular inflow (Video 20.10a). The doming of the thickened tricuspid leaflets is visualized. (**b**)/***Upper right panel,*** Apical 4-chamber view showing the thickened and hypomobile tricuspid valve leaflets (Video 20.10b). (**c**)/***Lower left panel***, Apical 4-chamber view with color Doppler showing the severe tricuspid regurgitation with a large vena contracta width (Video 20.10c). (**d**)/***Lower right panel,*** three-dimensional echocardiography with volume rendering of the tricuspid valve from the ventricular perspective. The *en-face* view of the valve allows the visualization of the thickened leaflets, the fused commissures and the size of the residual opening orifice (Video 20.10d). *ATL* anterior tricuspid leaflet, *LA* left atrium, *LV* left ventricle, *MV* mitral valve, *PTL* posterior tricuspid leaflet, *RA* right atrium, *RV* right ventricle, *RVOT* right ventricular outflow tract, *STL* septal tricuspid leaflet, *TV* tricuspid valve

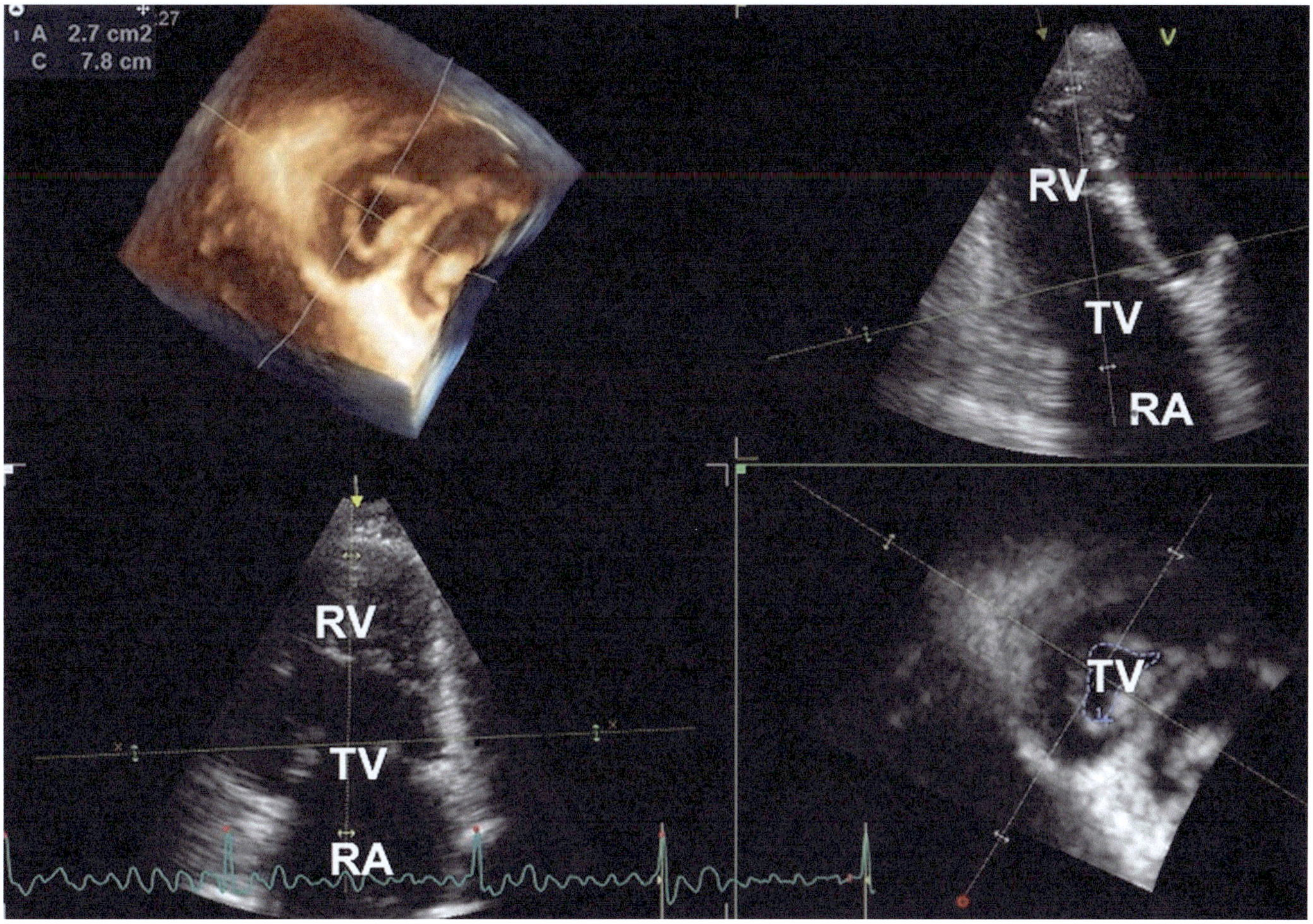

Fig. 20.11 Quantitative assessment of the severity of the tricuspid stenosis using three-dimensional echocardiography. Similarly to what is done for the mitral stenosis, a cut plane (green line) is positioned at the tip of the tricuspid leaflets in open position and oriented perpendicular to the opening axis of the valve (yellow line) to obtain a short axis view of the tricuspid orifice (right lower panel) that can be planimetered. *RA* right atrium, *RV* right ventricle, *TV* tricuspid valve

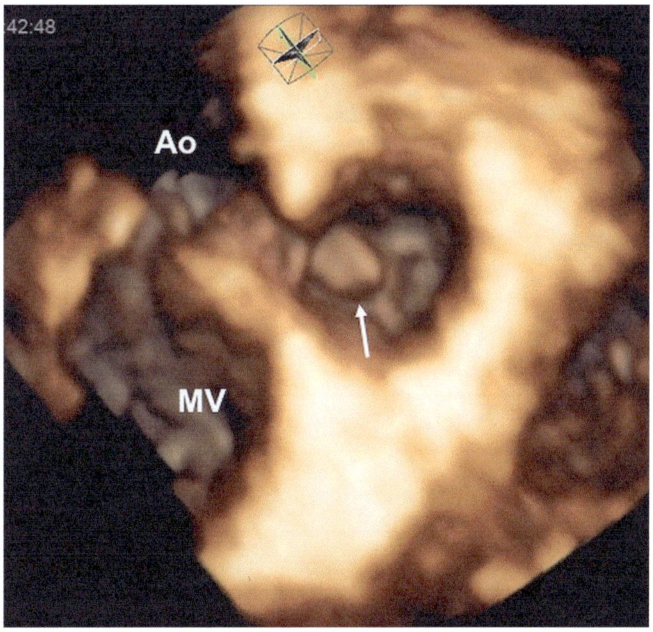

Fig. 20.12 Degenerative tricuspid regurgitation. Prolapse (white arrow) of the septal tricuspid leaflet (Video 20.11). *Ao* aortic valve, *MV* mitral valve

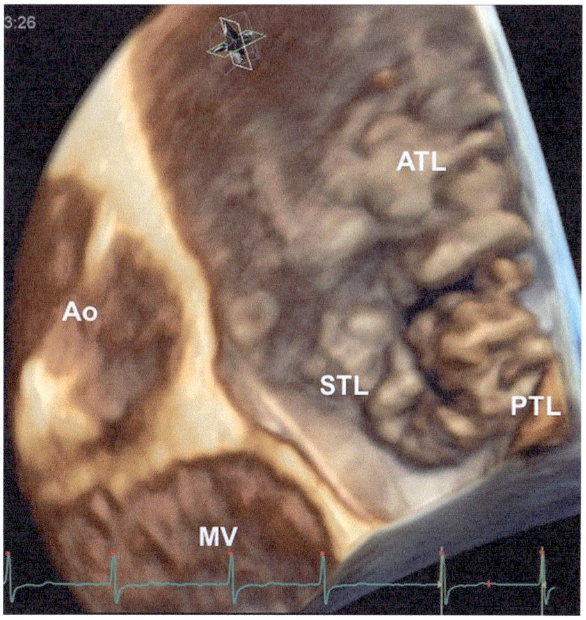

Fig. 20.13 Volume rendering of the tricuspid valve seen from the atrial perspective in a patient with Barlow disease. The bubble like morphology of the tricuspid valve leaflet and the enlarged tricuspid annulus were well visualized (Video 20.12). *Ao* aortic valve, *ATL* anterior tricuspid leaflet, *MV* mitral valve, *PTL* posterior tricuspid leaflet, *STL* septal tricuspid leaflet

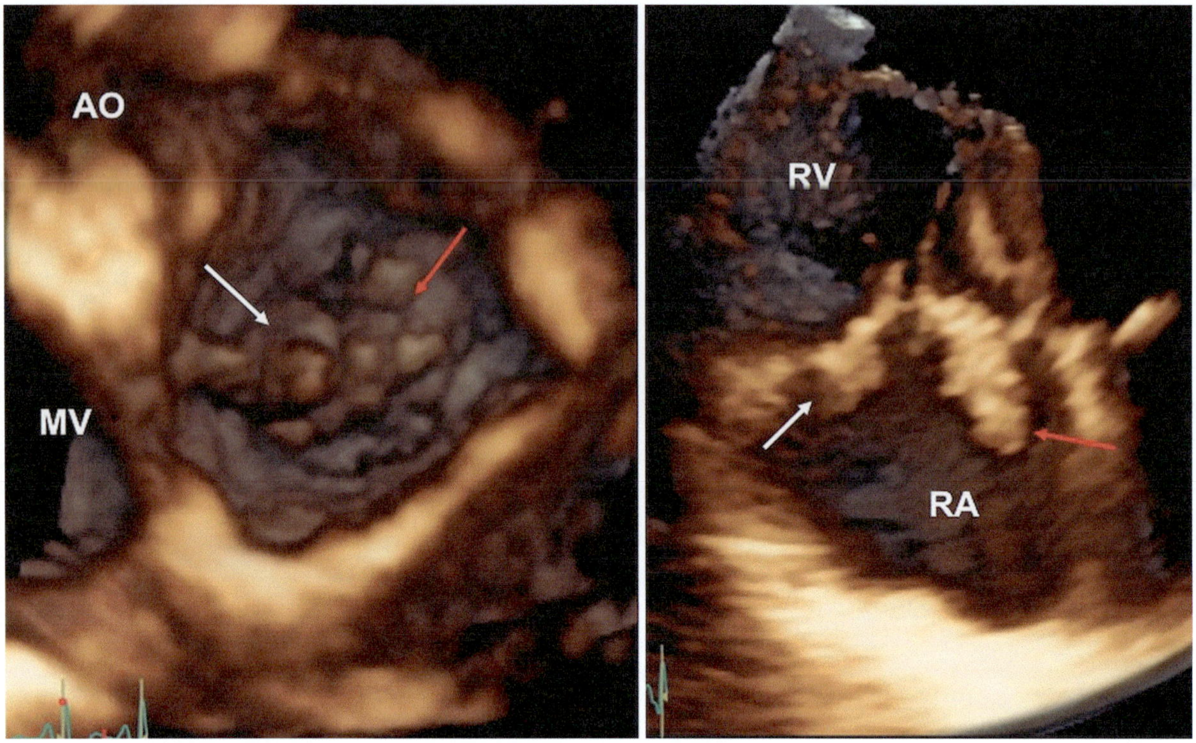

Fig. 20.14 Infective endocarditis of the tricuspid valve in a drug abuser. Two large vegetation were visualized on the septal (red arrow) and anterior (white arrow) leaflets of the tricuspid valve. Transthoracic 3DE and volume rendering of the tricuspid valve displayed from the atrial perspective (*left panel*, Video 20.13a left) and using a longitudinal cut plane at the level of the valve (*right panel*, Video 20.13b right). The site of attachment and the size of the vegetations as well as their functional interference with the valve function can be appreciated. *Ao* aortic valve, *MV* mitral valve, *RA* right atrium, *RV* right ventricle

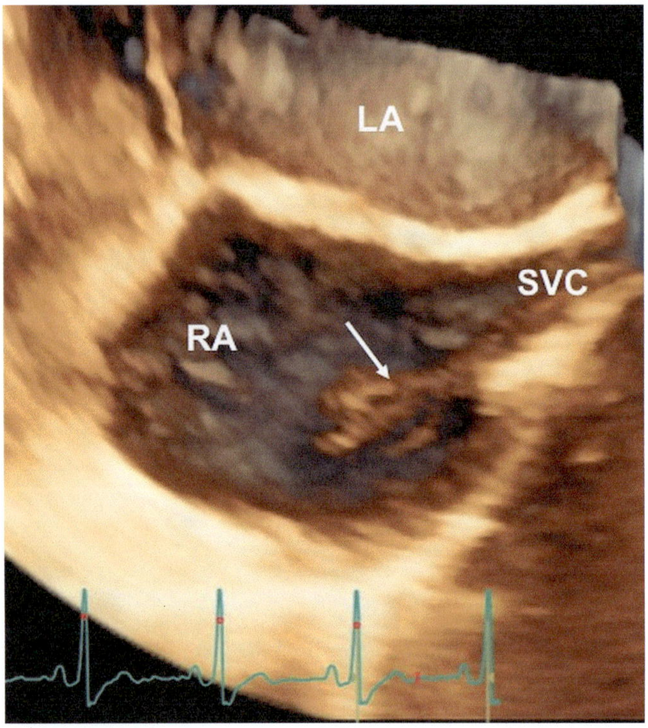

Fig. 20.15 Infective endocarditis localized at the origin of the superior vena cava after removal of infected pace-maker lead. Transesophageal 3DE with the volume rendering of the right atrium and origin of the superior vena cava (Video 20.14). A long and floating vegetation is attached at the origin of the superior vena cava (with arrow). *LA* left atrium, *RA* right atrium, *SVC* superior vena cava

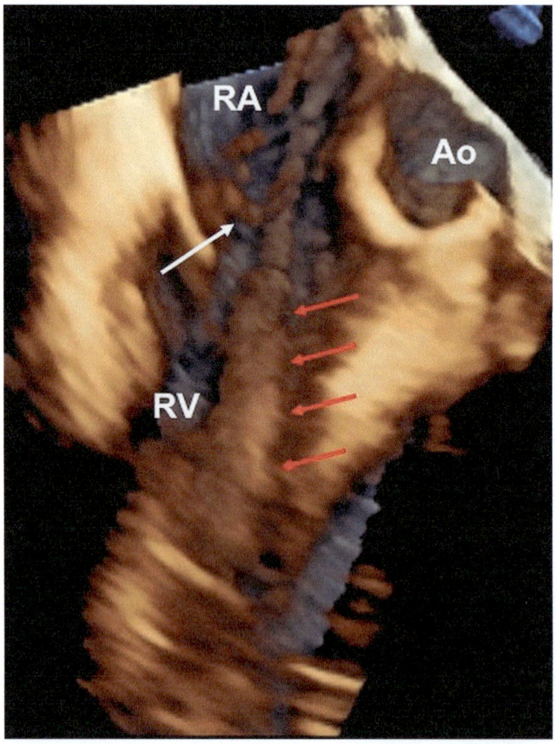

Fig. 20.16 Lead-dependent infective endocarditis. Transesophageal 3DE and volume rendering display of a large endocarditis mass wrapped around the ventricular portion of the lead of an implantable intracardiac defibrillator (red arrows). A mobile vegetation attached to the tricuspid valve is also visualized (white arrow). (Video 20.15). *Ao* aortic valve, *RA* right atrium, *RV* right ventricle

their mobility, due to its high temporal and spatial resolution. However, its tomographic nature and limited views induce the inherent risk of missing the diagnosis when the vegetations develop outside the standard two-dimensional views of the TV, as well as uncertainties and errors regarding their true size and precise insertion. Vegetation size is an important predictor for embolic events and for response to treatment. The measurements of the maximum dimension(s) by two-dimensional echocardiography are routinely used to quantify the vegetation size. However, most vegetations are irregularly shaped and highly mobile, making it difficult to accurately image them in one tomographic view or select the largest diameter. The selection of a diameter that is not truly the largest may lead to the underestimation of the vegetation size and to the misinterpretation of patient prognosis. 3DE images the entire volume of the vegetation mass, allowing for accurate measurements from multiple planes, properly aligned to delineate the true largest dimensions.

References

1. Muraru D, Badano LP, Sarais C, Solda E, Iliceto S. Evaluation of tricuspid valve morphology and function by transthoracic three-dimensional echocardiography. Curr Cardiol Rep. 2011;13:242–9.
2. Badano LP, Agricola E, Perez de Isla L, Gianfagna P, Zamorano JL. Evaluation of the tricuspid valve morphology and function by transthoracic real-time three-dimensional echocardiography. Eur J Echocardiogr. 2009;10:477–84.
3. Stankovic I, Daraban AM, Jasaityte R, Neskovic AN, Claus P, Voigt JU. Incremental value of the en face view of the tricuspid valve by two-dimensional and three-dimensional echocardiography for accurate identification of tricuspid valve leaflets. J Am Soc Echocardiogr. 2014;27:376–84.
4. Addetia K, Yamat M, Mediratta A, et al. Comprehensive two-dimensional interrogation of the tricuspid valve using knowledge derived from three-dimensional echocardiography. J Am Soc Echocardiogr. 2016;29:74–82.
5. Anwar AM, Geleijnse ML, Soliman OI, et al. Assessment of normal tricuspid valve anatomy in adults by real-time three-dimensional echocardiography. Int J Cardiovasc Imaging. 2007;23:717–24.
6. Muraru D, Hahn RT, Soliman OI, Faletra F, Badano LP. Three-dimensional echocardiography in imaging the tricuspid valve. JACC Cardiovasc Imaging. 2019;12:500–15.
7. Greutmann M, Buechel ERV, Jost CA. The caveats of cardiac imaging in Ebstein anomaly. 2018. pii: S1050-1738(18)30030-6. https://doi.org/10.1016/j.tcm.2018.02.007. [Epub ahead of print]
8. Patel V, Nanda NC, Rajdev S, et al. Live/real time three-dimensional transthoracic echocardiographic assessment of Ebstein's anomaly. Echocardiography. 2005;22:847–54.
9. Bharucha T, Anderson RH, Lim ZS, Vettukattil JJ. Multiplanar review of three-dimensional echocardiography gives new insights into the morphology of Ebstein's malformation. Cardiol Young. 2010;20:49–53.
10. van Noord PT, Scohy TV, McGhie J, Bogers AJ. Three-dimensional transesophageal echocardiography in Ebstein's anomaly. Interact Cardiovasc Thorac Surg. 2010;10:836–7.
11. Bhattacharyya S, Burke M, Caplin ME, Davar J. Utility of 3D transoesophageal echocardiography for the assessment of tricuspid and pulmonary valves in carcinoid heart disease. Eur J Echocardiogr. 2011;12:E4.
12. Bhattacharyya S, Toumpanakis C, Burke M, Taylor AM, Caplin ME, Davar J. Features of carcinoid heart disease identified by 2- and 3-dimensional echocardiography and cardiac MRI. Circ Cardiovasc Imaging. 2010;3:103–11.
13. Muraru D, Tuveri MF, Marra MP, Badano LP, Iliceto S. Carcinoid tricuspid valve disease: incremental value of three-dimensional echocardiography. Eur Heart J Cardiovasc Imaging. 2012;13:329.
14. Chang JD, Manning WJ, Ebrille E, Zimetbaum PJ. Tricuspid valve dysfunction following pacemaker or cardioverter-defibrillator implantation. J Am Coll Cardiol. 2017;69:2331–41.
15. Lin G, Nishimura RA, Connolly HM, Dearani JA, Sundt TM III, Hayes DL. Severe symptomatic tricuspid valve regurgitation due to permanent pacemaker or implantable cardioverter-defibrillator leads. J Am Coll Cardiol. 2005;45:1672–5.
16. Seo Y, Ishizu T, Nakajima H, Sekiguchi Y, Watanabe S, Aonuma K. Clinical utility of 3-dimensional echocardiography in the evaluation of tricuspid regurgitation caused by pace-maker leads. Circ J. 2008;72:1465–70.
17. Schnabel R, Khaw AV, von Bardeleben RS, et al. Assessment of the tricuspid valve morphology by transthoracic real-time-3D-echocardiography. Echocardiography. 2005;22:15–23.
18. Mediratta A, Addetia K, Yamat M, et al. 3D echocardiographic location of implantable device leads and mechanism of associated tricuspid regurgitation. JACC Cardiovasc Imaging. 2014;7:337–47.
19. Addetia K, Maffessanti F, Mediratta A, et al. Impact of implantable transvenous device lead location on severity of tricuspid regurgitation. J Am Soc Echocardiogr. 2014;27:1164–75.
20. Looi JL, Lee AP, Wong RH, Yu CM. 3D echocardiography for traumatic tricuspid regurgitation. JACC Cardiovasc Imaging. 2012;5:1285–7.
21. Rashid MB, Parvin T, Ahmed CM, et al. Pattern and extent of tricuspid valve involvement in chronic rheumatic heart disease. Mymensingh Med J. 2018;27:120–5.
22. Faletra F, La Marchesina U, Bragato R, De Chiara F. Three dimensional transthoracic echocardiography images of tricuspid stenosis. Heart. 2005;91:499.
23. Naqvi TZ, Rafie R, Ghalichi M. Real-time 3D TEE for the diagnosis of right-sided endocarditis in patients with prosthetic devices. JACC Cardiovasc Imaging. 2010;3:325–7.

Functional Tricuspid Regurgitation

21

Jae-Kwan Song, Denisa Muraru, Andrada-Camelia Guta, and Luigi P. Badano

Abstract

Functional tricuspid regurgitation (FTR) is an important prognosticator in many cardiac diseases. Although surgical intervention has been being frequently applied, the success of current repair techniques is often uncertain and observation of residual or progressive FTR after tricuspid valve annuloplasty is not uncommon. Standard views obtained with two-dimensional transthoracic echocardiography, due to its inherent limitations, failed to evaluate geometric changes associated with FTR accurately. Transthoracic three-dimensional echocardiography (3DE) has revolutionized our approach for better understanding the 3D geometry of the tricuspid annulus both in normal subjects and in patients with FTR. The tricuspid annulus was found to be a non-planar structure with a distinct bimodal or saddle-shaped pattern like the mitral annulus, whereas, in patients with FTR, the annular area was larger and the annulus was flatter with markedly decreased annular height, which diminished the saddle shape. Potential contribution of right ventricular or right atrial geometric changes to the tricuspid annulus remodeling in FTR can also be evaluated using transthoracic 3DE data sets. 3DE, performed before and after the tricuspid annuloplasty, can provide an excellent opportunity to evaluate geometric changes associated with persistent or progressive FTR after the tricuspid annuloplasty. The current surgical approach can achieve tricuspid annulus size reduction at the expense of aggravation of leaflet tenting, which can explain suboptimal surgical results. 3DE color Doppler images can be adequately used for cross-sectional images of the vena contracta using multiplanar reconstruction images, which is useful to assess the severity of FTR. Thus, comprehensive and accurate evaluation of FTR is possible using 3DE and its impact to improve clinical outcome should be further tested.

Keywords

Functional tricuspid regurgitation · 3-Dimensional echocardiography · Tricuspid annulus · Leaflet tethering · Pathophysiology

Functional tricuspid regurgitation (FTR) is frequently caused by increased right ventricular (RV) pressure overloading and associated with advanced stages of left-sided valve, myocardial, or pulmonary diseases [1], and development of FTR has been proved to be an independent factor associated with increased mortality and morbidity [2–5]. Thus, there has been an increasing tendency to repair the tricuspid valve (TV) to abolish or decrease FTR at the time of concomitant surgery for left-sided disease [6, 7]. However, the outcome of the current TV repair procedures is sometimes unpredictable and residual or progressive TR after TV annuloplasty is not uncommon [8–10]. Although it is generally believed that FTR results from a combination of tricuspid annular dilatation and valve apparatus deformation, the inherent limitations of conventional two-dimensional imaging techniques used to assess patients with FTR have limited our understanding of the pathophysiology of this valve disease. Three-dimensional echocardiography (3DE), by allowing an anatomically sound visualization of the TV from any perspective as well as the measurement of the geometry of its components and of the size and function of the right atrium and RV, can contribute to

J.-K. Song (✉)
Department of Cardiology, Valvular Heart Disease Center, Asan Medical Center Heart Institute, Research Institute for Valvular Heart Disease, University of Ulsan College of Medicine, Seoul, South Korea
e-mail: jksong@amc.seoul.kr

D. Muraru · L. P. Badano
University of Milano-Bicocca, and Istituto Auxologico Italiano, IRCCS, San Luca Hospital, Milano, Italy
e-mail: denisa.muraru@unimib.it, denisa.muraru@unipd.it; luigi.badano@unimib.it

A.-C. Guta
Department of Cardiology, "Prof. Dr. C.C. Iliescu" Institute of Cardiovascular Diseases, Bucharest, Romania

L. P. Badano et al. (eds.), *Textbook of Three-Dimensional Echocardiography*, https://doi.org/10.1007/978-3-030-14032-8_21

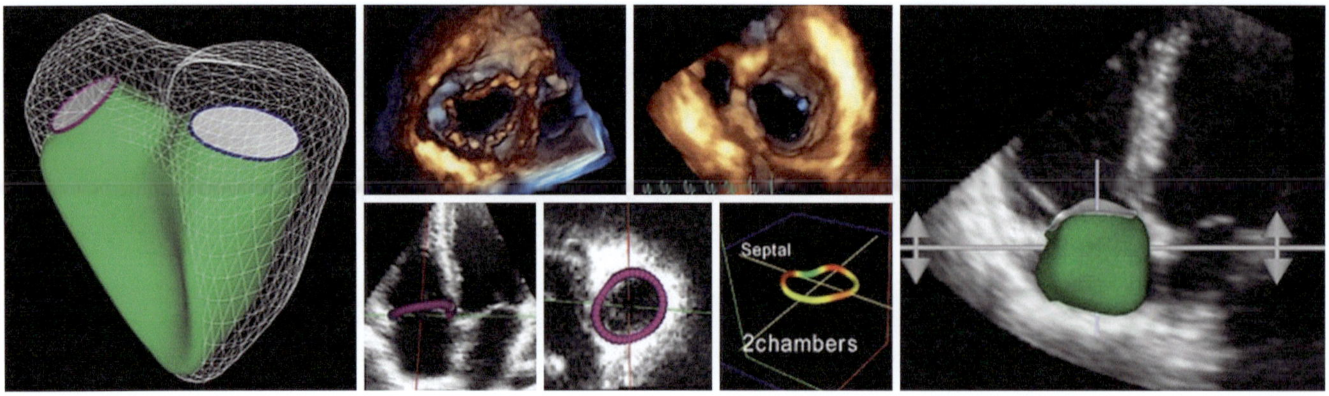

Fig. 21.1 Example of comprehensive assessment of the mechanism of functional tricuspid regurgitation. On the left, quantitative analysis of right ventricular volumes, shape and function. In the center, morphology of tricuspid leaflets and measurement of tricuspid annulus size and function. On the right, measurement of right atrial volumes and function

improve our understanding of the mechanisms leading to FTR in various cardiac conditions and thus providing better therapeutic options (Fig. 21.1).

Geometric Changes of Tricuspid Valve Complex in Functional Tricuspid Regurgitation

3DE has revolutionized our approach to assess the TV apparatus in normal subjects and in patients with FTR [11–13]. Transthoracic 3DE can visualize all three TV leaflets simultaneously (Fig. 21.2) and full volume datasets of the TV can be used to perform quantitative analysis of the various components of the TV (see Chap. 18).

Pathophysiology of Functional Tricuspid Regurgitation

The pathophysiology of FTR involves several mechanisms that may contribute, to different extents, in different cardiac conditions [1, 12]: (1) dilation of the tricuspid annulus secondary to RV and/or right atrial dilation; (2) distortion of the spatial relationships among leaflets, chordae and papillary muscles leading to leaflet tethering and malcoaptation; (3) changes in TA geometry (dilated, more circular and flatter) and dynamics (reduced area shortening and excursion).

The association between tricuspid dilation and FTR has been well established [14–18]. Tricuspid annulus dilation and right/left atrial enlargement are early and sensitive indicators of FTR [15]. Right atrial enlargement occurs before RV dilation, which occurs late and is associated with more severe TR. Studies of patients with isolated TR (i.e. without left heart disease or pulmonary hypertension) associated with atrial fibrillation have shown a close correlation between tricuspid annulus area and right atrial volume (and lower correlation with RV end-systolic volume), and between annular area and TR severity [18]. Despite the mounting evidence of the role played by the right atrium in determining tricuspid annulus dilation, the size and the function of the right atrium are almost systematically neglected when discussing the pathophysiology and management of FTR [19].

On the other hand, it is also a common observation that not all patients with tricuspid annulus dilation have FTR and, with the same extent of tricuspid annulus dilation, different degrees of FTR may be observed. This may be related to differential TV leaflet remodeling. Afilalo et al. [20] demonstrated that, in patients with pulmonary hypertension, TV leaflets remodel by increasing their area and both the occurrence and severity of FTR are related to the extent of leaflet adaptation to increased tricuspid annulus area expressed as the ratio between TV leaflet area/closure area. Nonetheless, annular dilatation has recently been associated with outcomes [21]. In 213 patients with moderate or severe TR secondary to left-sided valve diseases, nonvalvular disease, or isolated primary TR, an enlarged tricuspid annulus was positively associated with cardiovascular outcomes (composite of hospitalization for worsening heart failure, stroke, and cardiovascular death) irrespective of subgroups according to type or severity of TR.

Spinner et al. [14] demonstrated that both annular dilation and papillary muscle displacement contribute to FTR. Significant FTR occurs with only 40% dilation of tricuspid annulus area (compared to a 75% annulus area dilation needed to create functional mitral regurgitation). TA dilation caused the displacement of the anterior and posterior leaflets from the central coaptation line, with a progressive reduction of the leaflet coaptation surface until a gap occurred. In this experimental study, the minimum coaptation length to prevent regurgitation was 5 mm. The anterior leaflet was found to be the most affected by tricuspid annulus

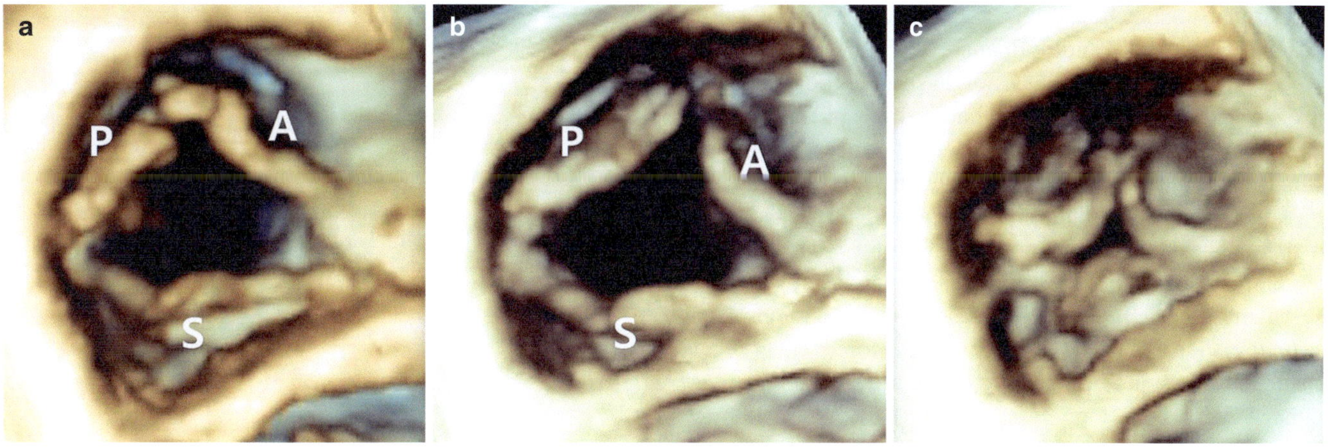

Fig. 21.2 The tricuspid valve obtained from transthoracic 3DE and visualized from the right ventricular perspective in normal control (**a**, diastole) and a patient with functional tricuspid regurgitation (**b**, **c**). Septal (S), anterior (A) and posterior (P) leaflets are simultaneously visualized. The coaptation gap in functional tricuspid regurgitation can be easily observed by comparing leaflet position during diastole (**b**) and systole (**c**)

dilation. The investigators demonstrated also that isolated papillary muscle displacement (i.e. without tricuspid annulus dilation) can cause FTR, and identified the septal as the most affected leaflet by papillary displacement. Of course, the concomitant presence of tricuspid annulus dilation and papillary muscle displacement produced the largest FTR.

The importance of RV geometry in the generation of tricuspid malcoaptation is supported by a number of other studies. Fukuda et al. [22] were one of the first to attribute changes in right-sided cavity size, RV sphericity and left ventricular function to tethering of the TV leaflets and consequent TR. These changes in ventricular geometry and function did not affect annular area. Topilsky et al. [23] studied patients with idiopathic FTR and compared them to patients with pulmonary hypertension with TR. Patients with idiopathic FTR had the largest basal RV diameter and annular area and lowest valvular/annular coverage ratio but normal valve tenting height and a conical RV shape. FTR associated with pulmonary hypertension had mild annular enlargement but excessive valve tenting height and an elliptical/spherical RV shape. Valvular changes were linked to specific RV changes: the largest basal dilatation, and normal length (RV conical deformation) in idiopathic functional TR versus longest RV with elliptical/spherical deformation (i.e. dilatation of the mid-ventricle) in pulmonary hypertension TR. Song et al. [24] reported that RV inlet dimension were the main determinants of TV geometry and severity of FTR. In particular, septal-lateral RV inlet dimension was the main determinant of the extent of TV leaflet tethering and septal-lateral tricuspid annulus diameter, whereas antero-posterior annulus diameter was determined by antero-posterior RV inlet dimension.

Accordingly, we can hypothesize two different pathophysiological models of FTR development in different cardiac conditions: a first model, where the starting mechanism is TA dilation, typical of patients with significantly dilated right atrium and normal or mildly dilated RV (e.g. chronic atrial fibrillation) [17, 18, 25]; and a second model, where the starting mechanism is the remodeling of the RV with the displacement of the papillary muscles and the tenting of TV leaflets, typical of patients with pulmonary hypertension, dilated RV and normal or mildly dilated right atrium [26, 27]. Once initiated, the RV and right atrium remodeling secondary to the volume overload may easily produce a further dilation of the tricuspid annulus, which aggravates the FTR starting a vicious circle in which FTR begets more FTR and both tricuspid annulus dilation and leaflet tethering coexist in the same patient.

Evaluation of Tricuspid Valve Apparatus

Evaluation of patients with FTR who are considered either for surgery or transcatheter procedures should include tricuspid annulus size, mode of leaflet coaptation, as well as the extent of leaflet tethering in addition to the severity of regurgitation [28].

Tricuspid Annulus

Current guidelines [29, 30] recommend two-dimensional echocardiography to size the tricuspid annulus. A cut-off value of 40 mm (or 21 mm/m^2 of body surface area) for the tricuspid annulus diameter obtained from an apical 4-chamber view, in diastole, has been selected to indicate the need of concomitant procedures on the TV when the patient needs surgery for left-sided heart valve diseases. However, two-dimensional echocardiography has several limitations in sizing the tricuspid annulus diameter.

Using a single linear dimension to size the tricuspid annulus is based on the assumptions that the tricuspid annulus is a flat structure, its shape is circular and the measured dimension is the actual diameter of the circle. In patients with severe FTR, the tricuspid annulus is more planar [31, 32]. However, in patients with mild or moderate FTR in whom surgical annuloplasty may be considered based solely on this measurement, it is a complex three-dimensional (3D) non-planar structure (See Fig. 18.4 in Chap. 18). Moreover, both the shape and the spatial orientation of the tricuspid annulus are quite variable [33]. Dreyfus et al. [33] found that, although tricuspid annulus shape was generally oval (mean eccentricity index = 1.35), there were large inter-individual differences from circular (eccentricity index = 1.07) to severely oval (eccentricity index 2.04) tricuspid annulus. Taking the vertical axis at the level of interventricular septum as the reference, the long axis of the tricuspid annulus can be positioned at a variable angle between 5° and 140° with a bimodal distribution with the most frequent orientations located at 40° and 140° [33]. Finally, the conventional apical 4-chamber view obtained with two-dimensional echocardiography does not have any anatomical landmark to allow a proper and reproducible orientation of the view [34]. Comparisons between the tricuspid annulus diameter obtained with two-dimensional echocardiography in apical 4-chamber view and anatomically oriented tricuspid annulus long-axis from 3DE showed an underestimation of 4–9 mm of the former, with wide limits of agreement (7 mm), reflecting also the variability of the differences related to the different shapes and orientations of the tricuspid annulus [33, 35]. Accordingly, 3DE, which allows acquisition of anatomically oriented tricuspid annulus measurements independent of assumptions about its shape and orientation, should be the first line imaging to size it. Tricuspid annulus measurements by 3DE are more accurate than those obtained by two-dimensional echocardiography, when compared with cardiac magnetic resonance [36], and the correlation between tricuspid annulus diameter obtained by two-dimensional echocardiography and severity of FTR is poor [35, 37]. In patients with insufficient acoustic window and in sinus rhythm, both 320-slices multislice computed tomography [38–40] and cardiac magnetic resonance [36, 41] can be used to measure the size of tricuspid annulus.

However, the current guidelines use a thresholds of ≥40 mm (or 21 mm/m^2 of body surface) obtained by two-dimensional echocardiography in the 4-chamber apical view in "diastole" without defining whether that measurement is taken in early, late or end-diastole. Tricuspid annulus area may change by 30% during the cardiac cycle [42, 43] and, within the diastolic time interval, the tricuspid annulus changes significantly [42–44] (Fig. 21.3). Current recommendations comes from a single study that identified a cut-off value of the stretched diameter of the tricuspid annulus ≥70 mm, measured intraoperatively, as an indication to perform concomitant tricuspid annuloplasty in patients undergoing mitral valve surgery independent on the severity of FTR [6]. Although this paper is consistently cited as support for the echocardiographically-measured tricuspid annulus end-diastolic 4-chamber diameter criteria of ≥40 mm [28, 29, 45], there is no echocardiographic data about the tricuspid annulus size in the original paper [6]. Moreover, it is unclear how a 40 mm diameter measured by two-dimensional echocardiography, in the beating heart, from the mid-septal to the mid-anterior (or mid-posterior) annulus could correspond to a 70 mm maximal diameter between the anteroseptal and anteroposterior commissure measured in the arrested heart. Finally, in healthy subjects the tricuspid annulus diameter is correlated to subject age, gender, right atrial and RV volume [46], and, in patients with FTR, tricuspid annulus diameter is also influenced by RV loading conditions. Using a 40 mm cutoff for diastolic tricuspid annulus diameter in 4-chamber view, 20% of healthy subjects would be classified as having "dilated" tricuspid annulus [46].

Since, 3DE is highly feasible and both the TV and the right heart are often better imaged by transthoracic than by transesophageal approach [11], we need dedicated software packages to measure the various components of the TV apparatus (Fig. 21.4). Then, outcome studies using 3DE to obtain anatomically sound measures, will be needed to identify the threshold of the tricuspid annulus dilation (taking into account patient age, gender, right heart chamber size and

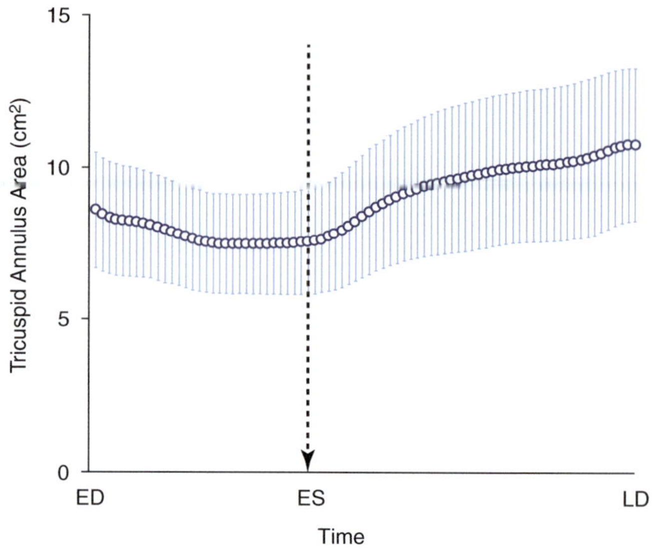

Fig. 21.3 Time course of tricuspid annulus area change during the cardiac cycle [43]. *ED* end-diastole, *ES* end-systole, *LD* late diastole. Modified from Addetia K, Muraru D, Veronesi F, et al. 3-Dimensional Echocardiographic Analysis of the Tricuspid Annulus Provides New Insights Into Tricuspid Valve Geometry and Dynamics. JACC Cardiovasc Imaging. 2019;12:401–412

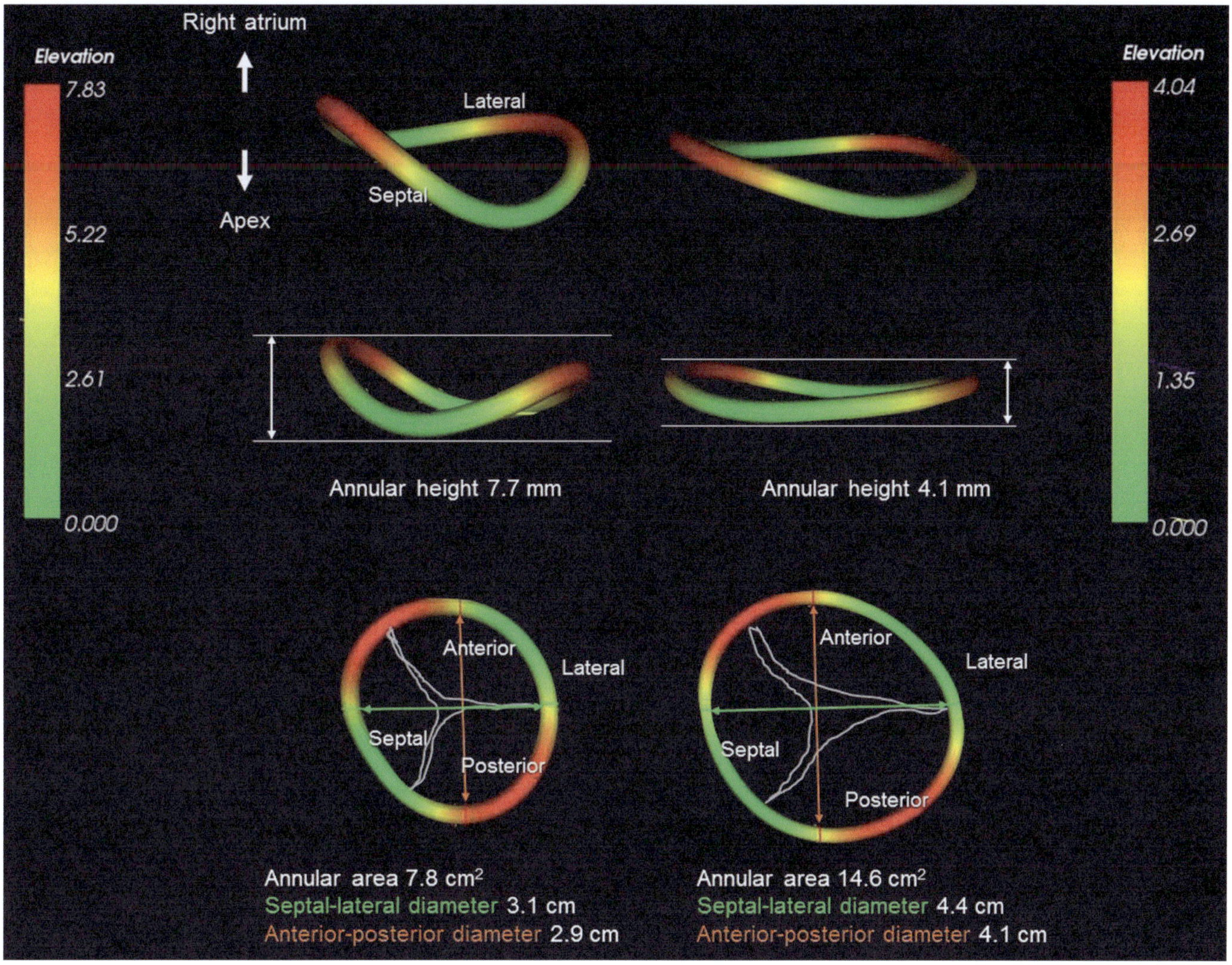

Fig. 21.4 Results of the 3D reconstruction of the tricuspid annulus geometry in a normal subject (left) and in a patient with functional tricuspid regurgitation (right) using a custom-made software package [43]. Normal tricuspid annulus is a non-planar structure with two high points (oriented superiorly toward the right atrium) and a bimodal or saddle-shaped pattern like the mitral annulus. In patients with functional tricuspid regurgitation, the tricuspid annulus is characterized by increased annular area and decreased annular height diminishing the saddle shape

loading conditions) which can indicate the need of concomitant tricuspid annuloplasty at the time of left heart surgery.

Tricuspid Valve Leaflet Coaptation

The extent and mode of leaflet coaptation is another important determinant of the presence and severity of FTR [28]. A coaptation of the body of the leaflet (body-to-body coaptation) guarantees TV sealing and absence of FTR. Normal coaptation of the TV leaflets takes place either at the TA level or more apically, just below it, with a 5–10 mm of the leaflets' body surfaces in contact during systole. When the coaptation surface decreases due to tricuspid annulus dilation and/or leaflets' tethering, the coaptation takes place on the free edges of the leaflets and FTR occurs. Current recommendations [47] suggest measuring the distance between the leaflet coaptation point and the annular plane (tethering distance) and the area between the closed leaflet and the annular plane (tenting area) to estimate the extent of leaflet tethering (Fig. 21.5). When the tethering distance is >8 mm and the tenting area is >1.6 cm^2, the extent of TV leaflet tethering is considered pathologic [10, 28]. However, these measurements obtained with two-dimensional echocardiography are based on the assumptions that tethering of the TV leaflets is symmetric and that the apical 4-chamber view allows the visualization of the highest coaptation point. Both conditions are unlikely to occur in patients with FTR and, not surprisingly, it has been reported that the tenting volume is a better predictor of FTR severity and of the occurrence of residual FTR after tricuspid annuloplasty [48] (Fig. 21.6).

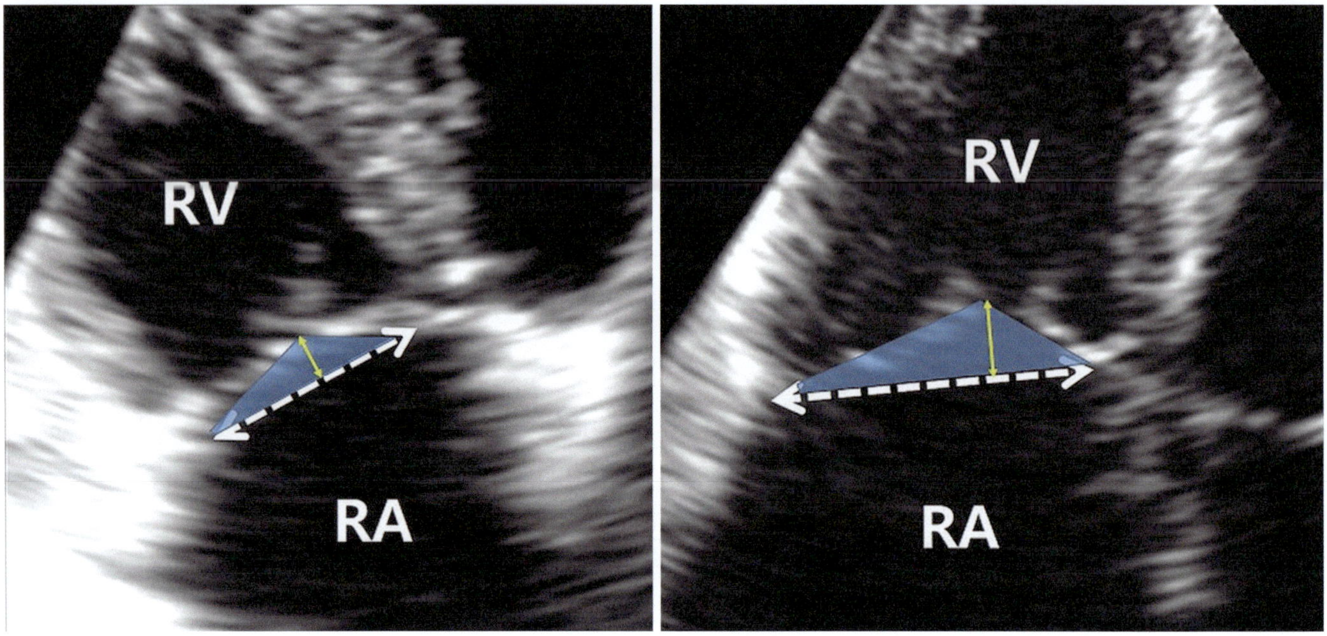

Fig. 21.5 Two-dimensional echocardiography assessment of the extent of the tethering of tricuspid valve leaflets in functional tricuspid regurgitation. Compared to normal control (*left*), in patients with functional tricuspid regurgitation (*right*), the annulus is dilated (double arrow white dashed line), the coaptation depth (double arrow yellow line) is more apically displaced and the tenting area (blue triangle) is larger. *RA* right atrium, *RV* right ventricle

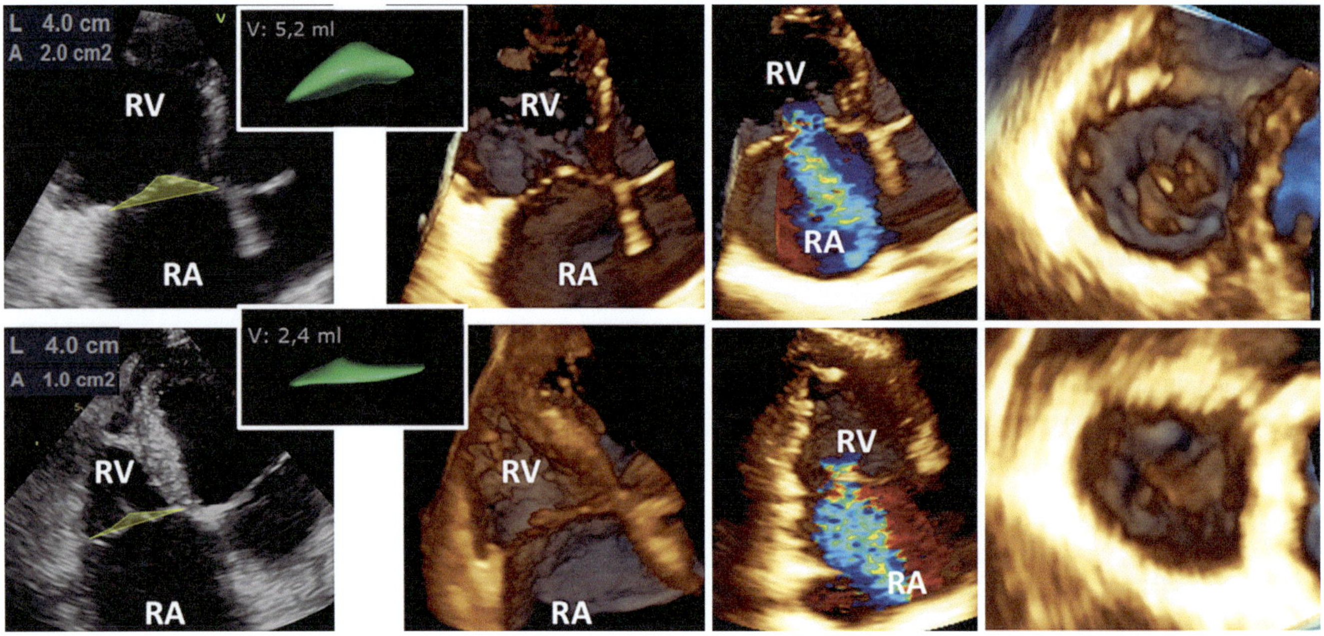

Fig. 21.6 Visualization and measurement of the tenting volume (V, green beutels) using three-dimensional echocardiography in two patients with similar dilatation of the tricuspid annulus (L). *Upper panels*, patient with dilatation of the right ventricle and tethering of the tricuspid leaflets. Lower panels, patient with dilatation of the right atrium, normal right ventricle and minimal tenting of tricuspid leaflets. From the left: two-dimensional echocardiography, apical 4-chamber view; transthoracic three-dimensional echocardiography, longitudinal cut-plane showing the right atrium (RA) and the right ventricle (RV); transthoracic three-dimensional color Doppler acquisition showing the extent of the tricuspid regurgitation jet; three-dimensional echocardiography, transversal cut-plane showing an "*en face*" view of the tricuspid valve from the ventricular perspective. *A* tenting area, *RA* right atrium, *RV* right ventricle

Evaluation of Tricuspid Regurgitation Severity

Because of the complexity for TR evaluation with invasive methods, echocardiography has always played a central role for TR assessment. The parameters used for this purpose range from qualitative to quantitative, and both of them are recommended by current American and European Guidelines [47, 49]. Among them, the measurement of the diameter of the vena contracta of the regurgitant jet and the calculation of the tricuspid effective regurgitation orifice area by the proximal isovelocity surface area (PISA) method are the most widely used, even if the final grading of the severity of TR should be further supported by other parameters.

The use of traditional quantitative parameters to assess the severity of TR is based on geometrical assumptions about the shape of the tricuspid regurgitant orifice and extrapolation of concepts learned from studying the mitral valve [50]. As the TV has unique features, being highly dynamic, with a complex coaptation among its three leaflets which determines complex geometric configurations of the regurgitant orifice, there is an urgent need for these parameters to be questioned [51, 52].

The basic geometrical assumptions in using the diameter of the vena contracta of the regurgitant jet are that the proximal part of the jet has a circular cross section and that the two-dimensional echocardiography view used to measure its diameter is passing though the actual diameter of the cross-sectional area of the vena contracta. Both of them are unlikely to occur in clinical practice where the regurgitant orifice assumes complex and unpredictable shapes (Fig. 21.7).

In addition to the fluidodynamic considerations about the TR jet [53], accurate calculations of the effective regurgitant orifice area using the PISA method are based on the following assumptions: (1) the regurgitant orifice is circular; (2) the regurgitant orifice is flat; (3) the PISA is a hemisphere and its area can be calculated by measuring the radius of the hemisphere. However, the regurgitant orifice is unlikely to be circular in FTR (Fig. 21.7). The regurgitant orifice is not flat, since a variable degree of tenting of the TV leaflets occurs according to the main mechanism determining the regurgitation (i.e. tricuspid annulus dilation and/or papillary muscle displacement) [14]. Finally, due to the variable shape of the regurgitant orifice of the TV, the large regurgitant orifice and relatively low velocity of regurgitant flow (when compared to mitral regurgitation) the hemispheric geometry of the PISA is unlikely to occur in real patients (Fig. 21.8).

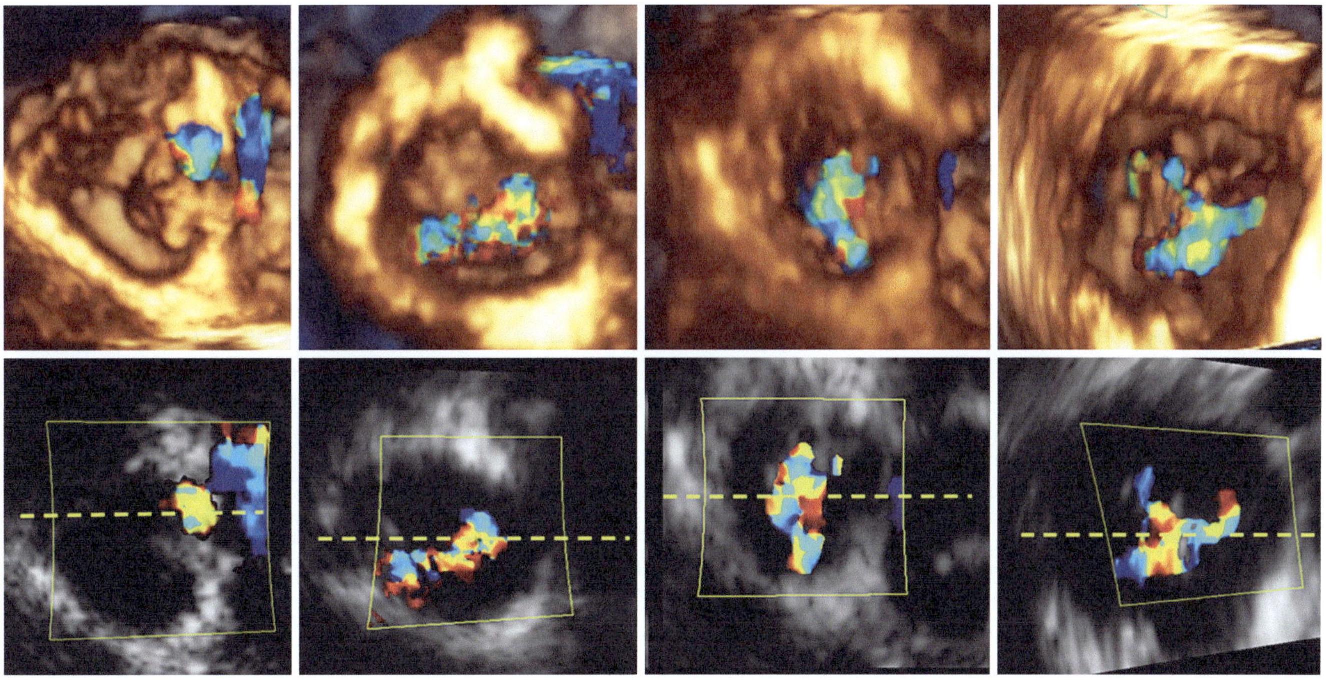

Fig. 21.7 Variable geometry of the tricuspid regurgitation orifice in different patients with functional tricuspid regurgitation. *Upper panels*, transthoracic three-dimensional color Doppler echocardiography. The data set has been cut transversally to show the regurgitant orifice from the ventricular perspective. *Lower panels*, the data sets have been sliced to allow the planimetry of the area of the vena contracta. The yellow dashed line shows the position of the apical 4-chamber view to allow to appreciate the lack of relationship between the vena contracta diameter and its actual shape and area

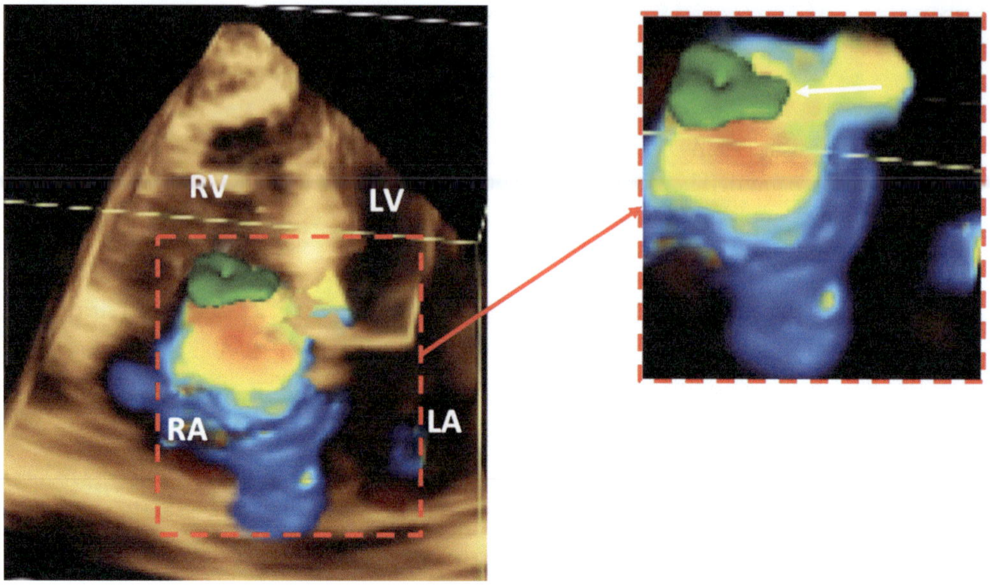

Fig. 21.8 Transthoracic three-dimensional color Doppler echocardiography obtained from a patient with functional tricuspid regurgitation. Three-dimensional reconstruction of the proximal isovelocity surface (green beutel shown by the white arrow in the magnified image) showing that its actual shape is quite far from that of a hemisphere

Interestingly, the partition values to define mild, moderate or severe the TR for the diameter of the vena contracta (<0.3 cm, 0.31–0.69 cm, and ≥0.7 cm, respectively) and the effective regurgitant orifice area (<0.2 cm^2, 0.2–0.39 cm^2, ≥0.4 cm^2, respectively) are similar to those identified to grade mitral regurgitation severity, despite the anatomical differences between the two valves and the different hemodynamic environment in which they operate.

The diameter of the vena contracta of the TR jet was validated by Tribouilloy et al. [50] in 71 patients with various degrees of TR. They measured it from a single 4-chamber apical view and used the effective regurgitant orifice area by PISA and hepatic venous flow as reference, both parameters having suboptimal accuracy and a number of limitation in patients with TR [49]. They found that a vena contracta diameter >6.5 mm identified severe TR with 88.5% sensitivity and 93.3% specificity. However, they tested the accuracy of the parameter on the same study population from which the parameter was derived and no other study has ever tested this cut-off value on any different population.

The effective orifice area calculated by means of the PISA method (used as the reference for the vena contracta diameter by Tribouilloy et al. [50]) was "validated" by Rivera et al. [54] in 45 patients using the Doppler 2DE volumetric method as reference. Notably, the Doppler 2DE volumetric method has shown to significantly overestimate the regurgitant volume and to have limited reproducibility in patients with mitral regurgitation [55], in whom the geometry of the annulus is more predictable than in TR, and there is no evidence for the partition values used to grade TR severity. They just adopted them in analogy with the mitral valve. However, it is unlikely that the same amount of regurgitation may have the same hemodynamic impact on a "pressure pump" (i.e. the left ventricle) and on a "flow pump" (i.e. the RV). Conversely, it is likely that the RV can handle larger regurgitant volumes than its left counterpart. Indeed, the need for a new TR grading scheme has recently been advocated [56]. However, the proposed partition values for "massive" and "torrential" TR were based "*…on the ranges of values for the current grades of mild or moderate*", with no outcome evidence supporting these cut-off values. Alternatively, we should consider the hypothesis that to be "clinically severe" (in terms of patient's morbidity and mortality) TR requires a larger regurgitant volume than mitral regurgitation.

Moreover, even if both the diameter of the vena contracta and the effective regurgitant orifice area were accurate estimates of TR severity in the frame they are calculated, it remains the problem of the actual hemodynamic and clinical significance of a static measure (in one frame) of a rapidly changing phenomenon throughout the cardiac systole like the TR. In patients with FTR, regurgitant flow is not constant (Fig. 21.9), but it varies continuously throughout systole, therefore a measurement taken in a single frame does not seem to be the ideal parameter to assess FTR severity.

Furthermore, both the regurgitant orifice area and the regurgitant volume across the TV are influenced by the respiratory cycle (Fig. 21.10) and loading conditions. Compared to expiration, during inspiration, TR presents a decrease in driving forces while the size of the regurgitant orifice increases by 69% [57]. During inspiration, as venous return to the right side of the heart increases, the RV and right atrium expand their width to accommodate a higher volume, without significantly changing their longitudinal dimensions. The increase in width of the right atrium and RV result in an increase of tricuspid annulus size. Moreover, the horizontal displacement of the papillary muscles [38] and the anatomical particularities of the TV (with the insertion of chordae tendineae to multiple papillary muscles and the RV

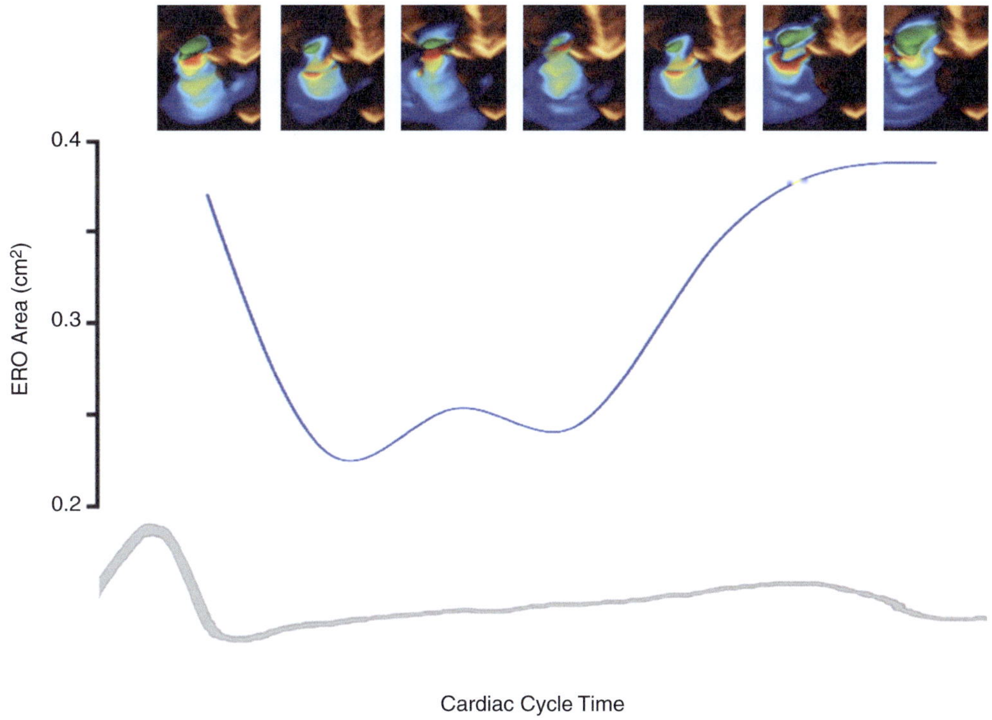

Fig. 21.9 Time course of tricuspid effective regurgitant orifice area during cardiac systole obtained from three-dimensional reconstruction of the proximal isovelocity surface area. Effective regurgitant orifice area is larger in proto- and end-systole and smaller in mid-systole when the contraction of the right ventricle pushes leaflets towards the annulus

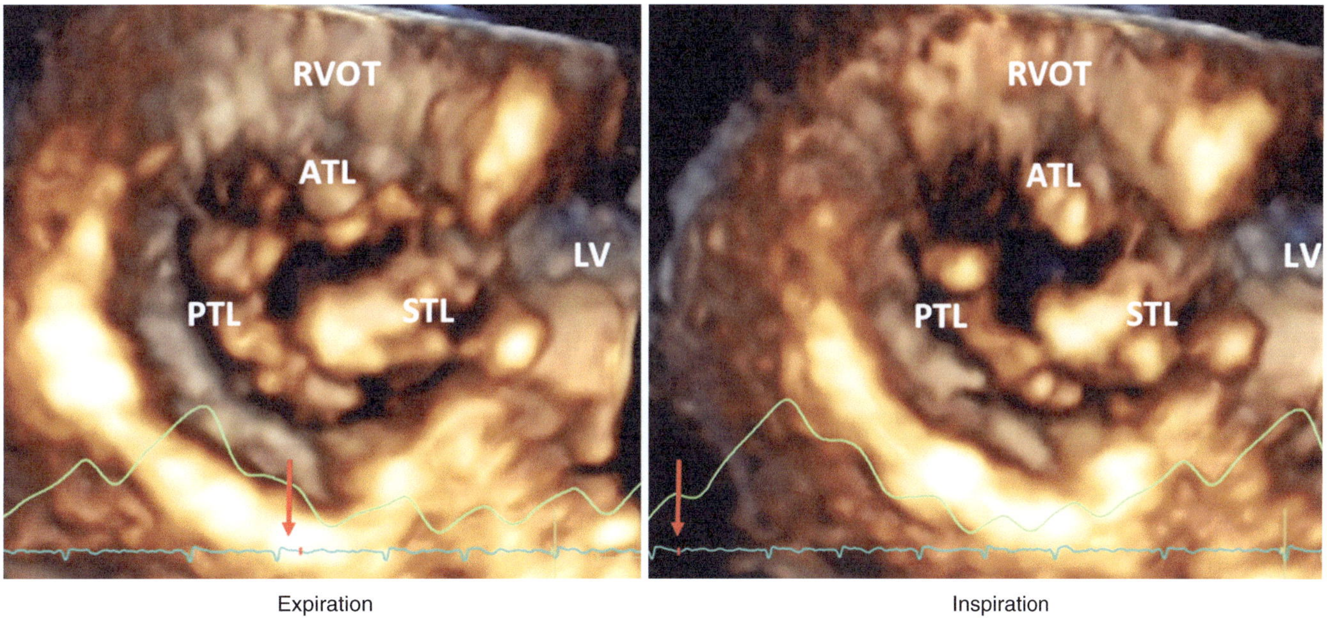

Fig. 21.10 *En-face* view of the tricuspid regurgitant orifice from the ventricular perspective obtained during quiet respiration by real-time transthoracic three-dimensional echocardiography showing the wide variation of the size of the regurgitant orifice from expiration (*left*) to inspiration (*right*) in a patient with functional tricuspid regurgitation. *ATL* anterior tricuspid leaflet, *LV* left ventricle, *PTL* posterior tricuspid leaflet, *RVOT* right ventricular outflow tract, *STL* septal tricuspid leaflet

free wall) determine an increase in leaflet coaptation height and tenting area. Consequently, tricuspid regurgitant orifice area increases (Fig. 21.10), ultimately resulting in an average increase in 20% of regurgitant volume during inspiration [57]. Currently, it remains to be determined which is the best moment to quantitate TR: during inspiration, during expiration, during halted respiration or, maybe, integrating the regurgitant volume over time throughout the respiratory cycle.

Finally, assessment of TR is further complicated by the fact that the right heart is more sensitive to both preload and afterload than its left counterpart. Within physiological limits, RV contractility can increase with increasing end diastolic volume, using the Frank Starling mechanism, translating in increased RV longitudinal function which can be measured using conventional two-dimensional echocardiography measurements [58]. Therefore, an increase in preload during inspiration will also increase RV contractility. However, in patients with severe TR, because of the increase of TR during inspiration, right atrial pressure also increases, approximating RV systolic pressure. Consequently, TR peak velocity measured by Doppler echocardiography decreases as well, and this decrease of peak velocity can variably affect effective orifice area calculations. An inspiratory decrease of TR peak velocity by 0.6 m/s or more has high specificity (94%), and negative predictive value (92%) for severe TR [59]. RV preload is also affected by treatment. Effective diuretic treatment at the time of the echocardiography study may dramatically decrease the estimate of TR severity.

The role of RV afterload as a mechanism contributing to FTR is also worth noting. The high prevalence of FTR in patients with pulmonary hypertension has been documented. However, the cause-effect relationship between pulmonary pressure and FTR is not that clear. Mutlak et al. [60] studied in a large cohort of patients divided in three groups according to pulmonary artery systolic pressure (<50 mmHg, 50–70 mmHg, >70 mmHg). Despite the fact that pulmonary systolic pressure (per 10 mmHg increase) was independently associated with significant TR (Odds Ratio = 2.26), not all patients with pulmonary hypertension had significant FTR. Sixty-five percent of patients with pulmonary systolic pressure between 50 and 70 mmHg, and 45% of those with pulmonary systolic pressure higher than 70 mmHg had only mild TR [60]. Extent of right atrial and RV remodeling was strongly associated with severe TR (Odds Ratio = 6.34 and 7.02, respectively) independent on pulmonary systolic pressure. In addition, this data supports the concept that even if RV afterload is related to FTR, this relationship is modulated by various other factors that affect the size of the TA or the extent of leaflet tethering.

Novel Echocardiographic Techniques to Assess Patients with Functional Tricuspid Regurgitation

3DE planimetry of the area of the vena contracta has been proposed as a method to overcome the problems related to the irregular shape of the regurgitant orifice in patients with FTR. This method solves the issues related to the irregular contour of the regurgitant orifice (Fig. 21.11). However, the regurgitant orifice is a curvilinear surface and, using a planimetry on a tomographic plane to measure it, will include the errors due to the fact that, on the atrial side, part of the jet is not yet contracted, whereas, on the ventricular side, part of the jet is not contracted anymore. Moreover, the size of the vena contracta is heavily dependent on color Doppler gain setting and does not overcome the fact that it is a static measure obtained in a single frame. In addition, a validated cut-off for the diagnosis of severe TR using 3DE planimetry of the vena contracta is still lacking. Velayudhan et al. [51] showed that a planimetered regurgitant orifice area >75 mm^2 was associated with severe TR, defined as a TR regurgitant jet larger than 10 cm^2 or a TR jet area/right atrial area ratio >34%. This cut-off was selected because of its high sensitivity and negative predictive value of 95%. Chen et al. [52] studied the role of 3DE planimetry of the vena contract to assess TR severity. In their study, both 3DE and 2DE acquisitions were performed during breath-holding. Influence of cardiac rhythm was also controlled by excluding patients with atrial fibrillation with more than 20% variation in R-R cycle length. They found a cut-off of 36 mm^2 to have a sensitivity of 89% and a specificity of 84% for predicting severe TR [52] defined using a multi-parameteric approach as indicated by ASE [49] and EACVI [47] guidelines. Another study in which 3DE planimetry of the area of the vena contracta has been explored identified a cut-off of >37 mm^2 for moderate TR (sensitivity 100%, specificity 69%), and >57 mm^2 for severe TR (sensitivity 100%, specificity 64%) defined using the effective regurgitant orifice area calculated with conventional PISA method [61]. Lacking an accepted reference method to quantitate FTR, the reported studies used different definitions of severe FTR and, as expected, found different cut-offs of 3DE vena contracta area to define severe FTR.

Another proposed method to assess the severity of TR using 3DE is to try to reconstruct the actual 3D volume of the PISA and to measure it independent of any geometric assumptions (Fig. 21.8). This technique is based on real-time (single-beat) 3DE acquisition of color Doppler data set using a vendor-specific equipment and, since it is supposed to allow a frame-by-frame measurement of the PISA volume, it can be applied to patients in atrial fibrillation. However, flow velocity measurements by color Doppler (as with any Doppler technique) are angle-dependent and, due to this angle-dependency, color Doppler displays only the vector velocity component (towards or away from the probe) and not the actual flow velocity. Therefore, color Doppler cannot show the "isovelocity surface" but only the "iso-Doppler surface" which cannot be a hemisphere and significantly underestimate the size of the proximal isovelocity surface [62, 63]. Thus, the 3DE PISA does not make any geometrical assumption about the shape of the iso-Doppler shell, but it assumes that color Doppler is angle independent. Moreover, only the peak velocity of TR jet is included in the formula for the calculation of the regurgitant orifice area. Therefore, the method

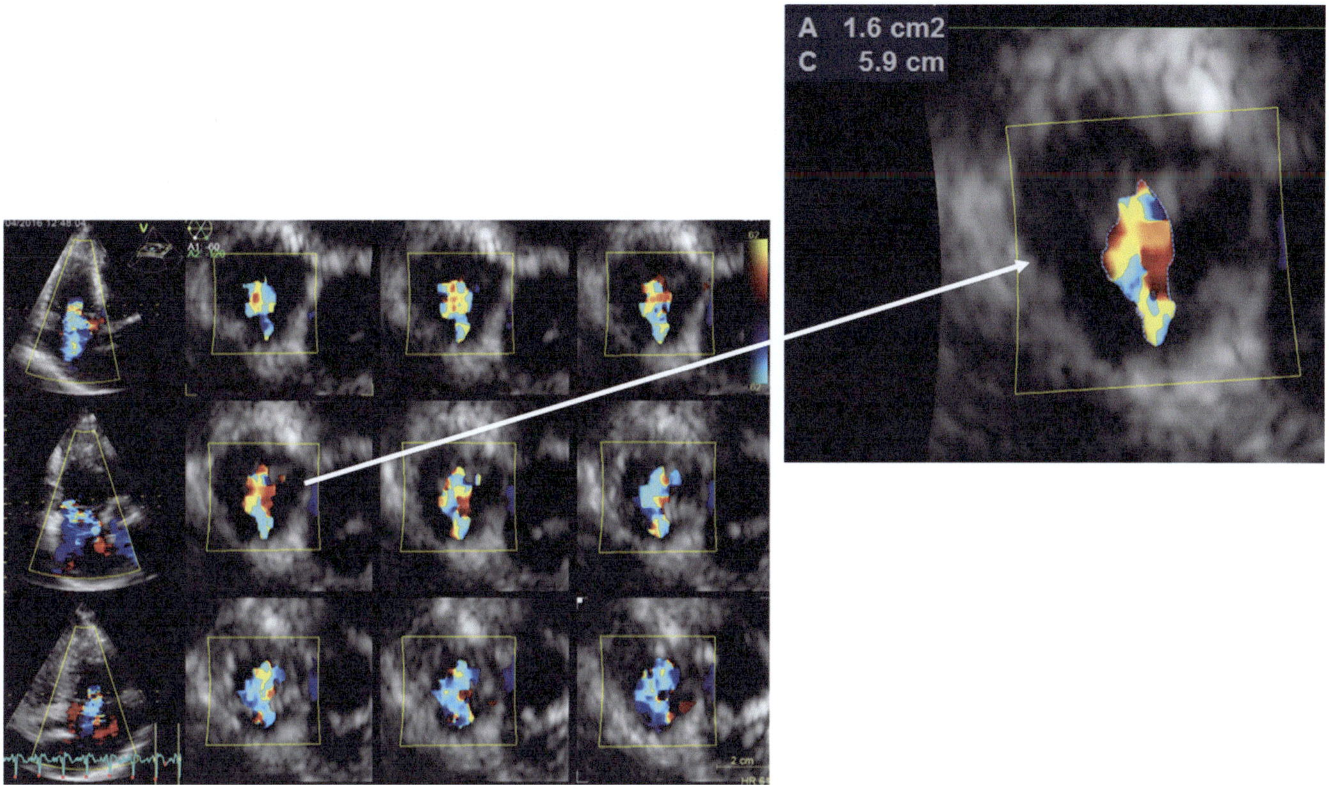

Fig. 21.11 Multislice display of a transthoracic 3DE color-Doppler data set of the regurgitant jet in a patient with functional tricuspid regurgitation. By slicing the proximal part of the jet with orientation of the cut planes perpendicular to the direction of the jet, the smaller cross-sectional area of the jet (vena contracta) can be identified and planimetered (see text for details). *A* area, *C* perimeter

cannot allow an actual measurement of frame-by-frame effective regurgitant orifice area change.

Finally, the 3DE PISA method has never been tested against any independent reference method to grade TR. De Agustin et al. [64] tested it against the effective regurgitant tricuspid orifice area calculated with 2DE and Doppler echocardiography volumetric method, and the 3DE planimetry of the vena contracta. Despite the known limitations of the volumetric method [55], the Authors found a very close correlation ($r = 0.97$) among the effective tricuspid regurgitant areas measured with the three echocardiographic methods [64], even higher than the correlations found during the in vitro testing of the 3DE PISA method ($r = 0.91$) [65].

Indeed, effective regurgitant orifice area may be a suboptimal parameter to estimate the severity of FTR. For the same effective regurgitant orifice area, the regurgitant volume can be quite different with different pressure gradients and we have discussed how the gradient between the RV and the right atrium can change throughout cardiac systole in patients with TR. Between a TR with an end-systolic effective regurgitant orifice area of 0.4 cm^2 and a TR with a holosystolic effective regurgitant orifice area of 0.3 cm^2—which would be more severe? The key parameter that best accounts for the volume overload on the right heart chambers is most likely the regurgitant volume, and not the single-frame regurgitant orifice area measurement.

Recently, a new software package has been released allowing to measure the regurgitant volume by tracking color flow during the whole cardiac cycle using real-time 3DE color flow acquisitions. Acquiring data sets of 3DE color flow at the level of the tricuspid and the pulmonary valves over 5–10 cardiac cycles and averaging the results allows the actual measurement of the TR volume independent on geometric assumptions about regurgitant orifice and/or proximal isovelocity surface shape, and taking into account intra-beat and respiratory variations of TR. Further studies about the feasibility and accuracy of these measurements are needed.

Conclusion

FTR is characterized by geometric changes of TV apparatus including leaflets and tricuspid annulus with associated RV and right atrial enlargement. Comprehensive evaluation of geometric changes of anatomical structures potentially involved in the pathophysiology of FTR can be possible using transthoracic 3DE. Moreover, 3D color Doppler imaging may help to overcome the limitations of conventional two-dimensional and Doppler echocardiography in the assessment of TR severity. Thus, transthoracic 3DE, including 3DE color Doppler imaging, should be the recommended technique for routine clinical practice for patients with FTR. Further investigations are necessary to evaluate whether certain measurements obtained from 3DE data set can affect the clinical outcomes in these patients.

References

1. Badano LP, Muraru D, Enriquez-Sarano M. Assessment of functional tricuspid regurgitation. Eur Heart J. 2013;34(25):1875–85.
2. Nath J, Foster E, Heidenreich PA. Impact of tricuspid regurgitation on long-term survival. J Am Coll Cardiol. 2004;43:405–9.
3. Calafiore AM, Gallina S, Iaco AL, et al. Mitral valve surgery for functional mitral regurgitation: should moderate-or-more tricuspid regurgitation be treated? a propensity score analysis. Ann Thorac Surg. 2009;87:698–703.
4. Varadarajan P, Pai RG. Prognostic implications of tricuspid regurgitation in patients with severe aortic regurgitation: results from a cohort of 756 patients. Interact Cardiovasc Thorac Surg. 2012;14:580–4.
5. Mascherbauer J, Kammerlander AA, Marzluf BA, Graf A, Kocher A, Bonderman D. Prognostic impact of tricuspid regurgitation in patients undergoing aortic valve surgery for aortic stenosis. PLoS One. 2015;10:e0136024.
6. Dreyfus GD, Corbi PJ, Chan KM, Bahrami T. Secondary tricuspid regurgitation or dilatation: which should be the criteria for surgical repair? Ann Thorac Surg. 2005;79:127–32.
7. McCarthy PM, Sales VL. Evolving indications for tricuspid valve surgery. Curr Treat Options Cardiovasc Med. 2010;12:587–97.
8. Bernal JM, Gutierrez-Morlote J, Llorca J, San Jose JM, Morales D, Revuelta JM. Tricuspid valve repair: an old disease, a modern experience. Ann Thorac Surg. 2004;78:2069–74.
9. McCarthy PM, Bhudia SK, Rajeswaran J, et al. Tricuspid valve repair:durability and risk factors for failure. J Thorac Cardiovasc Surg. 2004;127:674–85.
10. Fukuda S, Song JM, Gillinov AM, et al. Tricuspid valve tethering predicts residual tricuspid regurgitation after tricuspid annuloplasty. Circulation. 2005;111:975–9.
11. Muraru D, Hahn RT, Soliman IA, Faletra F, Basso C, Badano LP. Three-dimensional echocardiography in imaging the tricuspid valve. JACC Cardiovasc Imaging. 2019;12:500–15.
12. Muraru D, Surkova E, Badano LP. Revisit of functional tricuspid regurgitation; current trends in the diagnosis and management. Korean Circ J. 2016;46:443–55.
13. Badano LP, Agricola E, Perez de Isla L, Gianfagna P, Zamorano JL. Evaluation of the tricuspid valve morphology and function by transthoracic real-time three-dimensional echocardiography. Eur J Echocardiogr. 2009;10:477–84.
14. Spinner EM, Shannon P, Buice D, et al. In vitro characterization of the mechanisms responsible for functional tricuspid regurgitation. Circulation. 2011;124:920–9.
15. Nemoto N, Lesser JR, Pedersen WR, et al. Pathogenic structural heart changes in early tricuspid regurgitation. J Thorac Cardiovasc Surg. 2015;150:323–30.
16. Mutlak D, Lessick J, Reisner SA, Aronson D, Dabbah S, Agmon Y. Echocardiography-based spectrum of severe tricuspid regurgitation: the frequency of apparently idiopathic tricuspid regurgitation. J Am Soc Echocardiogr. 2007;20:405–8.
17. Najib MQ, Vinales KL, Vittala SS, Challa S, Lee HR, Chaliki HP. Predictors for the development of severe tricuspid regurgitation with anatomically normal valve in patients with atrial fibrillation. Echocardiography. 2012;29:140–6.
18. Utsunomiya H, Itabashi Y, Mihara H, et al. Functional tricuspid regurgitation caused by chronic atrial fibrillation: a real-time 3-dimensional transesophageal echocardiography study. Circ Cardiovasc Imaging. 2017;10(1). pii: e004897.
19. Prihadi EA, Delgado V, Hahn RT, Leipsic J, Min JK, Bax JJ. Imaging needs in novel transcatheter tricuspid valve interventions. JACC Cardiovasc Imaging. 2018;11:736–54.
20. Afilalo J, Grapsa J, Nihoyannopoulos P, et al. Leaflet area as a determinant of tricuspid regurgitation severity in patients with pulmonary hypertension. Circ Cardiovasc Imaging. 2015;8(5). pii: e002714.
21. Kim H, Kim IC, Yoon HJ, et al. Prognostic usefulness of tricuspid annular diameter for cardiovascular events in patients with tricuspid regurgitation of moderate to severe degree. Am J Cardiol. 2018;121:1343–50.
22. Fukuda S, Gillinov AM, Song JM, et al. Echocardiographic insights into atrial and ventricular mechanisms of functional tricuspid regurgitation. Am Heart J. 2006;152:1208–14.
23. Topilsky Y, Khanna A, Le Tourneau T, et al. Clinical context and mechanism of functional tricuspid regurgitation in patients with and without pulmonary hypertension. Circ Cardiovasc Imaging. 2012;5:314–23.
24. Song JM, Jang MK, Kim YJ, Kim DH, Kang DH, Song JK. Right ventricular remodeling determines tricuspid valve geometry and the severity of functional tricuspid regurgitation: a real-time 3-dimensional echocardiography study. Korean Circ J. 2010;40:448–53.
25. Rogers JH, Bolling SF. The tricuspid valve: current perspective and evolving management of tricuspid regurgitation. Circulation. 2009;119:2718–25.
26. Sukmawan R, Watanabe N, Ogasawara Y, et al. Geometric changes of tricuspid valve tenting in tricuspid regurgitation secondary to pulmonary hypertension quantified by novel system with transthoracic real-time 3-dimensional echocardiography. J Am Soc Echocardiogr. 2007;20:470–6.
27. Park YH, Song JM, Lee EY, Kim YJ, Kang DH, Song JK. Geometric and hemodynamic determinants of functional tricuspid regurgitation: a real-time three-dimensional echocardiography study. Int J Cardiol. 2008;124:160–5.
28. Dreyfus GD, Martin RP, Chan KM, Dulguerov F, Alexandrescu C. Functional tricuspid regurgitation: a need to revise our understanding. J Am Coll Cardiol. 2015;65:2331–6.
29. Nishimura RA, Otto CM, Bonow RO, et al. 2014 AHA/ACC guideline for the management of patients with valvular heart disease: a report of the American College of Cardiology/American Heart Association Task Force on Practice Guidelines. J Am Coll Cardiol. 2014;63:e57–185.
30. Baumgartner H, Falk V, Bax JJ, et al. 2017 ESC/EACTS guidelines for the management of valvular heart diseases. Eur Heart J. 2017;38(36):2739–91.
31. Ton-Nu TT, Levine RA, Handschumacher MD, et al. Geometric determinants of functional tricuspid regurgitation:insights from 3-dimensional echocardiography. Circulation. 2006;114:143–9.
32. Fukuda S, Saracino G, Matsumura Y, et al. Three-dimensional geometry of the tricuspid annulus in healthy subjects and in patients with functional tricuspid regurgitation: a real-time, 3-dimensional echocardiographic study. Circulation. 2006;114:I492–8.
33. Dreyfus J, Durand-Viel G, Raffoul R, et al. Comparison of 2-dimensional, 3-dimensional, and surgical measurements of the tricuspid annulus size: clinical implications. Circ Cardiovasc Imaging. 2015;8:e003241.
34. Stankovic I, Daraban AM, Jasaityte R, Neskovic AN, Claus P, Voigt JU. Incremental value of the en face view of the tricuspid valve by two-dimensional and three-dimensional echocardiography for accurate identification of tricuspid valve leaflets. J Am Soc Echocardiogr. 2014;27:376–84.

35. Anwar AM, Geleijnse ML, Ten Cate FJ, Meijboom FJ. Assessment of tricuspid valve annulus size, shape and function using real-time three-dimensional echocardiography. Interact Cardiovasc Thorac Surg. 2006;5:683–7.
36. Anwar AM, Soliman OI, Nemes A, van Geuns RJ, Geleijnse ML, Ten Cate FJ. Value of assessment of tricuspid annulus: real-time three-dimensional echocardiography and magnetic resonance imaging. Int J Cardiovasc Imaging. 2007;23:701–5.
37. Spinner EM, Lerakis S, Higginson J, et al. Correlates of tricuspid regurgitation as determined by 3D echocardiography: pulmonary arterial pressure, ventricle geometry, annular dilatation, and papillary muscle displacement. Circ Cardiovasc Imaging. 2012;5:43–50.
38. van Rosendael PJ, Joyce E, Katsanos S, et al. Tricuspid valve remodelling in functional tricuspid regurgitation: multidetector row computed tomography insights. Eur Heart J Cardiovasc Imaging. 2016;17:96–105.
39. Takaoka H, Funabashi N, Kataoka A, et al. Utilities of 320-slice computed-tomography for evaluation of tricuspid valve annular diameter before tricuspid-valve-plasty compared with the direct-measurement of tricuspid valve annular diameter during open heart-surgery. Int J Cardiol. 2013;168:2889–93.
40. Kabasawa M, Kohno H, Ishizaka T, et al. Assessment of functional tricuspid regurgitation using 320-detector-row multislice computed tomography: risk factor analysis for recurrent regurgitation after tricuspid annuloplasty. J Thorac Cardiovasc Surg. 2014;147:312–20.
41. Maffessanti F, Gripari P, Pontone G, et al. Three-dimensional dynamic assessment of tricuspid and mitral annuli using cardiovascular magnetic resonance. Eur Heart J Cardiovasc Imaging. 2013;14:986–95.
42. Tei C, Pilgrim JP, Shah PM, Ormiston JA, Wong M. The tricuspid valve annulus: study of size and motion in normal subjects and in patients with tricuspid regurgitation. Circulation. 1982;66:665–71.
43. Addetia K, Muraru D, Veronesi F, et al. 3-Dimensional Echocardiographic Analysis of the Tricuspid Annulus Provides New Insights Into Tricuspid Valve Geometry and Dynamics. JACC Cardiovasc Imaging. 2017;10. pii: S1936-878X(17)30902-6.
44. Miglioranza MH, Mihaila S, Muraru D, Cucchini U, Iliceto S, Badano LP. Variability of tricuspid annulus diameter measurement in healthy volunteers. JACC Cardiovasc Imaging. 2015;8:864–6.
45. Joint Task Force on the Management of Valvular Heart Disease of the European Society of Cardiology (ESC); European Association for Cardio-Thoracic Surgery (EACTS), Vahanian A, Alfieri O, Andreotti F, Antunes MJ, Barón-Esquivias G, Baumgartner H, et al. Guidelines on the management of valvular heart disease (version 2012). Eur Heart J. 2012;33:2451–96.
46. Miglioranza MH, Mihaila S, Muraru D, Cucchini U, Iliceto S, Badano LP. Dynamic changes in tricuspid annular diameter measurement in relation to the echocardiographic view and timing during the cardiac cycle. J Am Soc Echocardiogr. 2015;28:226–35.
47. Lancellotti P, Moura L, Pierard LA, et al. European Association of Echocardiography recommendations for the assessment of valvular regurgitation. Part 2: mitral and tricuspid regurgitation (native valve disease). Eur J Echocardiogr. 2010;11:307–32.
48. Min SY, Song JM, Kim JH, et al. Geometric changes after tricuspid annuloplasty and predictors of residual tricuspid regurgitation: a real-time three-dimensional echocardiography study. Eur Heart J. 2010;31:2871–80.
49. Zoghbi WA, Adams D, Bonow RO, et al. Recommendations for noninvasive evaluation of native valvular regurgitation: a report from the American Society of Echocardiography Developed in Collaboration with the Society for Cardiovascular Magnetic Resonance. J Am Soc Echocardiogr. 2017;30:303–71.
50. Tribouilloy C, Enriquez-Sarano M, Bailey K, Tajik A, Seward J. Quantification of tricuspid regurgitation by measuring the width of the vena contracta with Doppler color flow imaging: a clinical study. J Am Coll Cardiol. 2000;36:472–8.
51. Velayudhan DE, Brown TM, Nanda NC, et al. Quantification of tricuspid regurgitation by live three-dimensional transthoracic echocardiographic measurements of vena contracta area. Echocardiography. 2006;23:793–800.
52. Chen TE, Kwon SH, Enriquez-Sarano M, Wong BF, Mankad SV. Three-dimensional color Doppler echocardiographic quantification of tricuspid regurgitation orifice area: comparison with conventional two-dimensional measures. J Am Soc Echocardiogr. 2013;26:1143–52.
53. Hahn RT, Thomas JD, Khalique OK, Cavalcante JL, Praz F, Zoghbi WA. Imaging assessment of tricuspid regurgitation severity. JACC Cardiovasc Imaging. 2019;12:469–90.
54. Rivera JM, Vandervoort PM, Mele D, et al. Quantification of tricuspid regurgitation by means of the proximal flow convergence method: a clinical study. Am Heart J. 1994;127:1354–62.
55. Cawley PJ, Hamilton-Craig C, Owens DS, et al. Prospective comparison of valve regurgitation quantitation by cardiac magnetic resonance imaging and transthoracic echocardiography. Circ Cardiovasc Imaging. 2013;6:48–57.
56. Hahn RT, Zamorano JL. The need for a new tricuspid regurgitation grading scheme. Eur Heart J Cardiovasc Imaging. 2017;18:1342–3.
57. Topilsky Y, Tribouilloy C, Michelena HI, Pislaru S, Mahoney DW, Enriquez-Sarano M. Pathophysiology of tricuspid regurgitation. Quantitative Doppler echocardiographic assessment of respiratory dependence. Circulation. 2010;122:1505–13.
58. Haddad F, Hunt SA, Rosenthal DN, Murphy DJ. Right ventricular function in cardiovascular disease, part I: anatomy, physiology, aging, and functional assessment of the right ventricle. Circulation. 2008;117:1436–48.
59. Mutlak D, Carasso S, Lessick J, Aronson D, Reisner SA, Agmon Y. Excessive respiratory variation in tricuspid regurgitation systolic velocities in patients with severe tricuspid regurgitation. Eur Heart J Cardiovasc Imaging. 2013;14:957–62.
60. Mutlak D, Aronson D, Lessick J, Reisner SA, Dabbah S, Agmon Y. Functional tricuspid regurgitation in patients with pulmonary hypetension: is pulmonary artery pressure the only determinant of regurgitation severity? Chest. 2009;135:115–21.
61. Song JM, Jang MK, Choi YS, et al. The vena contracta in functional tricuspid regurgitation: a real-time three-dimensional color Doppler echocardiography study. J Am Soc Echocardiogr. 2011;24:663–70.
62. Francis DP, Willson K, Ceri Davies L, Florea VG, Coats AJ, Gibson DG. True shape and area of proximal isovelocity surface area (PISA) when flow convergence is hemispherical in valvular regurgitation. Int J Cardiol. 2000;73:237–42.
63. Moraldo M, Cecaro F, Shun-Shin M, et al. Evidence-based recommendations for PISA measurements in mitral regurgitation: systematic review, clinical and in-vitro study. Int J Cardiol. 2013;168:1220–8.
64. de Agustin JA, Viliani D, Vieira C, et al. Proximal isovelocity surface area by single-beat three-dimensional color Doppler echocardiography applied for tricuspid regurgitation quantification. J Am Soc Echocardiogr. 2013;26:1063–72.
65. Thavendiranathan P, Liu S, Datta S, et al. Quantification of chronic functional mitral regurgitation by automated 3-dimensional peak and integrated proximal isovelocity surface area and stroke volume techniques using real-time 3-dimensional volume color Doppler echocardiography: in vitro and clinical validation. Circ Cardiovasc Imaging. 2013;6:125–33.

Assessment After Surgery or Interventional Procedures on the Tricuspid Valve

22

Luigi P. Badano, Arnaldo Rabischoffsky, Marco Previtero, and Roberto Carlos Ochoa-Jimenez

Abstract

The association of better understanding of the role of tricuspid regurgitation (TR) as an independent predictor of patients' morbidity and mortality, and the advent of novel transcatheter devices to treat severe TR have contributed to increase the interest of cardiologists and cardiac surgeons about the tricuspid valve (TV). The number of transcatheter interventions for TR is growing, and procedural success relies significantly on the pre-procedural evaluation of the anatomy of the TV, etiology and severity of TR, right ventricular size and function, and importantly, the anatomic relationships of the TV. The role of three-dimensional echocardiography and multimodality imaging in patient selection and procedural planning for transcatheter TV repair is reviewed.

Keywords

Tricuspid valve · Three-dimensional echocardiography · Fusion imaging · Multimodality imaging · Tricuspid valve surgery · Transcatheter procedures · Tricuspid valve repair devices · Functional tricuspid regurgitation

Electronic Supplementary Material The online version of this chapter (https://doi.org/10.1007/978-3-030-14032-8_22) contains supplementary material, which is available to authorized users.

L. P. Badano (✉)
University of Milano-Bicocca, and Istituto Auxologico Italiano, IRCCS, San Luca Hospital, Milano, Italy
e-mail: luigi.badano@unimib.it

A. Rabischoffsky
Department of Echocardiography, Pro Cardiaco Hospital, Rio de Janeiro, Brazil

M. Previtero
Department of Cardiac, Thoracic and Vascular Sciences, University of Padua School of Medicine, Padua, Italy

R. C. Ochoa-Jimenez
Department of Internal Medicine, Mount Sinai St Luke and Mount Sinai West, New York, NY, USA

Introduction

Despite the fact that it is well known that tricuspid regurgitation can result in significant mortality and morbidity [1–7], it remains largely untreated [8]. Patients are rarely referred for isolated surgical repair, or replacement, and most surgeries are performed in the context of other planned cardiac surgeries. However, also surgical treatment of functional tricuspid regurgitation in the context of left-sided heart valve diseases remains a controversial issue, particularly about indications to surgery, surgical techniques and the late outcomes of surgical interventions. Indeed, all recommendations on the management of tricuspid valve disease in the 2014 joint ACC/AHA [9] and the 2017 joint ESC/EACTS [10] guidelines are based on expert opinions only.

Surgical Treatment of Tricuspid Valve Disease

Several techniques are available for a tailored surgical treatment of the tricuspid valve (Table 22.1). The "classic" De Vega annuloplasty consists of a plication of the posterior and anterior portion of tricuspid annulus with a double continuous suture, preserving the septal portion of the annulus which is inserted on the fibrous skeleton of the heart. Despite widely used, this technique is flawed by high incidence of regurgitation recurrence [11] (Fig. 22.1; Videos 22.1a, 22.1b, 22.1c, and 22.1d). Therefore, the most frequently performed surgical procedure, to repair functional tricuspid regurgitation secondary to annulus dilation, is undersized prosthetic tricuspid annuloplasty with devices such as flexible bands, rigid or semi-rigid annuloplasty prosthetic open rings. A frequent complication of this technique is the prosthetic annulus detachment and recurrence of the regurgitation (Fig. 22.2, Videos 22.2a and 22.2b).

L. P. Badano et al. (eds.), *Textbook of Three-Dimensional Echocardiography*, https://doi.org/10.1007/978-3-030-14032-8_22

Table 22.1 Current surgical techniques employed to treat tricuspid valve disease

Approach	Surgical techniques
Annuloplasty	De Vega annuloplasty Prosthetic band annuloplasty Prosthetic ring annuloplasty
Leaflet repair	Clover technique Tricuspid leaflet augmentation
Other	Double orifice valve technique Posterior annular bicuspidisation
Valve replacement	Prosthetic tricuspid valve replacement

The "clover technique" is similar to the Alfieri's stitch to repair the mitral valve. The central parts of the free edges of the tricuspid leaflets are sutured together to produce a clover-shaped valve. The procedure is always completed with a prosthetic ring annuloplasty. In case of leaflet tethering, in addition to tricuspid annulus dilation, as a cause of tricuspid regurgitation, the leaflet augmentation technique (enlargement of the anterior tricuspid leaflet by the use of an autologous pericardial patch) increases the surface of the leaflet coaptation by threefold and brings the coapta-

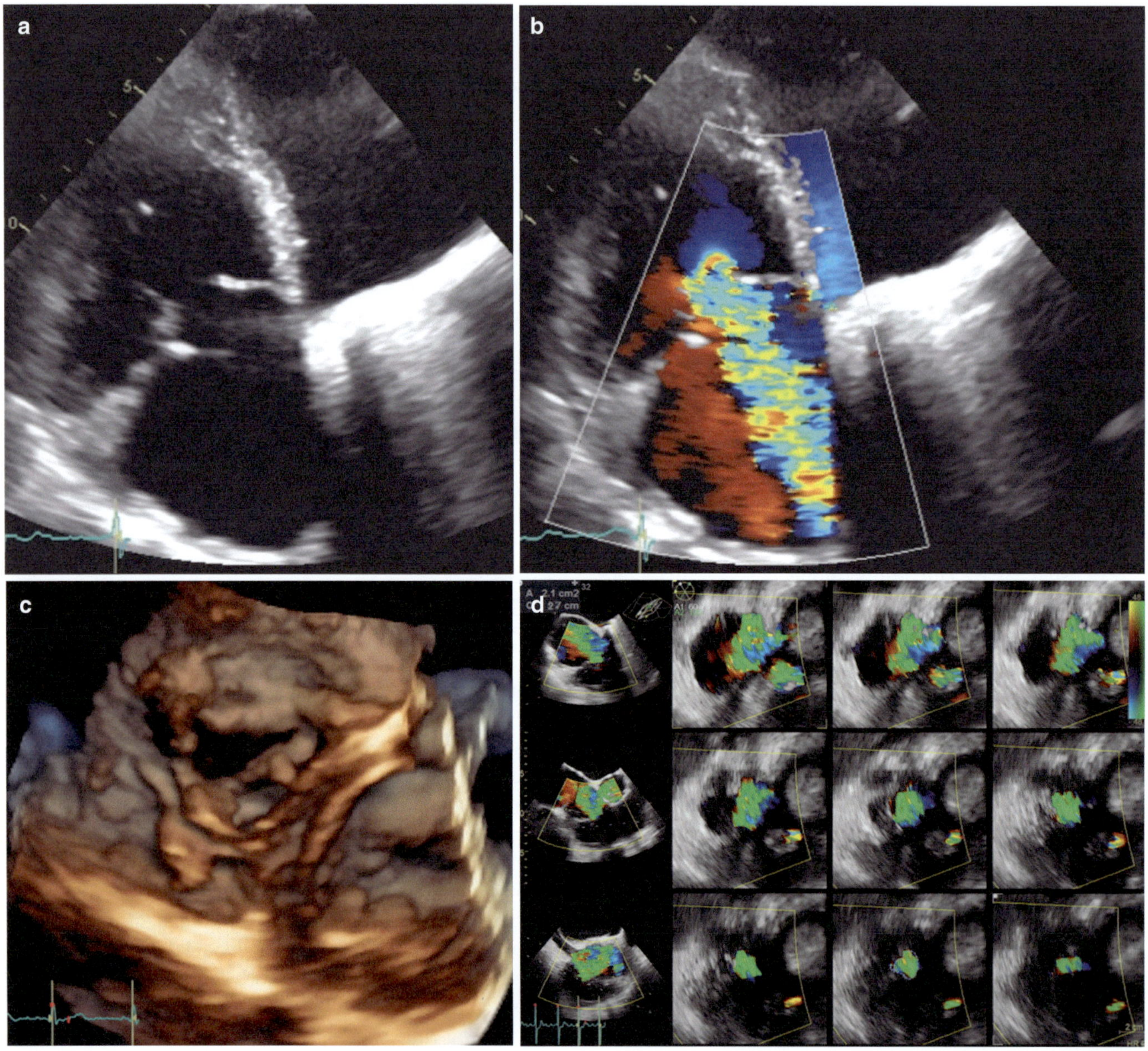

Fig. 22.1 De Vega annuloplasty failure with severe tricuspid regurgitation. (**a**) two-dimensional apical 4-chamber view showing lack of coaptation of the tricuspid leaflets (Video 22.1a); (**b**) two dimensional color Doppler showing a large vena contracta and regurgitant jet (Video 22.1b); (**c**) transesophageal three-dimensional volume rendering of the tricuspid valve seen from the atrial perspective (Video 22.1c); (**d**) multislice display of a 3DE color data set to identify and planimeter the area of the vena contracta (Video 22.1d)

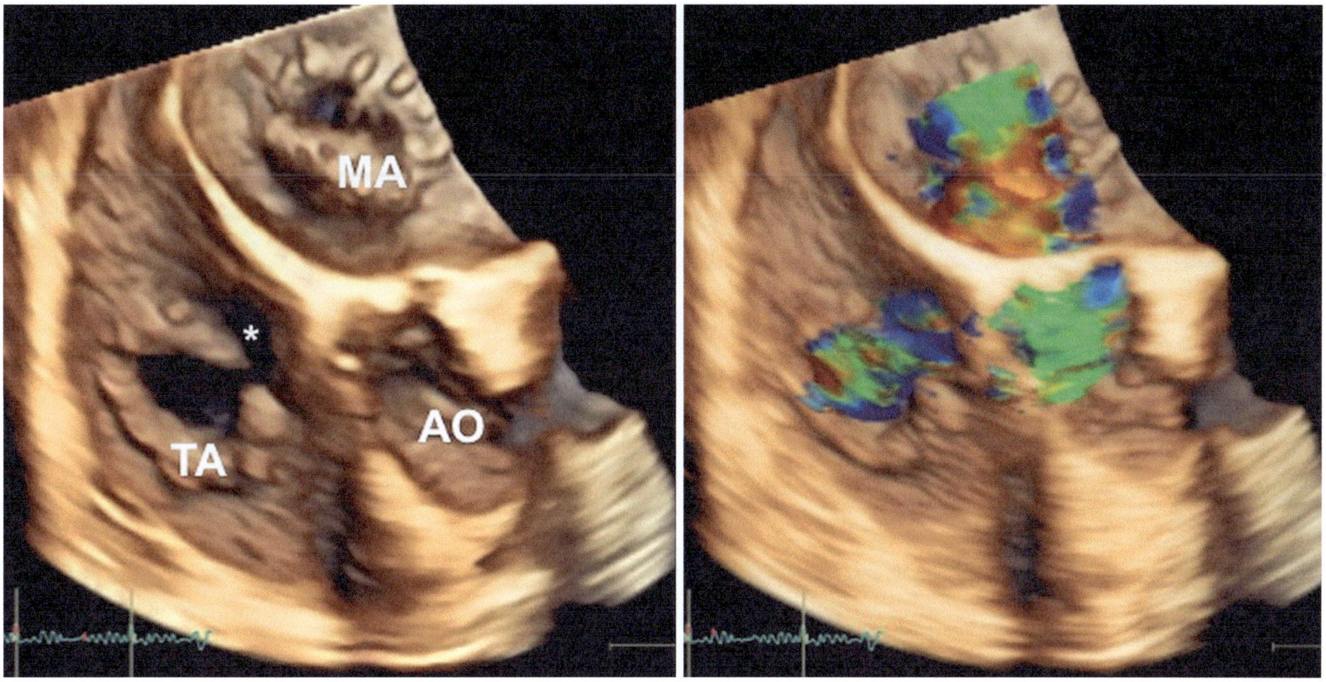

Fig. 22.2 Detachment of the prosthetic tricuspid annulus after surgical mitral and tricuspid annuloplasty. *Left panel*, three-dimensional volume rendering of the open prosthetic tricuspid annulus visualized from the atrial perspective with the site of detachment (asterisk) (Video 22.2a/left). Right panel, three-dimensional color flow showing the double regurgitant flow through the annulus and also through the perinannular orifice (Video 22.2b/right)

tion zone down into the right ventricle at the level of the tethered posterior and septal leaflets. The suture bicuspidisation is obtained by placing a double pledget-supported mattress suture from the anteroposterior to the anteroseptal commissure along the posterior annulus to reduce the extent of the dilation of the posterior tricuspid annulus. The double orifice technique is performed by passing two pledget supported mattress sutures from the center of the anterior annulus to the two thirds of the septal annulus, measured from the antero-septal commissure, to avoid the His bundle [12].

When valve repair is unlikely or when the results of a repair attempt are suboptimal, the tricuspid valve has to be replaced. The use of mechanical valve prostheses in the tricuspid position in multivalvular procedures has been associated to increased mortality and also to high incidence of thrombotic complications, valve dysfunction from tissue ingrowth and, in the case of cage and ball valves, incorporation of the cage into the wall of the right ventricle [13]. Therefore, the use of large size biological prostheses is favored over valve replacement with mechanical valves [9, 10] Among the most frequent complications of tricuspid valve replacement with bioprostheses, we can list: structural valve degeneration (Fig. 22.3), endocarditis (particularly frequent in intravenous drug abusers) (Fig. 22.4, Videos 22.3a and 22.3b), leaflet thrombosis, and valve detachment with significant paravalvular leak.

Transcatheter Approaches to Tricuspid Regurgitation

Despite the fact that tricuspid valve surgery combined with left heart surgery is not associated with a significant increase in mortality [14], re-operation, in patients with worsening or recurrent tricuspid regurgitation after previous surgery, is associated to high mortality [15]. Moreover, the increasing use of transcatheter procedures to treat left heart valve diseases leave a sizable number of high surgical risk patients with untreated tricuspid regurgitation who may eventually progress to severe regurgitation and right heart failure.

Accordingly, percutaneous transcatheter procedures are becoming more and more used as an attractive alternative for patients with symptomatic functional tricuspid regurgitation or severe deterioration of the tricuspid valve after surgical repair or replacement, and deemed to be high surgical risk candidates [16].

There are many issues that make the percutaneous implantation of a bioprosthesis in the tricuspid position very challenging: the dimensions and the angulation of the tricuspid

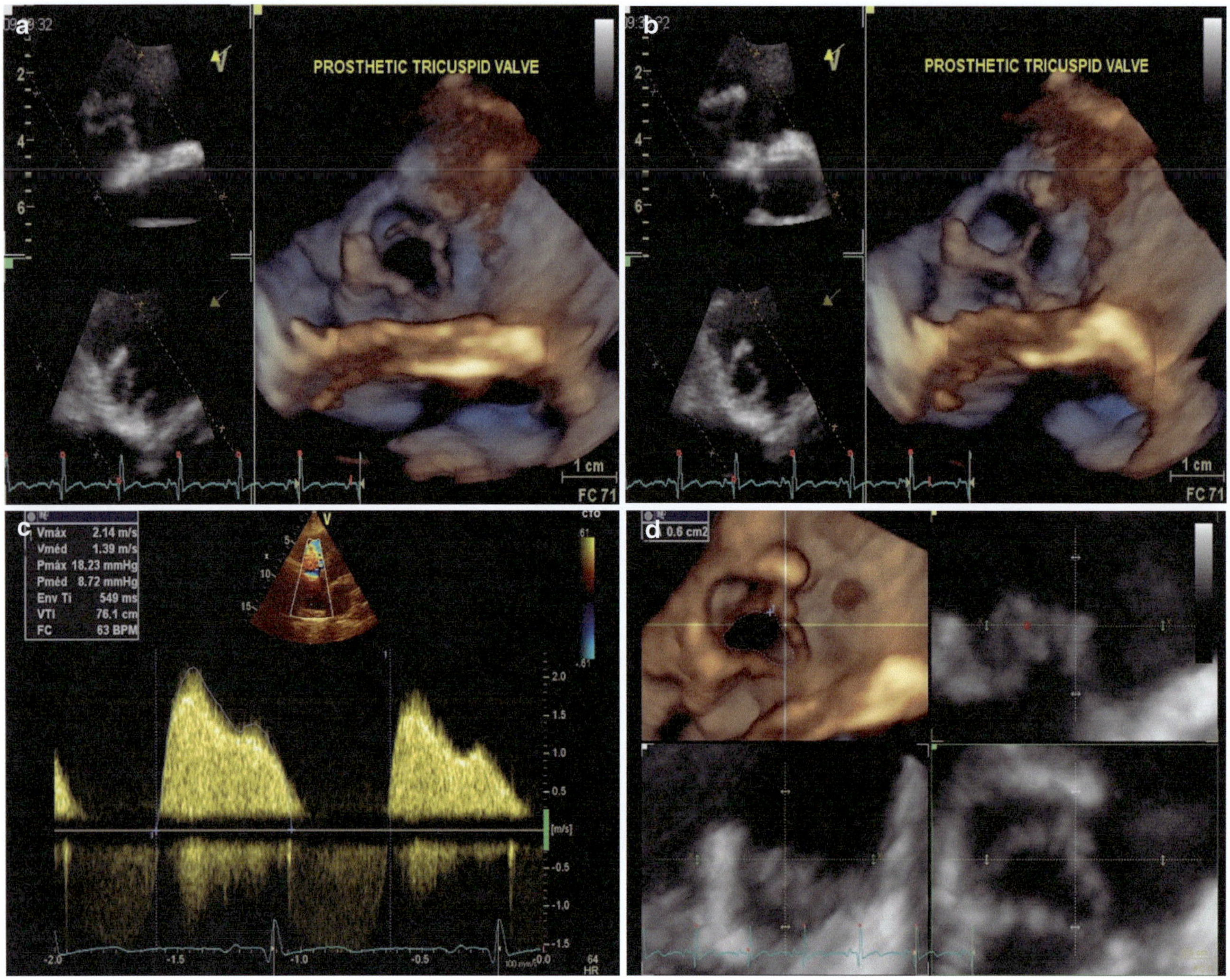

Fig 22.3 Structural degeneration of a bioprosthesis in tricuspid position. (**a**) Bioprosthesis in open position showing thickened leaflets and reduced anatomical orifice area; (**b**) Bioprosthesis in closed position; (**c**) continuous wave Doppler through the tricuspid valve to document high transprosthetic gradient; (**d**) planimetry of anatomical residual prosthetic orifice area

annulus in relation to the cava veins, the slow flow and the trabeculated structure of the right ventricle, the close relationship of the tricuspid annulus to atrtio-ventricular node and right coronary artery, and the lack of annular calcification. Therefore, percutaneous implantation of a bioprosthesis is usually performed only as valve-in-valve or valve-in-ring procedures [17].

On the other end, the following percutaneous options are under development to treat native tricuspid valve regurgitation [18]:

1. Implantation of a bioprosthetic valve in both caval veins [19]
2. Percutaneous tricuspid valve repair mimicking the surgical Kay procedure (TriCinch System, 4Tech Cardio Ltd, Galway, Ireland; Trialign System, Mitralign, Inc., Boston, MA) [20, 21]
3. Percutaneous tricuspid valve repair targeting leaflets (MitraClip System, Abbott Vascular, Abbott Park, IL) [22]
4. Direct percutaneous tricuspid annuloplasty (Cardioband, Edwards Lifesciences, Irvine, CA; Millipede, Millipede Inc., Santa Rosa, CA) [23]
5. Transcatheter delivery of a spacer providing a surface for leaflet coaptation (FORMA Spacer, Edwards Lifesciences, Irvine, CA) [24]
6. Tricuspid valve prosthesis implant

As for other transcatheter procedures, the role of imaging is pivotal for preprocedural planning and intraprocedural monitoring [25–27].

Pre-procedural evaluation focuses on the selection of potential candidates and of the most appropriate

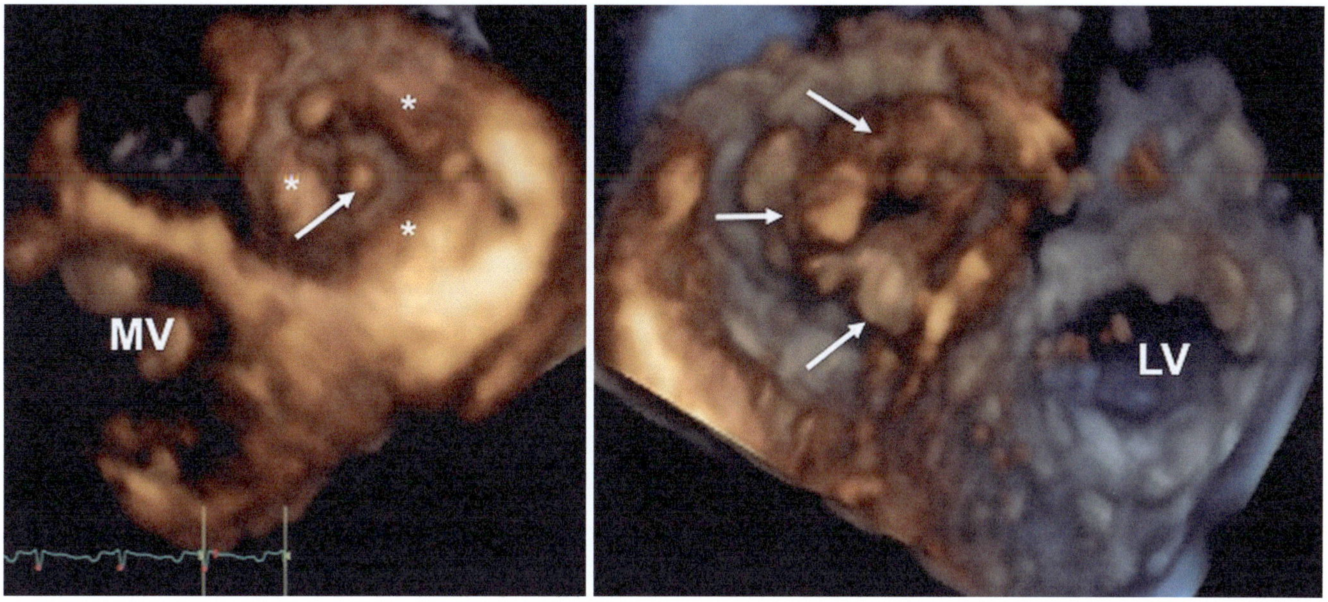

Fig. 22.4 Infective endocarditis on a bioprosthetic valve in tricuspid position. *Left panel*, transthoracic three-dimensional volume rendering of the prosthesis visualized from the atrial perspective. Extensive pannus overgrowth (asterisks) and the vegetation prolapsing in systole (arrow) can be seen (Video 22.3a/Left). *Right panel*, the same prosthesis visualized from the ventricular perspective showing multiple, large vegetations (arrows) (Video 22.3b/Right)

procedure/device. Pre-procedural planning mainly based on echocardiography and aims to: (1) define the mechanism of tricuspid regurgitation; (2) characterize tricuspid valve morphology and localization of commissures; (3) measure the tricuspid annulus perimeters and diameters; (4). define the spatial relationships between the tricuspid valve and surrounding cardiac structures (i.e. right coronary artery and atrio-ventricular node); and (5) size the inferior and superior vena cava. According to the concepts already discussed in Chaps. 18 and 21, it is clear the crucial role of 3DE in pre-procedural planning of transcatheter procedure to treat functional tricuspid regurgitation. A computed tomography scan may provide additional data about tricuspid annulus structure and size, quality of tricuspid annulus tissue, and spatial relationships with the right coronary artery.

Despite the relatively limited experience in treating functional tricuspid regurgitation has not allowed to define precise criteria for patient selection, suitable candidates with relatively high likelihood of clinical benefit seems to be patients with functional tricuspid regurgitation, normal tricuspid leaflet morphology and mobility, in whom the predominant mechanism of the regurgitation is the annulus dilation with limited tethering of the leaflets which maintain some degree of coaptation. The right ventricular geometry and function should be relatively preserved and pulmonary pressure not severely increased.

In patients in whom the tricuspid annulus dilation is the prevalent mechanism of the regurgitation, procedures/devices targeting the annulus emulating the surgical annuloplasty (Cardioband, Millipede) or the Kay procedure (Trialign, TriCinch) may be considered. In patients with normal or nearly normal annulus size, abnormal but relatively preserved leaflet coaptation between the septal and anterior leaflets (which are the usual target leaflets [28]) to allow valid tissue grasping by the clip, the MitraClip system may be a suitable option (Fig. 22.5, Videos 22.4b, 22.4c, and 22.4d).

In patients with severely enlarged annulus and wide leaflet coaptation gap, either the FORMA spacer or a bioprosthesis implant may be considered (Fig. 22.6, Videos 22.5a, 22.5b, 22.5c, and 22.5d).

A multimodality approach is usually needed to guide the procedure including two- and 3DE, fluoroscopy, angiography and, in some cases, intracardiac echocardiography. 3DE is pivotal to appreciate the spatial relationships between the tricuspid valve and surrounding structure, and to guide catheter navigation. In order to optimize the procedure and facilitate the interventionalist work, it is important to maintain the same orientation of the volume rendered cut planes in all procedural steps. Since conventional two-dimensional and biplane views have a higher spatial resolution than 3DE, they are used to visualize the devices and their fixation.

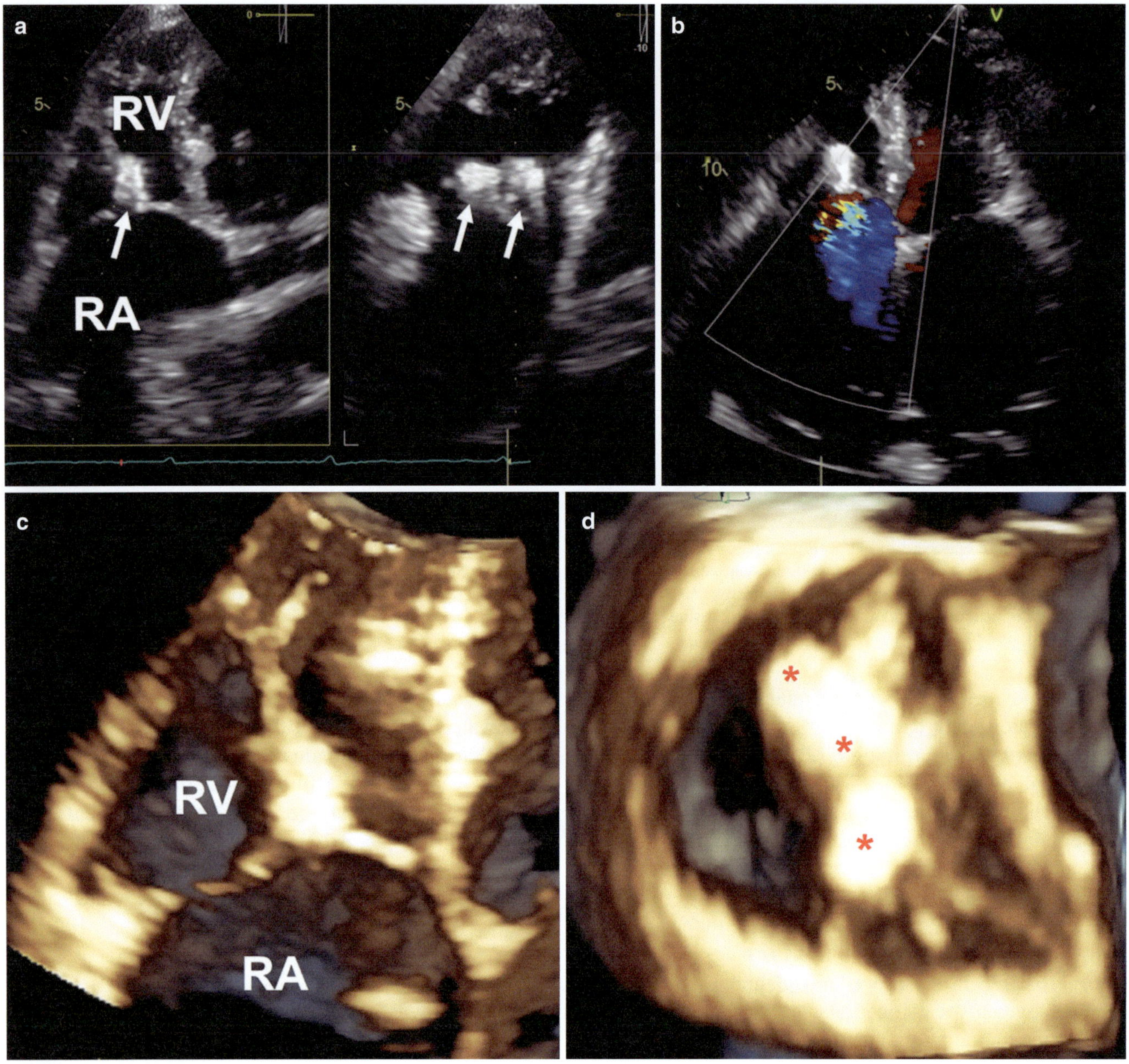

Fig 22.5 MitraClip transcatheter repair of severe tricuspid regurgitation. (**a**) Transthoracic biplane view showing the positions of the clips (arrows). In the 4-chamber view, only one clip has been visualized. Conversely, in the orthogonal view two clips are visible. (**b**) Transthoracic color flow imaging to assess the severity of residual regurgitation after the procedure (Video 22.4b). (**c**) Transthoracic three-dimensional volume rendering showing the position of the clips and their stability (Video 22.4c). (**d**) Transthoracic three-dimensional volume rendering using a transversal cut plane to visualize the clips from the ventricular perspective. Proper rotation of the cut plane reveals that three clips (red asterisks) have been implanted: two on the commissure between the septal and anterior leaflets, and one between the septal and posterior leaflets (Video 22.4d). *RA* right atrium, *RV* right ventricle

Transthoracic approach is sometimes needed also for the intraprocedural monitoring, because of the anterior position of the tricuspid valve in the chest (see Chap. 18). However, transthoracic echocardiography is quite challenging during the procedure because of the patient position, radiation exposure of the echocardiographer, and interference with the C-arm rotations. Therefore, the transesophageal approach is used in most of the procedures (Fig. 22.7, Videos 22.6a and 22.6b).

To avoid problems during the procedure, the quality of the images of the tricuspid valve using both the transthoracic

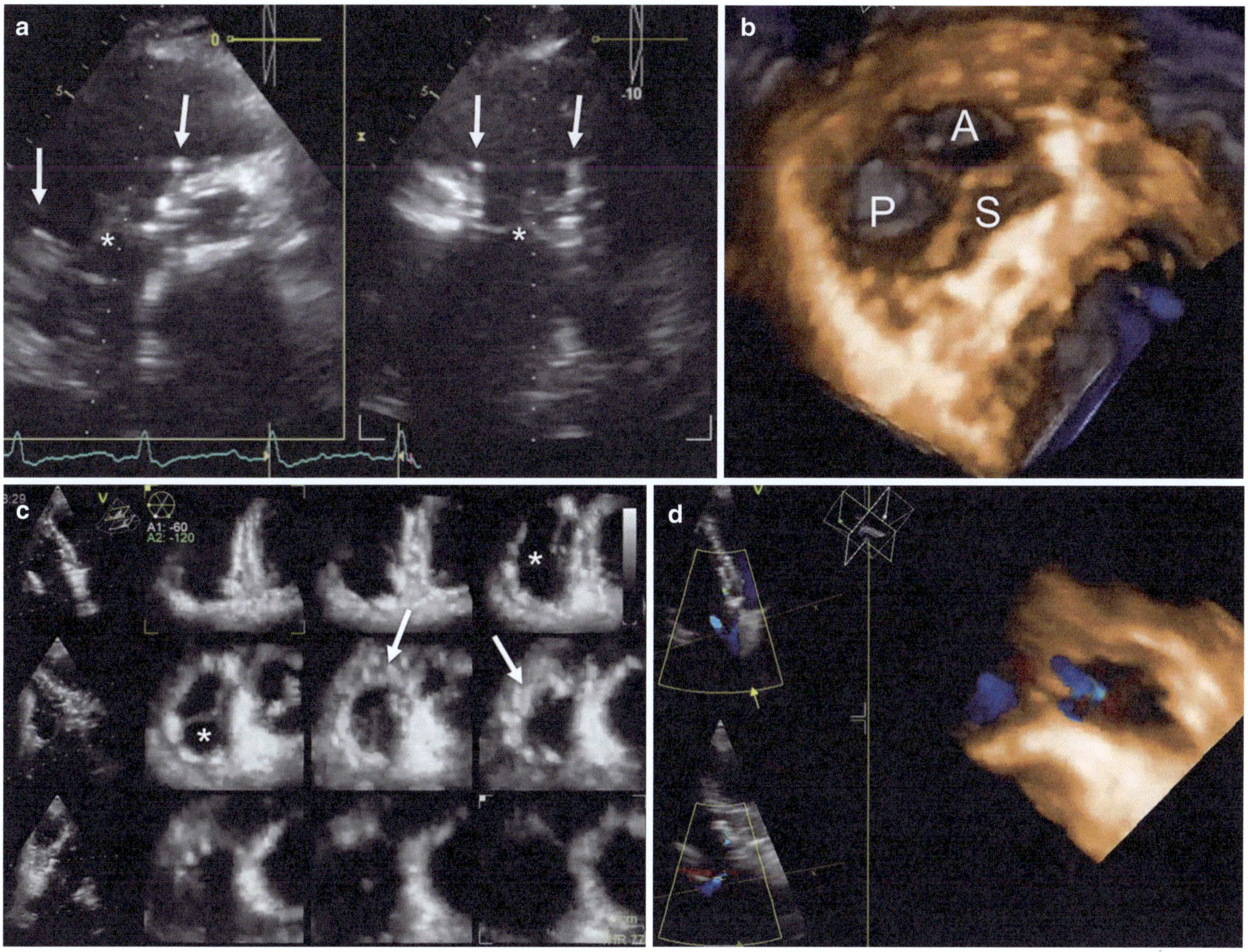

Fig 22.6 Transcatheter tricuspid valve implant using the Gate™ Tricuspid Valve Stent. (**a**) Biplane imaging of the implanted valve showing the metallic stents (arrows) and cusps (asterisks) (Video 22.5a). (**b**) Transthoracic three-dimensional volume rendering of the valve seen *en face* from the ventricular perspective (Video 22.5b). (**c**) Multislice display with the region of interest confined at the level of the valve to visualize the shape of the stent (arrows) and the motion of the leaflets (asterisks) (Video 22.5c). (**d**) Transthoracic three-dimensional color Doppler of the valve seen en face from the ventricular perspective to visualize the origin of the mild intraprosthetic jet (Video 22.5d)

and transesophageal approach with the patient laying supine on the bed (mimicking the position he/she will have in the catheterization laboratory) should always be checked during the echocardiographic study which qualifies the patient for the procedure.

Recently, a new imaging technique (fusion imaging) allows to superimpose on the same monitor patient-specific imaging data from both two- and 3DE transesophageal images and fluoroscopic projections, and to align them in the 3D space and in time (Fig. 22.8)

Echocardiographic-fluoroscopic fused images allow to put together the strengths of the two imaging modalities and reduce the impact of their limitations. The tissue of the various components of the tricuspid valve apparatus is soft and transparent to X-rays and, in patients with severe tricuspid regurgitation, only exceptionally there are calcium deposits on the tricuspid valve. Accordingly, the interventional cardiologist cannot rely on fluoroscopic imaging only to guide and monitor procedures on the tricuspid valve. However, fluoroscopy has its own strengths in the catheterization laboratory: interventional cardiologists are more familiar with fluoroscopy than with other imaging modalities; wires, guide catheters and devices have been designed to be radiopaque in order to optimize fluoroscopic guidance (conversely, they create artifacts when imaged with echocardiography); the system has a large field of view allowing the operator to follow long segments of catheters; the temporal resolution (up to 30 fps) is adequate to maneuver the catheters. On the other

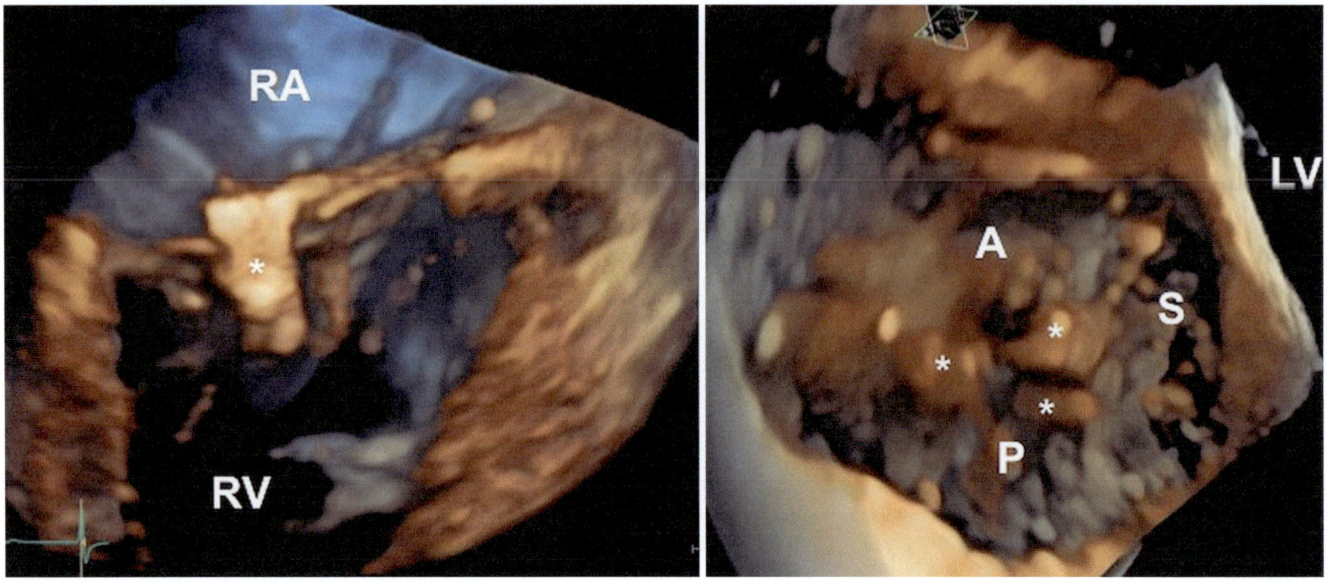

Fig. 22.7 Transesophageal three-dimensional echocardiography imaging during MitraClip position in a patient with severe tricuspid regurgitation. *Left panel*, volume rendered longitudinal cut plane to assess the grasping of both leaflets and the stability of the clip (asterisk) (Video 22.6a/Left). Right panel, volume rendered en face view of the valve from the ventricular perspective to localize the position of the clips (asterisks) (Video 22.6b/Right). *A* anterior tricuspid leaflet, *LV* left ventricle, *P* posterior tricuspid leaflet, *RA* right atrium, *RV* right ventricle, *S* septal tricuspid leaflet

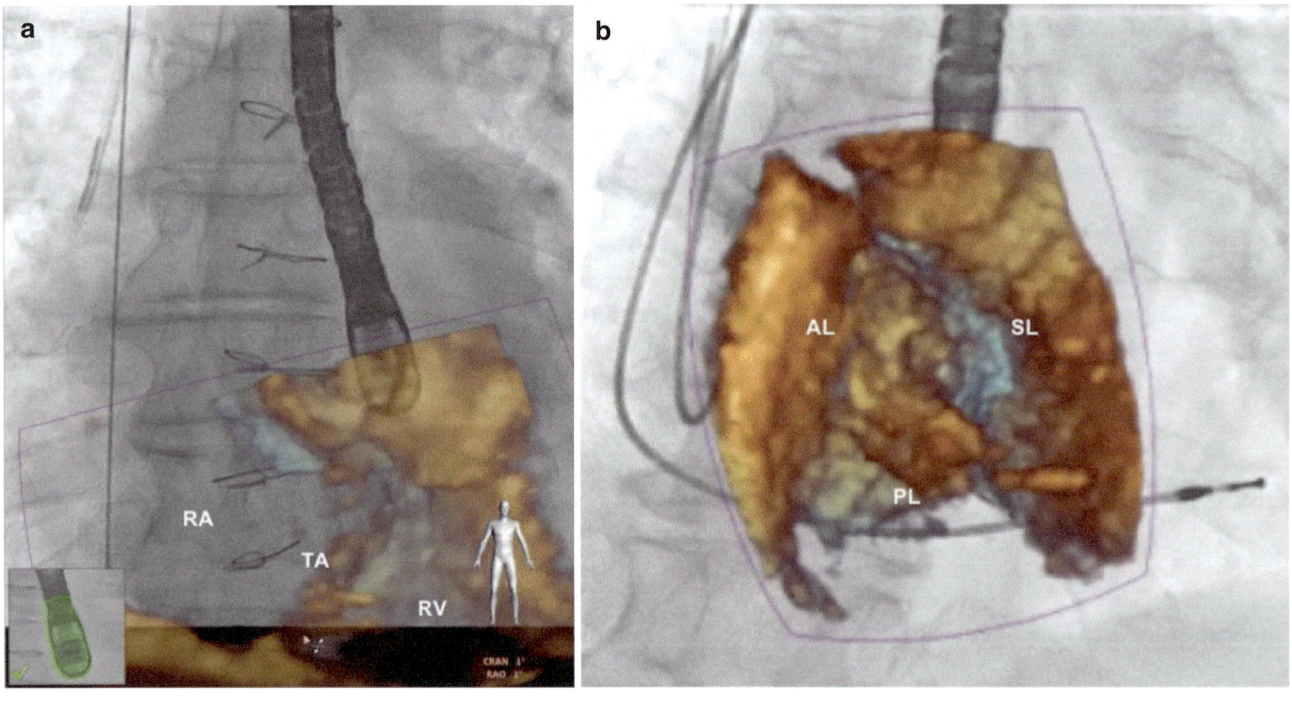

Fig. 22.8 Fusion imaging. (**a**) Three-dimensional frontal view of tricuspid valve superimposed on the antero-posterior fluoroscopic projection. (**b**) Three-dimensional *en face* view of the tricuspid valve superimposed on the left anterior oblique caudal fluoroscopic projection. The fused image shows the short axis of the TV, but from ventricular perspective. (**c**) Two-dimensional inflow-outflow view of the right chambers superimposed on the right anterior oblique cranial fluoroscopic projection during the transcatheter treatment of tricuspid regurgitation with MitraClip implantation. (**d**) Two dimensional 4-chamber view superimposed on left anterior oblique cranial fluoroscopic projection during the transcatheter treatment of tricuspid regurgitation with MitraClip implantation. (Courtesy of Dr. F. Ancona and Dr. E. Agricola, San Raffaele Scientific Institute, Milan, Italy). *AL* anterior leaflet, *PL* posterior leaflet, *RA* right atrium, *RV* right ventricle, *RVOT* right ventricular outflow tract, *SL* septal leaflet, *TA* tricuspid annulus, *TV* tricuspid valve

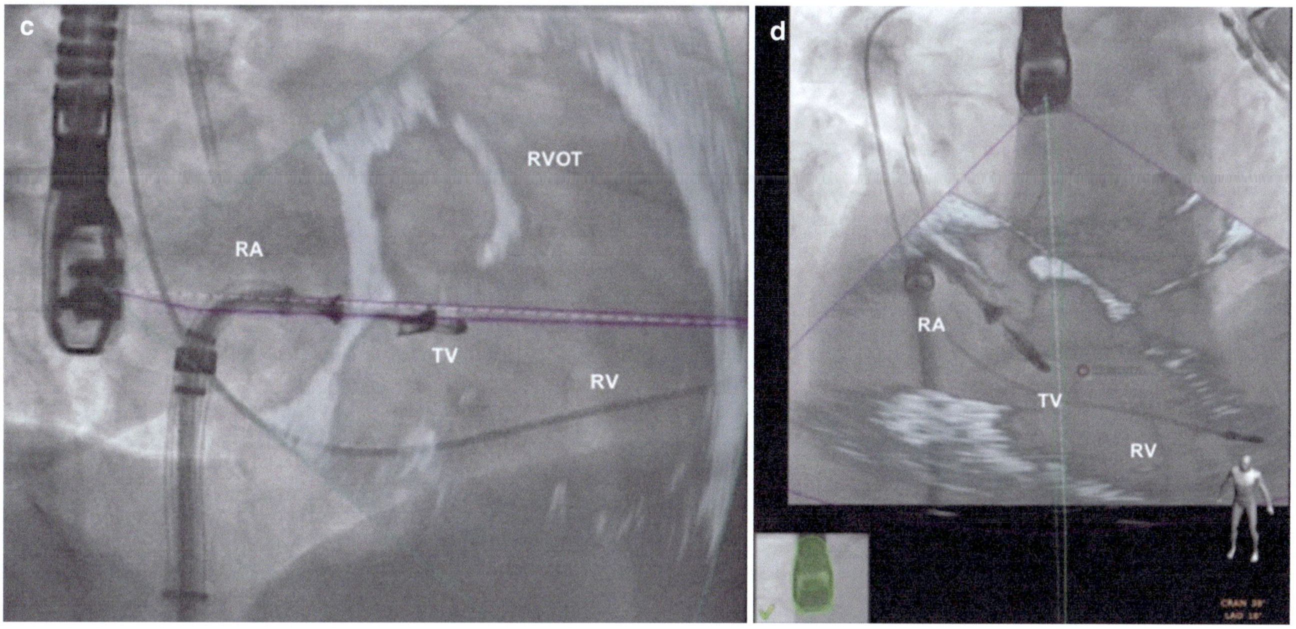

Fig. 22.8 (continued)

end, two- and 3DE can offer detailed anatomical assessment of the tricuspid valve structures and are pivotal for guiding catheter navigation during transcatheter procedures [29]. However, when images obtained from fluoroscopy (to manipulate catheters and devices) and echocardiography (to visualize the components of the tricuspid valve apparatus) are shown on to separate screens, the anatomical relationships between the position/orientation of the wires and catheters and the anatomy of the TV can be lost (also because, particularly for the tricuspid valve, the projections of the fluoroscopy seldom mimic the views of echocardiography). Echocardiography and fluoroscopic fused images are particularly useful during interventional procedures because they provide: (1) an easier localization of the anatomical structures of interest; (2) an improved localization of devices and an easier navigation inside the right-heart chambers; (3) a facilitated assessment of trajectories and axial alignment of catheter and devices; (4) more precise localization of the landing zone of devices [26].

References

1. Nath J, Foster E, Heidenreich PA. Impact of tricuspid regurgitation on long-term survival. J Am Coll Cardiol. 2004;43:405–9.
2. Badano LP, Muraru D, Enriquez-Sarano M. Assessment of functional tricuspid regurgitation. Eur Heart J. 2013;34(25):1875–85.
3. Neuhold S, Huelsmann M, Pernicka E, et al. Impact of tricuspid regurgitation on survival in patients with chronic heart failure: unexpected findings of a long-term observational study. Eur Heart J. 2013;34:844–52.
4. Calafiore AM, Gallina S, Iaco AL, et al. Mitral valve surgery for functional mitral regurgitation: should moderate-or-more tricuspid regurgitation be treated? a propensity score analysis. Ann Thorac Surg. 2009;87:698–703.
5. Mascherbauer J, Kammerlander AA, Marzluf BA, Graf A, Kocher A, Bonderman D. Prognostic impact of tricuspid regurgitation in patients undergoing aortic valve surgery for aortic stenosis. PLoS One. 2015;10:e0136024.
6. Varadarajan P, Pai RG. Prognostic implications of tricuspid regurgitation in patients with severe aortic regurgitation: results from a cohort of 756 patients. Interact Cardiovasc Thorac Surg. 2012;14:580–4.
7. Kalbacher D, Schafer U, von Bardeleben RS, et al. Impact of tricuspid valve regurgitation in surgical high-risk patients undergoing MitraClip implantation: results from the TRAMI registry. EuroIntervention. 2017;12:e1809–16.
8. Stuge O, Liddicoat J. Emerging opportunities for cardiac surgeons within structural heart disease. J Thorac Cardiovasc Surg. 2006;132:1258–61.
9. Nishimura RA, Otto CM, Bonow RO, et al. 2014 AHA/ACC guideline for the management of patients with valvular heart disease: a report of the American College of Cardiology/American Heart Association Task Force on Practice Guidelines. J Am Coll Cardiol. 2014;63:e57–185.
10. Baumgartner H, Falk V, Bax JJ, et al. 2017 ESC/EACTS guidelines for the management of valvular heart disease. Eur Heart J. 2017;38:2739–91.
11. Ren WJ, Zhang BG, Liu JS, Qian YJ, Guo YQ. Outcomes of tricuspid annuloplasty with and without prosthetic rings: a retrospective follow-up study. J Cardiothorac Surg. 2015;10:81.
12. Starck CT, Kempfert J, Falk V. Tricuspid valve interventions: surgical techniques and outcomes. EuroIntervention. 2015;11(Suppl W):W128–32.
13. Rizzoli G, Vendramin I, Nesseris G, Bottio T, Guglielmi C, Schiavon L. Biological or mechanical prostheses in tricuspid position? A meta-analysis of intra-institutional results. Ann Thorac Surg. 2004;77:1607–14.

14. Badhwar V, Rankin JS, He M, et al. Performing concomitant tricuspid valve repair at the time of mitral valve operations is not associated with increased operative mortality. Ann Thorac Surg. 2017;103:587–93.
15. Bernal JM, Morales D, Revuelta C, Llorca J, Gutierrez-Morlote J, Revuelta JM. Reoperations after tricuspid valve repair. J Thorac Cardiovasc Surg. 2005;130:498–503.
16. Rodes-Cabau J, Hahn RT, Latib A, et al. Transcatheter therapies for treating tricuspid regurgitation. J Am Coll Cardiol. 2016;67:1829–45.
17. Praz F, George I, Kodali S, et al. Transcatheter tricuspid valve-in-valve intervention for degenerative bioprosthetic tricuspid valve disease. J Am Soc Echocardiogr. 2018;31:491–504.
18. Hahn RT. Current transcatheter devices to treat functional tricuspid regurgitation with discussion of issues relevant to clinical trial design. Ann Cardiothorac Surg. 2017;6:240–7.
19. Lauten A, Dreger H, Laule M, Stangl K, Figulla HR. Caval valve implantation. Interv Cardiol Clin. 2018;7:57–63.
20. Rosser BA, Taramasso M, Maisano F. Transcatheter interventions for tricuspid regurgitation: TriCinch (4Tech). EuroIntervention. 2016;12:Y110–2.
21. Hahn RT, Meduri CU, Davidson CJ, et al. Early feasibility study of a transcatheter tricuspid valve annuloplasty: SCOUT trial 30-day results. J Am Coll Cardiol. 2017;69:1795–806.
22. Besler C, Orban M, Rommel KP, et al. Predictors of procedural and clinical outcomes in patients with symptomatic tricuspid regurgitation undergoing transcatheter edge-to-edge repair. JACC Cardiovasc Interv. 2018;11:1119–28.
23. Stephan von Bardeleben R, Tamm A, Emrich T, Munzel T, Schulz E. Percutaneous transvenous direct annuloplasty of a human tricuspid valve using the Valtech Cardioband. Eur Heart J. 2017;38:690.
24. Campelo-Parada F, Perlman G, Philippon F, et al. First-in-man experience of a novel transcatheter repair system for treating severe tricuspid regurgitation. J Am Coll Cardiol. 2015;66:2475–83.
25. Prihadi EA, Delgado V, Hahn RT, Leipsic J, Min JK, Bax JJ. Imaging needs in novel transcatheter tricuspid valve interventions. JACC Cardiovasc Imaging. 2018;11:736–54.
26. Ancona F, Agricola E, Stella S, et al. Interventional imaging of the tricuspid valve. Interv Cardiol Clin. 2018;7:13–29.
27. Ancona F, Stella S, Taramasso M, et al. Multimodality imaging of the tricuspid valve with implication for percutaneous repair approaches. Heart. 2017;103:1073–81.
28. Vismara R, Gelpi G, Prabhu S, et al. Transcatheter edge-to-edge treatment of functional tricuspid regurgitation in an ex vivo pulsatile heart model. J Am Coll Cardiol. 2016;68:1024–33.
29. Faletra FF, Pedrazzini G, Pasotti E, et al. 3D TEE during catheter-based interventions. JACC Cardiovasc Imaging. 2014;7:292–308.

The Right Atrium

23

Diletta Peluso and Marcelo Haertel Miglioranza

Abstract

Right atrium (RA) has been a neglected heart chamber for long time. Only recently, the recognition of its role in assisting right ventricular filling, the demonstration of the predictive value of RA size in various pathological conditions, and the identification of the RA as a target and transit chamber for many interventional procedures have raised clinical interest in RA assessment. Accordingly, three-dimensional echocardiography (3DE) has acquired an important role in RA evaluation. It allows to visualize internal structures of the RA with a richness of details that is comparable with the anatomical specimens. This capability is used more and more in the electrophysiology and catheterization laboratories and moreover it demonstrated to be useful in differentiating normal from pathological anatomical structures.

Recently, the updated guidelines on cardiac chamber quantification by echocardiography have introduced the RA volume as the recommended parameter to report RA size. 3DE demonstrated its capability to accurately measure RA volume, indipendently from any geometrical assumption about its shape, overcoming the limitations of two-dimensional echocardiography. Furthermore, 3DE enables measurement of RA volume in different moments of the cardiac cycle (maximum, minimum and pre-atrial contraction volumes), allowing evaluation of RA phasic function, in term of emptying volumes and fractions.

Keywords

Right atrium · Three-dimensional echocardiography · Right atrial volume · Right atrial function · Right atrial structures · Right atrial shape

Despite the fact that in 1628, William Harvey already identified the atrium as a "*receptacle and store-house*" and reported that the right atrium (RA) was "*the first to live, and the last to die*" [1], in modern clinical cardiology the RA has been a neglected heart chamber for long time.

Only recently, it has been realized the role of the RA to assist filling of the right ventricle by transferring a high volume of blood rapidly to the ventricle at low pressure, preventing peripheral edema and hepatic congestion.

Similar to the left atrium, RA mechanics is complex and three components can be identified: i. reservoir function, storing blood when the tricuspid valve is closed; ii. conduit function, passive blood transfer directly from the coronary and systemic veins to the right ventricle when the tricuspid valve is open; and iii. booster pump function, active atrial contraction in late diastole to complete ventricular filling [2–5]. Gaynor and coworkers [6] demonstrated that the RA can adjust its ability to act more as a reservoir than a conduit in a dynamic manner. The RA conduit-to-reservoir ratio was directly related to the right ventricular pressure-RA pressure gradient at the time of maximum RA volume, with increased ventricular pressures favoring conduit function, but it was inversely related to cardiac output, with an increase in the reservoir contribution favoring improved cardiac output.

RA remodel in different ways in different cardiac conditions [7] and, both in normal subjects and patients with atrial fibrillation, RA volumes measured with conventional two-dimensional echocardiography using the single-plane area-length algorithm are significantly underestimated compared with those measured by three-dimensional echocardiography (3DE) [8–10]. Finally, RA size has been reported to have an independent prognostic power in many diseases

D. Peluso (✉)
Cardiology Unit, Ospedale SS Giovanni e Paolo, Venice, Italy

M. H. Miglioranza
Cardiovascular Imaging Research and Innovation Lab, Institute of Cardiology - University Foundation of Cardiology, Porto Alegre, Rio Grande do Sul, Brazil

PREVENCOR—Mãe de Deus Hospital, Porto Alegre, Brazil

L. P. Badano et al. (eds.), *Textbook of Three-Dimensional Echocardiography*, https://doi.org/10.1007/978-3-030-14032-8_23

such as pulmonary hypertension [11, 12], congenital heart disease, heart failure, and the RA is the target or the transit heart chamber for many interventional procedure.

At the same time, the growing interest in RA evaluation [13] has been paralleled by the realization of the limitions of two dimensional echocardiography and of the potential of 3DE to assess RA geometry and function.

Acquisition and Display

3DE has been recently introduced for the evaluation of the RA size [10, 14] and morphology [15, 16]. To perform quantitative analysis of RA volumes and function, a full-volume 3D data set is usually acquired from the apical approach, adjusting depth and sector width in order to encompass the entire RA cavity in the data set (Fig. 23.1). The RA can be displayed either in the multi-slice or volume-rendered dispay modality. The multislice modality shows the RA data set as a series of orthogonal and parallel tomographic planes (Fig. 23.2) and it is mainly used to visualize the shape and the function of the RA. The tomographic planes can be freely oriented in order to achieve anatomically corrected cross-sections of the RA. Conversely, the volume-rendering modality displays the RA as a 3D structure (Fig. 23.3) and it can be cropped and oriented in order to visualize the anatomy of its internal structures and to assess their spatial relations. The management of the full-volume data set with a dedicated software package allows to measure RA phasic volumes and obtain functional parameters (e.g. emptying volumes and emptying fractions).

Real-time 3DE visualization of the RA is usually obtained by transoesophageal echocardiography and its main clinical application is the monitoring of electrophysiological and interventional procedures (Fig. 23.4).

Morphological Analysis

3DE is able to provide anatomical images of the RA structures with a richness of details that is comparable with the anatomical specimens [15]. This capability is used more and more in the electrophysiology and caheterization laboratories because the RA is the first entry point for most interventional procedures and is the target heart chamber of many electrophysiological procedures.

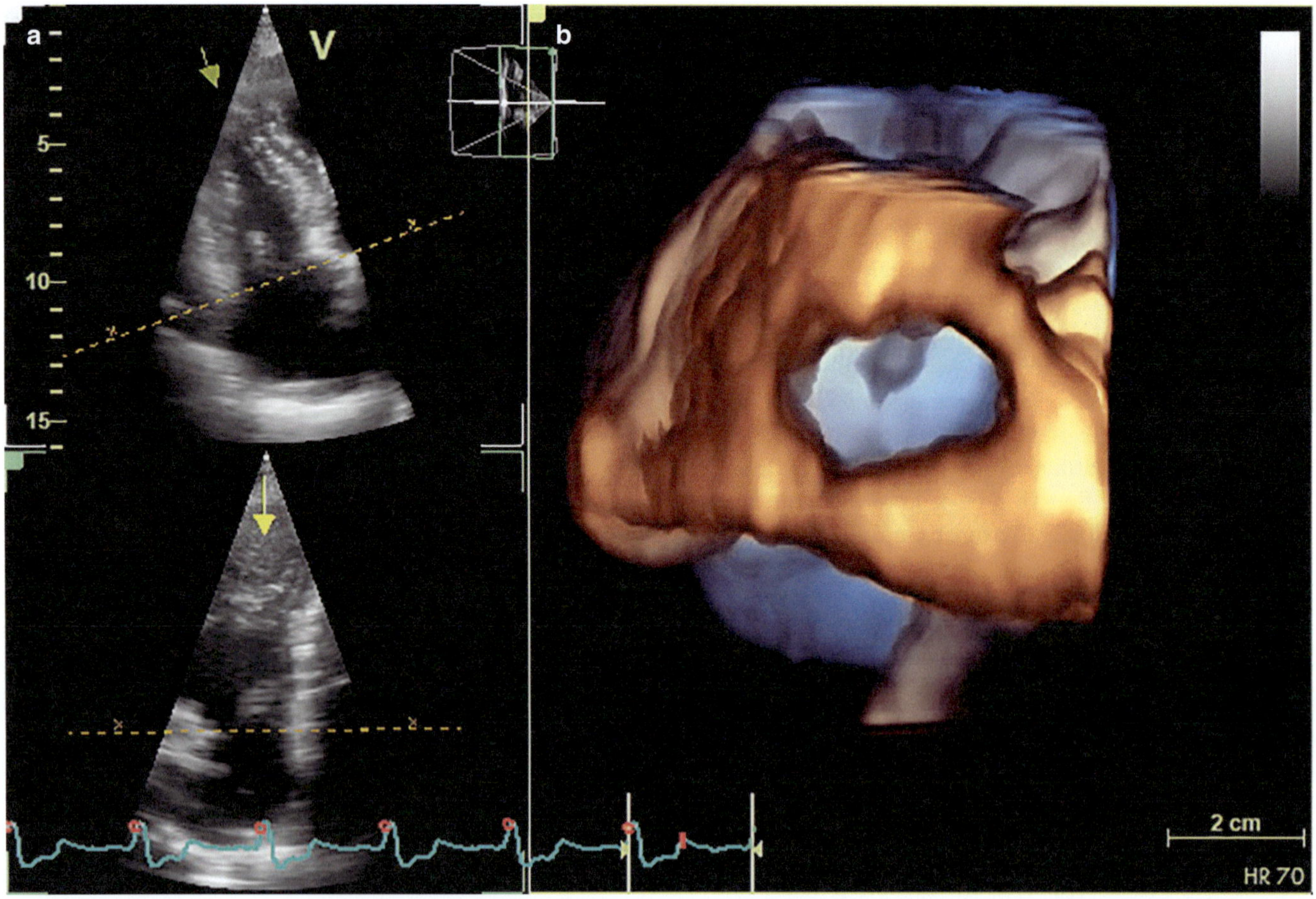

Fig. 23.1 Multi-beat full volume acquisition focused on the right atrium. (**a**) Two different apical planes were used as a reference to adjust the sector depth and width to encompass the entire right atrial cavity. (**b**) A full volume acquisition is displayed in volume rendering format and cropped at the tricuspid annulus plane

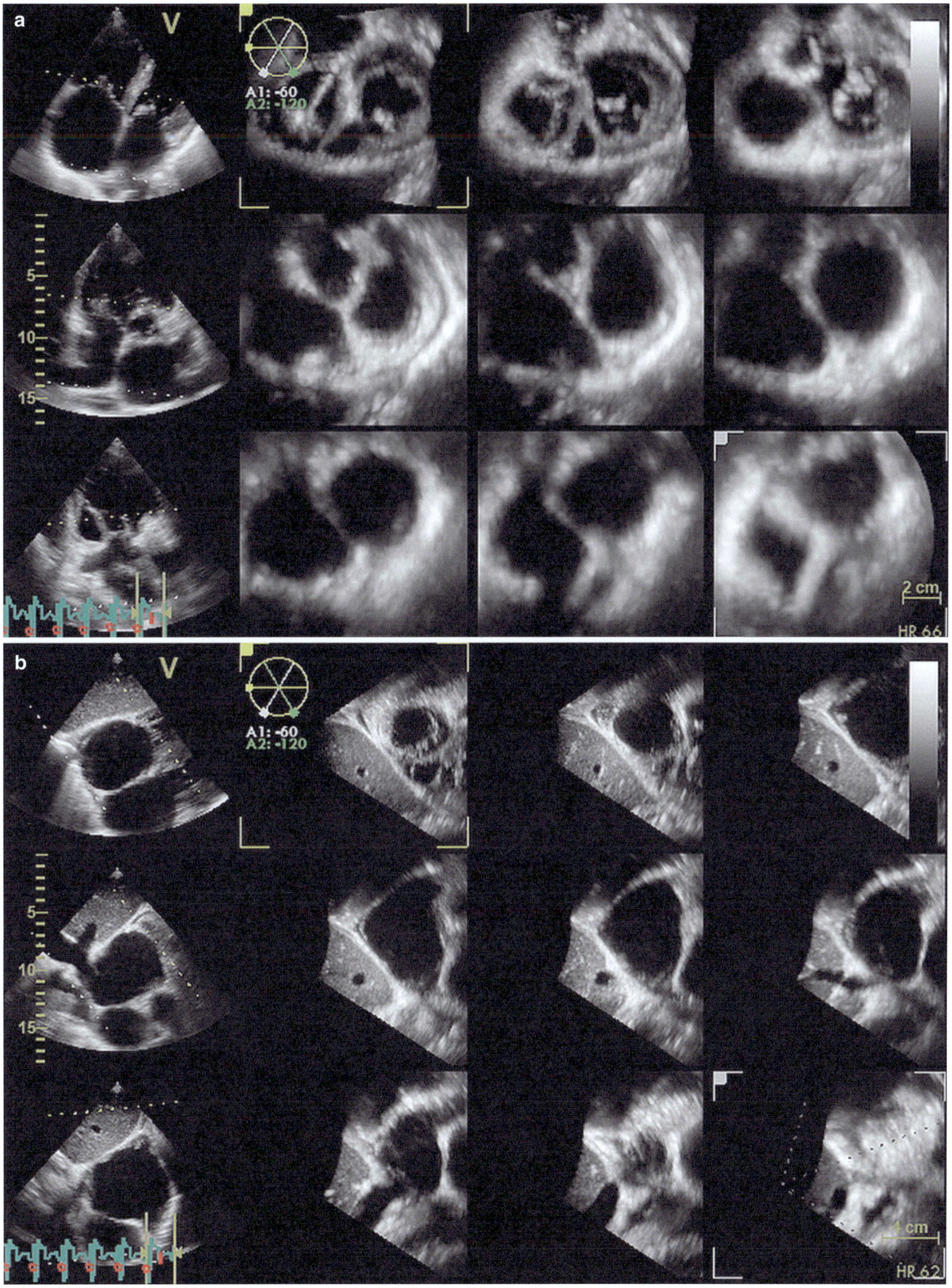

Fig. 23.2 Multi-slice evaluation of the right atrium. (**a**) Apical acquisition displaying three different longitudinal planes and nine transversal tomographic and parallel planes. (**b**) Subcostal acquisition displaying the right atrium, obtained rotating the transversal cutting planes parallel to the tricuspid valve and the roof of the right atrium

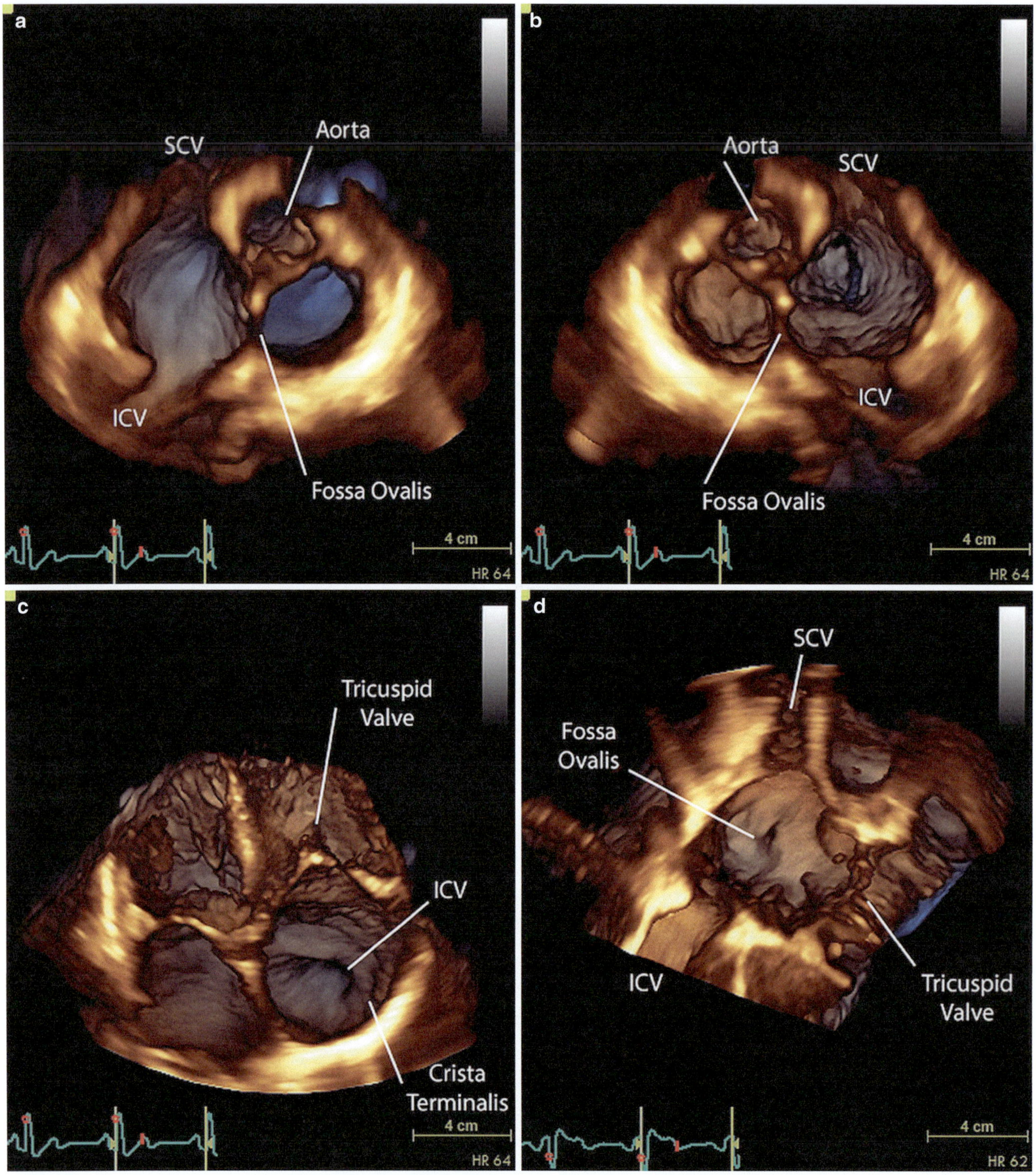

Fig. 23.3 Volume rendering allowing the complete analysis of the right atrial structure according to the posision of the cropping plane. (**a**) Transversal cropping plane at the level of the cavae veins displaying the right atrial roof; (**b**) Transversal cropping plane at the level of the cavae veins displaying the tricuspid valve; (**c**) Oblique cropping plane displaying the inferior cavae vein and the *Crista Terminalis*; (**d**) Longitudinal cropping plane showing the *Fossa Ovalis* en face. *ICV* inferior cavae vein, *SCV* superior cavae vein

Normal anatomical structures that characterize the RA are the crista terminalis, the cavotricuspid isthmus, the Chiari's network, the Eustachian valve, the ostium of the coronary sinus and the right side of interatrial septum.

Crista terminalis: it originates near the antero-medial wall of the RA, where it merges with the interatrial or Bachmann bundle. Then it passes along the anterior margin of the orifice of the superior vena cava, arcs later-

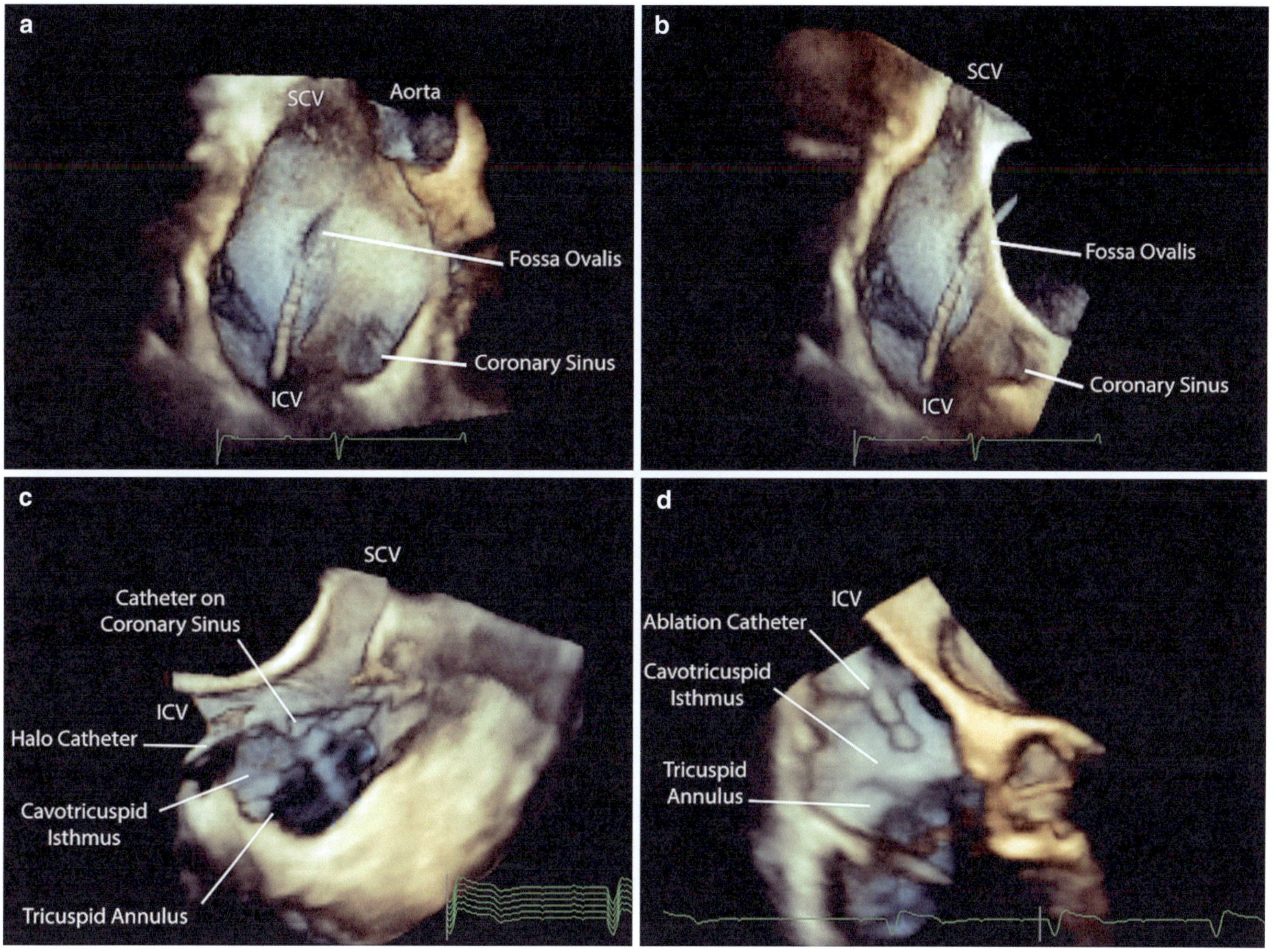

Fig. 23.4 Real-time three-dimensional visualization of the right atrium to monitor and guide interventional procedures. (**a**) and (**b**) Interatrial septal puncture; (**c**) and (**d**) Atrial flutter ablation. *ICV* inferior cavae vein, *SCV* superior cavae vein

ally, and descends towards the inferior vena cava, where it becomes rather indistinct as it branches into smaller bundles. Concern about this structure is related to its arrhytmogenic potential. Crista terminalis per se and the non-uniform architecture of myofibres at the junction of the crista with pectinate muscles is most likely the cause of the marked anisotropy observed, which may be the substrate for atrial arrhythmias [17]. 3DE allows to obtain an en-face view of the crista terminalis (Fig. 23.5). Sometimes, crista terminalis may appear in a conventional 4-chamber view as a mass attached to the roof of the right atrium. In this scenario, 3DE permits to define size, extension and spatial relationship of this 2DE finding, solving any problems of differential diagnosis towards pathological masses.

Cavotricuspid isthmus: it is a roughly quadrilateral-shaped endocardial region which is delimited anteriorly by the annular insertion of the septal and lateral leaflets of the tricuspid valve, posteriorly by the inferior cava vein border and the Eustachian valve/ridge. The lateral and medial borders are rather indistinctly marked by the final ramifications of the crista terminalis and the inferior border of the coronary sinus orifice, respectively [18]. The cavotricuspid isthmus may have a variable anatomy and many of its anatomical variants may create difficulties during ablation procedures [19]. Particularly, a pouch located in the middle part of the cavotricuspid isthmus may cause incomplete ablation of atrial flutter pathway for the difficulty to achieve an adequate catheter contact. Moreover, prominent pectinate muscles may encroach onto the cavotricuspid isthmus and cause the trapping of the catheter. 3DE enables the visualization of the cavotricuspid isthmus anatomy (Fig. 23.6) as well as its variants in order to correctly plan the ablation procedure and anticipate any issues.

Chiari's network: it is an embrionic remnant, first described in 1897 in an autopsy series, present in about 2–3% of the population [20]. It appears as a fenestrated or unfenestrated freely-mobile membrane that derives from the incomplete regression of the right valve of the sinus venosus [21] (Fig. 23.7). It can be confused with other pathological findings, such as tricuspid valve flail or veg-

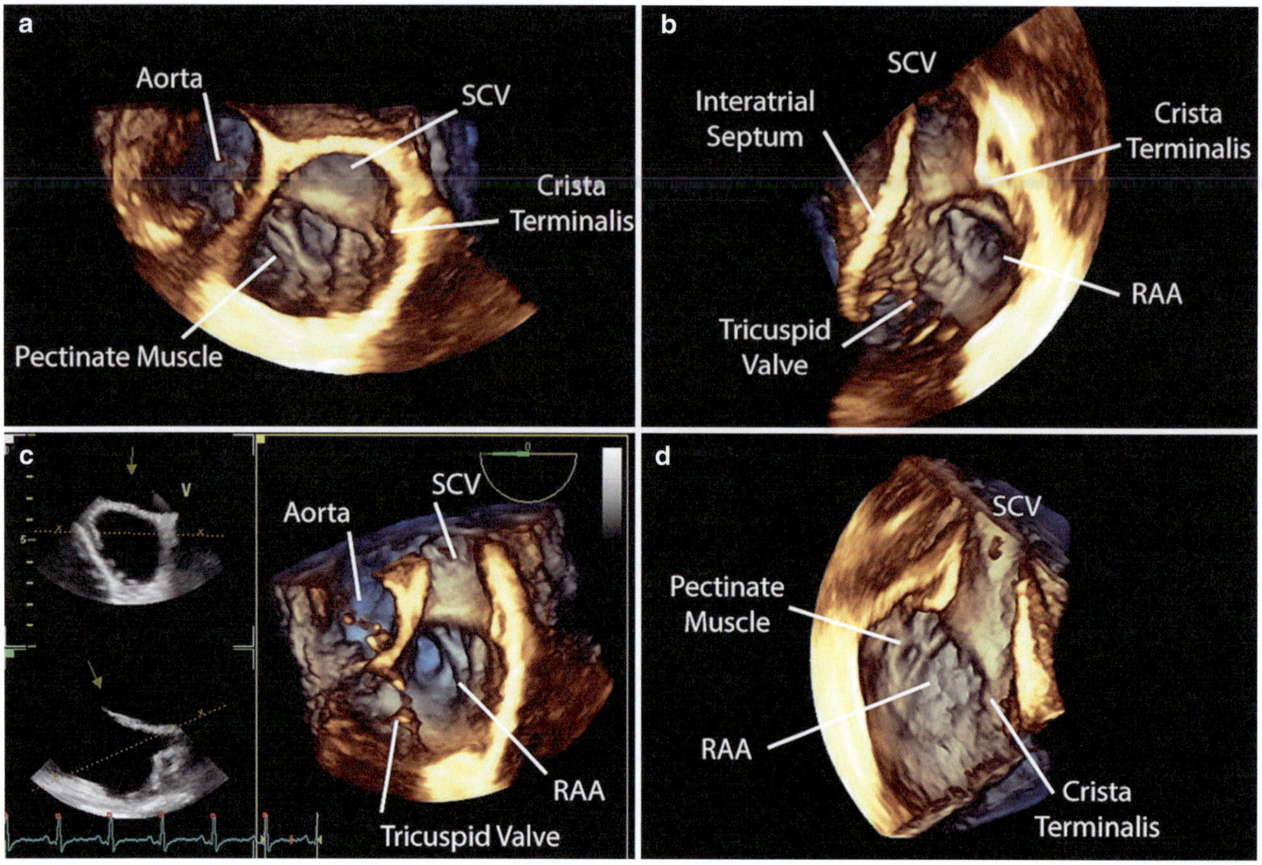

Fig. 23.5 Volume rendering of the right atrium, obtained by transesophageal acquisition displaying the *Crista Terminalis*, right atrial appendage (RAA) and pectinate muscle with their relation to the superior cavae vein (SCV) from different perspectives according to the cropping plane. (**a**) *en face* view of the superior cavae vein ostium showing the origin of the *Crista Terminalis* at the interatrial or Bachmann bundle on the antero-medial wall of the RA. Longitudinal views of the right atrial chamber visualizing the antero-medial wall (**b**), the anterior wall (**c**) and the lateral wall (**d**)

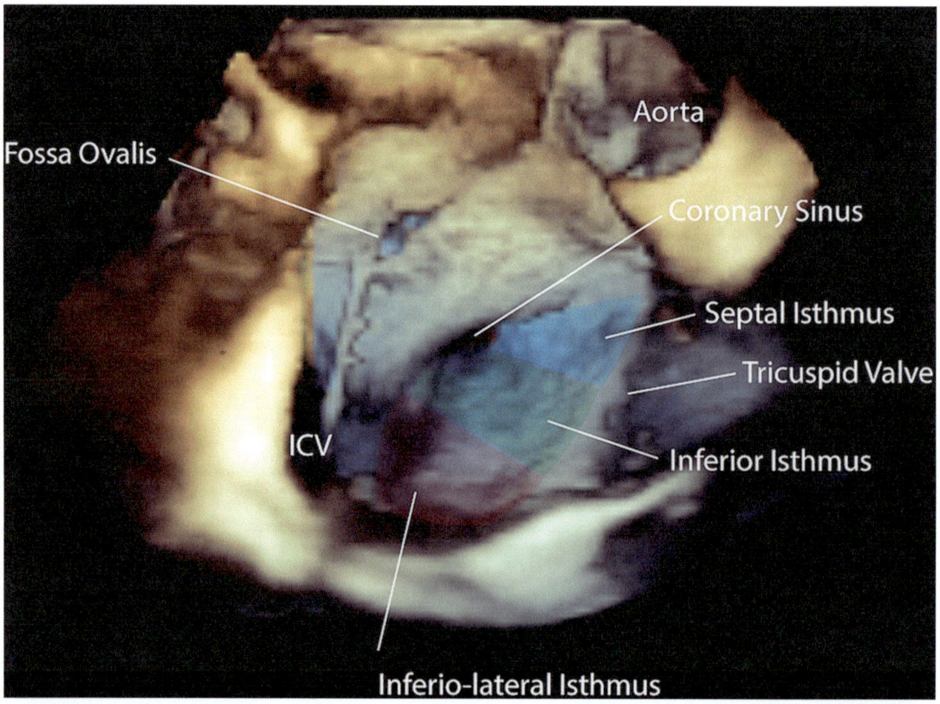

Fig. 23.6 *En face* view of the Cavo tricuspid isthmus and its relation with the tricuspid valve, inferior cavae vena (ICV) and coronary sinus

etations. 3DE may help in differential diagnosis thanks to its ability to define morphological features and spatial relationship [22]. Moreover, its identification is important because it might entangle catheter insertion into the RA.

Eustachian valve: it is an embronic structure that during the fetal life directs the blood flow from the inferior cava vein towards the interatrial septum and then the systemic circulation. After birth, it disappears or persists as thin filamentous structure originating fromt the inferior cava vein (Fig. 23.8). The degree of persistence is variable and sometimes it can appears as a large elongated structure mimicking the interatrial septum [23]. A redundant Eustachian valve may cause problematic catheter manipulation during electrophysiological procedures.

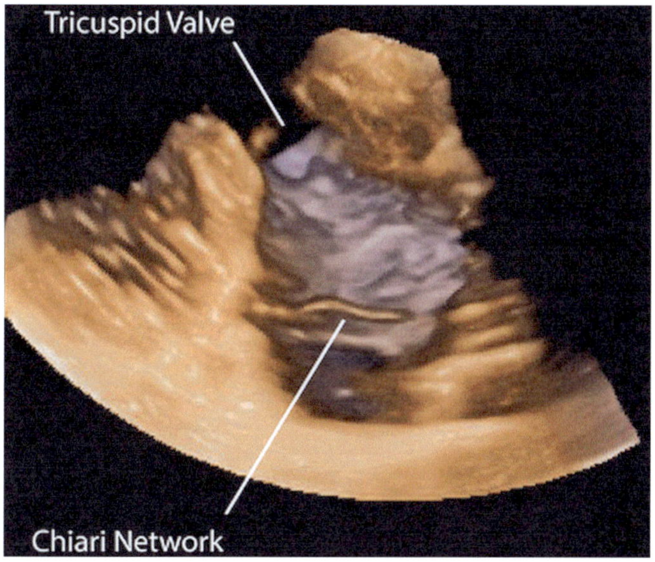

Fig. 23.7 Chiari's network

Coronary sinus ostium: it opens in the RA between the ostium of the inferior cava vein and the tricuspid orifice. In nearly 80% of cases, the ostium of the coronary sinus is guarded by a semilunar valve, the valve of the coronary sinus or the valve of Thebesius. The presence of this valve may make the cannulation of the coronary sinus very challenging. An 'en face' visualization of coronary sinus ostium from an atrial perspective is best achieved by 3D transoesophageal echocardiography (Fig. 23.9) [24] and can help in guiding coronary sinus cannulation.

Interatrial septum: its right side is characterized by the foramen ovale completely overlapped by its valve, which is a flap of tissue continuous with the left-atrial wall. The rim often appears as a thick or raised muscle that surrounds the oval-shaped depression of the foramen ovale. Because of this arrangement, the right side of the foramen ovale appears as a crater-like structure (Fig. 23.10). Two main anatomical variants of interatrial septum may make trans-septal crossing difficult: a small foramen ovale due to 'lipomatous' septum and large septal aneurysm [15].

Quantitative Analysis: Volumes, Shape and Emptying Fraction

Many pathological conditions may affect the RA size. In pulmonay hypertension, the degree of RA enlargement appeared to reflect the right heart pressure overload and subsequent RV remodeling and dysfunction [25]. Particularly, RA area demonstrated to be an outcome predictor in pulmonary hypertension [11, 12] as well as in Eisenmenger's syndrome [26]. Accordingly, in the current guidelines about pulmonary hypertension, RA area has been recognized as a prognostic determinants [27].

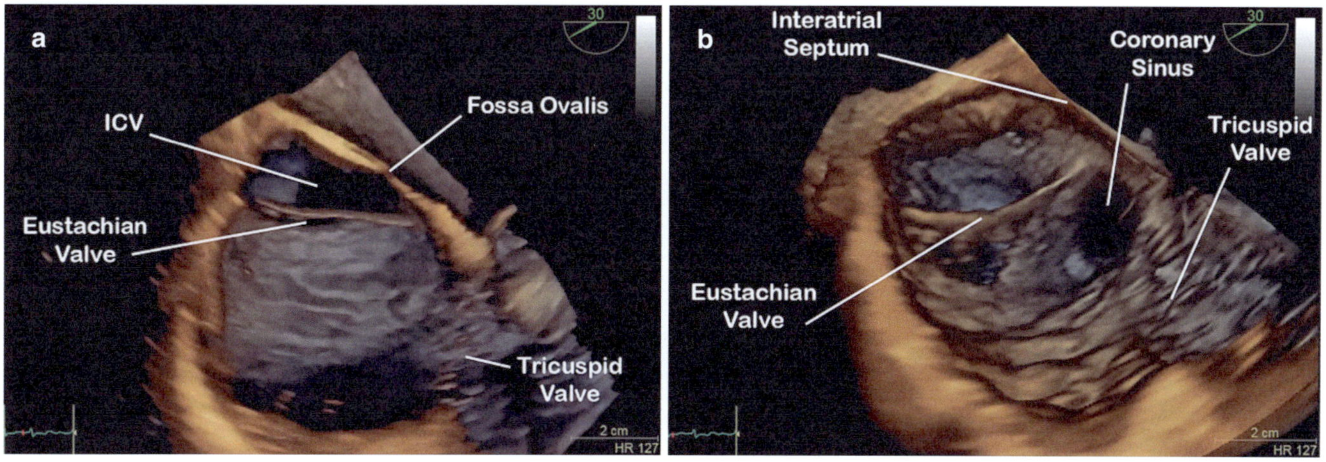

Fig. 23.8 Eustachian valve displayed from a transthoracic subcostal acquisition, demonstrating its relation with the inferior cavae vena (ICV), Eustachian ridge, superior cavae vena (SCV) in **a**, and coronary sinus in **b**

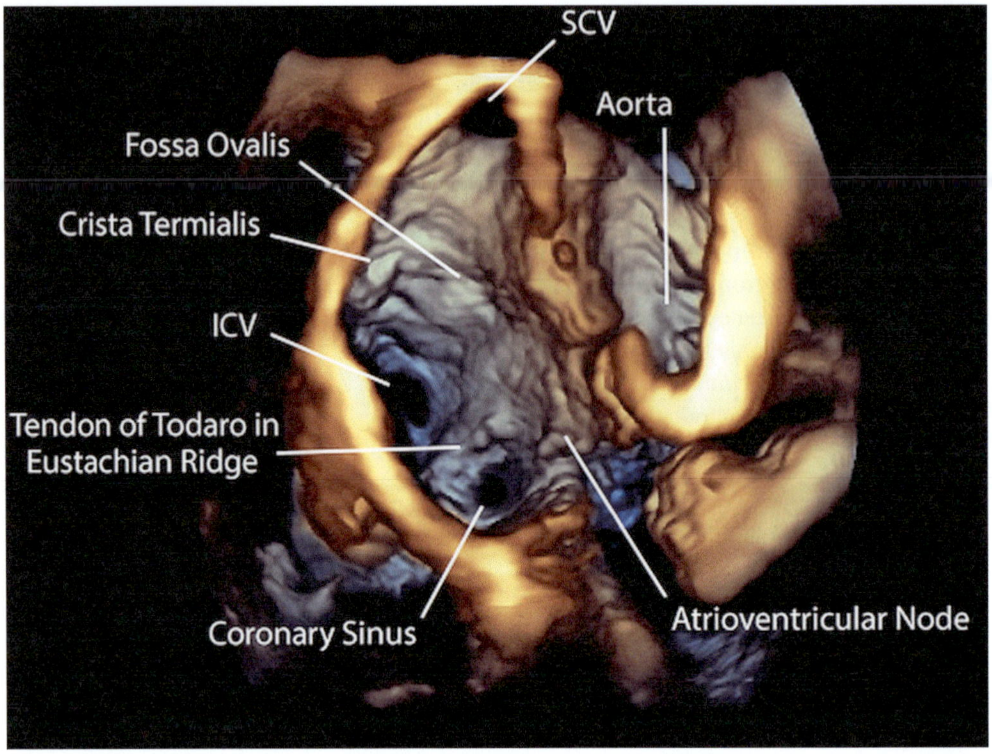

Fig. 23.9 *En face* view of the coronary sinus and its relation with the inferior cavae vena (ICV) and tendon of Todaro. *SCV* superior cavae vena

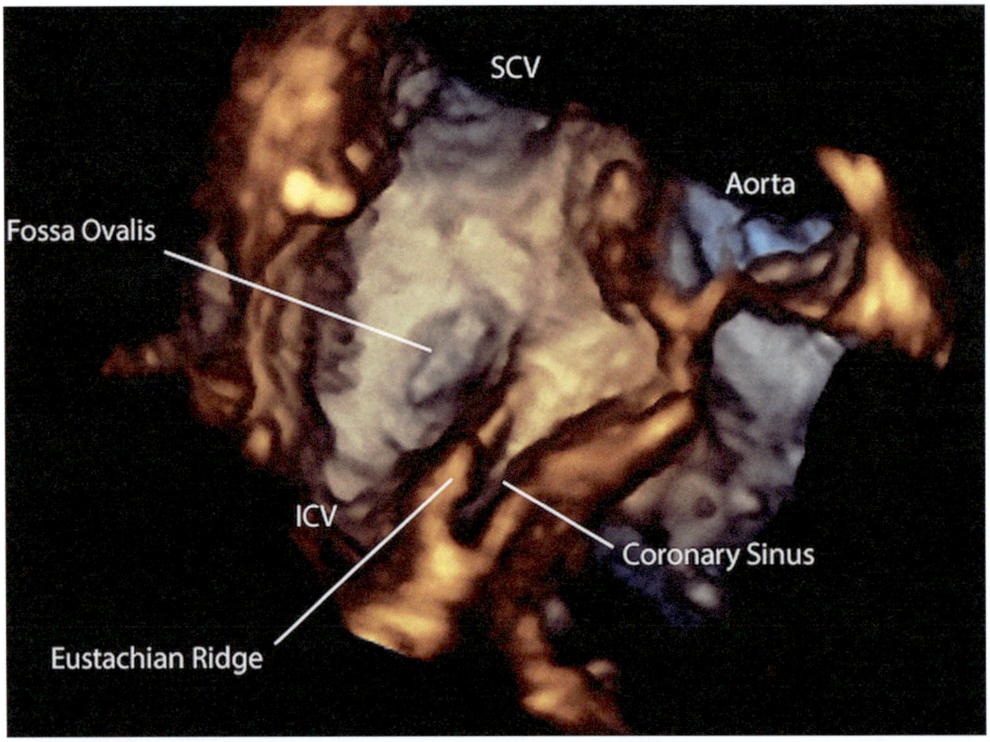

Fig. 23.10 *En face* view of the fossa ovalis and its anatomical relation with the superior cavae vena (SCV), inferior cavae vane (ICV), aorta and Eustachian ridge

In the clinical routine, the conventional assessment of RA size includes the calculation of the RA volume using the single-plane area-length algoritnm in a dedicated two-dimensional four-chamber apical view at the end-systolic frame, when the RA reaches its largest size [28]. However, two-dimensional calculation of RA volumes is limited by view dependency and geometric assumptions about its shape. A recent paper showed that the right atrial shape is related to the constitutional type, with the pyknic constitution associated to a more elongated RA [29]. Furthermore, in pathological conditions atrial remodelling is often asymmetric, rendering conventional volume measurements inadequate for the calculation of the real atrial size. Grapsa et al. [30] showed that in patients with pulmonary hypertension the RA enlarges predominantly along the transversal axis then the longitudinal one, with an increase in RA sphericity. RA remodeling appeared to be more related than right ventricular remodeling to clinical worsening [30]. Quraini et al. [31] applied 3DE to investigate which is the minimum number of planes for optimal assessment of RA volume, using eight-plane measurements as reference standard. They demonstated that the biplane method systematically underestimates RA volume size particularly in patients in whom atrial enlargement and remodeling occurred.

Despite the RA volume enlargement by two-dimensional echocardiography has been reported demonstrated to be an indipendent predictor of adverse outcome in chronic systolic heart failure [32], two-dimensional echocardiography underestimates RA volume. Due to its indipendence from any geometrical assumptions about RA shape, 3DE overcomes the limitations of two-dimensional echocardiography enabling accurate atrial volume measurement as well as quantitative assessment of RA shape [33–35] As shown in Fig. 23.11, even with an apparently correct apical 4-chamber view the RA area could be not fully maximized because the longitudinal plane is not crossing the RA through its major diameter. This is the most frequent cause of RA size underestimation.

At present, a dedicated software for RA volume measurements is not commercially available. Most of the authors who have investigated 3DE RA volumes have adapted to RA a vendor-specific software packages developed for left ventricular volume measurement [8, 14, 31]. Peluso, et al. [10] analyzed 3DE RA dataset using a dedicated non-vendor specific software designed for volumetric analysis of the left atrium (LA analysis, Tomtec Imaging Systems, Unterschleissheim, Germany). This software package has been validated against cardiac magnetic resonance [36] and its application for RA volume measurements demonstrated to be feasible and reproducible [10].

RA volumes obtained with 3DE demonstrated to be larger compared to 2DE derived volumes [10, 34], similar to RA volumes obtained with cardiac magnetic resonance [34] and smaller compared to computed tomography derived volumes [37]. Moreno et al. [8] demonstrated a poor correlation between two- and 3DE RA volumes, underlying the limitation of two-dimensional echocardiography in terms of RA shape assumptions and foreshortening. Accordingly, two- and 3DE derived RA volumes cannot be used inter-changeably.

In healthy subjects, 3DE RA volumes demonstrated to be larger in men than in women, even after indexing for body surface area (Table 23.1). Then, reference values of 3DE RA volumes should be different according to gender. Ageing demonstrated to significantly affect RA preA volume, with no influence on maximum and minimum volumes [10].

Very few data are available about prognostic impact of RA volume derived from 3DE. Patel et al. [38] demonstrated the accuracy of 3DE RA volume index in detecting high RA pressure in patients with acutely decompensated heart failure. More studies are needed to demonstrate the added value of RA sizing by 3DE in the clinical routine.

Moreover, 3DE allows to investigate RA function by a volumetric method. The measurement of maximum, pre-atrial contraction and minimum RA volumes is automatically provided by the 3DE software package used to measure the atrial volumes (Fig. 23.12). It allows to calculate RA total, passive and active emptying volumes (EV) and fractions (EF) (Fig. 23.13), corresponding to reservoir, conduit and booster pump functions respectively, using the following equations:

- *RA total Emptying Volume = maximum Volume − minimum Volume*
- *RA passive Emptying Volume = maximum Volume − PreA Volume*
- *RA active Emptying Volume = preA Volume − minimum Volume*
- *RA total Emptying Fraction = (maximum Volume − minimum Volume)/maximum Volume*
- *RA passive Emptying Fraction = (maximum Volume − PreA Volume)/maximum Volume*
- *RA active Emptying Fraction = (preA Volume − minimum Volume)/preA Volume*

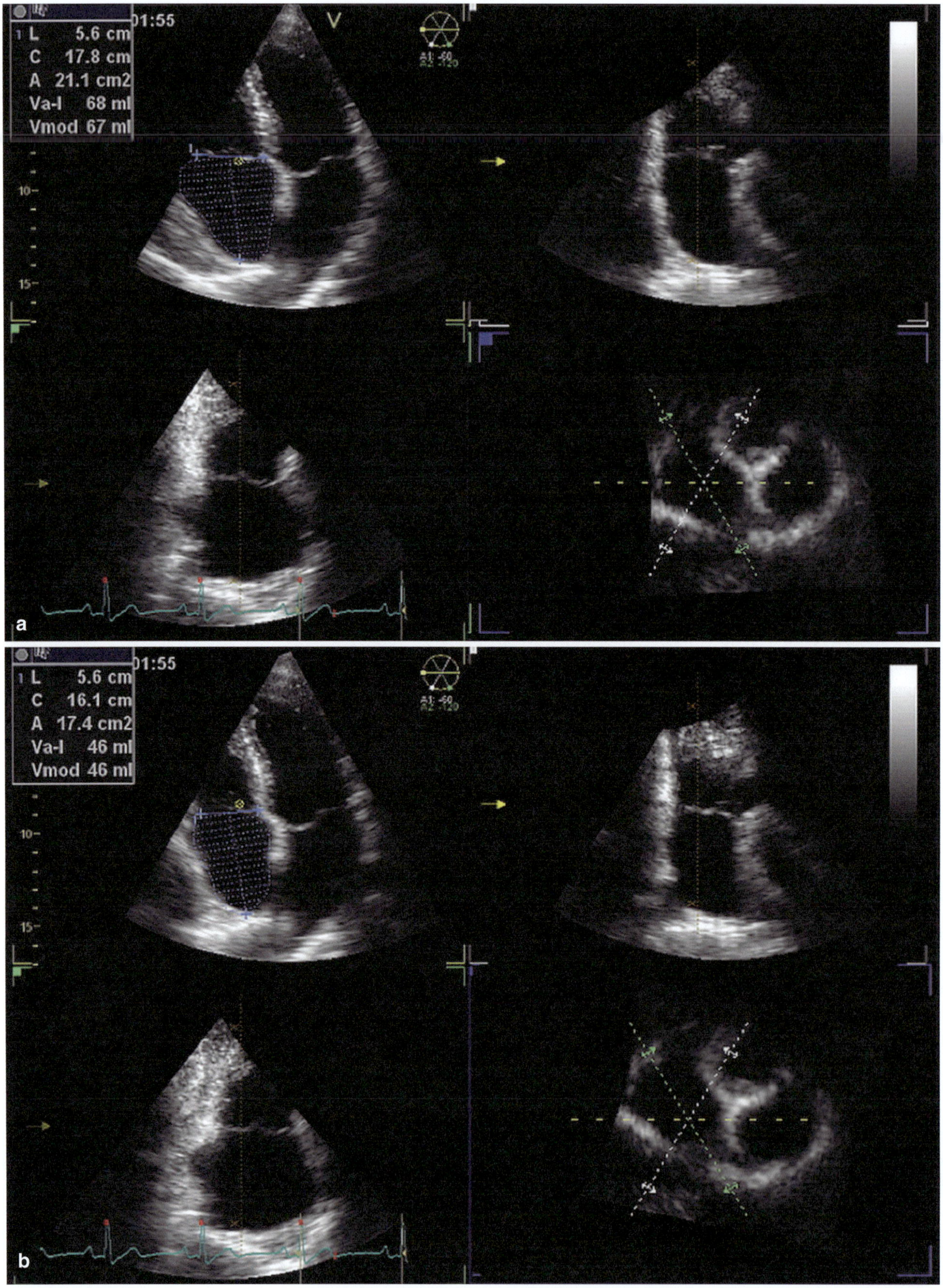

Fig. 23.11 Demonstration of how the two-dimensional planes position could affect the right atrial measurements. On (**a**) the longitudinal plane is positioned at the largest latero-medial diameter, resulting in a higher estimated right atrial area and volume whereas in (**b**) the longitudinal plane shortened the right atrial latero-medial diameter, resulting in a smaller right atrial size

Table 23.1 Studies reporting right atrial volume values in healthy subjects [8, 10, 14, 31]

Authors	N° healthy subjects	Year	Reference values (mL/m^2)				Echo system/software package for quantitation
Peluso et al. [10]	200	2013		All	Male	Female	GE Vivid E9/4D LA function
			Max V	29 ± 7	31 ± 8	27 ± 6	
			PreA V	16 ± 5	18 ± 5	14 ± 4	
			Min V	11 ± 4	12 ± 4	9 ± 3	
Aune et al. [14]	166	2009		All	Male	Female	Philips iE33/3D QLab
			Max V	18–47	18–50	17–41	
			PreA V	–	–	–	
			Min V	5–20	7–22	5–18	
Moreno et al. [8]	60	2013		All	Male	Female	Toshiba Artida system/Toshiba
			Max V	19 ± 7	–	–	
			PreA V	–	–	–	
			Min V	12 ± 6	–	–	
Quraini et al. [31]	35	2012		All	Male	Female	Philips iE33/4D LA function
			Max V	23 (10–33)	–	–	
			PreA V	–	–	–	
			Min V	–	–	–	

Max V maximum volume, *Min V* minimum volume, *PreA V* pre-atrial contraction volume

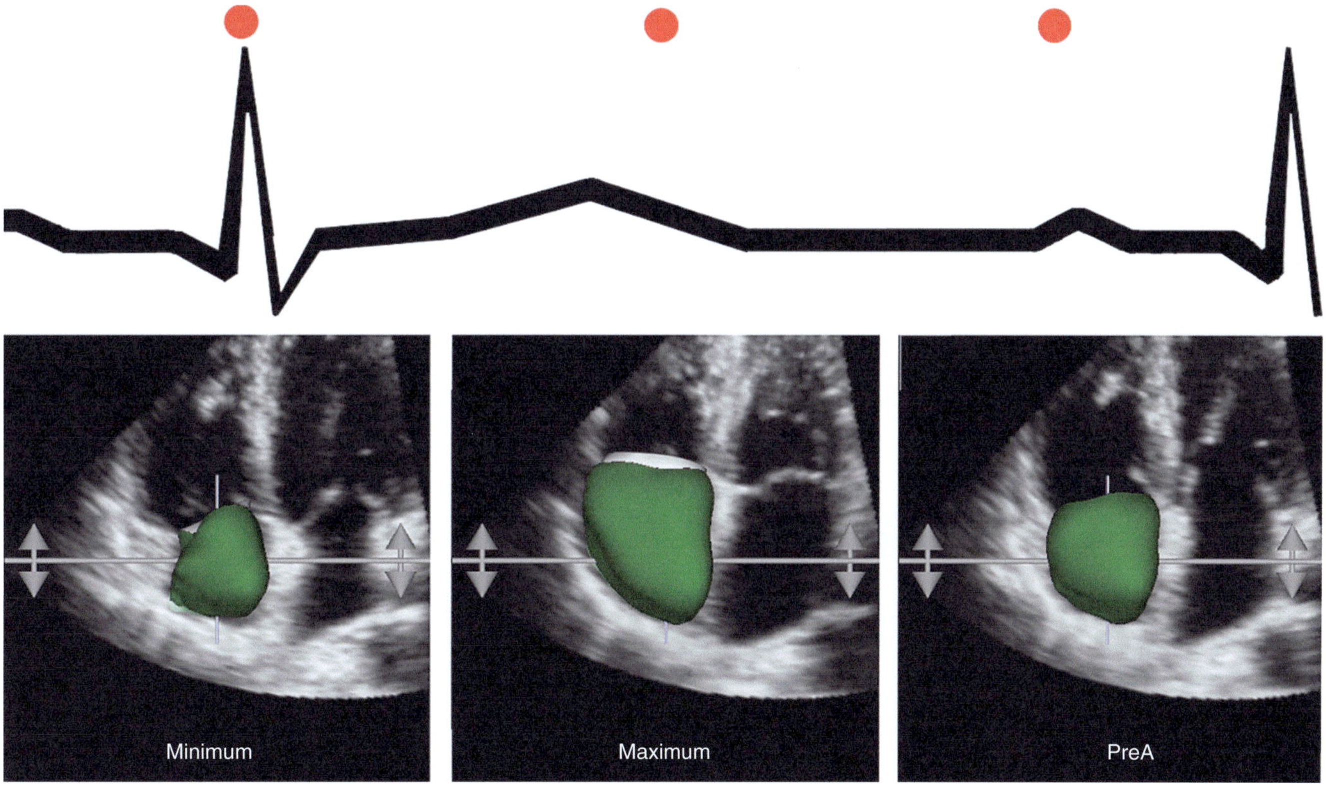

Fig. 23.12 Right atrial phasic volumes according with the cardiac cycle time

Normal values of all these three RA function components from a population of healthy volunteers have been provided by Peluso, et al. [10] and are summarized in Table 23.2. The authors showed that emptying volumes are larger in men than in women, but this difference disappeared after indexation for body surface area. Women showed higher values of emptying fraction. Conduit function appeared to decrease with ageing paralleled by a concomitant increase of booster pump function. Other data about normal values of RA function components are necessary for defining reference values.

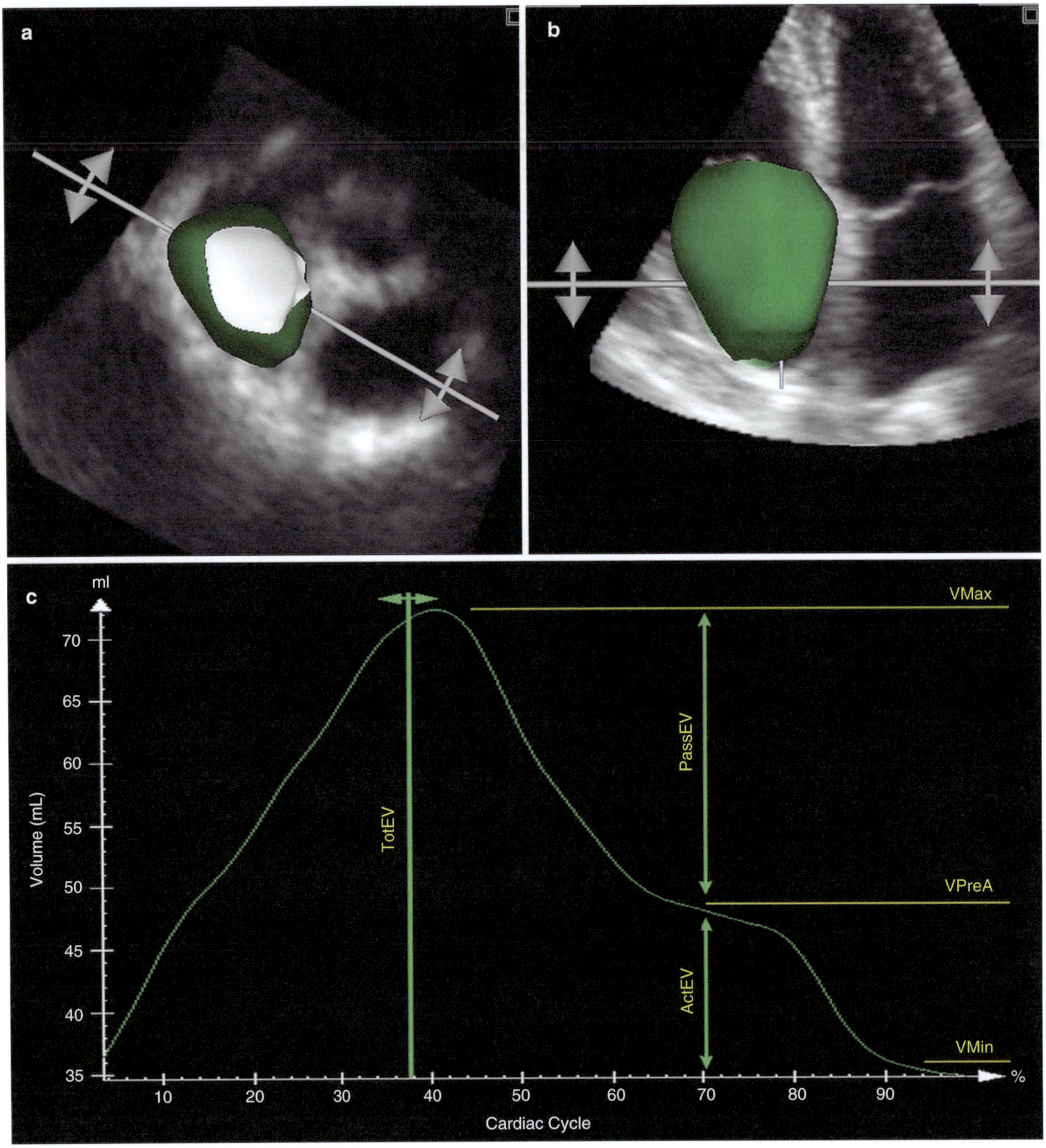

Fig. 23.13 Right atrial surface rendering in two different perspectives (**a** and **b**) from which a specific software can create a volume curve (**c**) obtaining the maximum, pre-atrial contraction and minimum volumes. Applying simple equations total, passive and active emptying volumes can also be calculated. ActEV active emptying volume; PassEV passive emptying volume; TotEV total emptying volume; VMax maximum volume; VMin minimum volume; VpreA pre-atrial contraction volume

Table 23.2 Values of right atrial volumetric functions in a healthy population [10]

	Overall	Men	Women	P
3D RA total emptying volume, mL	33 ± 10	37 ± 11	30 ± 8	<0.0001
3D RA total emptying volume/BSA, mL/m^2	18 ± 5	19 ± 5	18 ± 5	0.22
3D passive emptying volume, mL	24 ± 9	27 ± 10	22 ± 8	<0.0001
3D passive emptying volume/BSA, mL/m^2	13 ± 5	14 ± 5	13 ± 4	0.34
3D active emptying volume, mL	9 ± 4	10 ± 4	8 ± 4	0.001
3D active emptying volume/BSA, mL/m^2	5 ± 2	5 ± 2	5 ± 2	0.37
3D total emptying fraction, %	63 ± 9	61 ± 8	65 ± 8	<0.0001
3D passive emptying fraction, %	46 ± 11	44 ± 10	48 ± 12	0.013
3D active emptying fraction, %	31 ± 8	29 ± 7	33 ± 9	0.002

BSA body surface area

References

1. Harvey W. An anatomical study of the movement of the heart and blood in animals (translated by Leake CD, 1628). Baltimore: Thomas; 1928, p. 123.
2. Carlson DE, Burchard KW, Gann DS. Right atrial volume during hemorrhage in the dog. Am J Physiol Heart Circ Physiol. 1986;250(6 Pt 2):H1136–44.
3. Ferguson JJ III, Miller MJ, Aroesty JM, Sahagian P, Grossman W, McKay RG. Assessment of right atrial pressure-volume relations in patients with and without an atrial septal defect. J Am Coll Cardiol. 1989;13(3):630–6.
4. Maniar HS, Prasad SM, Gaynor SL, Chu CM, Steendijk P, Moon MR. Impact of pericardial restraint on right atrial mechanics during acute right ventricular pressure load. Am J Physiol Heart Circ Physiol. 2003;284(1):H350–7.
5. Miller MJ, McKay RG, Ferguson JJ, Sahagian P, Nakao S, Come PC, Grossman W. Right atrial pressure-volume relationships in tricuspid regurgitation. Circulation. 1986;73(4):799–808.
6. Gaynor SL, Maniar HS, Prasad SM, Steendijk P, Moon MR. Reservoir and conduit function of right atrium: impact on right ventricular filling and cardiac output. Am J Physiol Heart Circ Physiol. 2005;288(5):H2140–5.
7. Nemes A, Domsik P, Kalapos A, Kormanyos A, Ambrus N, Forster T. Three-dimensional speckle-tracking echocardiography detects different patterns of right atrial dysfunction in selected disorders: a short summary from the MAGYAR-Path Study. Quant Imaging Med Surg. 2018;8(2):182–6.
8. Moreno J, Perez de Isla L, Campos N, Guinea J, Dominguez-Perez L, Saltijeral A, et al. Right atrial indexed volume in healthy adult population: reference values for two-dimensional and three-dimensional echocardiographic measurements. Echocardiography. 2013;30(6):667–71.
9. Muller H, Reverdin S, Burri H, Shah D, Lerch R. Measurement of left and right atrial volume in patients undergoing ablation for atrial arrhythmias: comparison of a manual versus semiautomatic algorithm of real time 3D echocardiography. Echocardiography. 2014;31(4):499–507.
10. Peluso D, Badano LP, Muraru D, Dal Bianco L, Cucchini U, Kocabay G, et al. Right atrial size and function assessed with three-dimensional echocardiography in 200 healthy volunteers. Eur Heart J Cardiovasc Imaging. 2013;14(11):1106–14.
11. Raymond RJ, Hinderliter AL, Willis PW, Ralph D, Caldwell EJ, Williams WG, et al. Echocardiographic predictors of adverse outcomes in primary pulmonary hypertension. J Am Coll Cardiol. 2002;2002(39):1214–9.
12. Bustamante-Labarta M, Perrone S, De La Fuente RL, Stutzbach P, De La Hoz RP, Torino A, et al. Right atrial size and tricuspid regurgitation severity predict mortality or transplantation in primary pulmonary hypertension. J Am Soc Echocardiogr. 2002;15:1160–4.
13. Tadic M. The right atrium, a forgotten cardiac chamber: an updated review of multimodality imaging. J Clin Ultrasound. 2015;43(6):335–45.
14. Aune E, Baekkevar M, Roislien J, Rodevand O, Otterstad JE. Normal reference ranges for left and right atrial volume indexes and ejection fractions obtained with real-time three-dimensional echocardiography. Eur J Echocardiogr. 2009;10:738–44.
15. Faletra FF, Muzzarelli S, Dequarti MC, Murzilli R, Bellu R, Ho SY. Imaging-based right-atrial anatomy by computed tomography, magnetic resonance imaging, and three-dimensional transoesophageal echocardiography: correlations with anatomic specimens. Eur Heart J Cardiovasc Imaging. 2013;14(12):1123–31.
16. Faletra FF, Ho SY, Auricchio A. Anatomy of right atrial structures by real-time 3D transesophageal echocardiography. JACC Cardiovasc Imaging. 2010;3(9):966–75.
17. Loukas M, Tubbs RS, Tongson JM, Polepalli S, Curry B, Jordan R, Wagner T. The clinical anatomy of the crista terminalis, pectinate muscles and the teniae sagittalis. Ann Anat. 2008;190(1):81–7.
18. Cabrera JA, Sanchez-Quintana D, Ho SY, Medina A, Anderson RH. The architecture of the atrial musculature between the orifice of the inferior caval vein and the tricuspid valve: the anatomy of the isthmus. J Cardiovasc Electrophysiol. 1998;9(11):1186–95.
19. Ho SY, Ernst S. The right atrium relevant to supraventricular tachycardia. In: Anatomy for cardiac electrophysiologists. A practical handbook. Cardiotext; 2012. p 97–127.
20. Chiari H. Ueber Netzbildungen im rechten Vorhof des Herzens. Beitr Path Anat. 1897;22:1–10.
21. Lanzarini L, Lucca E, Fontana A, Foresti S. Cor triatriatum dextrum resulting from the persistence of embryonic remnants of the right valve of the sinus venosus: prevalence and echocardiographic aspects in a large consecutive non-selected patient population. Ital Heart J Suppl. 2001;2(11):1209–16.
22. Betrián Blasco P, Sarrat Torres R, Pijuan Domènech MA, Marimón Blanch C, Pérez Herrera V, Girona Comas J. Three-dimensional Imaging of Redundant Chiari's Network Prolapsing into Right Ventricle. J Am Soc Echocardiogr. 2008;21(2):188.e1–2. Epub 2007 Jul 23.
23. Iida R, Vonder Muhll I. A prominent eustachian valve dividing the right atrium imaged by three-dimensional transesophageal echocardiography. J Clin Ultrasound. 2013;41(8):514–6.
24. Kalman JM, Olgin JE, Karch MR, Hamdan M, Lee RJ, Lesh MD. Cristal tachicardias': origin of right atrial tachicardias from crista terminalis identified by intracardiac echocardiography. J Am Coll Cardiol. 1998;31(2):451–9.
25. Sato T, Tsujino I, Oyama-Manabe N, Ohira H, Ito YM, Yamada A, et al. Right atrial volume and phasic function in pulmonary hypertension. Int J Cardiol. 2013;168(1):420–6.
26. Moceri P, Dimopoulos K, Liodakis E, Germanakis I, Kempny A, Diller GP, et al. Echocardiographic predictors of outcome in Eisenmenger syndrome. Circulation. 2012;126(12):1461–8.
27. Galiè N, Humbert M, Vachiery JL, Gibbs S, Lang I, Torbicki A, et al. 2015 ESC/ERS guidelines for the diagnosis and treatment of pulmonary hypertension. Eur Heart J. 2016;37:67–119.

28. Lang RM, Badano LP, Mor-Avi V, Afilalo J, Armstrong A, Ernande L, et al. Recommendations for cardiac chamber quantification by echocardiography in adults: an update from the American Society of Echocardiography and the European Association of Cardiovascular Imaging. Eur Heart J Cardiovasc Imaging. 2015;16(3):233–70.
29. Chaplygina EV, Kornienko NA, Kaplunova OA, Kornienko AA. Peculiarities of the anatomical structure of the posterior-lower part of the right atrium in people of various constitutional types. Morfologiia. 2013;144(6):32–5.
30. Grapsa J, Gibbs JS, Cabrita IZ, Watson GF, Pavlopoulos H, Dawson D, et al. The association of clinical outcome with right atrial and ventricular remodeling in patients with pulmonary arterial hypertension: study with real-time three-dimensional echocardiography. Eur Heart J Cardiovasc Imaging. 2012;13(8):666–72.
31. Quraini D, Pandian NG, Patel AR. Three-dimensional echocardiographic analysis of right atrial volume in normal and abnormal hearts: comparison of biplane and multiplane methods. Echocardiography. 2012;29(5):608–13.
32. Sallach JA, Tang WH, Borowski AG, Tong W, Porter T, Martin MG, et al. Right atrial volume index in chronic systolic heart failure and prognosis. JACC Cardiovasc Imaging. 2009;2(5):527–34.
33. Kleijn SA, Aly MF, Terwee CB, van Rossum AC, Kamp O. Comparison between direct volumetric and speckle tracking methodologies for left ventricular and left atrial chamber quantification by three-dimensional echocardiography. Am J Cardiol. 2011;108(7):1038–44.
34. Keller AM, Gopal AS, King DL. Left and right atrial volume by freehand three dimensional echocardiography: in vivo validation using magnetic resonance imaging. Eur J Echocardiogr. 2000;1(1):55–65.
35. Badano LP, Boccalini F, Muraru D, Dal Bianco L, Peluso D, Bellu R, et al. Current clinical applications of transthoracic three-dimensional echocardiography. J Cardiovasc Ultrasound. 2012;20(1):1–22.
36. Mor-Avi V, Yodwut C, Jenkins C, Kühl H, Nesser HJ, Marwick TH, et al. Real-time 3D echocardiographic quantification of left atrial volume: multicenter study for validation with CMR. JACC Cardiovasc Imaging. 2012;5(8):769–77.
37. Takahashi A, Funabashi N, Kataoka A, Yajima R, Takahashi M, Uehara M, et al. Quantitative evaluation of right atrial volume and right atrial emptying fraction by 320-slice computed tomography compared with three-dimensional echocardiography. Int J Cardiol. 2011;146(1):96–9.
38. Patel AR, Alsheikh-Ali AA, Mukherjee J, Evangelista A, Quraini D, Ordway LJ, et al. 3D echocardiography to evaluate right atrial pressure in acutely decompensated heart failure correlation with invasive hemodynamics. JACC Cardiovasc Imaging. 2011;4(9):938–45.

The Role of 3DE in the Evaluation of Cardiac Masses

24

Francesco Fulvio Faletra, Romina Murzilli, Laura Anna Leo, and Denisa Muraru

Abstract

Echocardiography is the most frequently used imaging modality to assess intra-cardiac masses. Two-dimensional echocardiography uses orthogonal tomographic planes obtained from several acoustic windows to try to mentally reconstruct a model of how the mass would actually appear in three dimensions and how it would relate to the adjacent cardiac structures. Three-dimensional transthoracic and transesophageal echocardiography have revolutionized the echocardiographic assessment of intracardiac masses. A single acquisition of a three-dimensional data set can be post-processed to show the actual size and shape of the mass and characterize its volume, location, point of attachment, relationships with adjacent structures empowering the echocardiographer with a new level of confidence in the diagnosis, follow-up and management of patients with intracardiac masses.

In the first part of the chapter, we will describe how the most frequent benign and malign tumors appear on 3DE imaging. The second part of the chapter will cover *non-tumor* masses, in particular thrombi and vegetations. The last part will describe some normal intracardiac structures that may protrude in the heart cavities and appear as cardiac masses when exuberant.

Electronic Supplementary Material The online version of this chapter (https://doi.org/10.1007/978-3-030-14032-8_24) contains supplementary material, which is available to authorized users.

F. F. Faletra (✉) · R. Murzilli · L. A. Leo
Department of Cardiology, Fondazione Cardiocentro Ticino, Lugano, Switzerland
e-mail: francesco.faletra@cardiocentro.org; romina.murzilli@cardiocentro.org; lauraanna.leo@cardiocentro.org

D. Muraru
University of Milano-Bicocca, and Istituto Auxologico Italiano, IRCCS, San Luca Hospital, Milano, Italy
e-mail: denisa.muraru@unimib.it, denisa.muraru@unipd.it

Keywords

Intracardiac masses · Primary cardiac tumors · Secondary cardiac tumors · Myxoma · Lamb's excrescences · Non-tumor masses

General Concepts

The term "cardiac masses" refers to a heterogeneous group of abnormal structures within or adjacent to the heart. Primary cardiac tumors (benign and malign), metastasis from extra-cardiac tumors, and "*non-tumor* masses", such as intracardiac thrombi and vegetations, are the most common types of cardiac masses.

Primary cardiac tumors are rare (less than 0.1% in a large series of autopsies) and nearly 75% of them are benign [1]. Cardiac myxoma is the most common in the adults accounting for more than 50% of benign tumors while rhabdomyoma is the most frequently encountered benign tumor in children [2]. Despite being "benign", primary cardiac tumors may cause several functional impairments such as valve obstruction or regurgitation (due to interference of the tumor with valve function) impaired contractility, arrhythmias, conduction disorders (due to the extension of the tumor through the myocardium), pericardial effusion and systemic embolisms. However, more often, clinical findings and/or symptoms are vague or even completely absent. In such cases the tumor is occasionally discovered during an examination (usually echocardiography) required for other reasons.

The remaining 25% of cardiac tumors are *malignant neoplasms*. Among them, the most common are sarcomas and lymphomas. *Malignant tumors* from other organs may metastasize to the heart by continuity or through vascular channels. Their frequency is 20–40 times higher than primary tumors [3]. The most common extra-cardiac tumors invading the heart are lung cancer followed by melanoma and lymphoma.

L. P. Badano et al. (eds.), *Textbook of Three-Dimensional Echocardiography*, https://doi.org/10.1007/978-3-030-14032-8_24

Two-dimensional transthoracic and transesophageal echocardiography are the first line imaging techniques in the diagnosis of cardiac masses. Sensitivity of transthoracic two-dimensional echocardiography in detecting cardiac tumors varies from 55 to 90% depending on size and site of the mass. Two dimensional transesophageal echocardiography yields a higher sensitivity, approaching 97% [4].

Three-dimensional transthoracic and transesophageal echocardiography (3DE) has three advantages when compared with two-dimensional imaging. *First,* 3DE provides a better understanding of the shape and location of the tumor along with its spatial relationship with the surrounding structures in a single perspective without the need of acquiring multiple tomographic planes from different acoustic windows and performing a mental reconstruction of how the mass would actually appear in three dimensions and how it would relate to the adjacent cardiac structures. *Second,* 3DE is more precise in defining the size of tumor since it can measure the volume of the mass independent on geometric assumptions about its shape. The size of any cardiac mass (tumor, endocarditis or thrombi) is "*per se*" predictor of embolic events and death. *Third,* being included into a three-dimensional data set, the tumor can be visualized from different perspectives and "cropped" in any plane. This possibilities allows to identify the site of attachment, its extension and to explore the internal structure of the mass and distinguish between solid and cystic or mixed using a single acquisition.

In the first part of the chapter, we will describe how the most frequent benign and malign tumors appear on 3DE imaging. The second part of the chapter will cover *non-tumor* masses, in particular thrombi and vegetations. The last part will describe some normal intracardiac structures that may protrude in the heart cavities and appear as cardiac masses when exuberant.

Acquisition and Display

There is no specific approach or acoustic window that can be recommended to acquire 3DE data sets of the various cardiac tumors or masses. The acoustic window which allows to include the whole mass in the data set with the best image quality and border definition is usually used to acquire the 3DE data set. Multislice display of the data set is used to ensure that the whole mass and surrounding structures are included in the data set. Since the mass are usually large and hypomobile, single- or multi-beat acquisitions with a limited number of heart beats are usually enough to obtain good quality data sets.

Different display modalities can be used for different purposes. *Volume rendering*, to visualize the shape of the mass, its motion, and its anatomical relationships with adjacent cardiac structures (Fig. 24.1a, Video 24.1a). Adding color will provide information about the impact of the mass on intracardiac hemodynamics (Fig. 24.1b, Video 24.1b). Multislice, to identify the point of attachment and (particularly, for masses infiltrating the ventricular or atrial walls) to define their extension (Fig. 24.1c, Video 24.1c). *Surface rendering*, to visualize the shape of the mass and measure its volume (Fig. 24.1d).

Careful cropping and slicing of the 3DE data set can provide additional information about the structure of the mass and its anatomical relationships with the surrounding cardiac structures (Fig. 24.2, Videos 24.2a, 24.2b, 24.2c, and 24.2d).

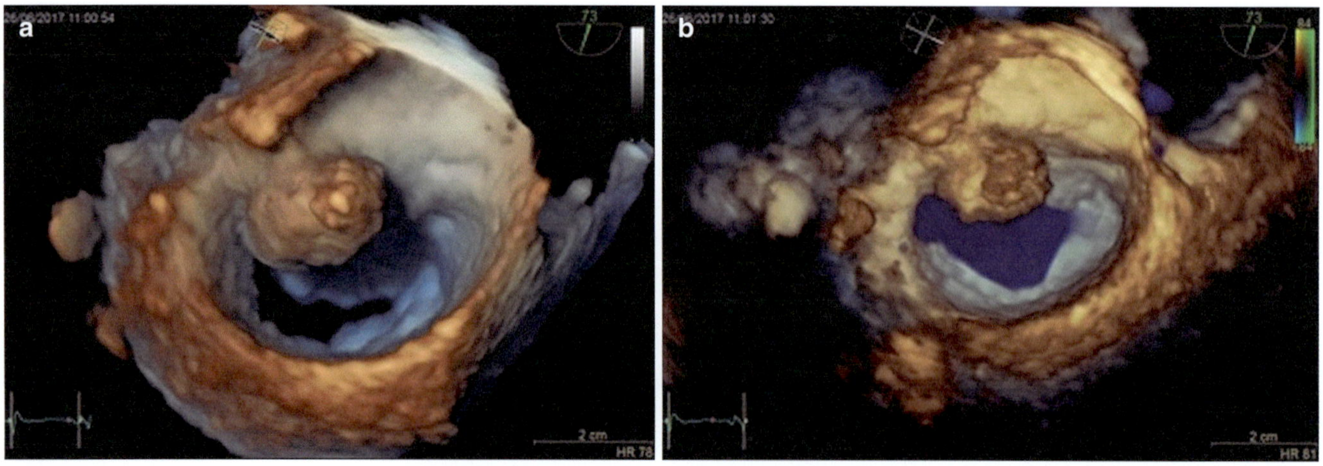

Fig. 24.1 Various display modes of cardiac masses (left atrial myxoma) imaged by three-dimensional echocardiography. (**a**) Volume rendering (Video 24.1a). (**b**) Color volume rendering (Video 24.1b). (**c**) Multiplane (biplane) (Video 24.1c). (**d**) Surface rendering. See text for details

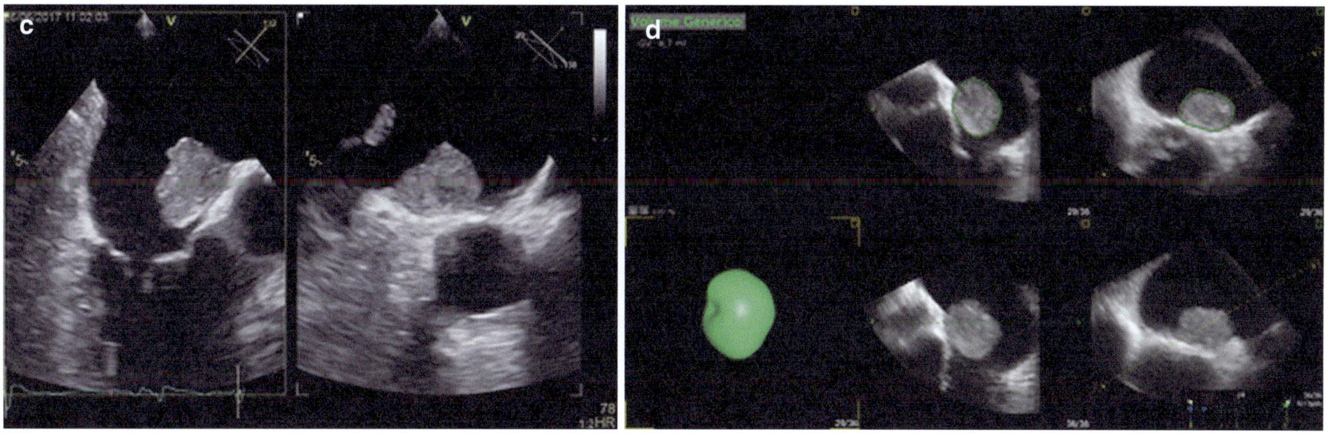

Fig. 24.1 (continued)

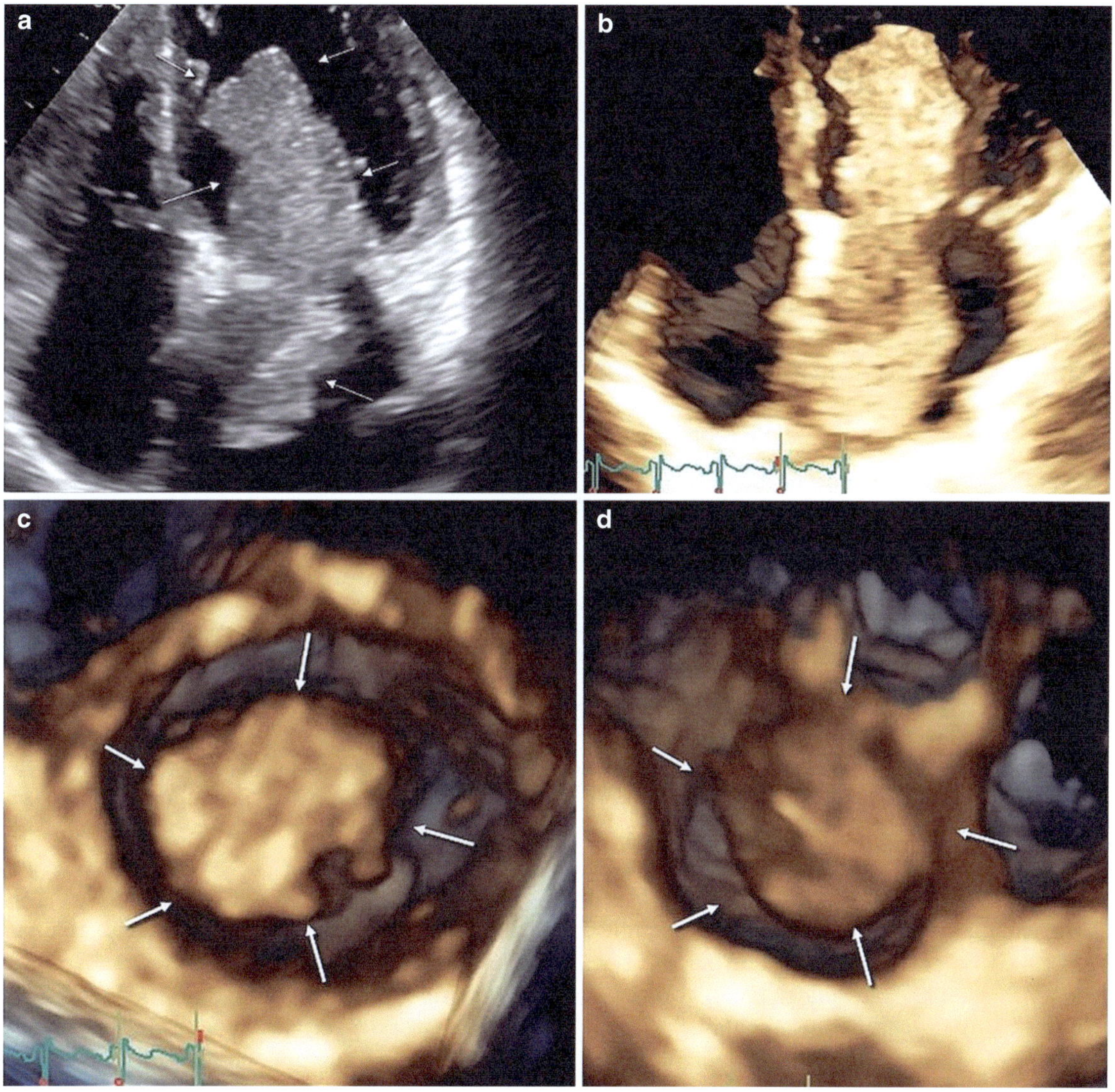

Fig. 24.2 Left atrial myxoma. (**a**) Conventional two-dimensional image of left atrial myxoma (white arrows) in diastole occluding the mitral orifice and falling deep in the left ventricle seen from 4-chamber view (Video 24.2a). (**b**) Transthoracic 3DE and volume rendering of left atrial mixoma visualized in longitudinal cut plane to show the point of attachment to interatrial septum and its prolapse into the left ventricle through the mitral orifice (Video 24.2b). (**c**) Transthoracic 3DE and volume rendering of left atrial mixoma visualized from left ventricular perspective, using a transversal cut plane, to examine its protrusion through the mitral annulus (Video 24.2c). (**d**) The same mixoma visualized from the atrial perspective using a transversal cut plane to show the large stalk and the point of attachment to interatrial septum (Video 24.2d)

Cardiac Tumors

Cardiac Myxoma

King, et al. first described left atrial myxoma in 1845 [5]. In 1952, Goldberg and al. first illustrated a left atrial myxoma in a patient presenting with a clinical diagnosis of mitral stenosis and peripheral emboli using angiography [6]. Since then and for several years, angiography was the only imaging modality for the "*in vivo*" diagnosis of atrial myxoma. At the beginning of the echocardiography era, the "classic" M-mode image of a left atrial myxoma (a cloud of linear echoes filling the left cavity and falling in diastole through the mitral orifice behind the anterior mitral leaflet) was so characteristic, that Feigenbaum chose it as the cover of the second edition of his book. Today two- and 3DE are the techniques of choice in the diagnosis of atrial myxoma providing a complete set of morphological and functional data.

Cardiac myxomas usually arise from atrial wall. Seventy-five per cent of myxomas develop in the left atrium (with a favorite site around the border of fossa ovalis), most of the remaining (18%) develop in the right atrium and very few (6%) in both left and right ventricles [7, 8].

Histologically myxoma is composed of neoplastic primitive multipotential mesenchymal cells, often stellate, imbibed in a loose connective tissue composed of proteoglycans, collagen, and elastin with a variable number of lymphocytes and plasma cells [9]. Macroscopically, cardiac myxoma may have a round or ovoid shape with a smooth or lobulated surface or (more rarely) an irregular aspect consisting of very fine multiple villous excrescences. The tumor may be either pedunculated or sessile and often contains cysts or areas of necrosis and hemorrhage. The size varies from few millimeters to several centimeters and the mobility depends on the consistency of the tumor, on its attachment and on the length of the stalk [8].

Depending of the size, location, consistency and mobility, cardiac myxomas may present with a wide spectrum of clinical findings ranging from the complete absence of symptoms to the sudden death. Small and sessile tumors may be completely silent.

Patients with a large ovoid or round compact myxoma may complain symptoms similar to that caused by the mitral stenosis and due to partial obstruction of the mitral orifice (Fig. 24.2). Complete obstruction of the valve orifice may lead to syncope or even sudden death. Symptoms referred to mitral orifice obstruction are the most common, accounting for more than 50% of patients with cardiac myxoma.

Myxomas with multiple excrescences are gelatinous and fragile and tend to break into small pieces that embolise. Hence, systemic embolisms are the second most common symptom of myxoma.

Not rarely patients with myxoma have a specific clinical manifestations (constitutional symptoms) such as fatigue, fever, arthralgia, loss of weight, and laboratory abnormalities.

Transthoracic two-dimensional echocardiography is the first line imaging technique. For decades, this technique has provided an accurate diagnosis and essential morphological and functional information (presence, location, size and mobility) for surgical management. Therefore, unless there is a suspicion of coronary artery disease, cardiologists avoid performing cardiac catheterization because of the risk of fragmentations of the tumor and patients with a diagnosis of atrial myxoma made by two-dimensional echocardiography usually undergo successful surgical resection based only on echocardiography data. Transthoracic 3DE provides additional information on the size and shape. In fact, once acquired the volumetric data set, the technique is able to provide images of the mass from a countless number of perspectives facilitating the assessment of its size and shape (Fig. 24.2).

Because of its superior spatial resolution, due to the higher frequencies used and proximity of tumor to the esophagus two-dimensional transesophageal echocardiography provides images of excellent quality allowing an accurate assessment of shape, surface, size, site and attachment to the atrial or septal wall (Fig. 24.3).

However, in case the tumor presents an irregular shape, it may be difficult to reconstruct the three-dimensional aspect of the mass, even using multiple planes. In fact, fringes of the tumor may appear and disappear during its motion through the echocardiographic plane (Fig. 24.4). Moreover, the size of an irregularly shaped tumor may be underestimate when using two-dimensional echocardiography.

3DE provides images of atrial myxoma of exquisite quality and, more important practically identical to the surgical or post-mortem specimen, allowing an immediate appreciation of its position, size and their macroscopic aspect (Fig. 24.5).

Since 3DE may show the myxoma from different perspectives, it provides a clear and immediate understanding of the shape, surface irregularity, maximum size and spatial relationships with the surrounding structures (Figs. 24.2 and 24.6, Video 24.4).

Myxomas with multiple excrescences are usually fragile and gelatinous, changing continuously their shape during

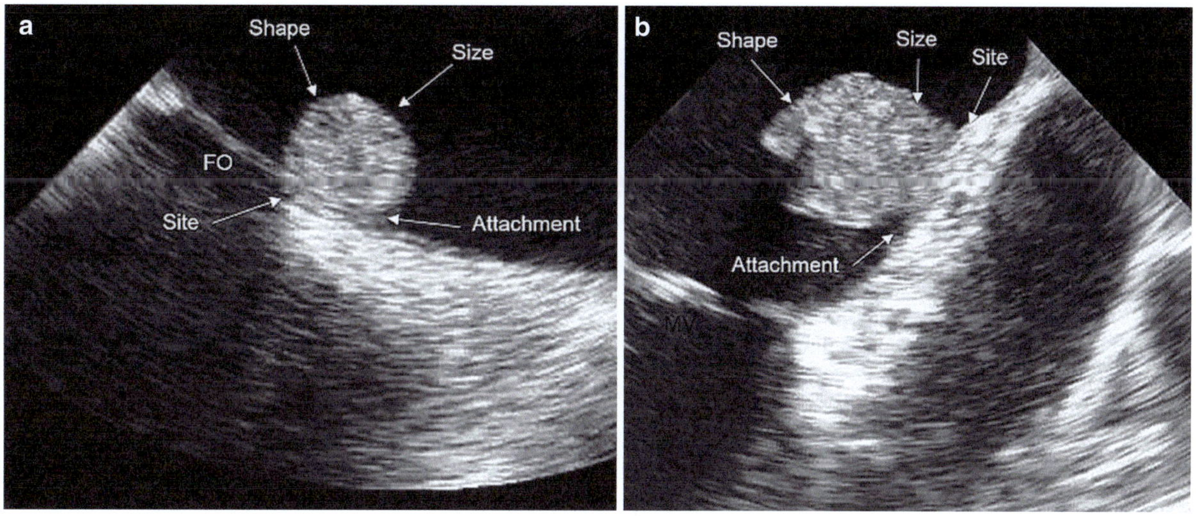

Fig. 24.3 Two-dimensional transesophageal echocardiography imaging of left atrial myxomas. (**a**) A small, round sessile myxoma with a smooth surface. The shape, size, site (near the margin of the fossa ovalis (FO) are well defined. (**b**) A larger, near-elliptic, sessile myxoma with a more irregular surface

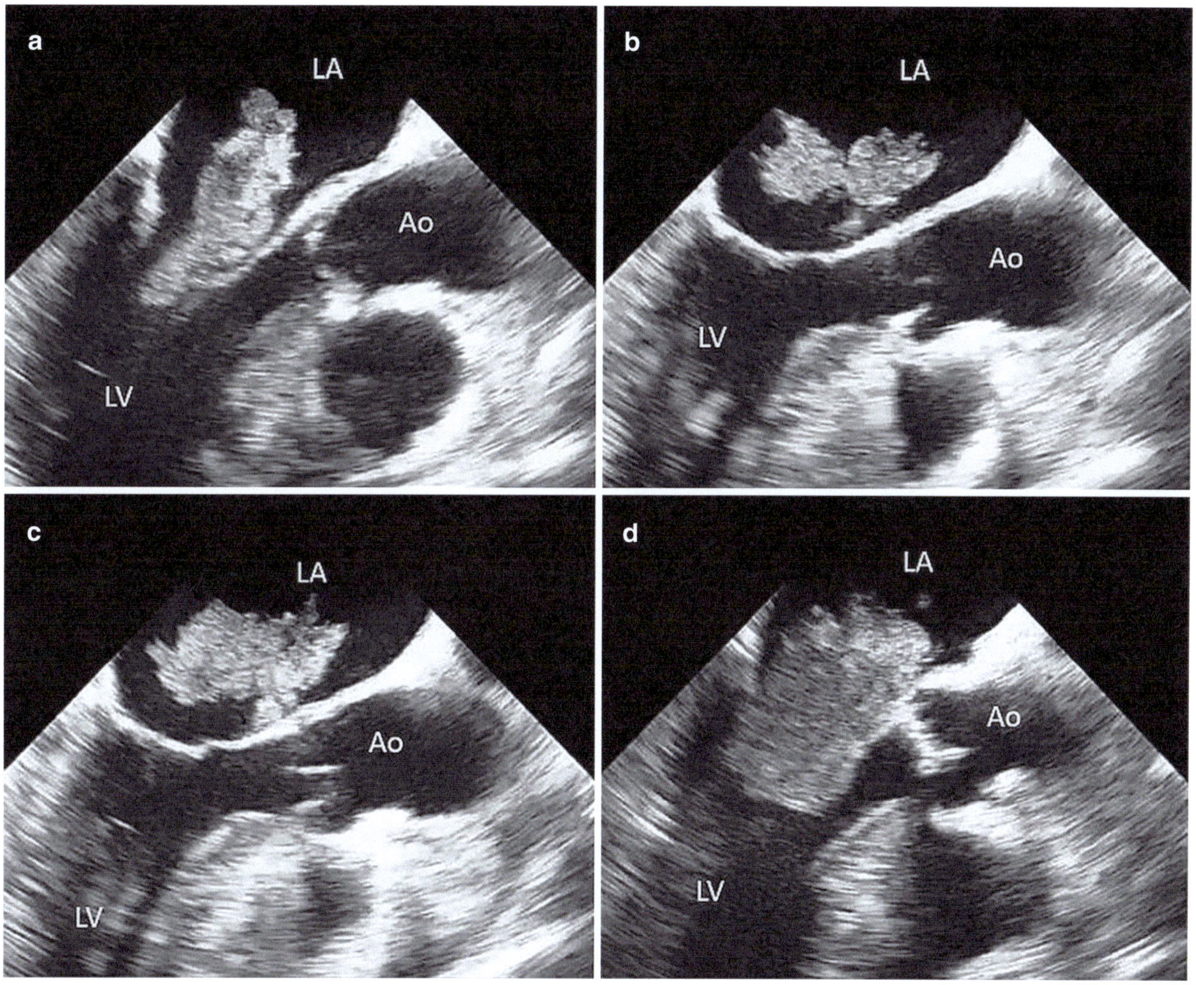

Fig. 24.4 Two-dimensional echocardiography of left atrial myxoma with irregular shape (**a–d**). Although the diagnosis of myxoma is unquestionable, the precise size and shape of the tumor is difficult to define since during the cardiac cycle parts of the tumor appear and disappear as it moves through the echocardiographic plane (Video 24.3)

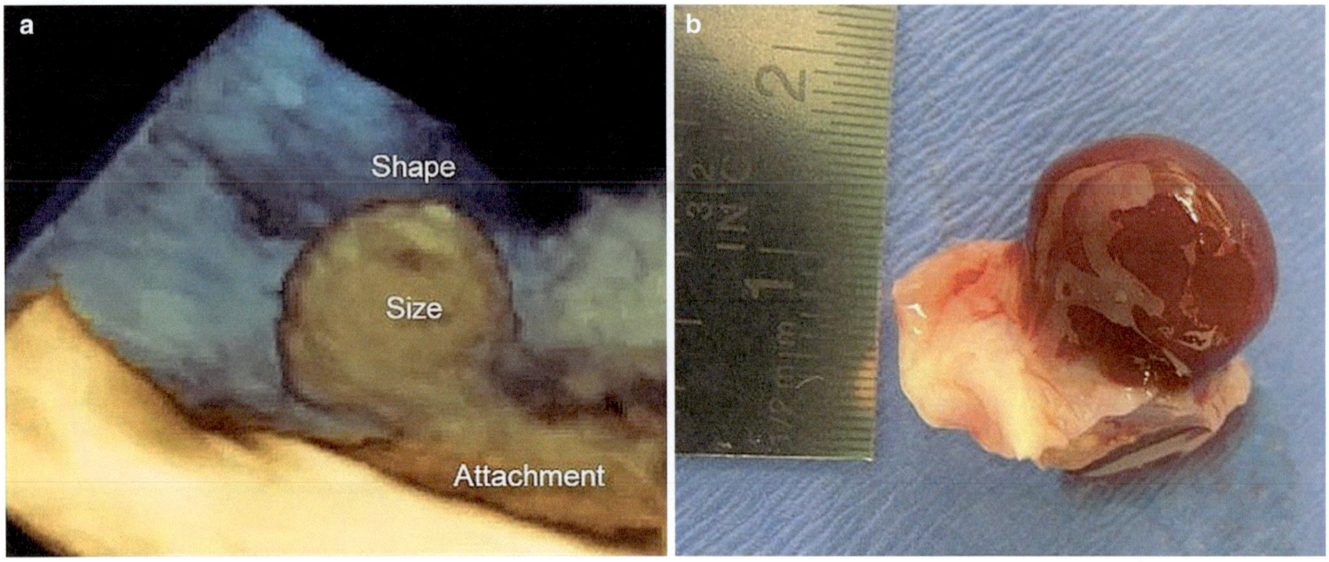

Fig. 24.5 Transesophageal 3DE volume rendering (**a**) and surgical specimen (**b**) of the case illustrated in Fig 24.3a. 3DE provides anatomically sound images of exquisite quality and practically identical to the surgical specimen

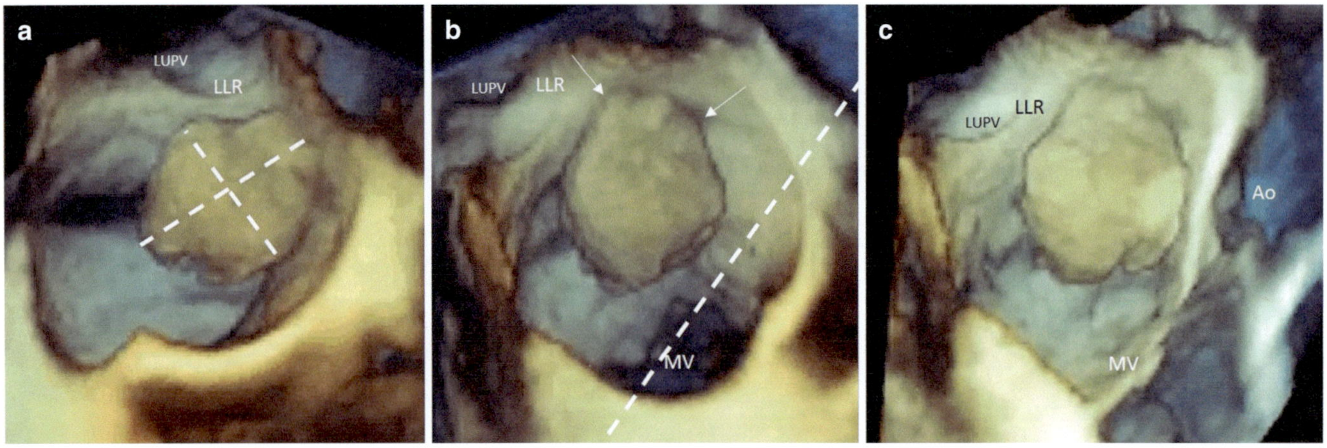

Fig. 24.6 Transesophageal 3DE image showing volume rendering display of the same case of Fig. 24.3b from different perspectives. (**a**) Medial-to-lateral perspective that provides the maximum size (dashed lines) and the spatial relationship between the tumor, the left lateral ridge (LLR) and the left upper pulmonary vein (LUPV). (**b**) The tumor seen from above showing the margins (arrows) of the tumor attached on the atrial wall and its spatial relationships with the mitral valve (MV) (Video 24.4). (**c**) Same perspective as in (**b**) after having cropped along the white dashed line shown in (**b**). The cropped image shows the spatial relationship of the tumor with the aortic valve (Ao)

the cardiac cycle. In such cases, 3DE provides in a single three-dimensional perspective the entire aspect of the mass showing the changes in shape occurring during the cardiac cycle in real time. By comparing the images in Figs. 24.4 and 24.7 (Video 24.5) the echocardiographer can appreciate the added value of 3DE when imaging a myxoma with multiple excrescences.

Interestingly, despite the fact that 3DE has suboptimal utility in tissue characterization (in 3DE the different shades of color mainly represent different depths rather than different types of tissue, see also Chap. 2), marked differences in tissue compactness may produce detectable differences in color shades. The weak consistence of the gelatinous myxoma produces a brown color, which is clearly different from the beige/yellow color of the atrial wall. Conversely, the compact, ovoid myxoma produces shades of beige/yellow color indistinguishable from the atrial wall (Fig. 24.8).

Right atrial myxoma account for 15–20% of all cardiac myxomas and, like its left counterpart, the preferred location of right atrial myxoma is the atrial septum at the border of the fossa ovalis. When the tumor consists of multiple frag-

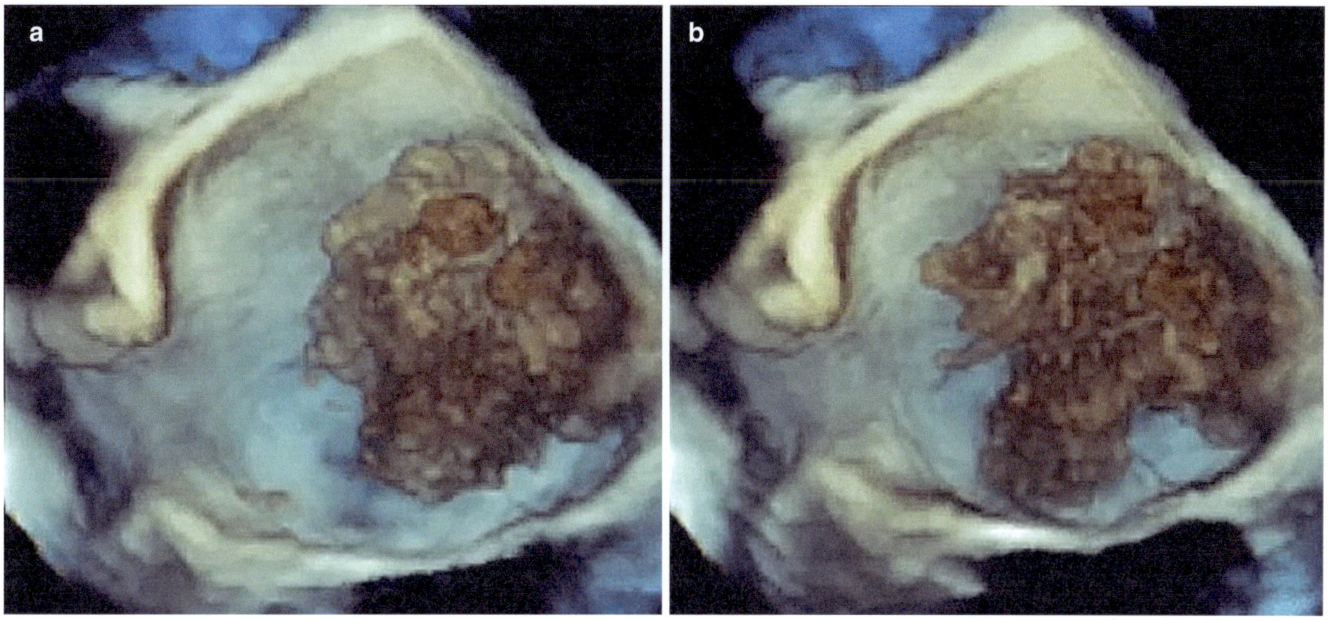

Fig. 24.7 Transesophageal 3DE volume rendering of a myxomas with multiple excrescencies (**a**, **b**). These tumors are gelatinous and fragile, continuously changing their shape during the cardiac cycle (Video 24.5)

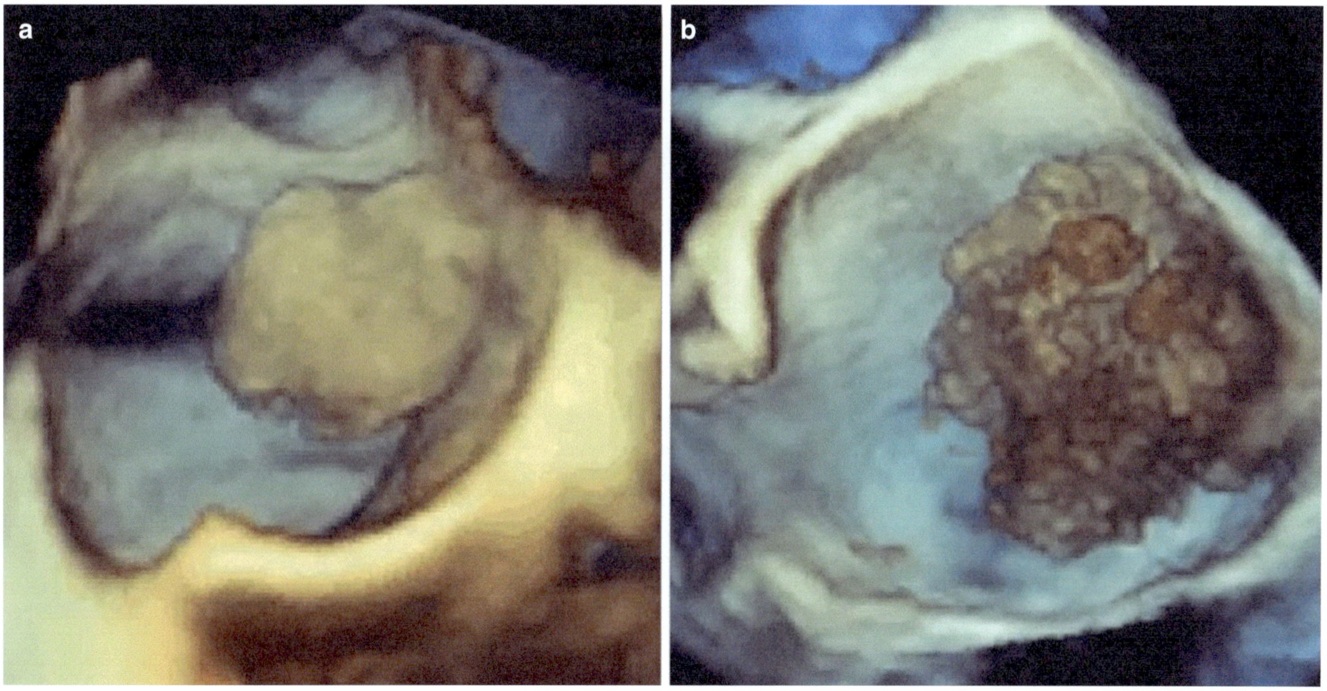

Fig. 24.8 Transesophageal 3DE images of the two most frequent types of myxomas. (**a**) Round, compact myxoma. The consistence of this tumor is similar to the atrial wall and consequently the shades of colors are similar. (**b**) Irregular, gelatinous, high mobile myxoma. In this case, the myxomas has a lower compactness than the atrial wall resulting in different shades of color

ile excrescencies, it tends to embolise causing pulmonary embolism with cyanosis and hypoxia. Massive right atrial myxoma may occlude the tricuspid orifice causing syncope or right heart failure (Fig. 24.9).

Conversely, small compact right atrial myxoma are usually asymptomatic and may be found accidentally on cardiac imaging (Fig. 24.10).

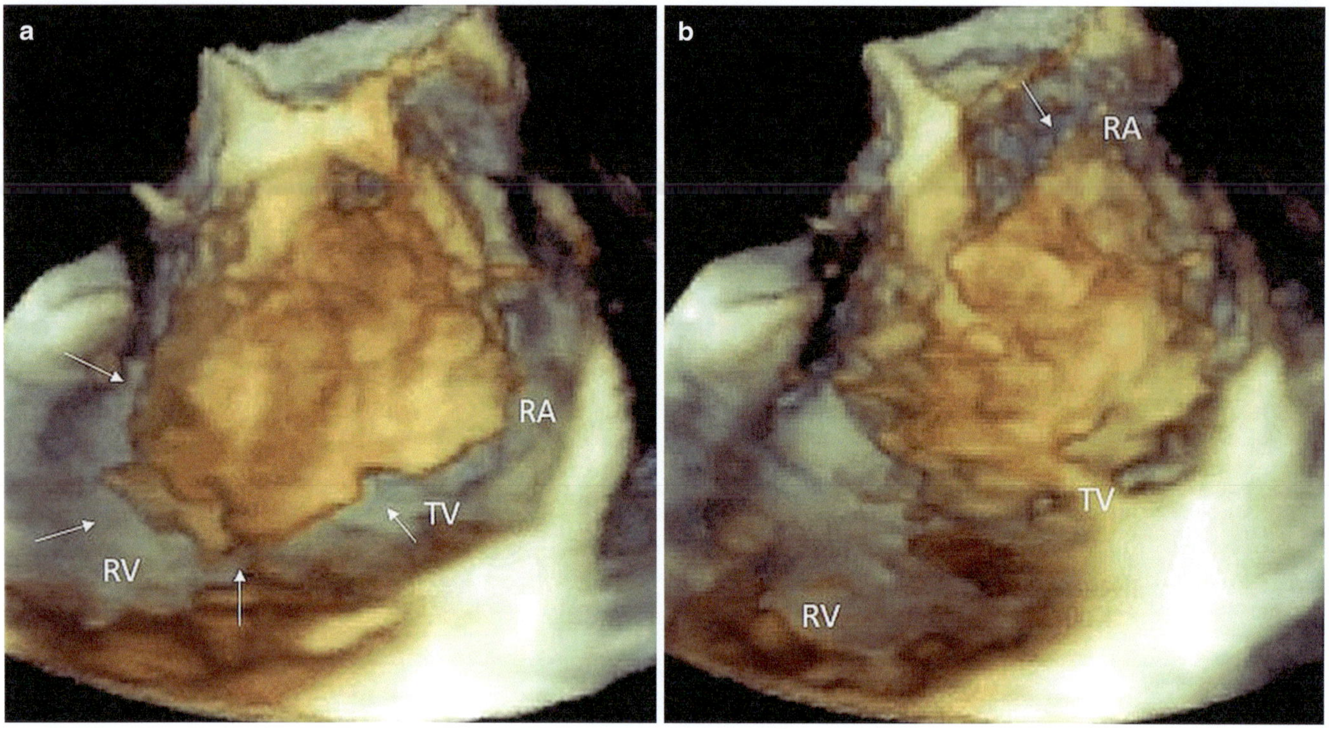

Fig. 24.9 Huge and mobile right atrial myxoma visualized by transesophageal 3DE. (**a**) Volume rendering of the tumor showing a huge cardiac myxoma (white arrows) almost occluding the tricuspid orifice and protruding in right ventricle in diastole. (**b**) During systole, the myxoma almost fills the entire right atrial cavity. *Ra* right atrium, *RV* right ventricle, *TV* tricuspid valve

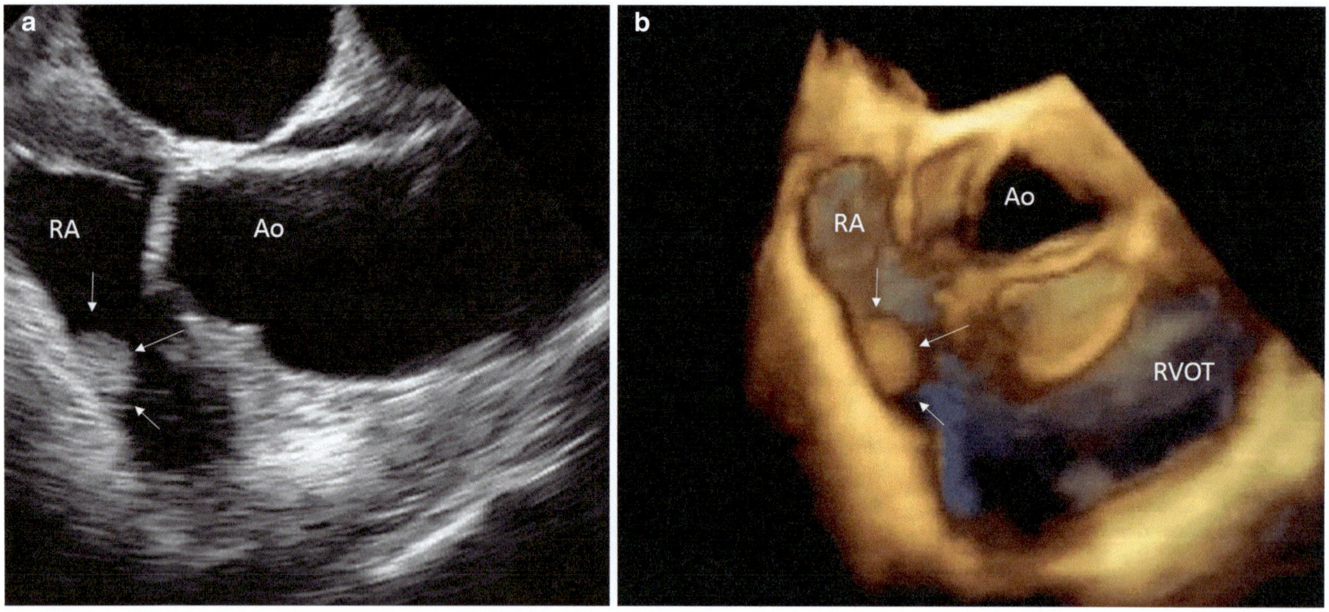

Fig. 24.10 Small and sessile right atrial myxoma visualized by transesophageal 3DE. Two- (**a**) and 3DE (**b**) transesophageal images of a small right atrial myxoma located on the hinge line of the tricuspid valve. *RA* right atrium, *AO* aorta, *RVOT* right ventricular outflow tract

Papillary Fibroelastoma

Papillary fibroelastoma is the third most common benign cardiac tumor (surpassed only by myxomas and fibromas) with a predilection for valvular endocardium: up to 75% of papillary fibroelastomas are located on one of the cardiac valves (50% on the aortic leaflets and 30–35% on mitral valve) while nearly 20% on "non valvular" endocardium. Over the years, this tumor has been increasingly detected, because of the improvement of resolution of transthoracic echocardiography and the introduction of transesophageal echocardiography. Histologically, papillary fibroelastoma has an inner dense fibrous core, covered by a layer of loose connective tissue and elastic fibers, walled by a monolayer of endothelial cell that is continuous with the endothelium of underlying leaflet. Macroscopically the papillary fibroelastoma tends to be relatively small, usually not larger than 20 mm in length and 15–20 mm in width. The papillary fibroelastoma is highly mobile with a pedunculated or stalk attachment to leaflets. The shape of papillary fibroelastoma may vary from ones with a well-defined "head" to ones with elongated, strand-like projections resembling to a "sea anemone" [10].

Often the tumor is asymptomatic and hence discovered incidentally during an echocardiographic examination (quite often during a routine intraoperative transesophageal echocardiography in patients scheduled for cardiac surgery). More rarely, papillary fibroelastoma can result in life-threatening complications such as chest pain or ventricular fibrillation, due to transient occlusion of left main coronary artery or systemic embolism due to fragments of papillary fronds.

Echocardiography

The two-dimensional transthoracic echocardiography appearance is usually that of a small round, ovoid or irregular mass with a homogeneous texture (Fig. 24.11a). 3DE may provide a better assessment of the position and the attachment of papillary fibroelastoma (Fig. 24.11b, c).

However, two-dimensional transthoracic echocardiography may fail to detect very small papillary fibroelastomas. In one of the largest echocardiographic series (48 patients with pathologically confirmed papillary fibroelastoma), the sensitivity and specificity of two-dimensional transthoracic echocardiography for detection of papillary fibroelastoma larger than 2 mm were 88.9% and 87.8% respectively, with an overall accuracy of 88.4%. When the papillary fibroelastoma was smaller than 2 mm were included in the analysis, the sensitivity of transthoracic echocardiography dropped to 61%. Because of its superior spatial resolution, two-dimensional transesophageal echocardiography may improve accuracy (indeed in the same series the sensitivity of two-dimensional transesophageal echocardiography in detecting papillary fibroelastoma smaller than 2 mm was 76.6%). Transesophageal 3DE may provide a finer definition of the edges, size and location of the tumor [11] (Figs. 24.11 and 24.12).

Lambl's Excrescences

Lambl's excrescences are filiform fronds attached along the line of valve closure at the atrial surface of mitral valve and on the ventricular surface of aortic valve. Vilem Dusan Lambl first identified these valvular strands in 1856. Macroscopically Lambl's excrescences may occur as single strand, in rows or even in clusters. They can vary in length from 1 to 10 mm and they are usually less than 1 mm in thickness. When larger and longer they take the name of "giant Lambl's excrescences" and are difficult to distinguish from papillary fibroelastoma. Histologically LE consists of an acellular central elastic connective-tissue core that forms a continuum with the connective tissue of the valve, covered by a single layer of endothelium. Lamb's excrescencies may occur either in normal or in calcified leaflets.

The most accepted hypothesis of their pathogenesis is that LE are simply organized thrombi. Along the line of coaptation, wear and tear may cause endothelial damage that pro-

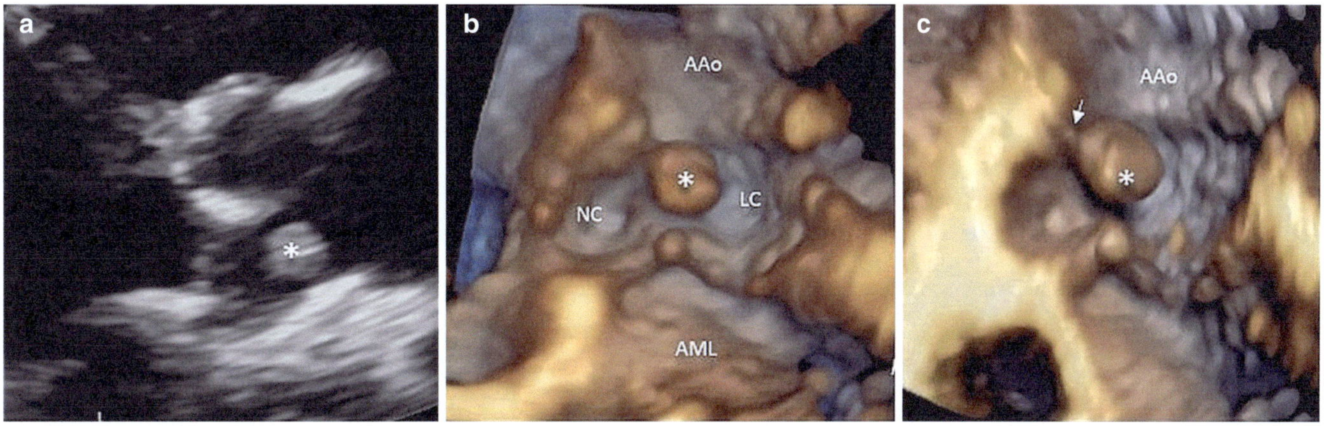

Fig. 24.11 Papillary fibroelastoma attached on the endocardium of the aortic root. (**a**) Classic transthoracic two-dimensional transesophageal echocardiography appearance (asterisk) (Video 24.6a). (**b**) Transesophageal 3DE volume rendering of the same case providing a better assessment of its shape and position (near the sino-tubular junction on the commissure between the non-coronary (NC) and left coronary (LC) leaflets (Video 24.6b). (**c**) A slight rotation allows visualization the thin attachment of the mass to the aortic root (arrow) (Video 24.6c)

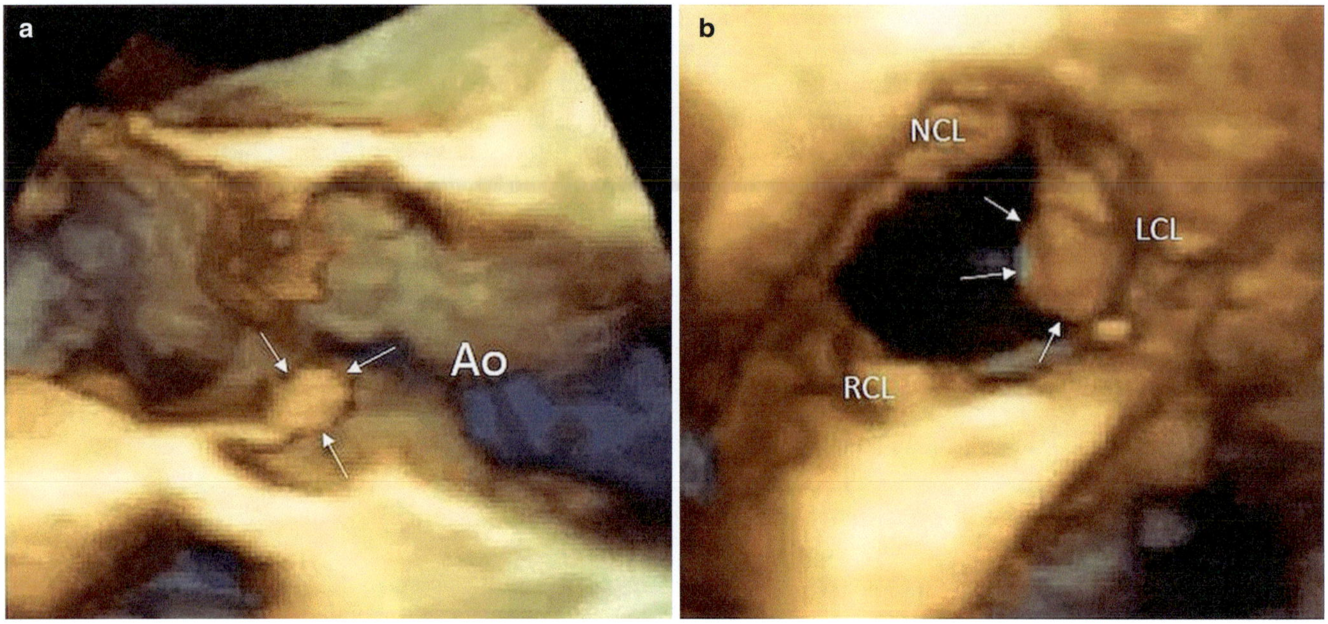

Fig. 24.12 Papillary fibroelastoma attached on the aortic valve. Transesophageal 3DE longitudinal (**a**) and transversal (**b**) cut planes at the level of the aortic valve showing a small round fibroelastoma (white arrows) attached to the left coronary leaflet (LCL). *NCL* non-coronary leaflet, *RCL* right coronary leaflet

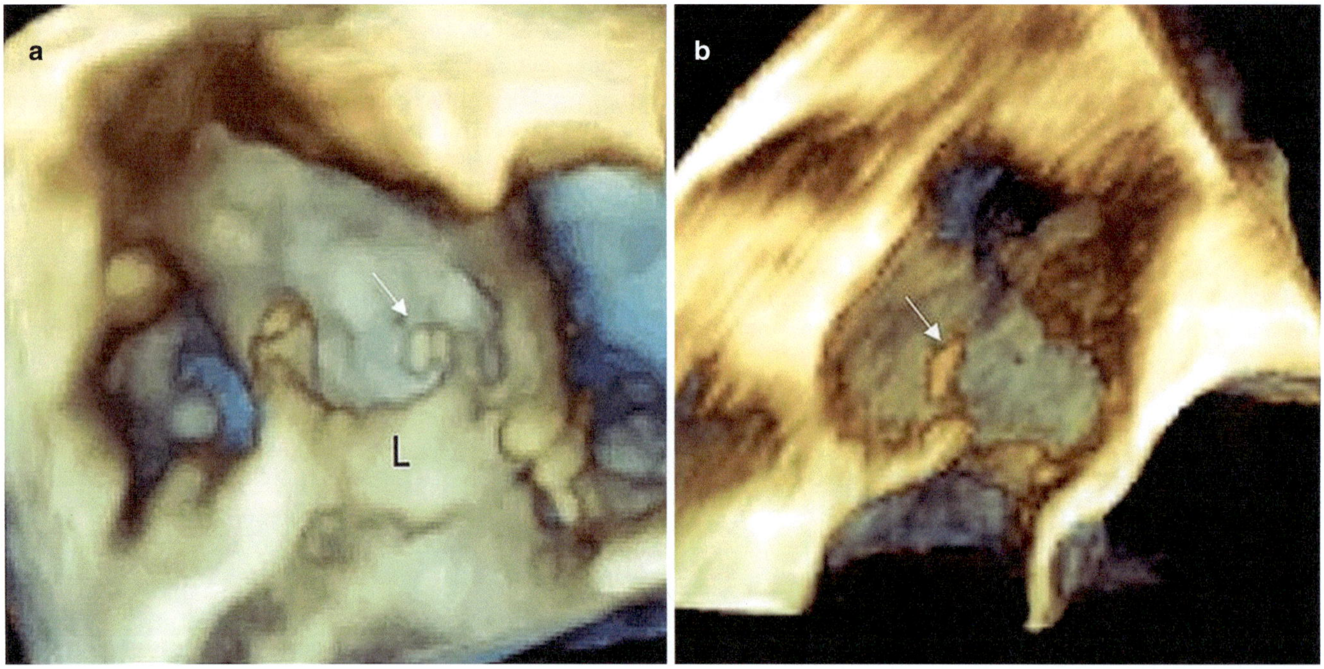

Fig. 24.13 Transesophageal 3DE volume rendering display of Lambl's excrescencies on aortic leaflets free margin (**a**, **b** white arrows)

motes fibrin and small thrombi formation, which eventually forms collagen filiform organization.

Typically, large Lambl's excrescencies can be detected by transthoracic two-dimensional echocardiography, while the smaller ones can only be discovered in vivo by transesophageal two-, 3DE (Fig. 24.13).

Usually asymptomatic and present in older individuals Lamb's excrescencies are considered benign age-related variants. However occasionally, these excrescencies may embolise. In such cases, treatment consists on anticoagulation while surgical excision may become a therapeutic option in patients suffering of multiple embolic strokes.

Malignant Primary Cardiac Tumors

Nearly 25% of all tumors and cysts of the heart and pericardium are malignant [1]. The most common is the angiosarcoma (33% of all malignant cardiac tumors are angiosarcomas). This tumor originates from the vascular endothelium and it is usually located in the right side of the heart. Often large and infiltrative, the tumor causes cardiac failure or pericardial effusion. Rhabdomyosarcomas accounts for 20% of all malignant cardiac tumors. The majority of patients with rhabdomyosarcomas have aspecific findings. Other malignant cardiac tumors are mesothelioma and other sarcomas, which have the propensity to cause pericardial involvement. Surgical excisions associated with chemotherapy may prolong survival but the outcome is often disappointing.

Metastatic Tumors

Metastatic tumors are more frequent than primary ones [12]. Nearly 9% of patients with known malignancies have cardiac metastases and up to 14% of patients with metastases have cardiac or pericardial involvement. Metastases may reach the heart through several pathways: vascular and lymphatic channels, transvenous or by direct extension. The ways used by the tumors to reach the heart may reveal their origin. Certain tumors such as renal cell or hepatocellular carcinomas can extend into the inferior vena cava and grow into the right atrium via transvenous extension (Fig. 24.14a, b, Videos 24.7a and 24.7b). Epithelial pulmonary tumor may reach the left atrium through pulmonary veins. Mesothelioma usually invades the pericardium by continuity. Pericardium represents the most frequently involved site of cardiac metastasis, followed by epicardial and myocardial involvement (Fig. 24.14c, d).

Symptoms depend on their location and tumor burden and invasiveness ranging from completely silent to life-threatening manifestations. For instance, involvement and disruption of conduction system may lead to lethal arrhythmias; metastatic involvement of coronary arteries may result in angina or in acute coronary syndrome; invasion of pericardial sack may cause pericardial effusion and cardiac tamponade; fragmentation of intracardiac metastases may cause pulmonary or systemic embolisms.

Echocardiography is the initial imaging modality and allows obtaining data on localization, size and mobility of the mass. Posterior mass are better identified with two-dimensional transesophageal echocardiography. As for other non-tumor or benign masses, transesophageal 3DE allows a better assessment of site, size and shape.

The limited field of view of echocardiography allows exploring only the heart cavities and valves, while both computed tomography and cardiac magnetic resonance, having a larger field of view, may explore extra-cardiac tissue thus identifying direct extension from the mediasti-

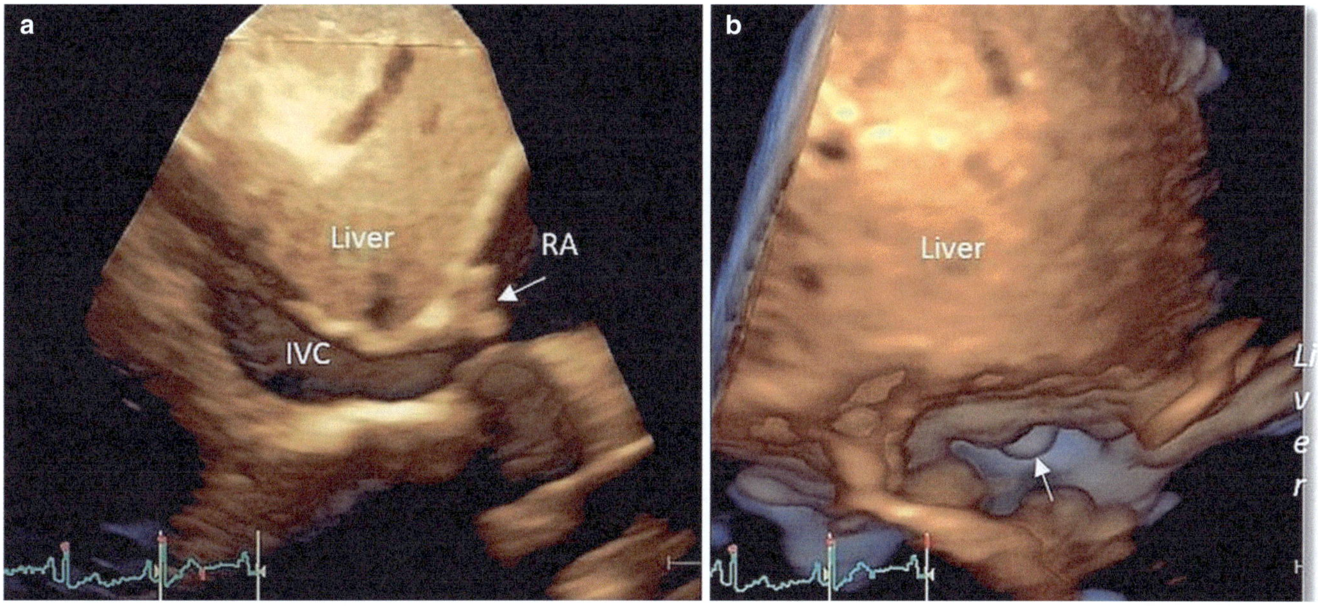

Fig. 24.14 Metastatic tumors. Renal cell carcinoma. The tumor is seen emerging from the inferior vena cava. (**a**) Transthoracic 3DE data set obtained from a subcostal approach with a longitudinal cut of the inferior vena cava (Video 24.7a). (**b**) Same 3D data set rotated in "en face" view. The white arrow points at the part of the tumor protruding into the right atrium (Video 24.7b). (**c**) Metastasis of colon adenocarcinoma invading the apex of left ventricle and the entire lateral wall of the right ventricle (**d**). In (**c**), the arrows delimit the intracavitary borders of the tumors. In (**d**), the arrows delimit the tumors invading the entire wall of the right ventricle

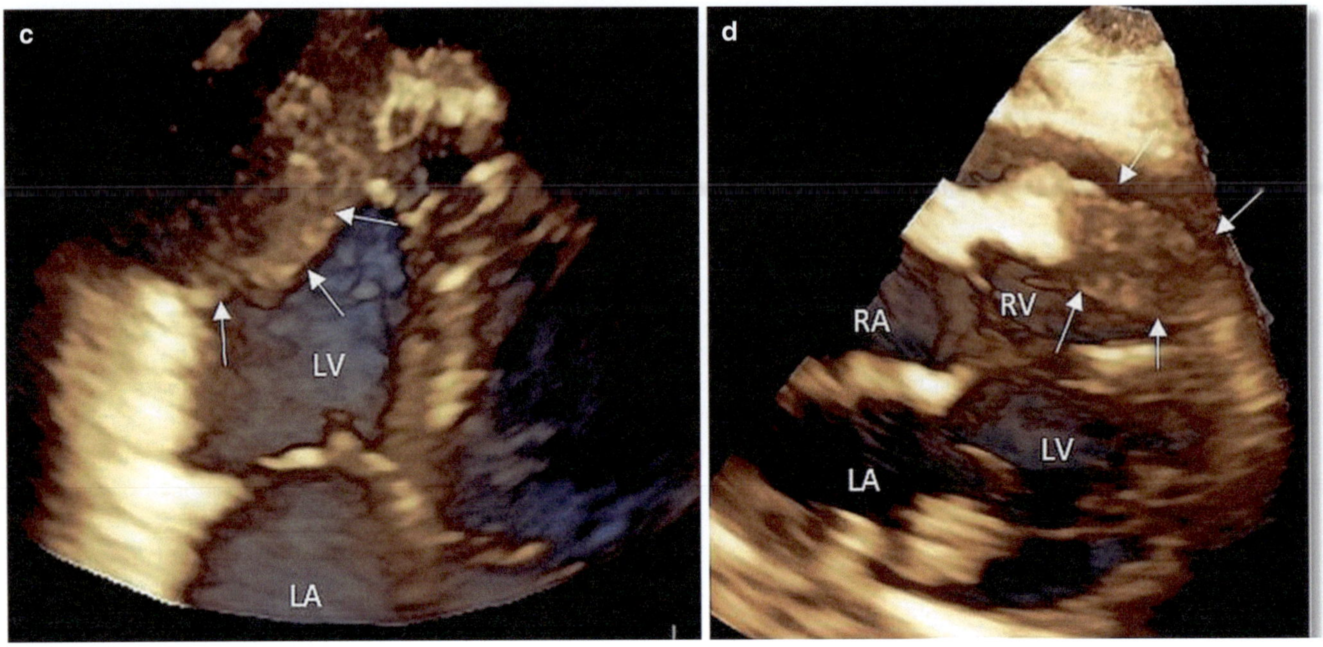

Fig. 24.14 (continued)

num or inferior vena cava. Moreover, the excellent tissue characterization of magnetic resonance imaging allows defining intra-myocardial masses not always visible with echocardiography.

Non-tumor Masses

Intracardiac Thrombi

Intracardiac thrombi may be located in any of the four cardiac chambers in different clinical settings. All pathological conditions that promote blood stasis may cause thrombus formation. Thus, within atria, thrombi are usually located in the left atrial appendage in patients with atrial fibrillation and in left atrial appendage and left atrium in patients with mitral stenosis. Thrombi migrating from systemic veins may cross the right atrium and ventricle to reach the pulmonary arteries. Thrombi in the right atrium may also originate "in situ" in case of permanent intra-atrial devices. Within the left ventricle thrombi occur in patients with large myocardial infarction (both in acute and chronic phase) or in patients with end-stage dilated cardiomyopathy. Thrombi may embolize causing severe morbidities and even death. Major clinical presentations of left side embolisms are acute neurological attack (transient ischemic attack or stroke) and acute peripheral vascular obstruction. Right side clots usually lead to pulmonary embolism and pulmonary infarcts.

Left ventricular thrombi tend to occur in areas of blood stasis such as aneurysm, apical dyskinesia or in ventricles with diffuse hypokineasia and severe pump dysfunction. A combination of blood stasis, endothelial injury and a state of hypercoagulability predisposes thrombus formation in a setting of acute myocardial infarction [13]. Actually, thrombus formation is a physiological response to the acutely infarcted myocardium and may play a protective role. In fact, a thick thrombotic layer acts as support to the infarcted myocardium protecting against wall rupture. The fibrin mesh favors the collagen fibers repair. Moreover, by restoring the wall thickness, the thrombus may limit myocardial expansion. On the other hand, the embolic potential of thrombus may have disastrous effects. For this reason, left ventricular thrombus is considered one of the most feared complications after acute myocardial infarction rather than a simple physiological response to injured myocardium [14]. Thrombi prone to embolization are those that protrude in the left ventricular cavity (in fact, these thrombi are exposed to the blood flow on several sides), and have a free mobility (which indicates thrombus friability) [15].

Usually, left ventricular thrombi are located at the apex, although they may also occur at the septal region and less frequently at the infero-posterior regions.

Left ventricular thrombi may also occur in presence of chronic ventricular aneurysm and in ischemic or idiopathic cardiomyopathies. In the latter cardiac conditions, thrombus formation is due to the blood stasis, as documented by the presence of spontaneous echo-contrast often visible in the apical and periapical regions.

The echocardiographic appearance of a thrombus is that of a discrete echo-dense mass with well definite margins. They can have different shape, size and mobility ranging from a thin layer of immobile mural thrombus to a large protruding mass oscillating into the ventricular cavity. Usually they have a homogeneous texture with an echo density softer than that of myocardium. Occasionally they may have echolucent central areas, which suggest that the thrombus is relatively recent and still "in a growing phase".

When located in the apex probably transthoracic echocardiography is the best technique, as with the transesophageal approach the LV apex is usually foreshortened and in the far field. 3DE has the advantage of a "*panoramic*" view, compared to the tomographic nature of two-dimensional echocardiography, allowing a more precise assessment of size, shape, mobility and number of thrombi especially when mobile and protruding. Moreover, cropping and rotating the volumetric data set allow obtaining the perspective that best visualizes the thrombi and their attachment of the ventricular wall. Finally, the possibility to re-align the tomographic planes obtained from a 3DE data set reduces the risk of missing small apical thrombi due to foreshortening of apical views with two-dimensional echocardiography. However, while using two-dimensional echocardiography the texture of the thrombus appears softer than the surrounding myocardium, allowing an easy distinction between thrombus and myocardial tissue, it is known that with 3DE the different shades of blue/brown color give a visually perception of the depth of different structures rather than their texture. As consequence, both thrombus and surrounding myocardial tissue have similar shades of blue/bronze color if they are at the same distance from the transducer (Fig. 24.15, Video 24.8).

Left Atrial Thrombi

Atrial fibrillation consists of rapid and uncoordinated contractions of atrial fibers that cause blood stasis. Because of its complex anatomical configuration (multilobulated, narrow entry orifice), blood stasis is particularly marked within left atrial appendage. In fact, in patients with atrial fibrillation more than 90% of thrombi are located in left atrial appendage. However, patients with mitral stenosis may have thrombi both in left atrial cavity and in left atrial appendage even with sinus rhythm.

Discovering thrombi in left atrial appendage requires the transesophageal approach. As for the left ventricular thrombi, 3DE is unable to distinguish between thrombi and the surrounding atrial wall based on tissue characterization. In case of large thrombi, usually transesophageal 3DE provides a correct evaluation despite the lack of tissue characterization. Moreover, the technique allows cropping and rotating the image in any direction, obtaining the most favorable perspectives (Fig. 24.16).

However, small or flat thrombi adherent to myocardial wall may be difficult to detect using transesophageal 3DE without the help of two-dimensional imaging (Fig. 24.17).

Right Atrial Thrombi

Thrombus formation is less common in the right sided cardiac chambers compared with the left counterpart. Right atrial thrombosis may occur in presence of atrial fibrillation. However, the relatively flat configuration of the right atrial appendage, with a large orifice opened in the right atrial cavity, the absence of tortuous lobes and the presence of the blood stream from the superior vena cava flow, (which flashes the right atrial appendage), are factors that prevent the formation of blood stasis due to atrial fibrillation. Thus, thrombus formation in right atrial appendage is less common than in its left counterpart (Fig. 24.18a–d).

Right atrial thrombosis is also relatively frequent in presence of foreign bodies such as central venous line or pacemaker leads. The occurrence of thrombosis after implantation may occur in almost 20–40% of patients although most of them remain clinically silent [16].

Peripheral venous clots may lodge in the right atrial cavity on their way to the pulmonary arteries. This usually occurs in patients with a venous thromboembolic disease. These floating thrombi are accidentally discovered during an echocardiographic examination performed in a patient with suspected pulmonary embolism.

Both two- and 3DE are effective in diagnosis, although transesophageal 3DE may provide a better understanding of the site and size of thrombus (Fig. 24.19, Video 24.9).

Infective Endocarditis

Infective endocarditis (bacterial or fungal) is an infection of the endothelial surface of the heart that occurs on valvular tissue (leaflets or chordae), mural endocardium, site of septal defects or arteriovenous shunts, or on paraprosthetic tissue and is one of the most harmful diseases [17]. Several reasons may explain the difficulties in management of this, often fatal, condition. First, contemporary patients with infective endocarditis are older, sicker, and affected by other comorbidities than in the early antibiotics era. Second, bacteria are more virulent and resistant to antibiotics than they were decades ago. Third, degenerative heart valve diseases, diabetes, intravenous drug abuse, immuno-deficiency, valve prostheses, permanent intracardiac foreign bodies, both electronic devices and catheters, have replaced rheumatic heart disease as the major predisposing factors [18]. Finally, establishing an accurate diagnosis early in the course of the disease, when an appropriate medical or surgical treat-

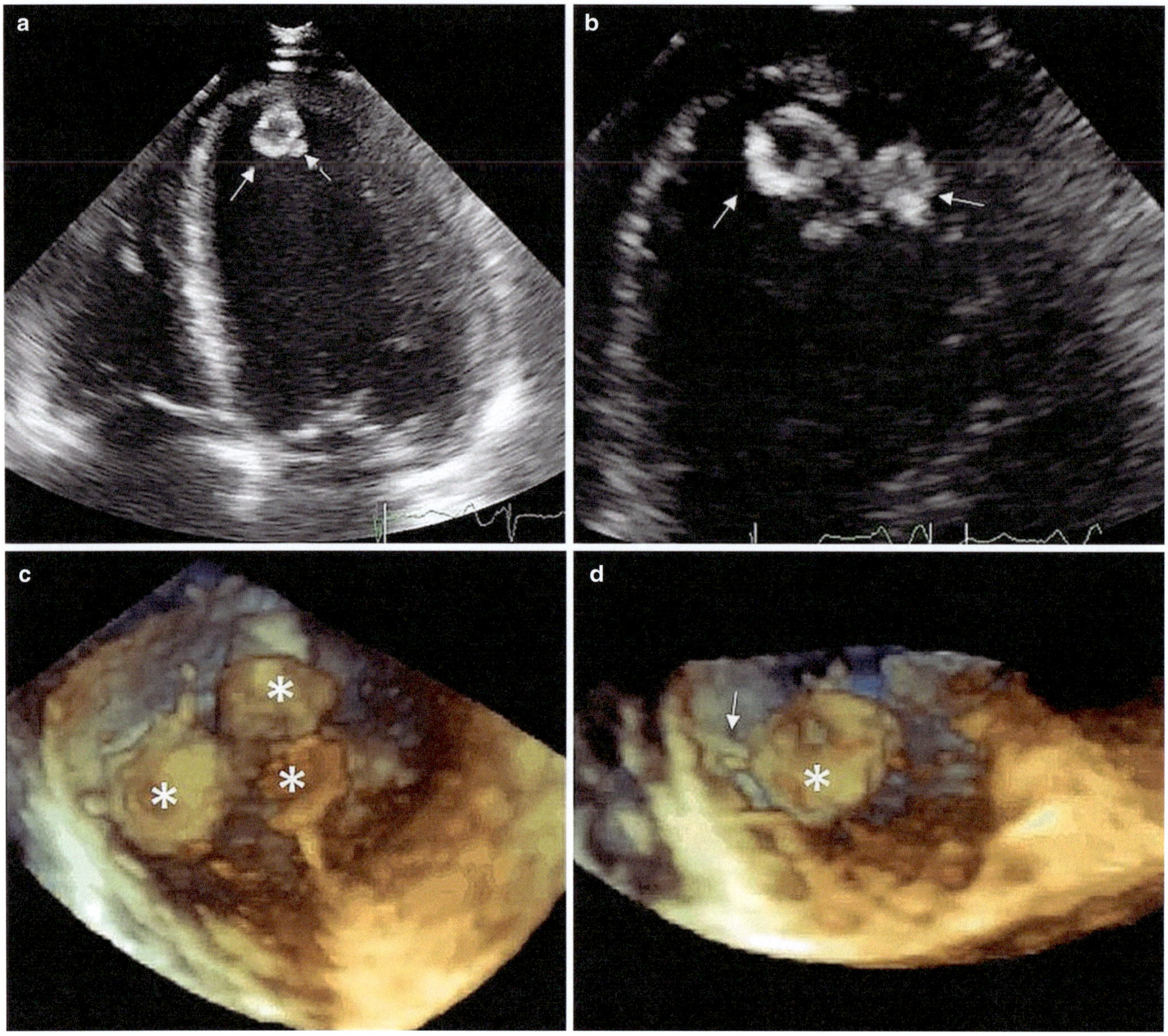

Fig. 24.15 Left ventricular thrombi. (**a**) Two-dimensional transthoracic echocardiography showing a round-shaped thrombus (arrows) in the apex in a patient with severe dilated cardiomyopathy. The central part of the thrombus appear echo lucent being constituted by blood. (**b**) Magnified image of the apex showing in a different still frame three masses. Because of the thin slice of two-dimensional echocardiography, mobile masses may appear and disappear from the tomographic plane. (**c**) Transthoracic 3DE of the same case. Perspective is from above, slightly oblique. Three well-defined thrombi are visible (asterisks). (**d**) A slight modified perspective showing a thin peduncle (arrow) of one of the thrombi (Video 24.8)

ment would be more effective, is difficult. Thus, despite major advances in medical and surgical treatment, infective endocarditis remains a "malignant" disease, as defined by William Osler in his Gulstonian lecture in 1885, with high mortality rate and prolonged hospitalization.

Endothelium lesions associated with bacteremia, and an immunological predisposition to the disease are the primary causal factors. High-velocity turbulent jets that accompany valvular dysfunction, valve prostheses and congenital defects, hitting against the endothelium leads to the endothelial damage. This first lesion releases inflammatory tissue factors that in turn trigger the event cascade leading to a sterile platelets-fibrin-thrombus vegetation. Transient or persistent bacteremia is the events that ultimately converts the sterile vegetation into infective endocarditis. However not always the coincidence between bacteremia and endothelial lesions leads to infective endocarditis. Bacteria able to colonize sterile vegetations must have a specific resistance to host defense and peculiar adherence capabilities [19]. Usually, a colony of bacteria embedded in a meshwork of fibrin, platelets and inflammatory cells forms a vegetation of variable shape, size and mobility is the patho-morphological hallmark of infec-

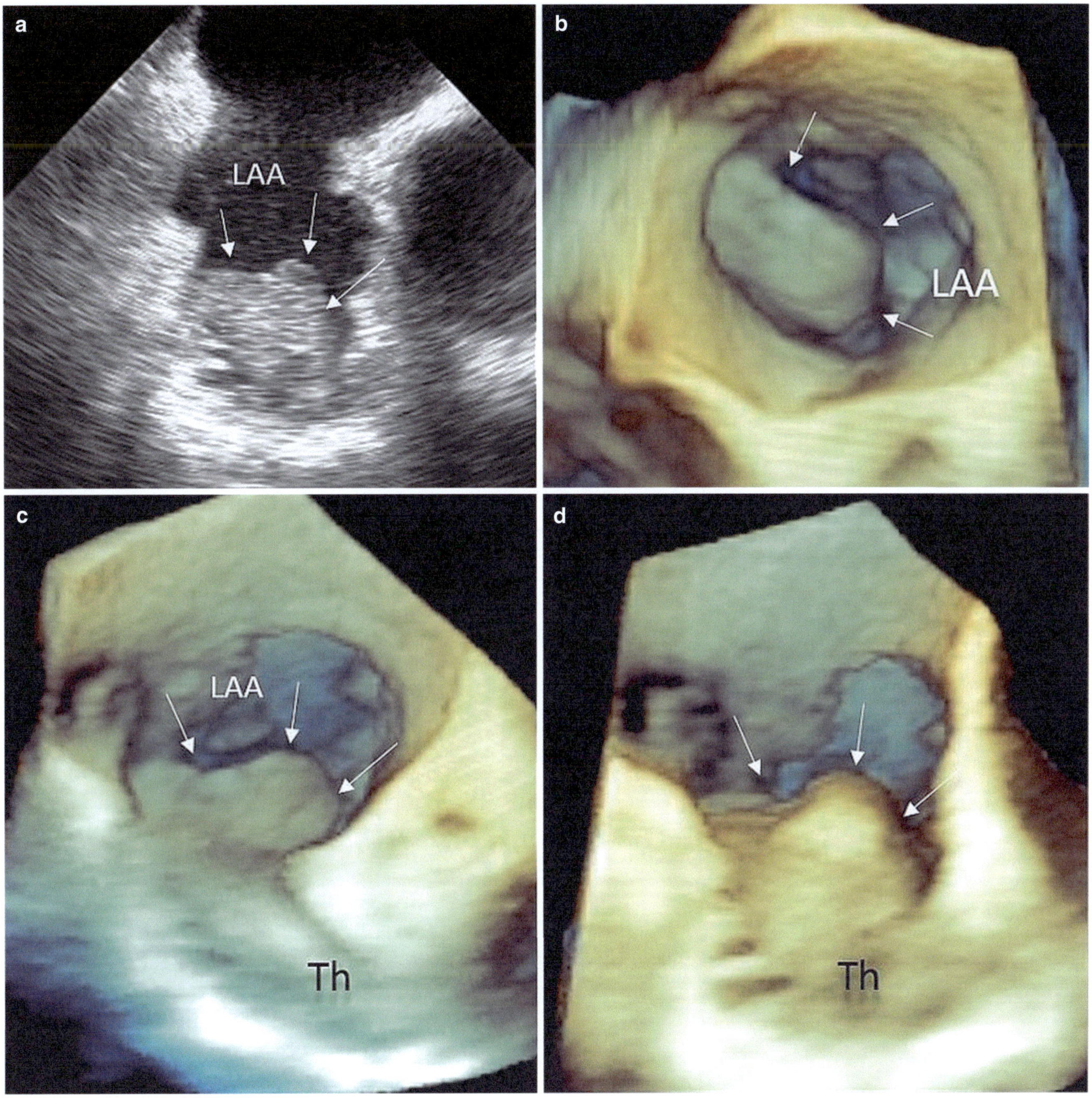

Fig. 24.16 Huge thrombus (arrows) in left atrial appendage visualized by two-dimensional transesophageal echocardiography (**a**) and transesophageal 3DE image. Volume rendering transversal cut plane from above (**b**) and oblique perspectives. (**c**, **d**) Volume rendered longitudinal cut planes showing how the thrombus is deep implanted into the left atrial appendage. *LAA* left atrial appendage, *th* thrombus

tive endocarditis. Although the endothelial damage is often the "primum mover", particularly virulent microorganisms such as Staphylococcus Aureus may directly infect healthy valve tissue.

Currently the diagnosis of infective endocarditis is based on the modified Duke criteria that incorporate clinical findings, microbiological analysis and imaging data, assigning at each one of these three domains minor or major diagnostic relevance [20]. A definitive diagnosis requires either two major, one major and three minor, or five minor criteria [21]. Although other imaging techniques such as computed tomography or cardiac magnetic resonance may contribute to the diagnosis and risk stratification of patients with infective endocarditis, both transthoracic and transesophageal two-dimensional echocardiography remain the first-line diagnostic techniques in patients with suspected infective

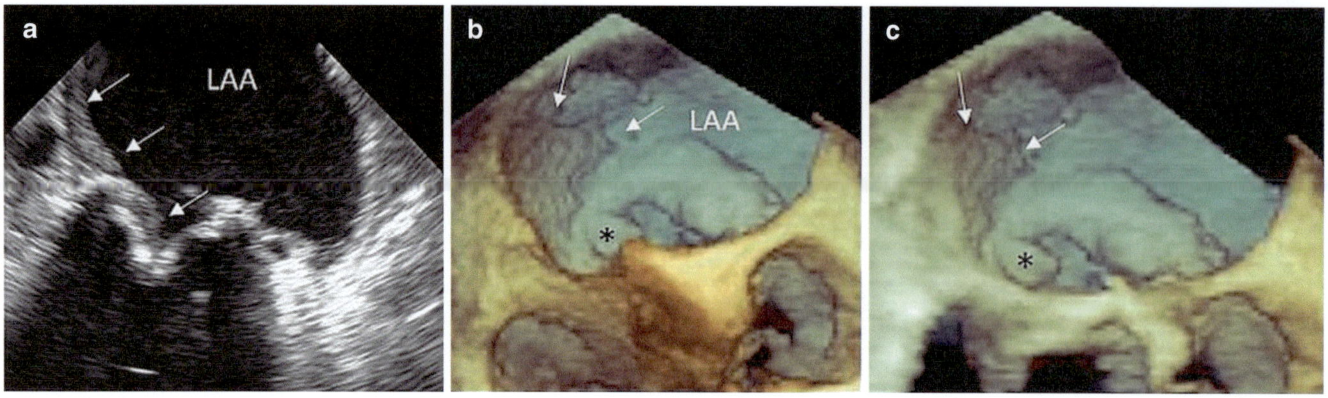

Fig. 24.17 Flat thrombus (white arrows) that adheres to the posterior wall of the left atrium and extents to one of the prosthetic leaflets of a biological prosthesis in mitral position. (**a**) Two-dimensional transesophageal image showing the different texture of the thrombus compared with that of atrial wall which is a key feature for the diagnosis. (**b**) Transesophageal 3DE volume rendering to visualize the position and extension of the thrombotic mass. Arrows delimit the edges of the thrombus adhering to the atrial wall. Asterisk points at the portion of the thrombus extending to the prosthetic leaflet. The absence of differences in texture makes the differential diagnosis of thrombus difficult if based only on 3DE images. (**c**) A minimum cropping in z direction allows to better visualize the portion of thrombus on the prosthetic leaflet

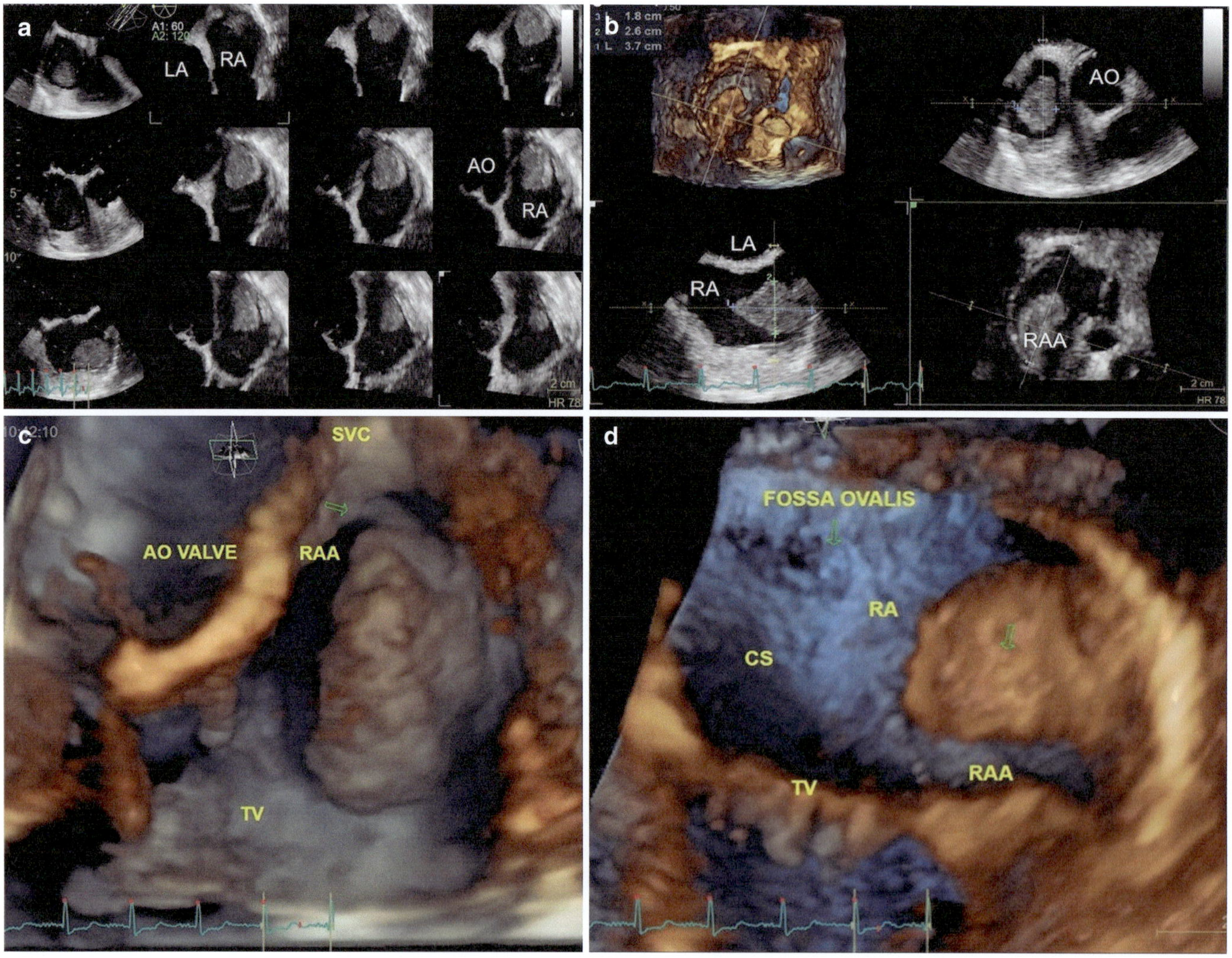

Fig. 24.18 Thrombus in right atrial appendage. Left upper panel/(**a**), Transesophageal 3DE volume rendering of a large thrombus in the right atrium. Right upper panel/(**b**), slight rotation and cropping of the data set to show that the origin of the thrombus is from the right atrial appendage. Left lower panel/(**c**), Multislice display of the 3D data set to show anatomical relationships of the mass, its shape and size. Right lower panel/(**d**), slice and quantitative assessment of the mass (Courtesy of Alex Felix, MD, Department of Echocardiography, National Institute of Cardiology, Laranjeiras, Rio de Janeiro, Brazil). *AO* aortic, *CS* coronary sinus, *LA* left atrium, *RA* right atrium, *RAA* right atrial appendage, *SVC* superior vena cava, *TV* tricuspid valve

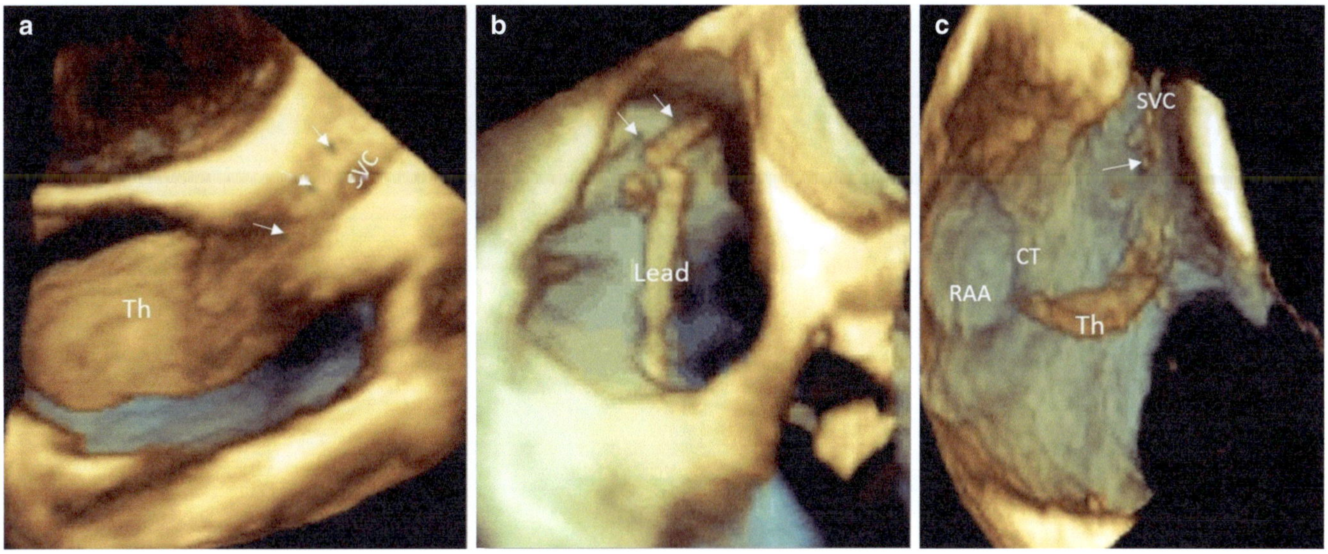

Fig. 24.19 Thrombi in the right atrium. (**a**) Transesophageal 3DE volume rendering of a huge thrombus (white arrows) originating form superior vena cava, which appears obstructed, and protruding into the right atrium. (**b**) Small thrombus (white arrows) attached on a pacemaker lead. (**c**) Residual thrombus (Th) attached to SVC endothelium, after having the pacemaker lead removed (Video 24.9)

endocarditis. The echocardiographic appearance of an oscillating intracardiac mass and/or valvular disruptions, as consequence of bacteria invasiveness, such as annular abscesses, prosthetic valve partial dehiscence, or new valvular regurgitations represent, in an appropriate clinical context, a major Duke criteria [22]. However, because a vegetation starts as a microscopic nidus, its presence may not be visualized at an early echocardiographic examination and additional, sequential studies may be needed to clarify the diagnosis.

At echocardiography, vegetations appear as irregularly shaped, low echogenic masses that can be either sessile or pedunculated, and are usually attached to the upstream side of valve leaflets. Their chaotic motion differs from that of the leaflets themselves. Their "shaggy" appearance may help distinguishing them from more organized and compact masses such as intracardiac tumors or thrombi. However, it must be emphasized that no a single echocardiographic characteristic allows to label any mass as vegetation.

The term "endocarditis" may suggest that the infection involves only the endocardium. However, infective endocarditis spreads through the entire thickness of the valve leaflet causing destructive effects such as leaflet perforation, chordal rupture or dissection of the mitral-aortic curtain.

Several echocardiographic features of infective endocarditis may identify patients at risk for life-threatening complications. Large and highly mobile vegetations are strong predictors of peripheral embolic events. Severe regurgitation due to chordal rupture or leaflets perforation identifies patients at risk of heart failure. Para-prosthetic abscesses may cause prosthetic dehiscence, paravalvular fistulae and atrio-ventricular block.

Transesophageal 3DE refines the diagnosis providing a more precise assessment of the site, size and relationship with adjacent structures. Moreover, the volumetric data set may be cropped and rotated to obtain the most useful and diagnostic perspectives (Fig. 24.20, Video 24.10).

The term mitral "*kissing*" vegetation defines a propagation of a vegetation from the aortic leaflets to healthy mitral leaflet. The "kissing" effect occurs when an aortic vegetation attached to the ventricular side of the leaflet, protrudes into the left ventricular outflow tract, "physically" hitting the anterior mitral leaflet. This mechanism of propagation explains why the vegetation is attached on the ventricular surface of anterior mitral leaflet rather than on its atrial surface (Fig. 24.21).

Paravalvular aortic and mitral abscesses are among the most feared complications of infective endocarditis. More often caused by aggressive bacteria such as staphylococci or enterococci, their presence complicates the course of the disease. Antibiotic therapy usually fails to sterilize the abscesses and once detected, surgical repair is mandatory. The most common sites of abscess are the annular regions.

From an echocardiography viewpoint abscess presents as an echo-lucent pocket, around the mitral or aortic annulus. Often its aspect is inhomogeneous being partially filled by echo-dense material and divided by fibrous septa in a multi-chambered cavity. An abscess may rupture allowing a communication with one of the surrounding cavities. The rupture of a mitral annular abscess may cause a fistulous communication between right and left ventricle, while a rupture of an aortic abscess may result in a communication between aorta and left of right atrium or between the aorta and left ventricle (Fig. 24.22a, b). When the rupture occurs, the color flow may demonstrate flow within the abscess cavity. Particularly frequent are abscesses localized around the aortic annulus in patients with aortic prosthesis. In such a case, the abscess dissects the intervalvular fibrosa, resulting in a pseudo aneurysm formation. Transesophageal 3DE allows unusual

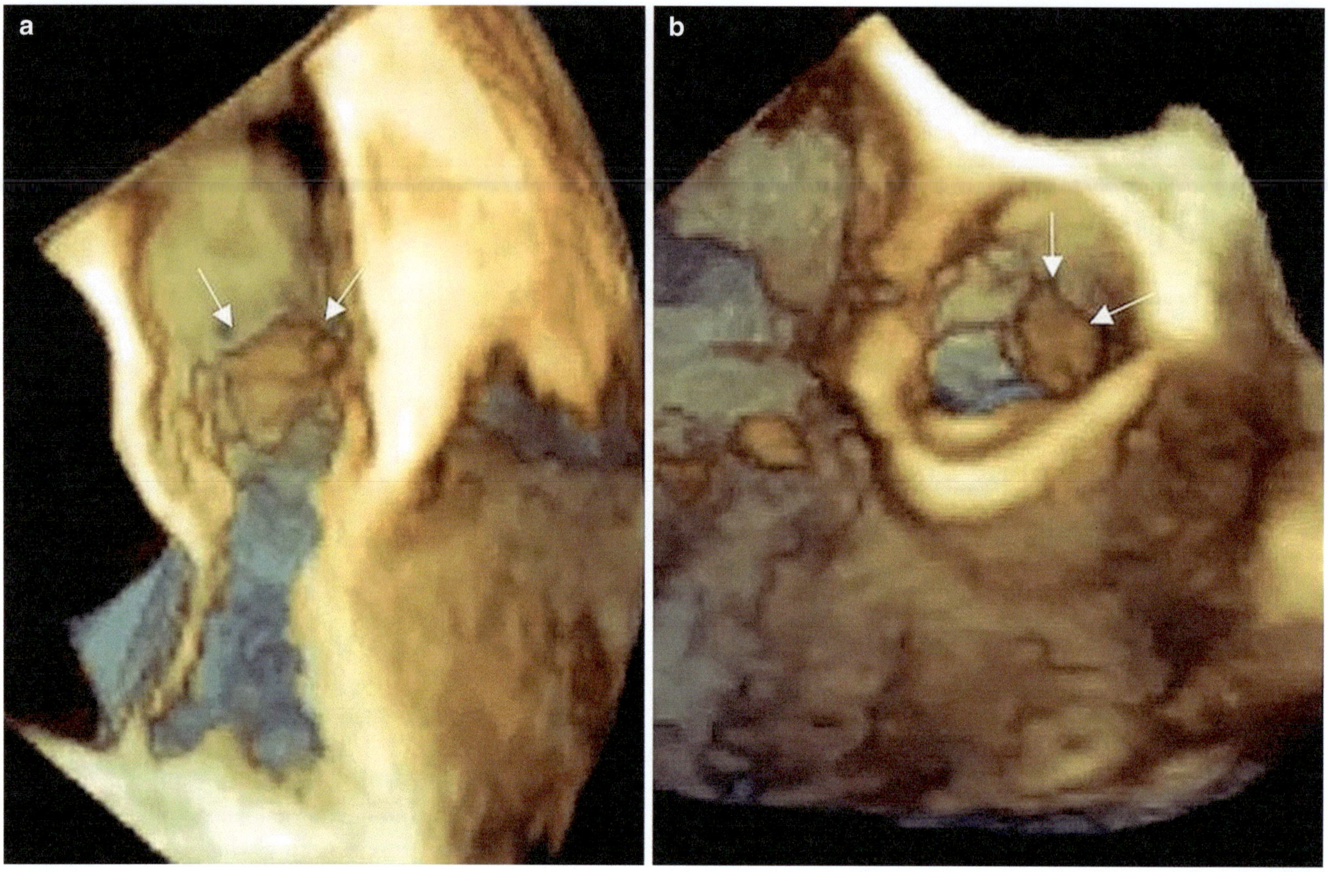

Fig. 24.20 Transesophageal 3DE volume rendering of a large endocarditis vegetation (white arrows) attached at the ventricular surface of the left coronary aortic leaflet. (**a**) Longitudinal cut plane. (**b**) Slightly oblique cut plane from the aortic perspective (Video 24.10)

views: from an atrial perspective, the aortic abscess appears as a mass protruding into the left atrium and is indistinguishable from a dilatation of the Valsalva's sinuses, which causes a similar bulging (Fig. 24.22c). From an aortic perspective, the shape and size of the communication between the abscess cavity and the left ventricular outflow tract is often visible (Fig. 24.22d).

Right Side Infective Endocarditis

Right side infective endocarditis is today a well-defined clinical entity in intravenous drug abusers or in patients having a pacemaker leads or other intracardiac device. The clinical course is more favorable since patients with right side infective endocarditis can have a benign evolution with medical therapy alone or device extraction. Vegetations can be located on tricuspid and pulmonary leaflets or attached to the catheters/devices. Symptoms are similar to those of respiratory infection (fever, dyspnea, and pulmonary infiltration), making diagnosis difficult. As for other left side masses, despite the fact that transthoracic echocardiography can detect the majority of right side infective endocarditis, the transesophageal approach can increase the sensitivity of the technique due to its higher spatial resolution. Transesophageal 3DE allows more precise definition of the size and site of the mass and its relation-ship with surrounding structures (Fig. 24.23).

Aortic Atheroma

Protruding atheroma within the aorta may be source of cerebral and systemic embolization especially in the elderly [23–25]. The organ/s target of embolism is related to the positon of the plaque within the aorta. Plaques located in the ascending aorta will mainly cause cerebral embolism, while those located in the descending aorta will be more related to systemic embolism, respectively. However, Harloff, et al. [26] raised the hypothesis that, despite their distal position, atheromatous complex plaques in the proximal descending aorta may also be source of cerebral embolism. Using a special protocol magnetic resonance imaging sequence (multidirectional 3D velocity mapping), the authors found a significant retrograde diastolic flow and a strong association between complex plaques in descending aorta and cerebral ischemic lesions. Further studies need to confirm this hypothesis.

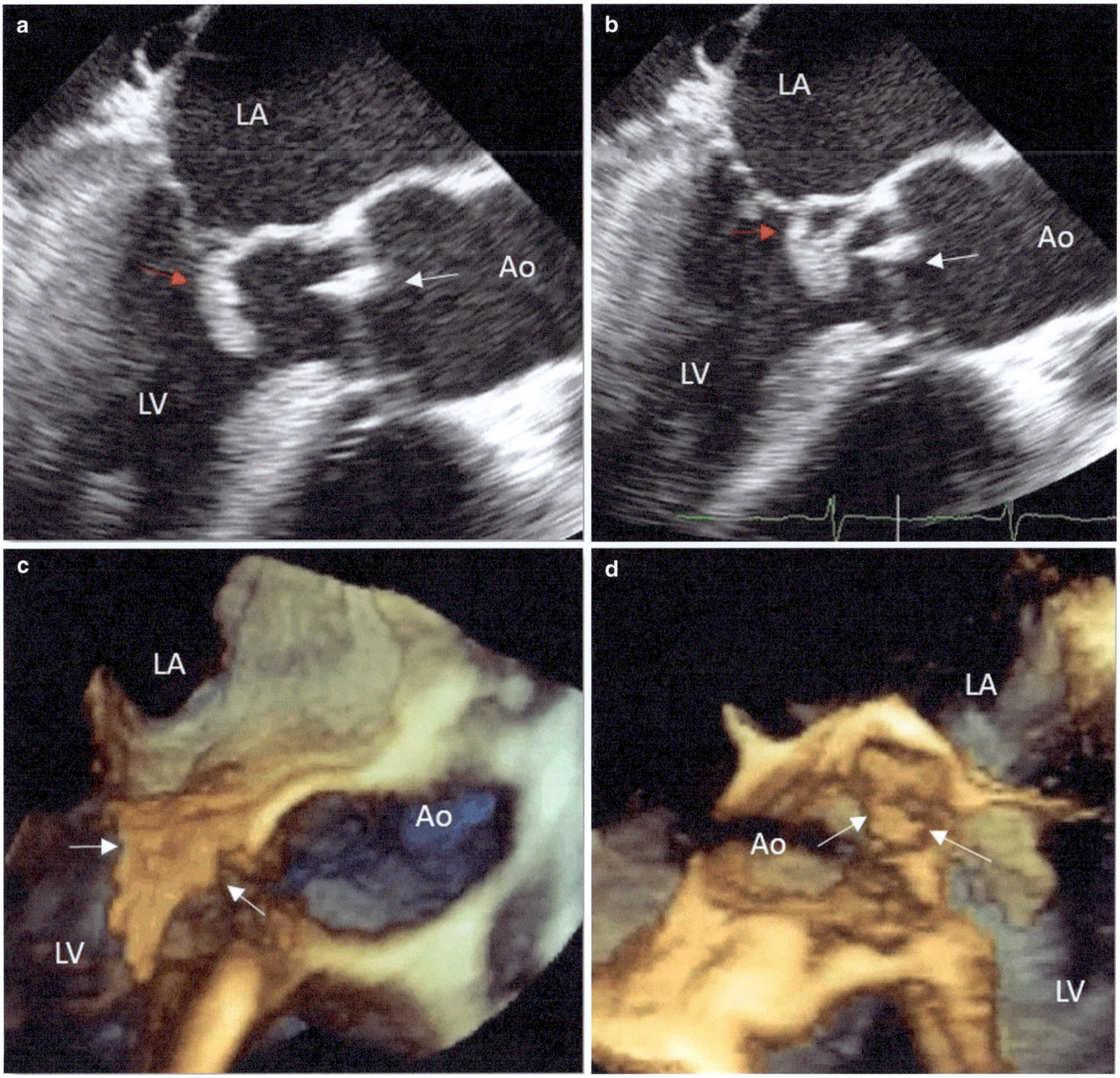

Fig. 24.21 Kissing propagation of aortic valve infective endocarditis on the mitral valve. (**a**, **b**) Two-dimensional transesophageal echocardiography showing a mitral, oblong, highly mobile (note the position of the vegetation in two different still frames) vegetation (red arrow) attached on the ventricular surface of the anterior mitral leaflet. This atypical site id due to a "kissing" propagation from an apparently small vegetation on the ventricular site of the right coronary aortic cusp (white arrow). (**c**, **d**) Transesophageal 3DE volume rendering of the same case. Both mitral (white arrows, **c**) and aortic (white arrows, **d**) vegetations appear larger than it was supposed with two-dimensional imaging. *Ao* aorta, *LA* left atrium, *LV* left ventricle

Atheroembolism may also occur during cardiac catheterization. Large guide catheters may dislodge atherosclerotic debris from the aorta by physical abrasion. In one study of 1000 consecutive guiding catheter removed after PCI revealed the presence of macroscopic aortic debris within the guide lumen in more than 50% of cases [27].

Two-dimensional transesophageal echocardiography remains the first line and the most versatile technique for imaging aortic atheromatous plaques. With the exception of aortic segment at the junction of the aortic arc and descending aorta (that is hidden by the tracheal air), two-dimensional transesophageal echocardiography allow visualization of the entire thoracic aorta providing high-resolution "real time" images of aortic atheromatous plaques and allowing a fine characterization of the shape and size of the atheroma. Complex plaques, i.e. plaques large more of 4 mm and those that with evidence of ulceration or mobile components, revealed by two-dimensional transesophageal echocardiography have been shown

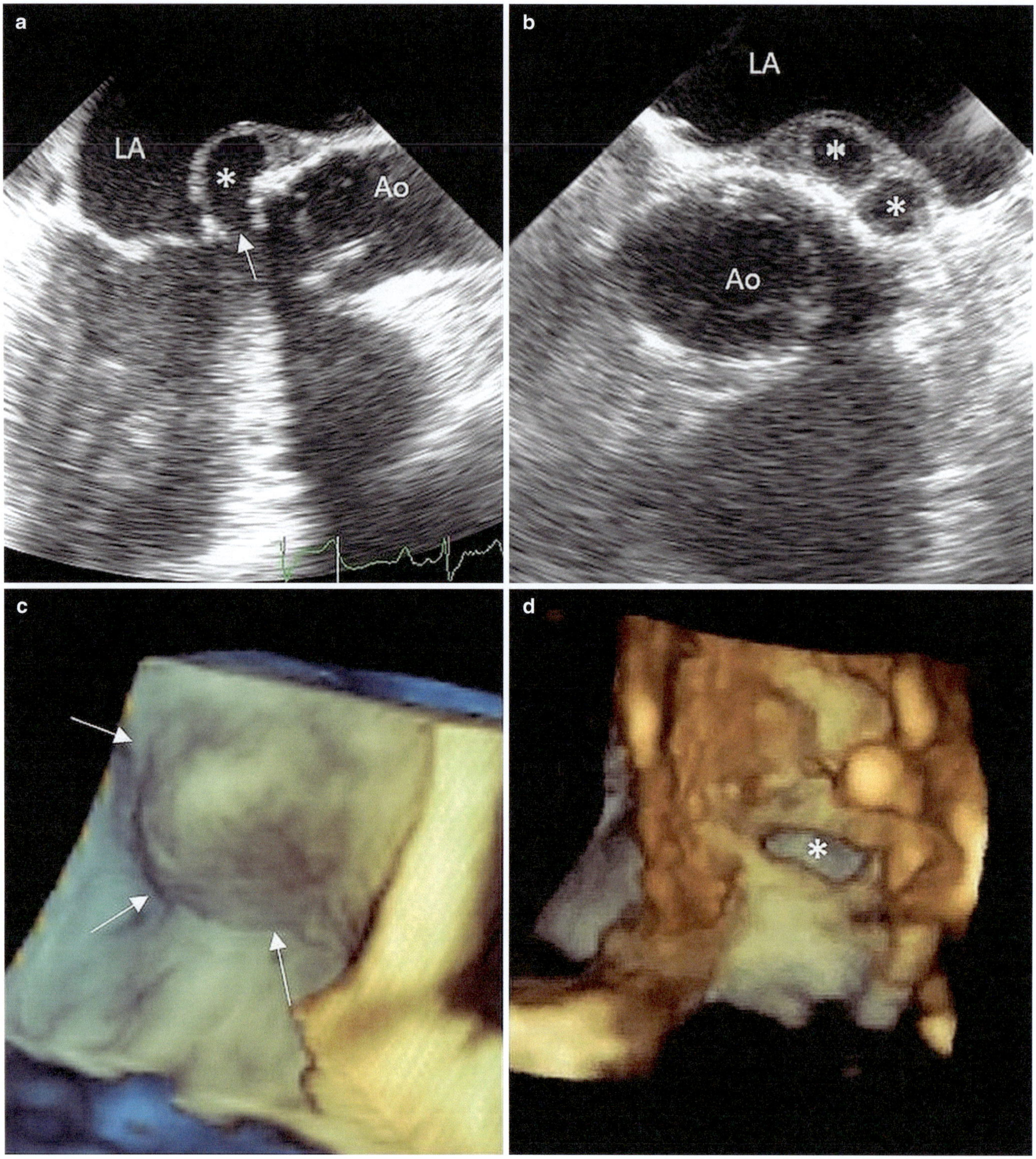

Fig. 24.22 Para-aortic abscess. (**a**) Two-dimensional transesophageal long axis view showing an para-aortic abscess in a patient with a biological prosthesis in aortic position. The asterisk marks the cavity. The arrow points at the hole on the mitral-aortic curtain. (**b**) Two-dimensional transesophageal short axis view showing the bilobed configuration of the cavity (asterisks). (**c**) Transesophageal 3DE volume rendering of the abscess from the atrial perspective. The abscess appears as a mass (arrows) protruding into the atrial cavity. (**d**) By cropping from the aortic perspective, the hole on the mitral aortic curtain (asterisk) can be visualized "en face". *Ao* aorta, *LA* left atrium

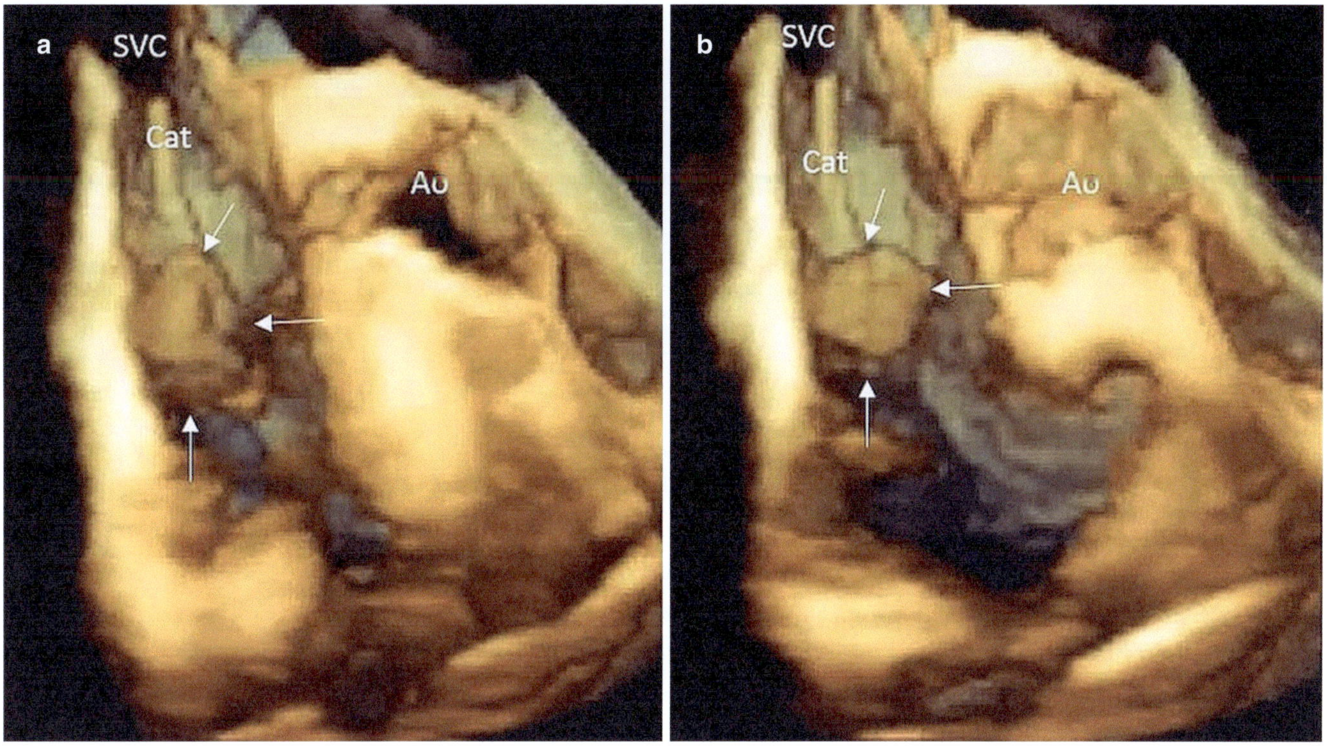

Fig. 24.23 Right side infective endocarditis. Transesophageal 3DE volume rendering of a large vegetation (**a**, **b**, arrows) attached on the atrial surface of tricuspid leaflet in patient with a permanent intracardiac catheter. *Ao* aorta, *Cat* intracardiac catheter, *SVC* superior vena cava

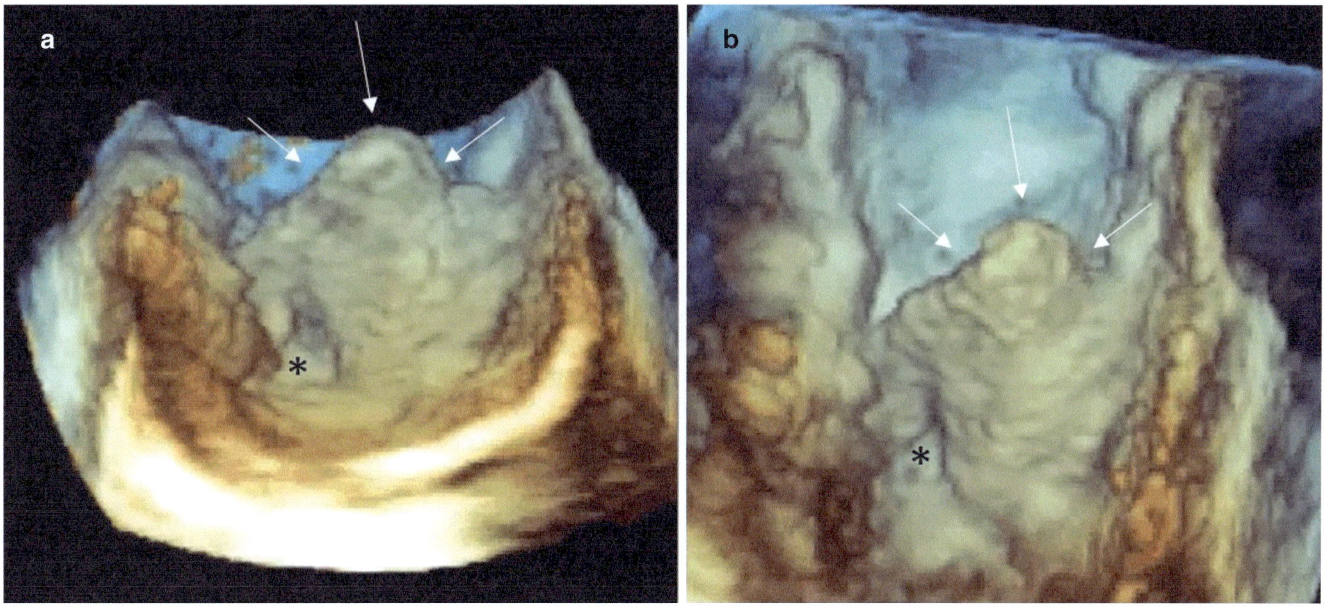

Fig. 24.24 Transesophageal 3DE volume rendering of a huge and complex atheromatous plaque (**a**, **b**, arrows) in descending aorta seen from two different perspectives The asterisk points at one ulceration

to be independent risk factors for ischemic stroke [24, 25]. Transesophageal 3DE provides a more accurate definition of irregularities, protrusions, ulcerations and mobile segments which are shown as in a topographic map (Fig. 24.24).

Moreover, since transesophageal 3DE provides a more "panoramic" view, it allows a more precise definition of the size, contours and irregularities of the plaque compared to the two-dimensional technique (Fig. 24.25).

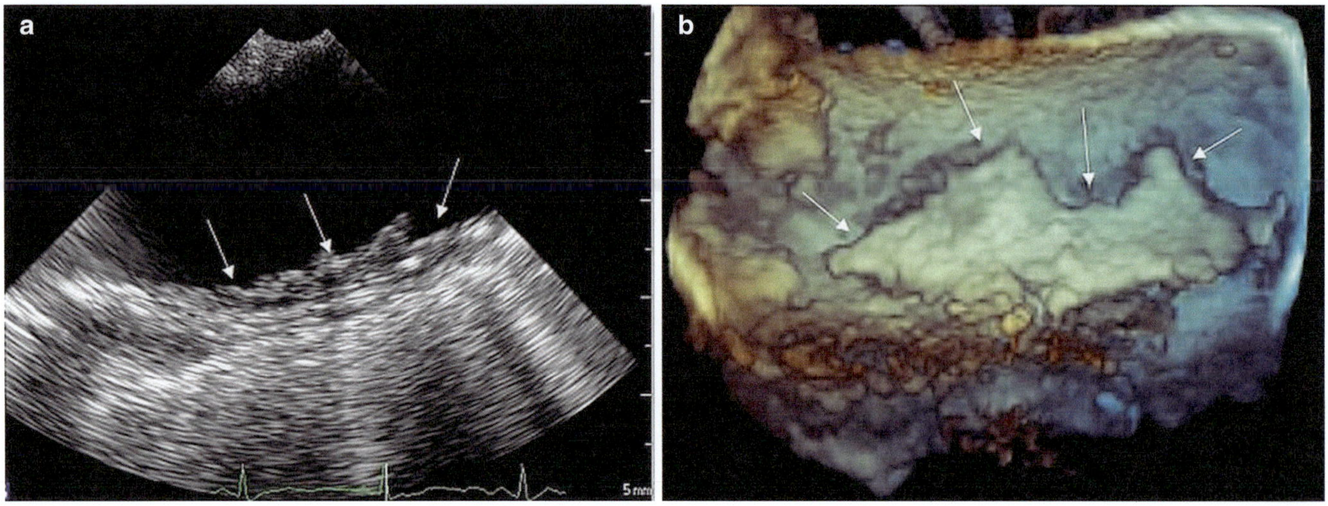

Fig. 24.25 Two- (**a**) and 3DE (**b**) visualization of an atheromatous plaque (arrows) in the descending aorta. In comparison to the two-dimensional view, the 3DE image provides a more precise assessment of the size, contours and irregularities of the atheromatous plaque

Other Pseudo Masses

Knowledge the anatomy of normal intracardiac structures and normal variants is a prerequisite for correctly diagnosing an intracardiac mass. Indeed, several normal intracardiac structures can mimic abnormal masses. In this paragraph, we will illustrate the 3DE features of normal variants of some anatomical structures that can be mistaken for abnormal masses (and indeed, in the early era of transesophageal echocardiography this happened): the Eustachian valve, the crista terminalis or terminal crest, the lipomatous septum, and the left lateral ridge.

Eustachian Valve

The Eustachian valve is an embryogenic remnant of the valve of inferior vena cava. In the fetal life, the inferior vena cava is partially partitioned from the remaining right atrium, by a large flap of tissue encircling the orifice of inferior vena cava extending into the right atrial cavity a sometimes continuing around the fossa ovalis as Eustachian ridge [28]. This valve directs the oxygenated blood returning via the umbilical veins into the left atrium and systemic fetal circulation through the foramen ovalis. In the newborn or childhood period, the valve gradually regresses, disappearing or becoming a thin flap of tissue attached on the anterior-medial border of the orifice of inferior vena cava in adult life.

Absent resorption, lead to a prominent Eustachian valve while incomplete resorption to a reticular network of fine strands called Chiari's network. Either large Eustachian valve or Chiari's network can be mistaken for an abnormal mass [29]. Despite the fact that both of them are "benign" anatomical variants, they may be associated with various clinical manifestations. A large Eustachian valve, for instance, by guiding the inferior vena cava flow against the fossa ovalis may interfere with the spontaneous closure of the patent foramen ovalis, facilitating the persistence of patent foramen ovalis. Both Chiari's network and a large and rigid Eustachian valve may interfere with electrophysiological procedures such as ablation of cavo tricuspid isthmus or with structural heart disease procedures such as percutaneous closure of patent foramen ovalis and atrial septal defect. Finally, Chiari's network may predispose to thrombus formation "in situ" or may capture transient thrombi formed elsewhere in the body (in that case acting like a filter).

Two-dimensional transthoracic and transesophageal echocardiography show a prominent Eustachian valve as a thin "line" of tissue arising from the anterior border of inferior vena cava. Because of its ability to visualize the Eustachian valve from multiple perspectives, transesophageal 3DE provides an accurate imaging of the valve "en face" (i.e. a flap of tissue circling the anterior border of the inferior vena cava similar to the anatomical specimen (Fig. 24.26).

Probably the best perspective to imaging the entire extension of a large EV is an "en face view" from the right atrium (Fig. 24.27).

Crista Terminalis

The internal aspect of the right atrium consists of several components particularly relevant for electrophysiologists. The crista terminalis or terminal crest is one of them. The

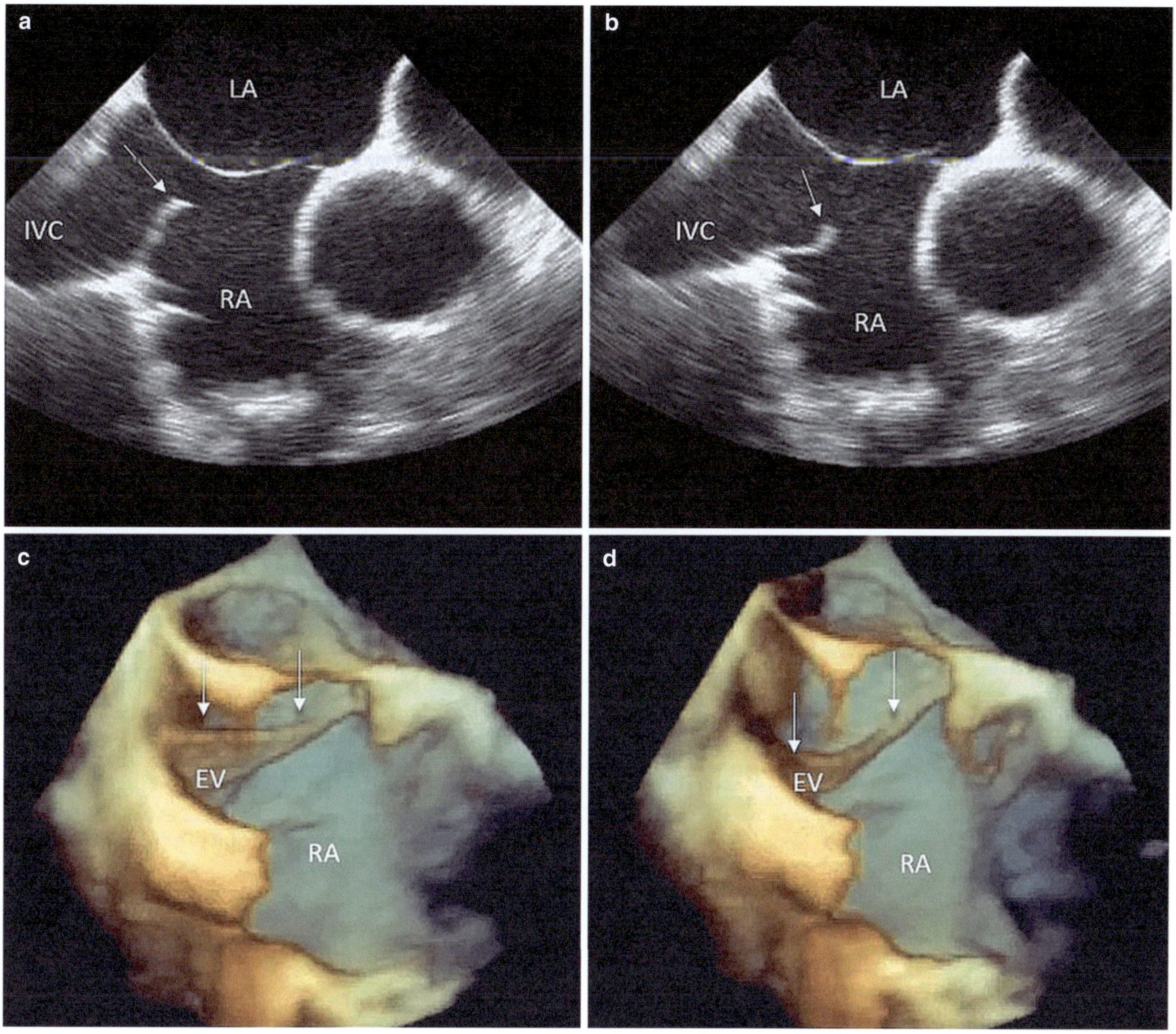

Fig. 24.26 Eustachian valve. (**a**, **b**) Two-dimensional echocardiography of a long Eustachian valver (arrow). (**c**, **d**) Transesophageal 3DE volume rendering of the same Eustachian valve. The Eustachian valve (white arrows) is much larger than hypothesized looking at the tomographic images. *IVC* inferior vena cava, *LA* left atrium, *RA* right atrium

terminal crest is a muscular ridge that divides the smooth wall of sinus venous from the trabeculated surface of the right atrial appendage. Externally the terminal crest corresponds to the sulcus terminalis. The terminal crest originates from the anteromedial wall of the right atrium and descends towards the inferior vena cava, where ends into fine trabeculations. When particularly hypertrophic two-dimensional transthoracic echocardiography may show a bump in four-chamber view that may be easily mistaken for an abnormal mass (Fig. 24.28a, Video 24.11a). In particularly echogenic cases, transthoracic 3DE may show the course of the terminal crest from superior vena cava towards the tricuspid orifice (Fig. 24.28b, Video 24.11b). Transesophageal 3DE shows the terminal crest in "en face" perspective (Fig. 24.28c) where the terminal crest appears as an elongated protrusion, or in lateral perspective (Fig. 24.28d) where it shows its arcuate aspect.

The Lipomatous Atrial Septum

One of the first necropsy descriptions dating back to 1964 [28] describes the lipomatous infiltration of interatrial septum as an abnormal accumulation of fat inside the septum.

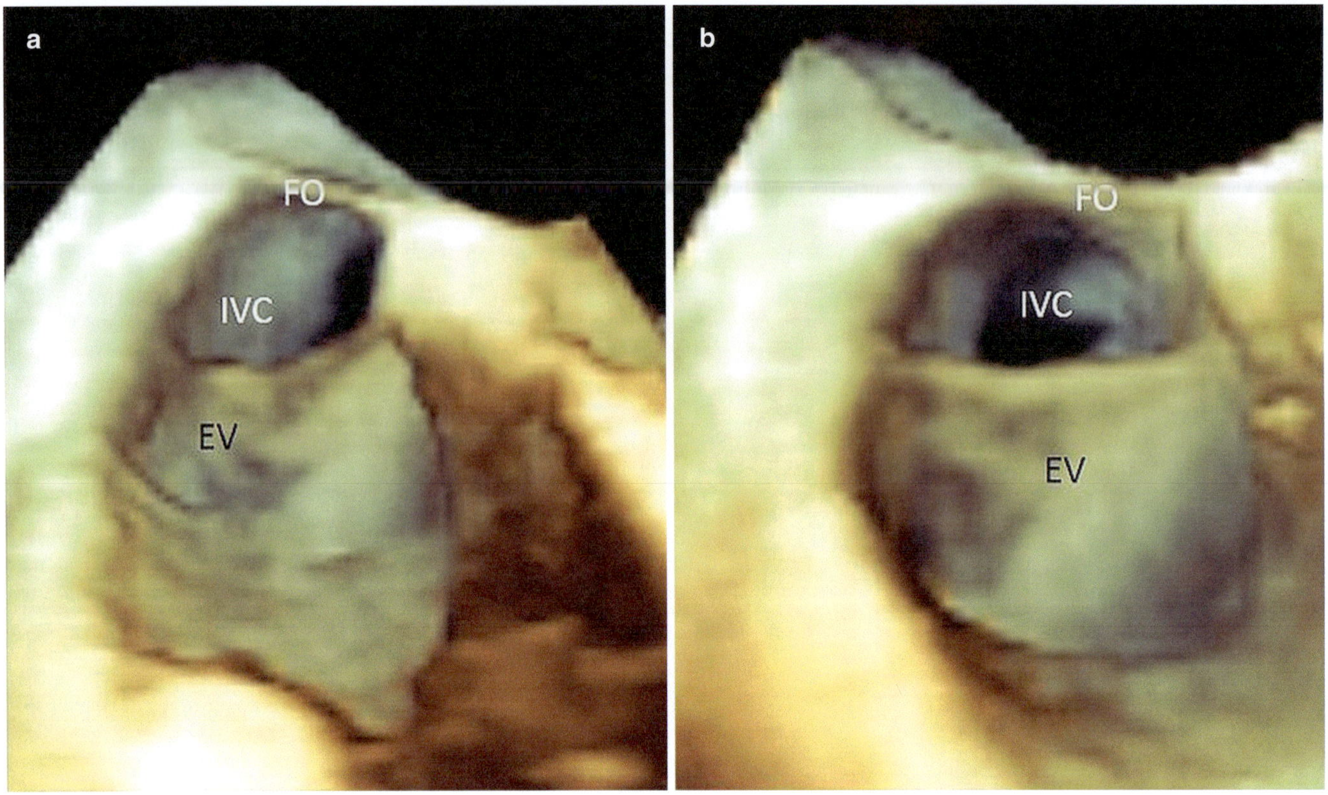

Fig. 24.27 Transesophageal 3DE volume rendering of large Eustachian valve visualized "en face" from a right atrial perspective (**a**, **b**). The valve is a flap of tissue inserted of the anteromedial border of inferior vena cava. *EV* Eustachian valve, *FO* fossa ovalis, *IVC* inferior vena cava

Since then and for several years the lipomatous interatrial septum was considered a benign tumor-like mass, similar to a lipoma.

A more modern anatomical approach describes the interatrial septum as a fibrous partition that separates the right and left atrial cavity. Based on this definition the interatrial septum appears to be limited to the fossa ovalis and to the immediate surrounding muscular rims. Indeed, the so-called "septum secundum", is not a partition between the two atria but rather an enfolding of the superior and posterior atrial wall. Externally, this enfolding, called Waterson's groove is filled with epicardial fat [30].

According to this specific atrial arrangement the lipomatous interatrial septum is nothing else than an unusual accumulation of epicardial fat within this enfolding as consequence of a generalized increased deposit of subepicardial adipose tissue. Since both atrial wall and fat have similar acoustic impedance, both two and 3DE are unable able to delineate this specific septal arrangement. Thus, a lipomatous interatrial septum appears at two- and 3DE as a dumbbell-shaped structure well distinct from the thin flap of the fossa ovalis (Fig. 24.29).

Left Lateral Ridge

A muscular ridge, currently called left lateral ridge, divides the orifices of the left upper pulmonary vein and left atrial appendage. This ridge may have different shapes ranging from a bulbous tip to large muscular band, to a thin partition between the left upper pulmonary vein and the left atrial appendage. When particularly prominent, this ridge protrudes deeply on the left atrial cavity. Because of this, in the early era of two-dimensional transesophageal echocardiography, it was frequently mistaken for a mass or for a thrombus. Thus, not rarely, the patient was treated with anticoagulant unnecessarily. For this reason, the left lateral ridge is also known as "Coumadin ridge". In reality, the left lateral ridge is not a muscular crest arising from the atrial wall but rather an enfolding of lateral atrial wall extending into the left

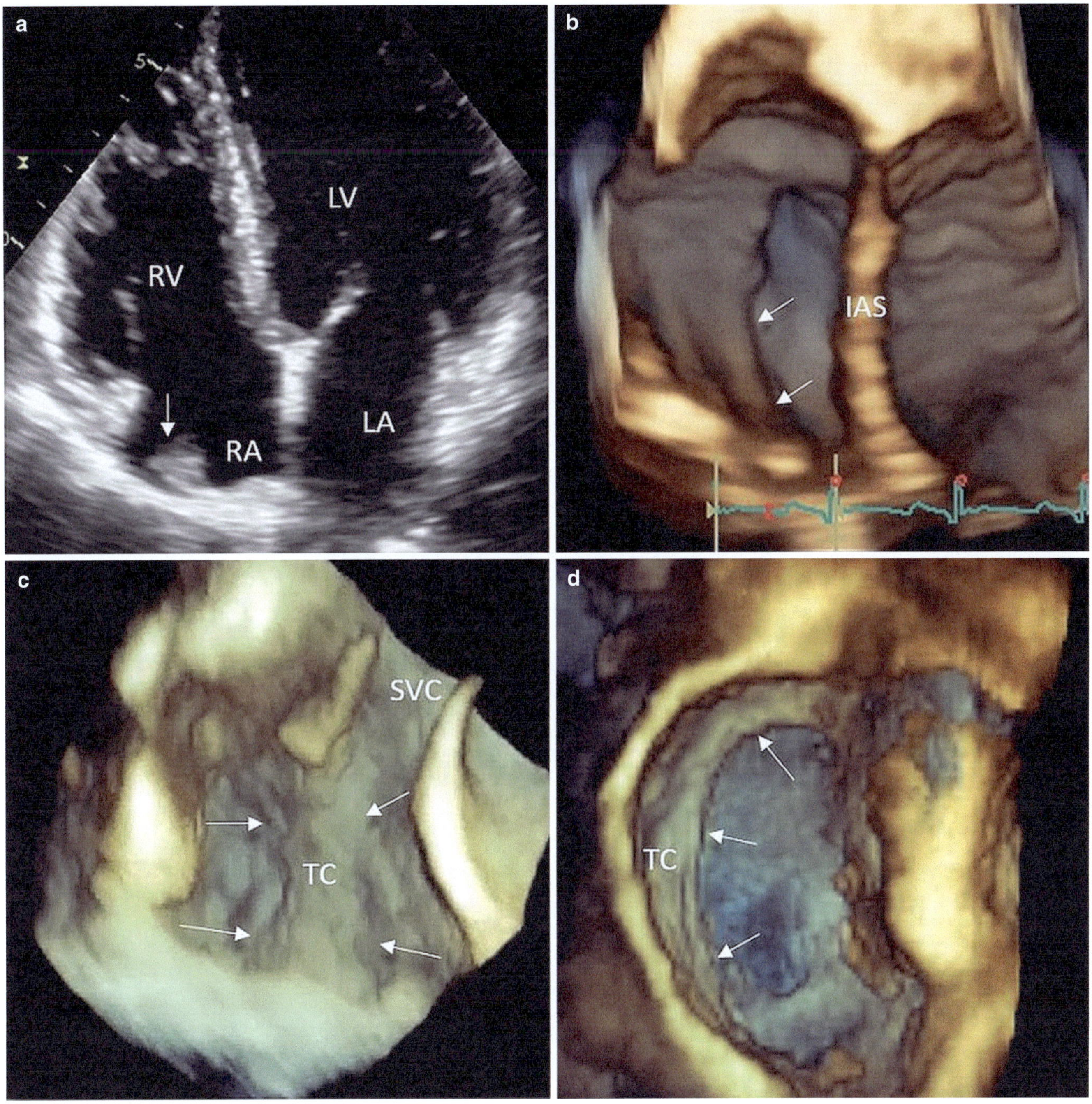

Fig. 24.28 *Crista terminalis* or terminal crest. (**a**) Two-dimensional transthoracic four-chamber view showing an "abnormal" structure (arrow) that may easily be misdiagnosed for a tumor or thrombus attached to the superior wall of right atrium (Video 24.11a). (**b**) Transthoracic 3DE reveals that the "mass" is actually the terminal crest extending from the superior vena cava (not seen in the image) towards the tricuspid orifice (Video 24.11b). (**c**) Transesophageal 3DE volume rendering of a large and thick terminal crest (arrows) visualized "*en face*". (**d**) Transesophageal 3DE image showing the terminal crest (arrows) from a lateral perspective. This perspective enables to appreciate the "arcuate" aspect of the terminal crest

atrial cavity [31]. The epicardial site of this enfolding contains fat, nerve bundles, small atrial arteries, and the remnant of Marshal's vein. Because of the presence of the Marshal's vein, electrophysiologists named the left lateral ridge "ligament of Marshall".

The enfold aspect of the ridge may be visualized with 2D TE (Fig. 24.30), However, more often, the space of the fold is virtual and the ridge appears as a compact muscular protrusion.

Transesophageal 3DE nicely shows the variable shape of the left lateral ridge [32] (Fig. 24.31).

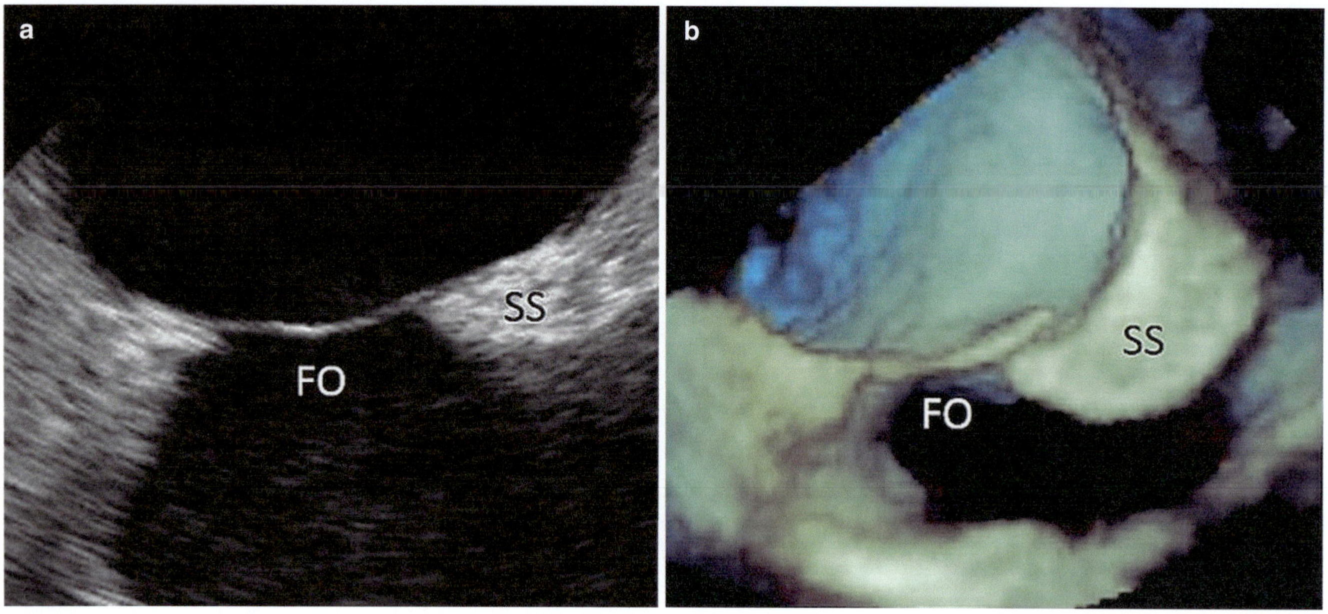

Fig. 24.29 Lipomatous atrial septum visualized using two- (**a**) and 3DE (**b**) transesophageal echocardiography. Both techniques are unable distinguishing the fat within the septum secundum). The dumbbell-shaped structure is well distinct from the thin fossa ovalis. *FO* fossa ovalis, *SS* septum secundum

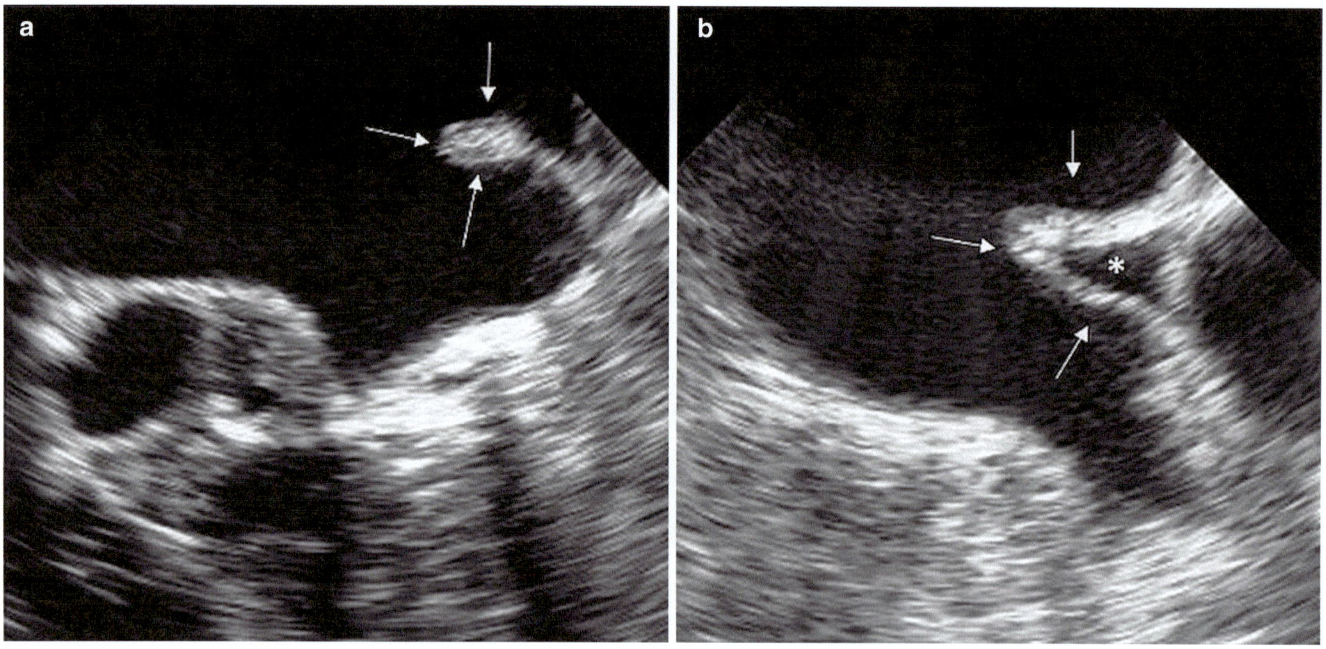

Fig. 24.30 Left lateral ridge with a bulbous tip (arrows, **a**). (**b**) Two-dimensional transesophageal image showing that the left lateral ridge is an enfolding of the atrial wall (arrows). The asterisk marks the space inside the enfolding that contains fat, nerves bundles, small atrial arteries, and the remnant of Marshal's vein

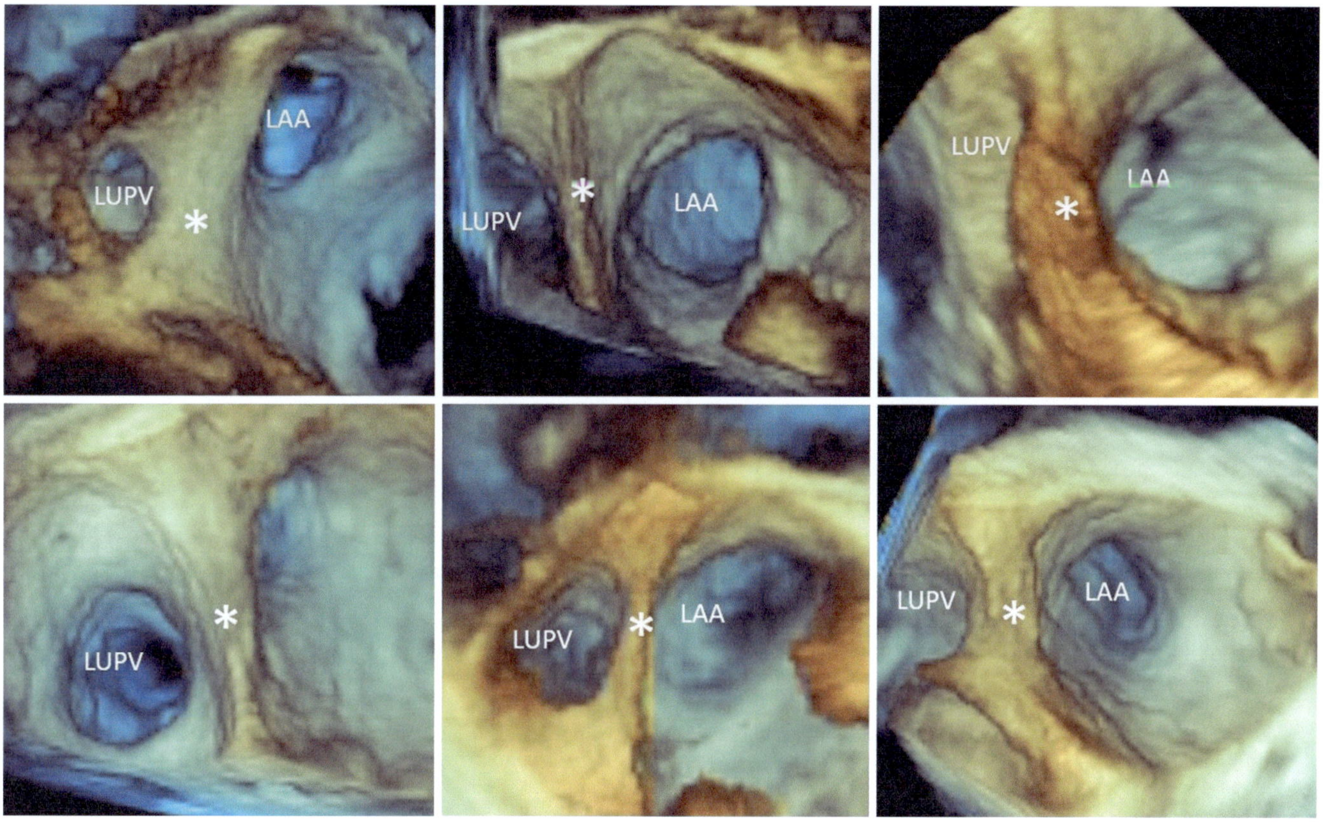

Fig. 24.31 Transesophageal 3DE volume rendering of various left lateral ridges (asterisks) showing its wide variability in shape. *LUVP* left upper pulmonary vein, *LAA* left atrial appendage

Conclusions

Since the days of the M-mode, echocardiography has had an essential role in the diagnosis of intracardiac masses. The appearance in the clinical arena of the two-dimensional transthoracic first, and then of transesophageal have enhanced our ability in detecting and characterizing mass size, shape, location and motility. For many years, two-dimensional echocardiography has been the first line technique in the diagnosis of cardiac mass, providing a complete set of information. However, the tomographic nature of the technique has always "forced" images of the mass within a thin white/gray cross-echocardiographic slice. We call this modality "section-oriented approach". Only the advent of 3DE in the recent years has made possible a new paradigm: shifting from "section-oriented approach" of two-dimensional echocardiography to "anatomy oriented approach" of 3DE. Indeed, once acquired the 3DE data set, the operator are able to image the intracardiac mass from a countless number of perspective. Useful tools allow, on and off-line, rotating, angulating and removing the redundant tissues from the image. The result is a 3D volume rendering of mass that are similar to the anatomic specimen.

References

1. Lam KY, Dickens P, Chan AC. Tumors of the heart. A 20-year experience with a review of 12,485 consecutive autopsies. Arch Pathol Lab Med. 1993;117:1027–31.
2. Burke A, Virmani R. Tumors of the heart and great vessels. In: Atlas of tumor pathology. 3rd ed. Washington, DC: Armed Forces Institute of Pathology; 1996. p. 79–90.
3. Salcedo EE, Cohen GI, White RD, Davison MB. Cardiac tumors: diagnosis and management. Curr Probl Cardiol. 1992;17:73–137.
4. Mugge A, Daniel WG, Haverich A, Lichtlen PR. Diagnosis of noninfective cardiac mass lesions by two-dimensional echocardiography. Comparison of the transthoracic and transesophageal approaches. Circulation. 1991;3:70–8.
5. King TW. On simple vascular growths in the left auricle of the heart. Lancet. 1845;2:428–9.
6. Goldberg HP, Glenn F, Dotter CT, Steinberg I. Myxoma of the left atrium: diagnosis made during life with operative and postmortem findings. Circulation. 1952;6:762–7.
7. HA MA Jr, Fenoglio JJ Jr. Tumors of the cardiovascular system. Atlas of tumor pathology. 2nd series. Fascicle 15. Washington, DC: Armed Forces Institute of Pathology; 1978. p. 1–20.
8. Prichard RW. Tumors of the heart: review of the subject and report of one hundred and fifty cases. Arch Pathol. 1951;51:98–128.
9. Lie JT. The identity and histogenesis of cardiac myxomas: a controversy put to rest. Arch Pathol Lab Med. 1989;113:724–6.
10. Klarich KW, Enriquez-Sarano M, Gura GM, Edwards WD, Tajik AJ, Seward JB. Papillary fibroelastoma: echocardiographic char-

acteristics for diagnosis and pathologic correlation. J Am Coll Cardiol. 1997;30(3):784–90.
11. Sun JP, Asher CR, Yang XS, Cheng GG, Scalia GM, Massed AG, et al. Clinical and echocardiographic characteristics of papillary fibroelastomas: a retrospective and prospective study in 162 patients. Circulation. 2001;103(22):2687–93.
12. Goldberg AD, Blankstein R, Padera R. Tumors metastatic to the heart. Circulation. 2013;128:1790–4.
13. Keren A, Goldberg S, Gottlieb S, Klein J, Schuger C, Medina A, et al. Natural history of left ventricular thrombi: their appearance and resolution in the post-hospitalization period of acute myocardial infarction. J Am Coll Cardiol. 1990;15:790–800.
14. Vaitkus PT, Barnathan ES. Embolic potential, prevention and management of mural thrombus complicating anterior myocardial infarction: a meta-analysis. J Am Coll Cardiol. 1994;22(4):1004–9.
15. Haugland JM, Asinger RW, Mikell FL, Elsperger J, Hodges M. Embolic potential of left ventricular thrombi detected by two-dimensional echocardiography. Circulation. 1984;70:588–98.
16. Oginosawa Y, Abe H, Nakashima Y. The incidence and risk factors for venous obstruction after implantation of transvenous pacing leads. Pacing Clin Electrophysiol. 2002;25:1605–11.
17. Moreillon P, Que YA. Infective endocarditis. Lancet. 2004;363:139–49.
18. Correa de Sa DD, Tleyjeh IM, Anavekar NS, Schultz JC, Thomas JM, Lahr BD, et al. Epidemiological trends of infective endocarditis: a population-based study in Olmsted County, Minnesota. Mayo Clin Proc. 2010;85:422–6.
19. Werdan K, Dietz S, Löffler B, Niemann S, Bushnaq H, Silber RE, et al. Mechanisms of infective endocarditis: pathogen-host interaction and risk states. Nat Rev Cardiol. 2014;11:35–50.
20. Prendergast BD. Diagnostic criteria and problems in infective endocarditis. Heart. 2004;90:611–3.
21. Li JS Sexton DJ, Mick N, Nettles R, Fowler VG Jr, Ryan T, et al. Proposed modifications to the Duke criteria for the diagnosis of infective endocarditis. Clin Infect Dis. 2000;30:633–8.
22. Habib G, Badano L, Tribouilloy C, Vilacosta I, Zamorano JL, Galderisi M, et al. Recommendations for the practice of echocardiography in infective endocarditis. Eur J Echocardiogr. 2010;11:202–19.
23. Tunick PA, Perez JL, Kronzon I. Protruding atheromas in the thoracic aorta and systemic embolization. Ann Intern Med. 1991;115:423–7.
24. Amarenco P, Cohen A, Tzourio C. Atherosclerotic disease of the aortic arch and the risk of ischemic stroke. N Engl J Med. 1994;331:1474–9.
25. Jones EF, Kalman JM, Calafiore P. Proximal aortic atheroma: an independent risk factor for cerebral ischemia. Stroke. 1995;26:218–24.
26. Harloff A, Simon J, Brendecke S, Assefa D, Helbing T, Frydrychowicz A, et al. Complex plaques in the proximal descending aorta. An underestimated embolic source of stroke. Stroke. 2010;41:1145–50.
27. Keeley EC, Grines CL. Scraping of aortic debris by coronary guide catheters. A prospective evaluation of 1000 cases. J Am Coll Cardiol. 1998;32:1861–5.
28. Prior JT. Lipomatous hypertrophy of the cardiac interatrial septum. A lesion resembling hibernoma, lipoblastomatosis and infiltrating lipoma. Arch Pathol. 1964;78:11–5.
29. Faletra FF, Nucifora G, Ho SY. Imaging the atrial septum using real-time three-dimensional transesophageal echocardiography: technical tips, normal anatomy, ad its role in transseptal puncture. J Am Soc Echocardiogr. 2011;24:593–9.
30. Silbiger JJ, Bazaz R, Trost R. Lipomatous hypertrophy of the interatrial septum revisited. J Am Soc Echocardiogr. 2010;23:789–90.
31. Cabrera JA, Ho SY, Climent V, Sánchez-Quintana D. The architecture of the left lateral atrial wall: a particular anatomic region with implications for ablation of atrial fibrillation. Eur Heart J. 2008;29:356–62.
32. Faletra FF, HO SY, Regoly F, Acena M, Auricchio A. Real-time three-dimensional transoesophageal echocardiography in imaging key anatomical structures of the left atrium: potential role during atrial fibrillation ablation. Heart. 2013;99:133–42.

X-Ray-Echo Fusion Imaging in Catheter-Based Structural Heart Disease Interventions

25

Francesco Fulvio Faletra, Giovanni Pedrazzini, Elena Pasotti, Marco Moccetti, Tiziano Moccetti, and Mark J. Monaghan

Abstract

Currently, procedural guidance of catheter-based structural heart disease interventions depends on visual information obtained by fluoroscopy and echocardiography, which have their own projections and separate screens. The main disadvantage of this approach is the lack of precise temporal and spatial integration between catheter/devices, visualized in one screen, and the soft tissues of cardiac structures, visualized in a second screen. Therefore, during each catheter manipulation, interventional cardiologists have the need of interrogating repetitively and sequentially the two monitors. A novel imaging technique, called by the manufactures Echo-navigator©, merges soft tissue information from two- and three-dimensional echocardiography with the excellent catheters and devices visualization of X-ray fluoroscopy, introducing a new concept: all (images) in one (screen). In this chapter, we will describe some basic concepts about the X-ray/echocardiography fusion, potential role of the Echo-navigator© during SHD percutaneous interventions and current limitations

Keywords

Echo-navigator · Fusion imaging · X-ray-echocardiography fusion · Three-dimensional echocardiography · Two-dimensional echocardiography · Fluoroscopy

F. F. Faletra (✉) · G. Pedrazzini · E. Pasotti · M. Moccetti
T. Moccetti
Department of Cardiology, Fondazione Cardioicentro Ticino, Lugano, Switzerland
e-mail: francesco.faletra@cardiocentro.org; giovanni.pedrazzini@cardiocentro.org; elena.pasotti@cardiocentro.org; marco.moccetti@cardiocentro.org; tiziano.moccetti@cardiocentro.org

M. J. Monaghan
King's College Hospital, London, UK
e-mail: mark.monaghan@nhs.net

Introduction

Developments of new high-performance catheters and devices along with increasing dexterity and expertise of interventional cardiologists have made possible percutaneous, catheter-based, interventions for a wide spectrum of structural heart disease (SHD). A growing number of SHD that would have required open-heart surgery only few years ago, can now be effectively treated using catheter-based interventions.

Fluoroscopy remains the primary imaging modality for guiding catheter-based interventions. Several reasons may explain this "supremacy". Traditionally, fluoroscopy was the first (and, at that time, the only) imaging system used in the catheterization laboratory and the X-ray system was the "core" around which the catheterization laboratory was built and organized. The catheterization laboratory was the place where the original invasive cardiologists performed their first catheter-based procedures. In 1976, King et al. first published the "non-surgical" closure of a secundum atrial septal defect during cardiac catheterization [1]. Consequently, the modern interventional cardiologists are very familiar with this X-ray imaging based approach. Manufacturers purposely design guide wires, catheters and implantable devices to be radiopaque for optimizing fluoroscopic guidance. The system is easy to use. The large field of view allows the visualization of long segments of catheters. Finally, the high frame rate (up to 30 frames per second) allows a "fluid" and natural representation of the motion of catheters and devices.

However, detailed catheter "navigation" through the heart chambers or septa requires a meticulous knowledge of catheter position in a three-dimensional space. In this respect, there are several drawbacks to the sole use of X-ray fluoroscopy. First, fluoroscopic images are only a two-dimensional representation of a complex three-dimensional heart. A single plane flattens heart anatomy and overlaps cardiac structures on each other. Second, with the exception of transcutaneous

L. P. Badano et al. (eds.), *Textbook of Three-Dimensional Echocardiography*, https://doi.org/10.1007/978-3-030-14032-8_25

aortic valve implantation and balloon mitral valvuloplasty, where leaflet calcification makes them partially visible to fluoroscopy, most of the targets of SHD interventions are soft tissues, which are almost invisible to fluoroscopy. Third, the so-called "tactile feedback" (i.e. resistance to catheter movement felt by the operator as the catheter makes contact with the tissues) gives only an indirect awareness of the force of cardiac tissue contact, tissue proprieties and "environmental" conditions inside the heart. Fourth, although a skilled operator may use multiple projections and contrast angiography to mentally reconstruct the anatomy of cardiac structures and catheter localizations, in most cases interventional cardiologists, conduct these procedures using standard fluoroscopic angulations, without a precise knowledge of individual variations of the heart anatomy. Finally, the use of contrast may need to be limited in patients with renal insufficiency.

Today, the vast majority of interventional cardiologists agree that, at least for the most complex SHD interventions, a second imaging technique is necessary. For its real-time imaging capability, high spatial and temporal resolution, transesophageal echocardiography was the imaging technique most frequently used by interventional cardiologists as the companion of fluoroscopy. In 1996, Arora, et al. first described the role of two-dimensional transesophageal echocardiography in the catheterization laboratory [2]. Since then, echocardiography has played a major role either in pre-procedural, post-procedural assessment and/or in intra-procedural guidance of interventional procedures.

Consequently, over the past decade, a new player has appeared in the "domain" of catheter-based percutaneous SHD interventions: the "interventional echocardiographer". This new professional figure has novel and different competences: he/she has a clear notion of what an interventional cardiologist does at any step of a given procedure and which echocardiographic view must be used. He/she shares with the interventional cardiologist satisfaction for the success and responsibility for the failure of interventions and plays an important decision making role in the so-called "heart team". On the other hand, most modern interventional cardiologists are familiar with the standard echocardiographic views and use echocardiographic images as the primary guidance tool in many steps of complex interventional procedures. In the last 5 years, three dimensional transesophageal echocardiography (3D TEE) has gained acceptance amongst interventional cardiologists as an additional imaging technique in specific SHD interventions. Indeed, 3D TEE has the unique ability to depict cardiac structures as they actually are, allowing visualization of a panoramic three-dimensional view of the relevant structures with unprecedented anatomical accuracy and clarity. Moreover, a 3DE pyramidal data set easily visualizes relatively long segments of catheters and devices in a single real-time view, which facilitates catheter navigation [3]. There is therefore an increasing reliance on 3DE for the guidance of a growing number of catheter-based procedures. However, both echocardiographic techniques have their own limitations. Because of its tomographic nature, two-dimensional transesophageal echocardiography needs multiple views and adjustments to track catheter's motion. On the other hand, 3D TEE suffers from limited spatial and temporal resolution. With both techniques, catheters and devices can produce several disturbing artefacts such as reverberation and shadowing. Both techniques have a limited field of view. Finally, the usefulness of 2D/3D TEE images during the procedure depends upon image quality and operator's experience. Tables 25.1 and 25.2 summarize the advantages and limitations of fluoroscopy and echocardiography respectively as imaging technique during SHD interventions.

Table 25.1 Fluoroscopy

Advantages	Limitations
Interventional cardiologists are familiar with fluoroscopic projections	Poor soft tissue resolution
Fluoroscopy provides optimal definition of wire, catheters and devices	Single plane displaying overlapping anatomy
Good definition of calcified structures and contrast filled cavities	Difficulties in 3D space orientation
	No account of anatomical variability
	Use of ionizing radiation and contrast

Table 25.2 2D/3D TEE

Advantages	Limitations
Optimal visualization of soft tissue (2D and 3D TEE)	Narrow field of view
High frame rate and high spatial resolution (2D TEE)	Some interventionalists are not familiar with echocardiographic images (especially 3D TEE perspectives)
3D representation of the cardiac structures as they are in reality (3D TEE)	Relatively low temporal and spatial resolution
Panoramic 3D view of the "terrain" where the procedure takes place (3D TEE)	Worse definition of catheters and devices (due to reverberations, shadowing and other artefacts)
Easy tracking of catheters and devices (3D TEE)	Depends upon image quality and operator's experience

The Echo-Navigator©

All (Images) in One (Screen)

A novel imaging technique, called Echo-navigator©, has been developed to combines soft tissue information from two-dimensional or 3D TEE with the excellent catheter and device visualization of X-ray fluoroscopy, thereby introducing a new concept: all (images) in one (screen) [4]. In other words, this innovative technique merges in a single screen images provided by both modalities in a kind of "hybrid" image.

Both fluoroscopy and two-dimensional/3D TEE are well suited to "being displayed together" since both are real-time imaging modalities and have complementary abilities that offset their limitations: the larger field of view of fluoroscopy, for instance, counterbalances the narrow one of the two-dimensional/3D TEE data set. Soft tissues of cardiac structures are visible within the cardiac silhouette. Long segments of catheters (visible on fluoroscopy) cross soft tissues (visible on two-dimensional/3D TEE). Theoretically, there would be an enormous potential benefit in using this technique during SHD catheter-based procedures.

Basic Principles of the Echo-Navigator©

The success of the Echo-navigator© is based on so-called "co-registration" of the TEE probe within the fluoroscopy field. In order to determine the position of TEE probe in the fluoroscopic image, an image-based TEE probe-tracking algorithm localizes the spatial position and direction of the TEE probe within the X-ray coordinate system. This is done by computer recognition of the shape of the probe tip and the transducer elements, which are seen clearly on fluoroscopy. The co-registration algorithm automatically orients the 3D TEE volumetric data set within the fluoroscopic image. The boundaries of 3D data set, its location, orientation, and size are marked as a purple-violet 3D sector on the fluoroscopic image. A 3D digital green model of the probe, overlaying the live fluoroscopic image, ascertains that the co-registration is active and correct (Fig. 25.1). Whenever fluoroscopy is "on" the system overlaps the two- or 3DE images onto the fluoroscopic silhouette. Whenever the interventional cardiologist changes gantry angulation, the system immediately registers the new position of the gantry and updates the 3D image orientation on the screen [4].

The interventional cardiologist or the echocardiographer may split the display screen into one, two or four panels showing multiple 3D TEE perspectives and the fused image simultaneously (Fig. 25.2).

Displaying the entire ultrasound data set on the fluoroscopy may not be easily understandable for both interventionalists and echocardiographers and therefore procedurally useless. Various tools make the fused image more understandable.

(a) By means of a table-sided mouse, either interventional cardiologist or echocardiographer may "crop" the echocardiographic image, removing portions of the 3D image that are redundant and may cover the target structures (Fig. 25.3).
(b) Full opacity of the 3D TEE image may cover catheter(s) and device(s) and prevent their

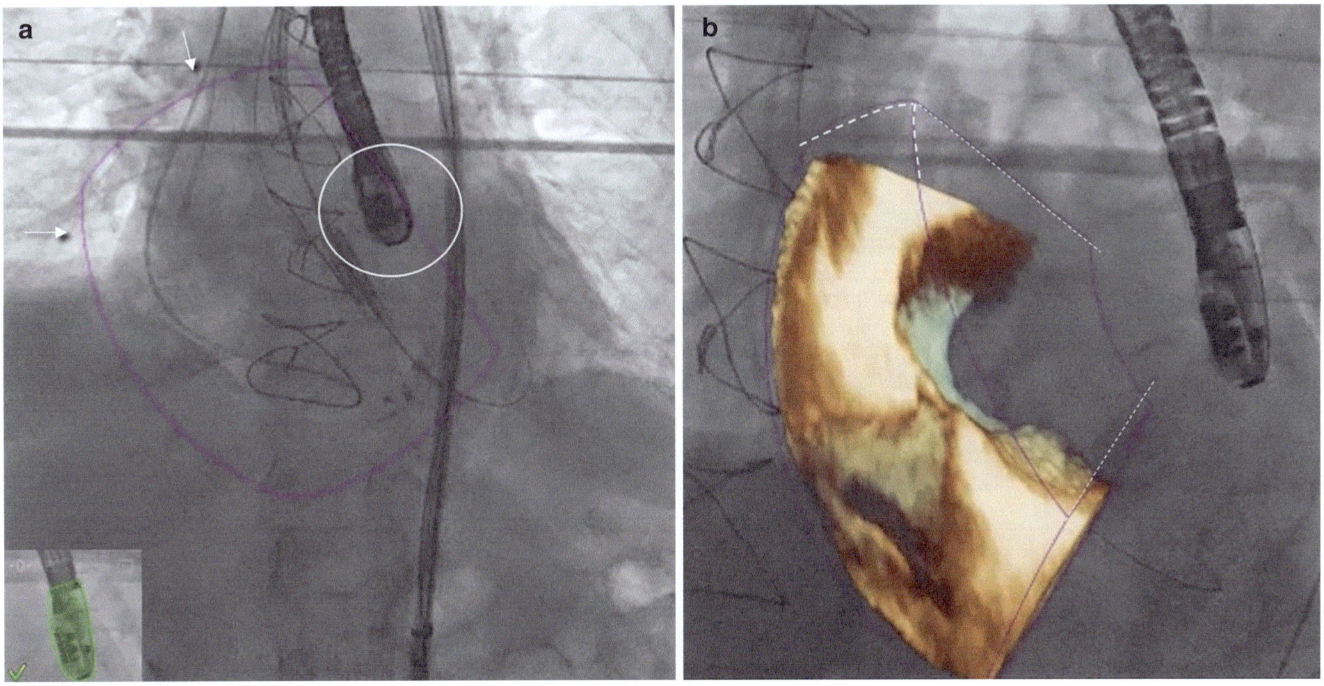

Fig. 25.1 (**a**) Fluoroscopic image showing the position of the TEE probe (white circle). A purple 3D sector (arrows) marks the direction and size of 3D pyramidal data set in the fluoroscopic image. The lower left corner shows the "green" probe that ascertains that co-registration is active and correct. (**b**) 3D images correctly oriented onto the X-ray coordinate system. The 3D sector is partially marked with white dotted lines

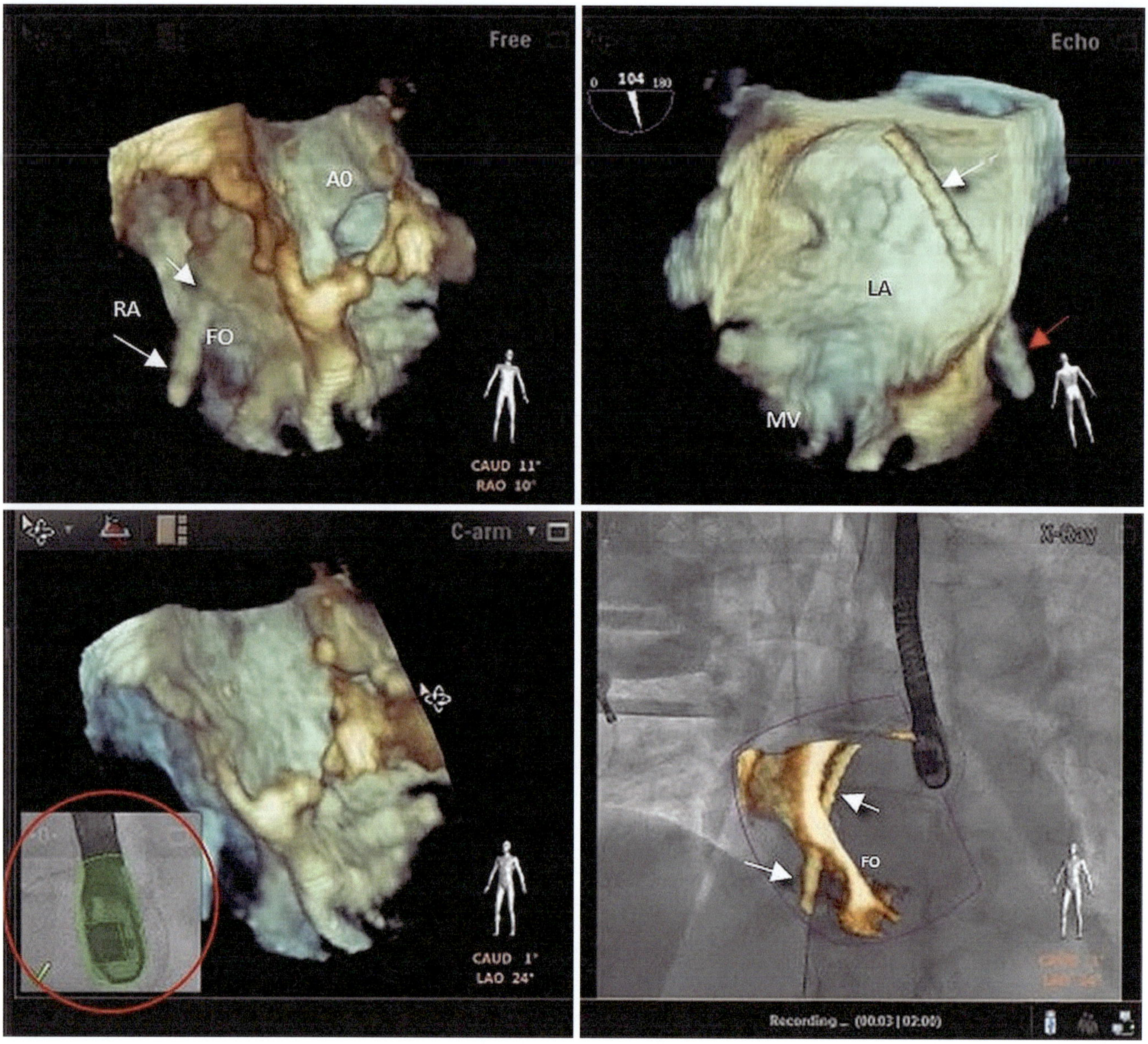

Fig. 25.2 "Four panel" screen. The first panel (upper right corner) shows 3D TEE images from a slightly right anterior oblique (RAO 10°) and cranial (11°) projection. The image shows the fossa ovalis (FO) a longitudinal cut of the aorta (Ao). A segment of catheter (arrows) is seen in right atrium (RA) pointing against the FO; the second panel shows the same image from an opposite perspective. Indeed, the image shows a segment of catheter (white arrow) in the left atrium (LA). The red arrow points to a segment of catheter in RA. The third panel shows the same image oriented in the equivalent perspective of fluoroscopy (i.e. LAO 24° and cranial 1°). In the left lower corner, a green digitalized model of the probe (red circle) ascertains the correctness of the co-registration. Panel 4 shows the X-ray-echo fused image. Please note that the 3D echo data displayed in the fused image are not the same as that shown in the third panel because the operator cropped the dataset until the catheter (arrows) is seen crossing the fossa ovalis (FO), to make guidance easier

visualization. Making soft structures (3D TEE images) more transparent relative to the fluoroscopic images allows one to follow the catheter or device movement (Fig. 25.4).

(c) Landmarks positioned on the two-dimensional/3D images are instantaneously visible on fluoroscopic screen allows visualizing the location of soft targets such as the fossa ovalis, mitral leaflets or paravalvular leaks. A red circle marks the precise ultrasound-determined position (Fig. 25.5).

Slicing the 3DE data set to obtain a two-dimensional view may better visualize the position of catheter(s) inside vessels or cavities (Fig. 25.6).

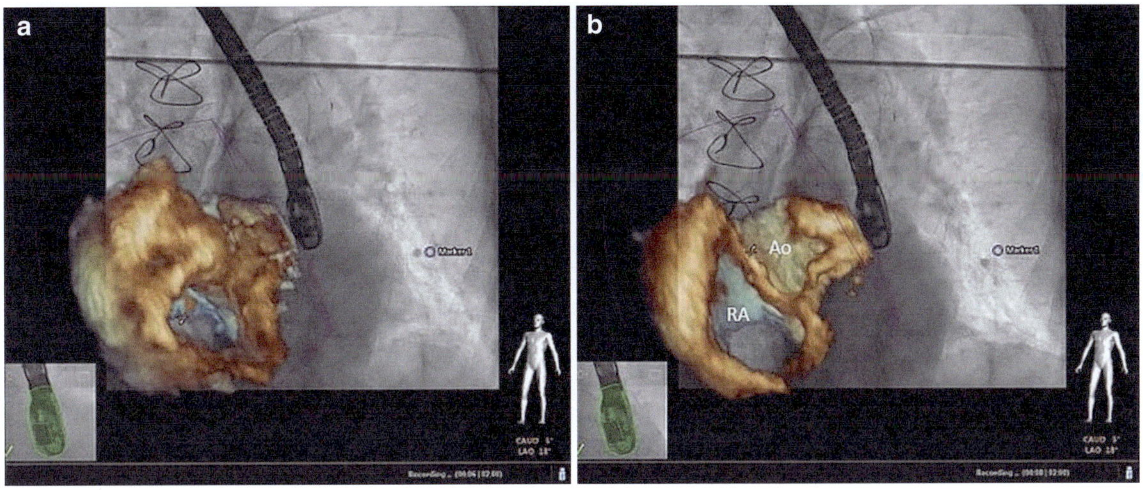

Fig. 25.3 (**a**) Fused image displaying the entire 3D data set. The fused image is incomprehensible for both interventional cardiologists and echocardiographers and therefore procedurally useless. (**b**) Same image after having cropped in antero-posterior (z-axis) direction. A longitudinal cut of the aorta (Ao) and the right atrium (RA) are clearly recognizable

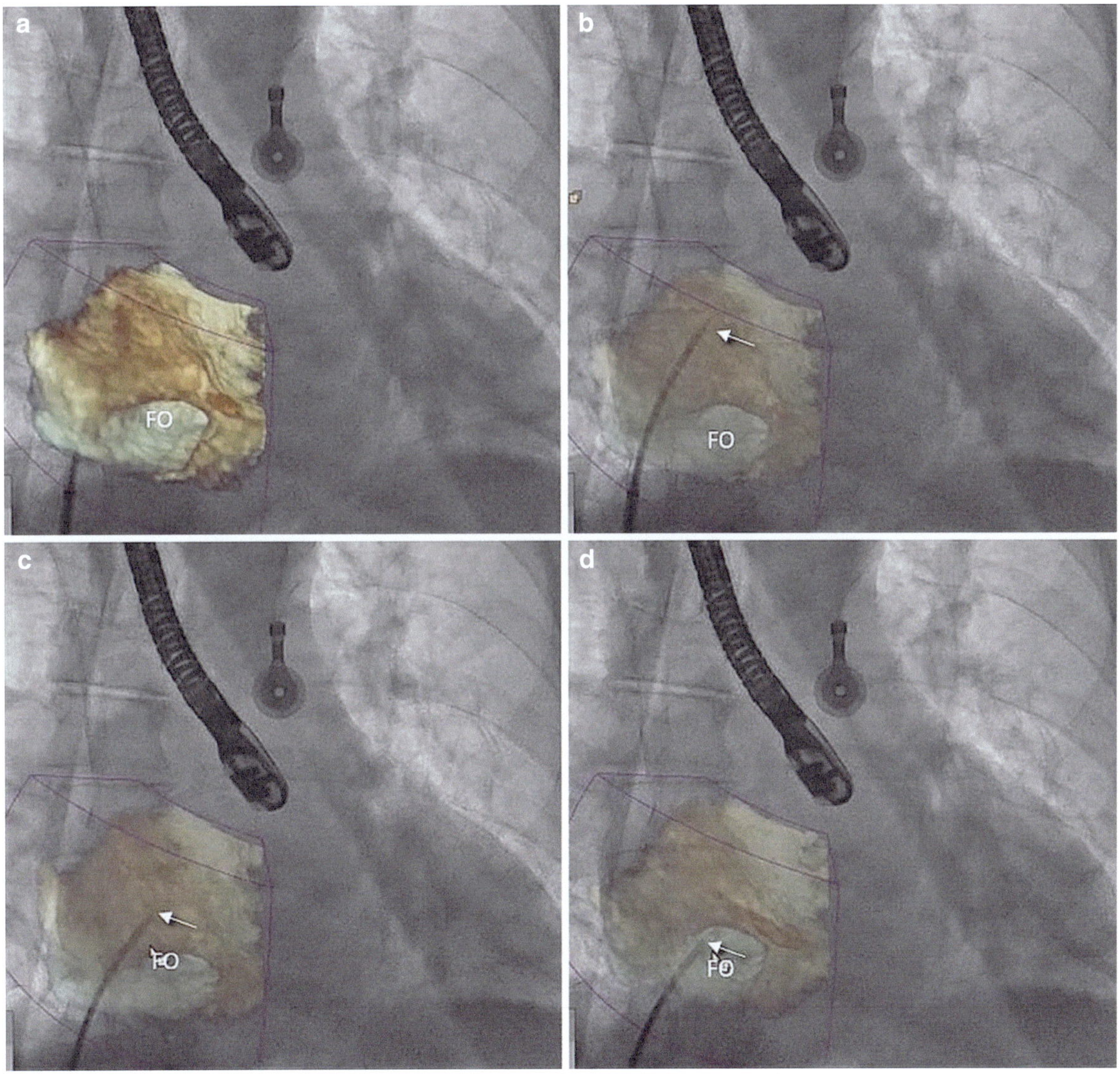

Fig. 25.4 (**a**) Fused image showing the fossa ovalis (FO) "*en face*". The full opacity of the 3D images covers the transseptal catheter. (**b**) Increasing the transparency of the tissue allows visualization of the tip of the catheter in the superior vena cava (arrow). (**c**, **d**) Two still frames showing the tip of the catheter (arrow) that moves in an up and down direction, eventually engaging the FO

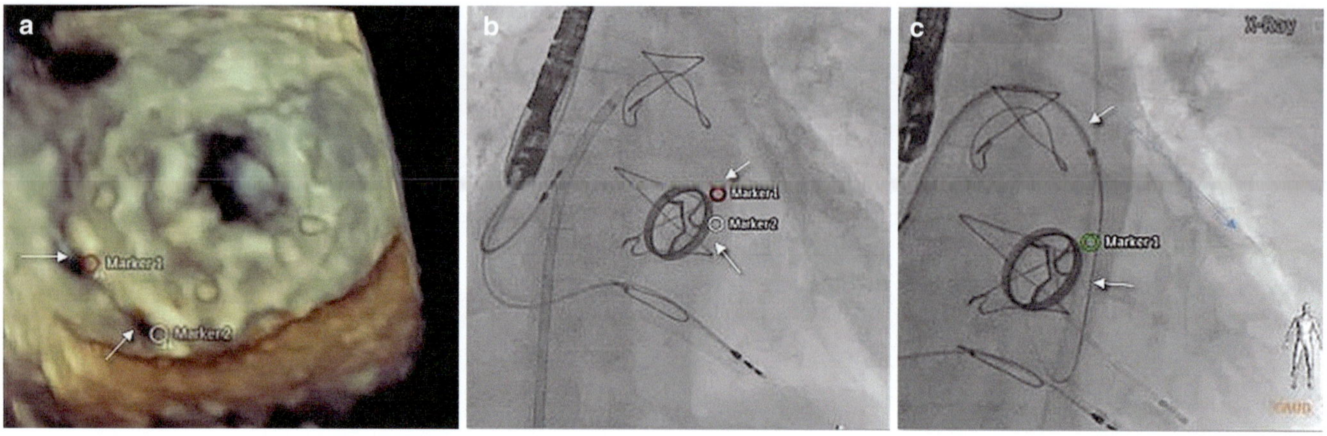

Fig. 25.5 (**a**) 3D TEE image showing two paravalvular leaks (arrows). The locations of the leaks are marked on the 3D image using an inbuilt tool. (**b**) The marks are automatically transferred onto the fluoroscopic image precisely showing the location of the leaks on the fluoroscopic plane. (**c**) A guide catheter (arrows) crossing one of the leaks

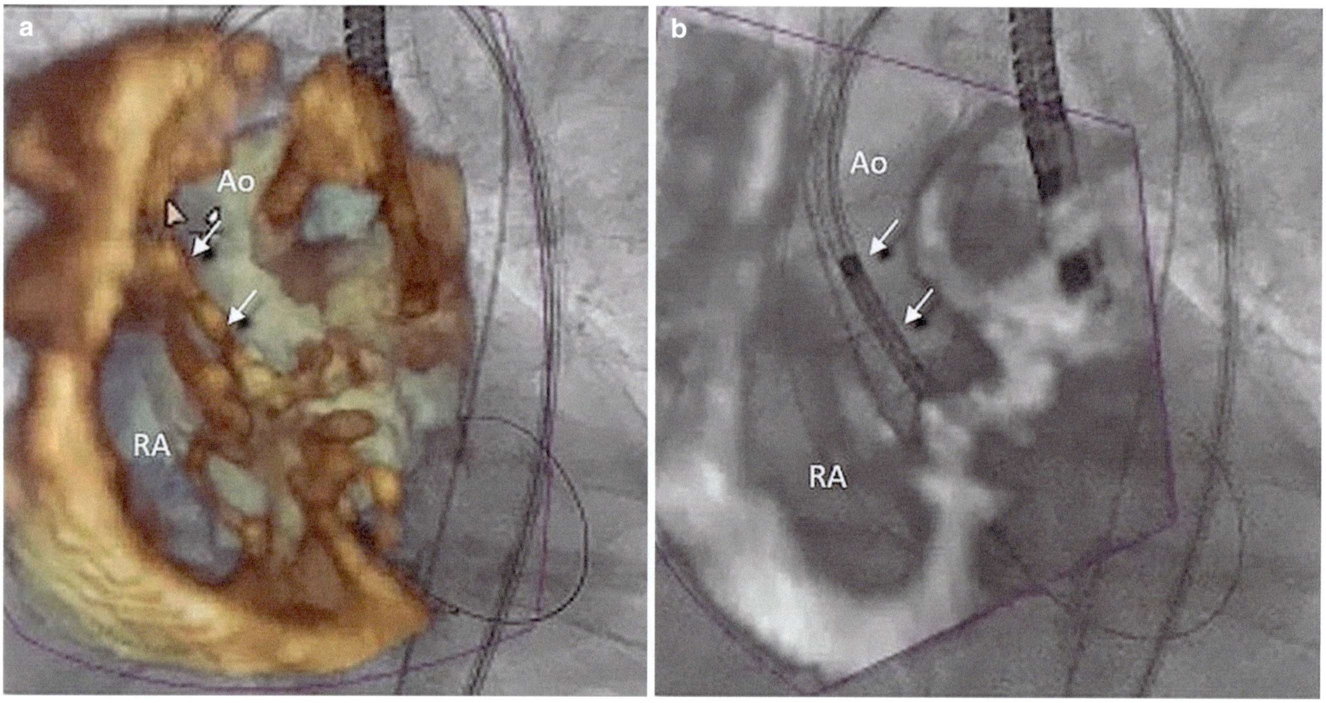

Fig. 25.6 (**a**) An X-ray-echo fused image showing the aorta in long axis view with a catheter (arrow) that crosses the aortic leaflets. However, the opacity of 3D image and the blooming artifact of catheter make this fused image difficult to understand. (**b**) The same image after having shifted from a 3D to 2D image derived from the 3D data set. The catheter (arrows) crossing the stenotic valve is now clearly visible in the center of the vessel

Potential Role of Echo-Navigator© in SHD Interventions

There are very few papers describing the use of this system during percutaneous procedures [5, 6]. In the following paragraphs, we therefore refer to our experience of the use of an X-ray-echocardiography fusion system in different procedures, underlining the advantages and current limitations.

Interatrial Septum Puncture

Although experienced operators can safely perform interatrial septum puncture with fluoroscopic guidance only, in patients with extreme rotation of cardiac axes, repeated transeptal punctores, small foramen ovalis, lipomatous or aneurysmal septum, the usual standard fluoroscopic projections, used alone, may be misleading and make the interatrial septum puncture potentially dangerous. In the

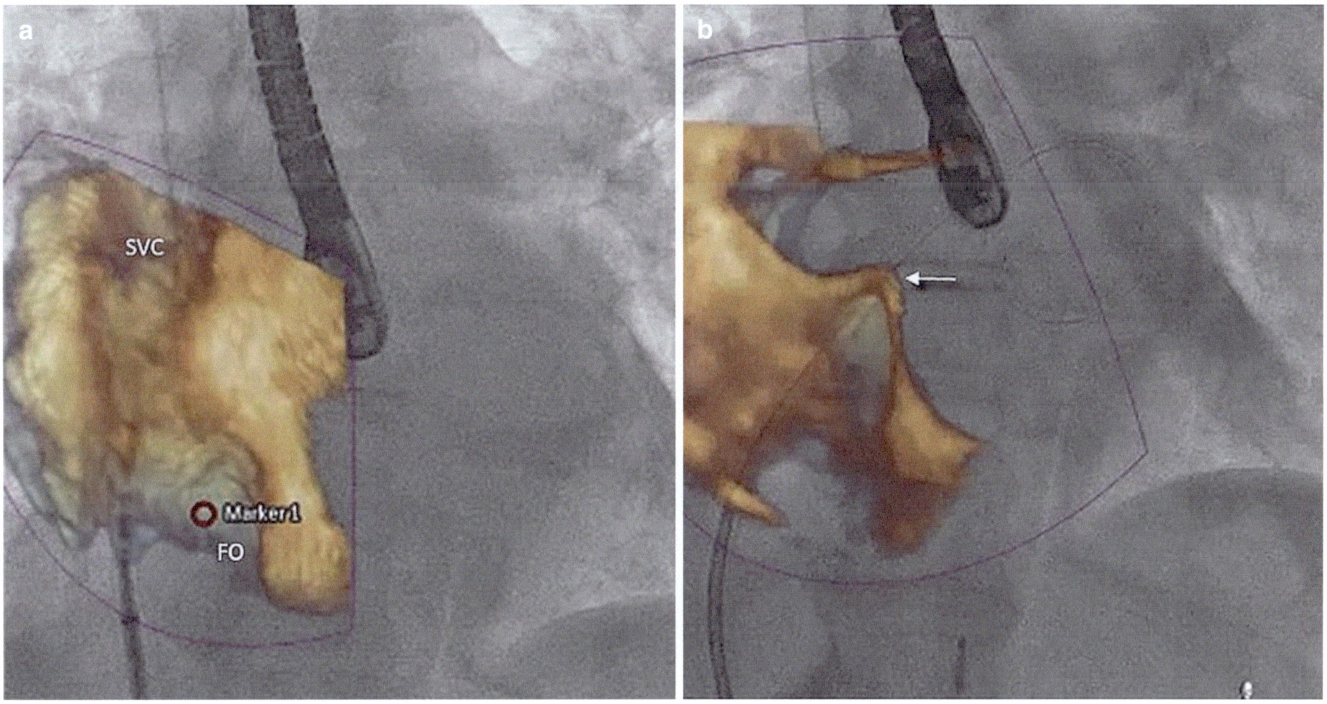

Fig. 25.7 X-ray-echo fused image from right anterior oblique (RAO) showing the fossa ovalis (FO) in "*en face*" view. (**a**) The red circle is the marker for the puncture. (**b**) The left oblique anterior (LAO) showing the septal tenting (arrow)

Mitra-clip© procedure, crossing the fossa ovalis at the highest and most posterior margin of the septum facilitates the steering of the Mitra-clip© delivery system within the left atrium. In these situations, the Echo-navigator© proves particularly useful. The right oblique anterior projection from 10° to 30° shows the foramen ovalis in an "en face" perspective within the cardiac silhouette. Thus, the correct site of the puncture may be marked and easily seen. The left anterior oblique projection (20–40°), displays the "side-on profile" of the foramen ovalis. This projection allows visualization of the "tenting" of the septum (Fig. 25.7).

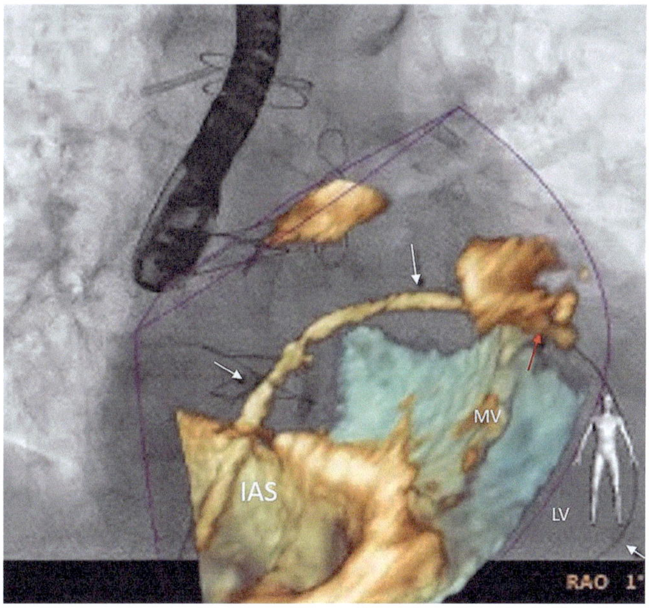

Fig. 25.8 X-ray-echo fused image showing a long segment of guide-wire (white arrows) crossing the interatrial septum (IAS) and the lateral commissure of the mitral valve (MV; red arrow) and looping (white arrow) in the left ventricle (LV). The simultaneous vision of guide wire and soft tissue guides the interventional cardiologists whilst they are advancing the guide-wire and catheters in the left atrium. Note the different thickness of the guide wire on 3D and in fluoroscopy due to 3D blooming artifacts

Mitra-Clip©

There are at least four steps of the procedure where X-ray-echo fusion imaging may be useful: trans-septal puncture (described above), navigation within the left atrium, localizing the origin of the regurgitant jet on the fluoroscopic screen, and guiding insertion of a second or third clip.

Navigation Within the Left Atrium

Advancing, withdrawing and steering the guide wire, guide catheter and mitral clip delivery system is safer if the soft tissues of the atrial wall, pulmonary veins and atrial septum are visible on the fluoroscopic image (Fig. 25.8).

Localizing the Origin of Residual Regurgitant Jet

When one or more clips are "in situ", localizing the site of any significant residual regurgitant jet is of paramount importance for implanting additional clips. Until recently, two-dimensional/3DE color Doppler provided this information on a separate screen. However, X-ray-echocardiography fusion imaging now projects the regurgitant jet onto the fluoroscopic image. Moreover, a marker, placed on the origin of the regurgitant jet, will be seen on fluoroscopic image and may guide navigation. In this context, the system proves extraordinarily useful for interventionalists, who may direct the clip exactly onto the regurgitant orifice (Fig. 25.9).

The Distance Between Clips

When there is the need to implant more than one clip, the distance between clips remains difficult to evaluate with two-dimensional/3D TEE alone because clips produce blooming artifacts. Thus, there may be the risk of impinging on or dislocating one clip during the maneuver. X-ray-echocardiography fusion imaging overcomes this difficulty by allowing assessment of the exact distance between the clips with fluoroscopy whilst maintaining visualization of soft tissues (Fig. 25.10).

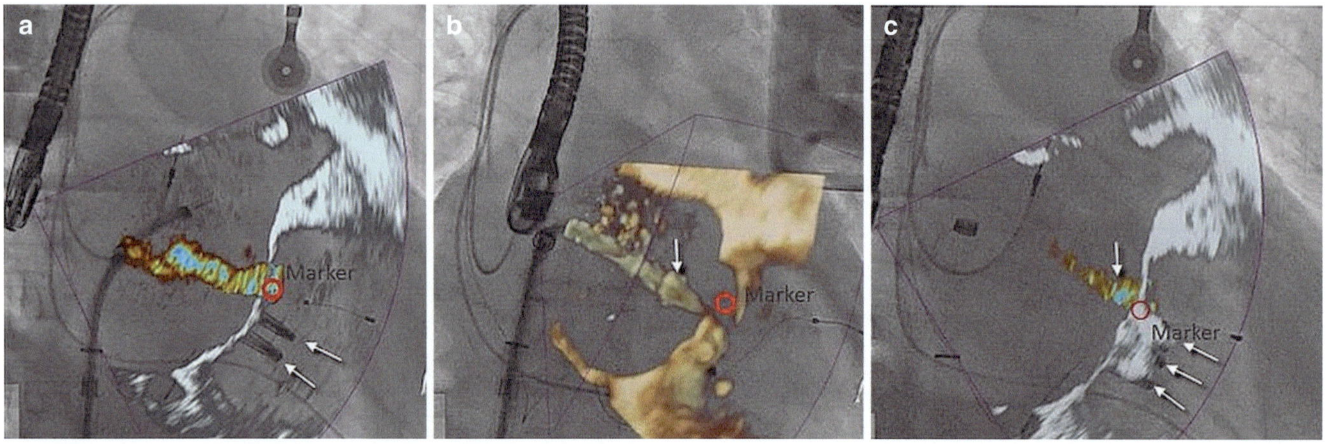

Fig. 25.9 (**a**) 2D TEE color flow fused image showing the site of significant residual regurgitant jet after having implanted two clips (arrows). The site is marked by an annotation (red circle). (**b**) 3D TEE fused image showing the mitral clip delivery system (arrow) advancing towards the annotation. (**c**) The residual regurgitant jet is significantly reduced after the implant of the third clip

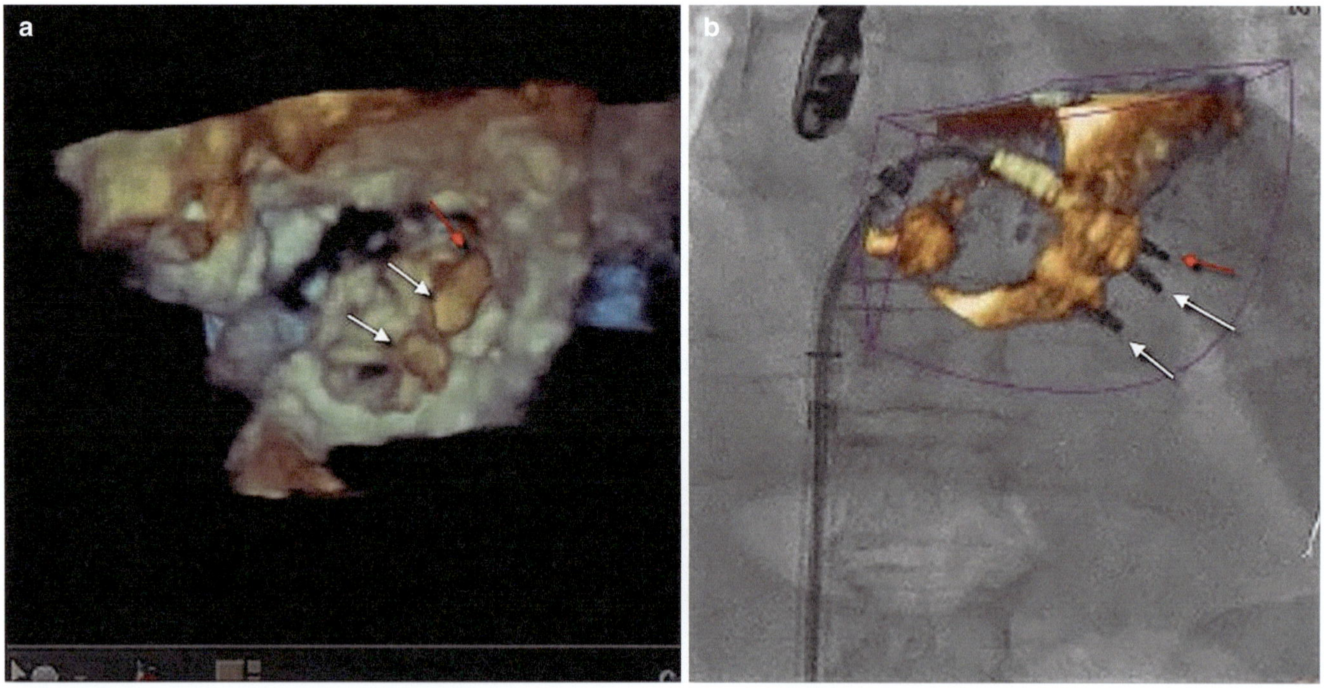

Fig. 25.10 (**a**) 3D TEE image showing three clips from the ventricular perspective. A third clip is still not released (red arrow). The white arrows point at the two clips already implanted. Because of blooming artifacts, the distance between clips cannot be well ascertained. (**b**) The X-ray-echo fused image clearly shows the spatial relationships between clips

Closure of Paravalvular Leak

Probably this is the procedure that most benefits from Echo-navigator©. Identifying on the fluoroscopic image the site of the leak is of invaluable help to interventionalists, who can concentrate more upon the fluoroscopy enhanced by color Doppler and markers/annotations (Fig. 25.11).

Transcutaneous Aortic Valve Implantation (TAVI)

For a safe and secure implantation, exact knowledge of the alignment of the three hinge points of the three cusps is crucial. Currently dedicated angiographic projections provide this information. However, a significant number of patients scheduled for TAVI are very old, fragile and suffer from renal insufficiency. In these patients, contrast may be harmful. The two-dimensional/3D TEE allows a precise delineation of the "virtual annulus". The three hinge points may be identified by two-dimensional/3D TEE and then transferred onto fluoroscopy. The fluoroscopic projection, where the three hinge points markers derived from two-dimensional/3D TEE create one orthogonal plane, may be used for implanting the valve (Fig. 25.12). This tool may make "zero-contrast" valve implantation possible. In addition, the technique can be used to identify the aortic valve orifice and this can greatly assist the process of crossing the aortic valve with a guide-wire. Finally, a semi-translucent 3D TEE image overlaid onto the Fluoroscopy can help guide valve positioning during deployment. This is particularly helpful when the aortic valve is not very calcified and is difficult to see on Fluoroscopy. It is also helpful when there is extensive calcification in the aortic root and/or on the anterior mitral valve leaflet since this may be misleading on Fluoro images alone.

Other Procedures

While is easily predictable that complex procedures may greatly benefit from the use of Echo-navigator©, it is unclear whether TEE echo-X-ray fusion may add an incremental value (with the exception of difficult trans-atrial crossing) in simple straightforward procedures such as patent foramen ovalis, atrial septal defect, closure or left atrial appendage occlusion (Figs. 25.13 and 25.14).

Limitations

One limitation of the Echo-navigator© system is the restricted rotation of the C-arm, which impedes merging onto the fluoroscopic background some very useful 3D TEE

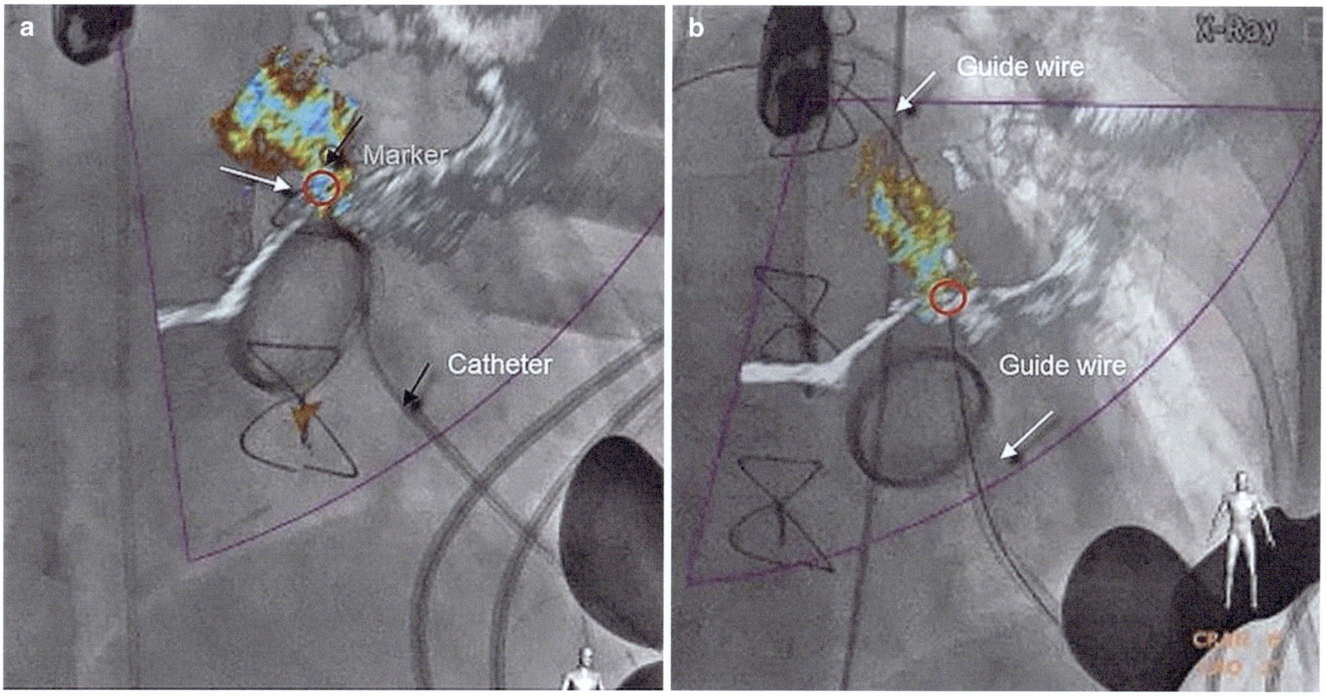

Fig. 25.11 (a) X-ray-echo fused image showing 2D TEE color Doppler TEE superimposed onto fluoroscopy. The regurgitant jet passing through the paravalvular leak is labeled (red circle and arrow). Interventional cardiologists may therefore direct the guidewire towards the annotated target and cross the leak (b)

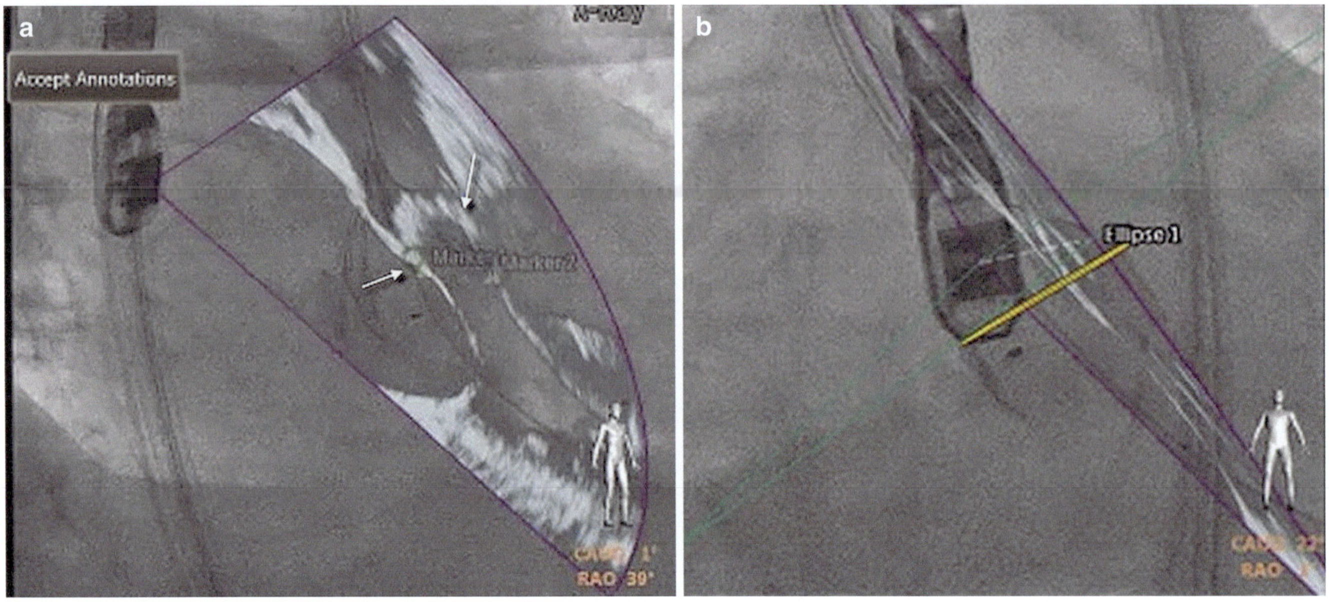

Fig. 25.12 (**a**) X-ray-echo fused image showing two markers (arrows) indicating two points of "virtual annulus". (**b**) X-ray-echo fused image showing the line indicating the virtual annulus

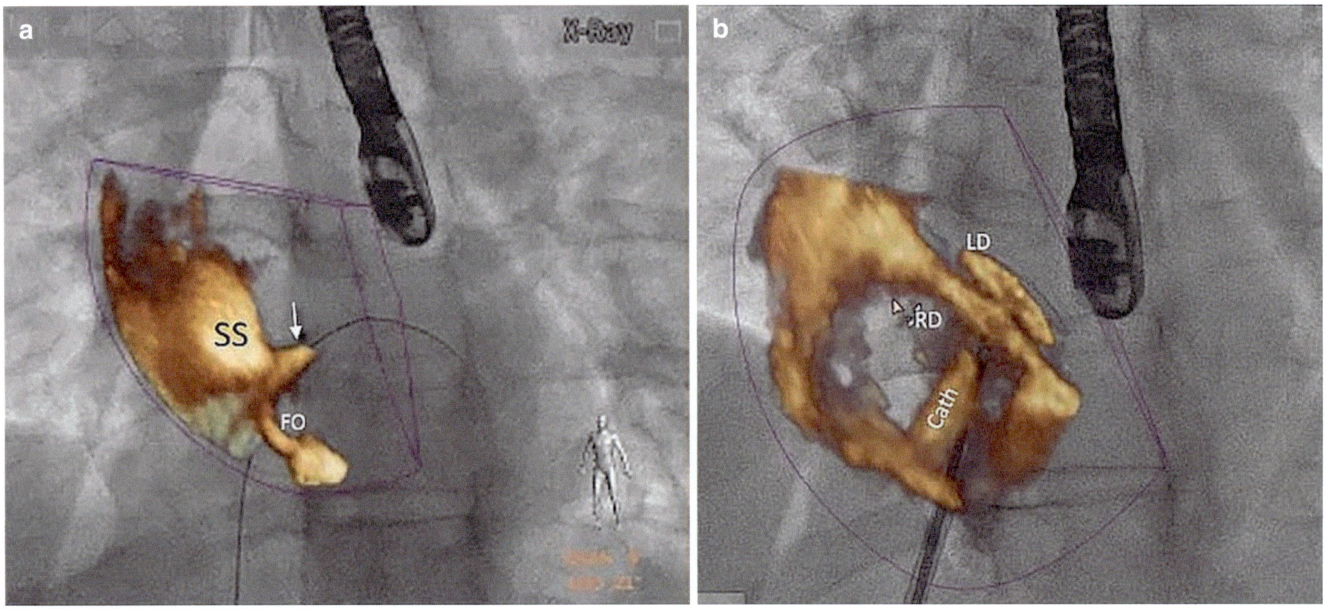

Fig. 25.13 X-ray-echo fused images during patent foramen ovale closure. (**a**) The arrow points at the guide wire crossing the fossa ovalis (FO). (**b**) Images of the left (LD) and right (RD) discs closing the PFO. *Cath* catheter

perspectives. One example: in the Mitra-clip© procedure, for instance, interventional cardiologists consider the 3D TEE overhead perspective the most useful for guiding the position of the arms perpendicular to the coaptation line of the leaflets. The same perspective cannot be merged with fluoroscopy. However, splitting the screen into two, three or four quadrants, allows visualization of a 3D TEE images from the overhead perspective along with the fused image (Fig. 25.15). A second limitation is the fact that, once positioned, annotations remain fixed on the screen and do not follow soft tissue motion. This limitation is particularly relevant when the virtual annulus of the aorta is annotated. Due to the longitudinal shortening of the ventricle, the aortic annulus moves in systole towards the apex. Thus, the location indicated by markers may be correct in one moment of the cycle and incorrect in another.

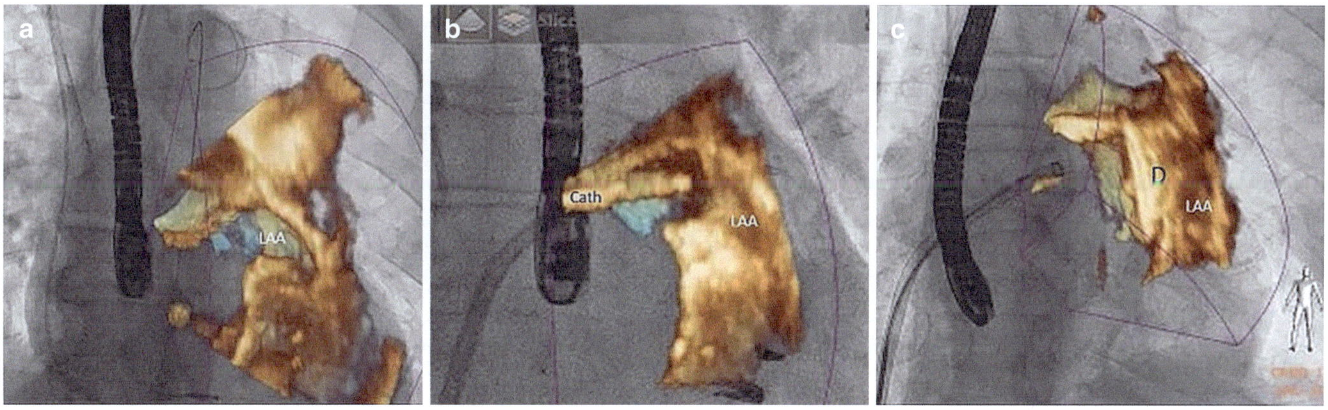

Fig. 25.14 X-ray-echo fused images showing the three main steps of left atrial appendage (LAA) occlusion. (**a**) the image shows the 3D TEE shape of the left atrial appendage (LAA) in the antero-posterior projection (**b**) the image shows the catheter (cath) engaging the LAA. (**c**) The image shows the device (**d**) positioned in LAA

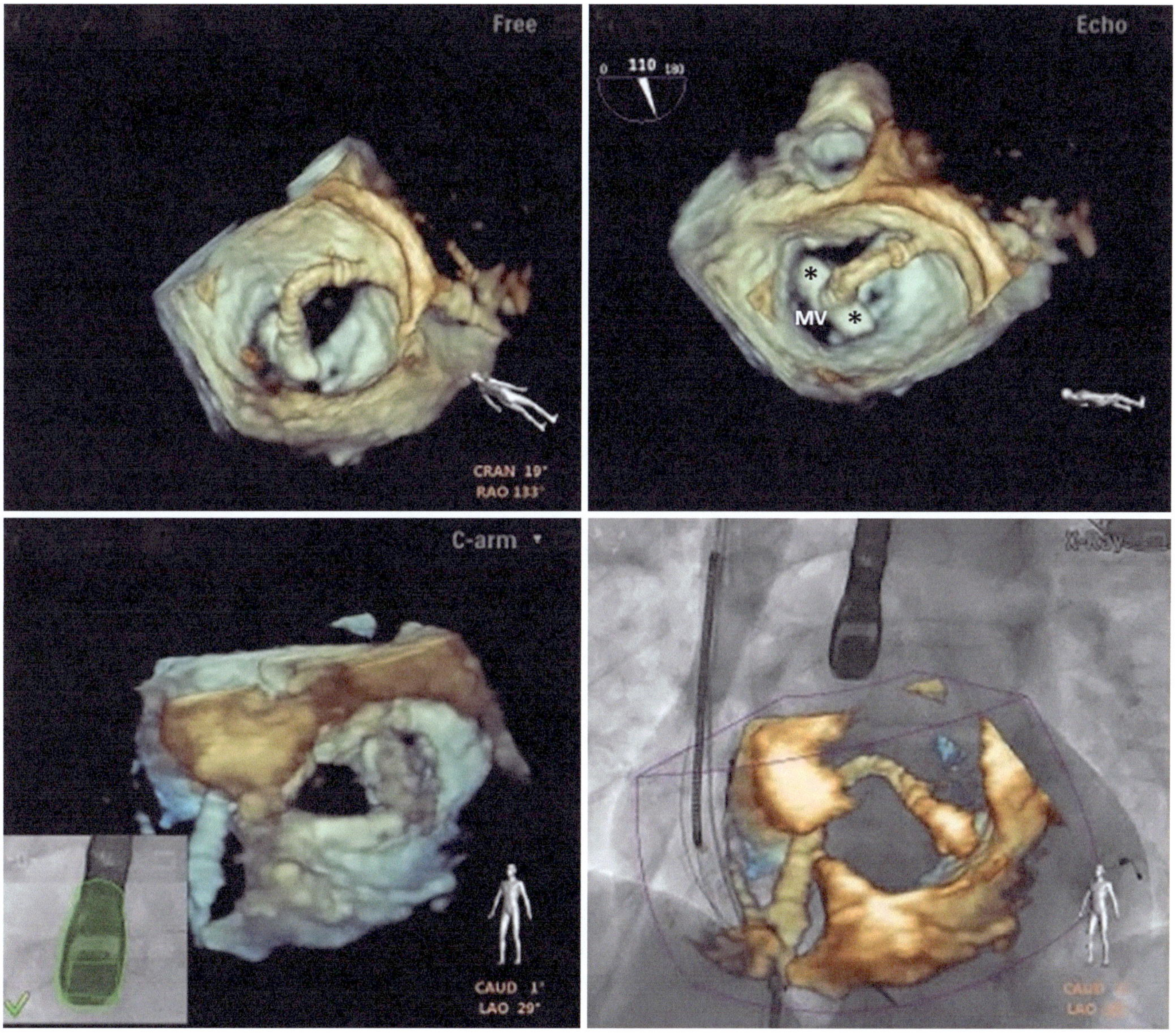

Fig. 25.15 Quad-screen format showing in the superior panel an overhead perspective of the arms (asterisks) and their spatial relationship with the coaptation line of mitral valve. The lower left panel shows the same 3D image from the ventricular perspective. Finally, the lower right panel shows the fused image in LAO projection

Conclusion

The Echo-navigator© tool is a new and extremely appealing system for guiding catheter-based SHD interventions. However, we currently lack data confirming that, in comparison with standard approaches, the system reduces procedural and fluoroscopic time, reduces intra-procedural risks, increases rate of success and safety of the intervention and finally improves outcomes. These data are difficult to collect since they depend on multiple variables. Thus, the cost/benefit ratio of introducing this new technology into an interventional Lab is uncertain. At this time, we can state that the main benefit of the procedure is the significantly better confidence of interventional cardiologists during the procedure and a more homogeneous communication between echocardiographers and operator.

There is still much to be learned and much to be improved.

References

1. King TD, Thompson SL, Steiner C, Mills NL. Secundum atrial septal defect. Non operative closure during cardiac catheterization. JAMA. 1976;235(23):2506–9.
2. Arora R, Trehan V. Role of echocardiography in cardiac catheterization laboratory. J Ind Acad Echocardiogr. 1996;1(2):68–75.
3. Faletra FF, Pedrazzini G, Pasotti E, Muzzarelli S, Dequarti MC, Murzilli R, et al. 3D TEE during catheter-based interventions. JACC Cardiovasc Imaging. 2014;7(3):292–308.
4. Gao G, Penney G, Ma Y, Gogin N, Cathier P, Arujuna A, et al. Registration of 3D trans-esophageal echocardiography to X-ray fluoroscopy using image-based probe tracking. Med Image Anal. 2012;16(1):38–49.
5. Clegg SD, Chen SJ, Nijhof N, Kim MS, Salcedo EE, Quaife RA, et al. Integrated 3D Echo-x-Ray to optimize image guidance for structural heart intervention. JACC Cardiovasc Imaging. 2015;8(3):371–4.
6. Balzer J, Zeus T, Hellhammer K, Veulemans V, Eschenhagen S, Kehmeier E, et al. Initial clinical experience using the EchoNavigator©-system during structural heart disease. World J Cardiol. 2015;7(9):562–70.

Index

L. P. Badano et al. (eds.), *Textbook of Three-Dimensional Echocardiography*, https://doi.org/10.1007/978-3-030-14032-8

MIX
Papier aus verantwortungsvollen Quellen
Paper from responsible sources
FSC® C105338

If you have any concerns about our products,
you can contact us on
ProductSafety@springernature.com

In case Publisher is established outside the EU,
the EU authorized representative is:
Springer Nature Customer Service Center GmbH
Europaplatz 3, 69115 Heidelberg, Germany

Printed by Libri Plureos GmbH
in Hamburg, Germany